LECTURE NOTES ON
PATHOLOGY

To Yvonne, Sheila
and our families,
Madeleine, Caroline, Ian and
Alison, Andrew and
Richard

LECTURE NOTES ON
PATHOLOGY

A.D. THOMSON

MA, MD, FRCP, FRCPath
Consultant Pathologist
60 Wimpole Street
London
Director of Pathology
Metpath (UK) Ltd

R.E. COTTON

MD, FRCPath
Consultant Pathologist
City Hospital, Nottingham
Special Professor of
Diagnostic Oncology
University of Nottingham

THIRD EDITION

BLACKWELL SCIENTIFIC PUBLICATIONS

OXFORD LONDON EDINBURGH

BOSTON MELBOURNE

© 1962, 1968, 1983 by Blackwell Scientific Publications
Editorial offices:
Osney Mead, Oxford OX2 0EL
8 John Street, London WC1N 2ES
9 Forrest Road, Edinburgh EH1 2QH
52 Beacon Street, Boston, Massachusetts 02108, U.S.A.
99 Barry Street, Carlton, Victoria 3053, Australia

First published 1962
Reprinted 1963, 1965, 1967
Second edition 1968
Reprinted 1970, 1974, 1976
Third edition 1983

Printed in Great Britain at the Alden Press, Oxford

DISTRIBUTORS

U.S.A.
  Blackwell Mosby Book Distributors, 11830 Westline
  Industrial Drive, St Louis, Missouri 63141

Canada
  Blackwell Mosby Book Distributors, 120 Melford
  Drive, Scarborough, Ontario, M1B 2X4

Australia
  Blackwell Scientific Book Distributors, 31 Advantage
  Road, Highett, Victoria 3190

British Library Cataloguing in Publication Data

Thomson, A.D.
  Lecture notes on pathology.—3rd ed.
  1. Pathology
  I. Title   II. Cotton, R.E.
  616.07   RB111

ISBN 0-632-00032-5

Contributors of Special Sections

C. W. Elston MD, FRCPath *Consultant Pathologist, City Hospital, Nottingham*
Chapters 43–44 Breast Diseases
Chapter 95 Lymph Nodes
Revision of Chapters 20, 21, 25–31

W. Jeffcoate MA, MRCP *Consultant Physician and Endocrinologist, City Hospital, Nottingham*
Chapters 55–58 Diseases of Endocrines

G. C. Jenkins PhD, MD, BS, FRCPath *Professor of Haematology, The London Hospital Medical College, Consultant Haematologist, The London Hospital*; with

R. G. Huntsman MD, FRCP, FRCPath *Professor of Pathology, Memorial University of Newfoundland, St John's, Newfoundland, Canada*; and

F. E. Boulton MD, BSc, MRCPath *Senior Lecturer, University of Liverpool, Consultant Haematologist, Liverpool Royal Infirmary*
Chapters 77–89 Haematology

Jane Johnson MB, BS, MRCPath *Consultant Pathologist, City Hospital, Nottingham*
Chapter 2 Cell Structure and Function
Revision of Chapters 5–7, 19, 23

W. G. Reeves MB, BS, BSc, FRCP *Consultant Immunologist and Senior Lecturer, University Hospital, Nottingham*
Chapters 16–18 Immunology

Joan Slack MD, FRCP *Senior Lecturer in Clinical Genetics, Royal Free Hospital, London*; and

N. C. Nevin MD, FRCP *Professor of Medical Genetics, Queen's University, Belfast*
Chapters 3–4 Genetics

A. M. J. Woolfson DM, MRCP *Consultant in Clinical Chemistry, City Hospital, Nottingham*
Chapter 15 Water, Electrolytes and Acid-Base Balance

CONTRIBUTORS TO SECOND EDITION

J. S. P. Jones MD, FRCPath, DMJ *Consultant Pathologist, City Hospital, Nottingham*
Illustrations

P. B. Schofield MRCS, LRCP, FRCPath *Formerly Senior Lecturer in Pathology, Institute of Ophthalmology, University of London, and Honorary Consultant Pathologist to Moorfield's Eye Hospital*
Chapters 59–61 Diseases of the Eye

Contents

Contents ix

List of Illustrations

Preface to Third Edition

Since the previous edition of the book was published, the pace of progress in pathological knowledge has markedly quickened. Techniques which were born in fields of basic research have been adapted to the investigation of human disease and are now often incorporated in regular diagnostic services.

Advances in immunology have been spectacular and the expansion of knowledge of cell ultrastructure and function demonstrated to be important in diseases of some organs. The techniques of chemical analysis have not only allowed more accurate estimations to be performed, but have enabled study of a very large range of substances present in very small quantities.

The decade has also seen significant changes in attitudes, not only by pathologists, but by others towards pathological sciences. The need for close clinical co-operation, so strongly demonstrated for many years by haematologists, has been increasingly advocated in the other disciplines and concepts of multidisciplinary team work have developed. The need for clinicians, immunologists, chemical pathologists and histopathologists in particular, to hold regular joint meetings to discuss management of problem cases, is well exemplified by the advances which are particularly well seen in respect of diseases of kidneys, liver and endocrine organs. This blending of the margins of traditionally separate disciplines has hopefully been universally accepted as advantageous, not only to the advancement of knowledge but also to the benefit of individual patients.

All this period of change is very much reflected in the alterations which have been made in this edition. Although the original format has been retained as a result of expressed wishes of readers, almost all chapters have been very extensively rewritten and some whole sections totally recast, with major changes of emphasis and incorporation of totally new concepts. This is perhaps best exemplified by the sections on liver and kidney diseases.

Where possible the World Health Organization's nomenclature for classification of tumours has been adopted and is strongly recommended as a means of standardization on a broad International basis.

At the same time many formerly common and important diseases, some world-wide in distribution, have been controlled or eliminated and have deserved, and been given, less prominent attention in this edition. This particularly applies to infective conditions such as tuberculosis and syphilis, although newly identified microbial diseases, e.g. legionnaires' disease, slow virus infections, have, in a way, taken their place.

We have been conscious of the need to keep the size of the book under control and have therefore, where it was thought appropriate, pruned hard. However, the explosion of knowledge has meant that there has been a modest increase in size for which we apologize, though there is only one wholly additional chapter, that on cell structure and function. The original intention was to produce a new edition at a shorter time interval from its predecessor, and though the spirit was willing, other factors and activities intervened. In the event this made the task harder, though it did perhaps give additional time to absorb the more recent advances.

It is a very great pleasure to record particular thanks to the many colleagues and friends who have been generous in help and constructive criticism. New major contributors have co-operated splendidly and are recorded on page v. They have our gratitude as do colleagues and our tolerant wives. To Drs Barbara and Alan Roper a specially warm thank you for allowing one author the advantages of the loan of their delightful and tranquil North Norfolk cottage. The atmosphere in these surroundings has made a major contribution to the completion of this edition. For this edition, the appalling task of translating almost illegible writing into immaculate manuscript has been most willingly and efficiently performed by Ann Booth, to whom we are doubly grateful, as she also prepared the index.

Many members of Blackwell Scientific Publications have shown their considerable expertise and understanding during the preparation of this book.

We would especially like to thank two members of the Saugman family, Per and Peter, as well as our faithful supporters Keith Bowker and John Robson; to them all we extend our sincere gratitude and thanks for their forbearance over the years.

A. D. Thomson
60 Wimpole Street, London W1

R. E. Cotton *The Grange,*
Normanton-on-the-Wolds, Nottingham NG12 5NN

POSTSCRIPT

As joint author, it is my pleasure to confess that Roger Cotton has shouldered the major role in the preparation of this book. My function has been mainly editorial and I do wish to record my sincere thanks to my co-author for all the very considerable time and effort spent by him and which has culminated in the emergence of this new edition. To him personally my sincere gratitude, but to myself, a full share of responsibility for any errors.

A. D. Thomson
Director of Pathology, The Churchill, Cromwell,
Royal Masonic and Wellington Hospitals

Preface to First Edition

This book is based on Lectures in Pathology which we give to the Students at the Middlesex Hospital Medical School, London.

Appreciating the already heavily burdened curriculum of medical students, we have endeavoured to present a comprehensive and yet concise account of the important pathological features of disease and to link, where possible, the pathological changes with the effects on the patient.

With a view to clarity, liberal use of headings and sub-headings has been employed in the layout of the book and the text is purposely written in a didactic manner for brevity. Some abbreviations, e.g. polymorphs for polymorphonuclear leucocytes, have been used in an attempt to limit the length of the text; we apologize to those who may find this a source of annoyance. Each chapter starts with a tabulated summary sheet of the entire contents of the section which lays out the subject matter in a classified form for clarity of presentation, ease of understanding and speed of revision. We have endeavoured to give a figure in respect of the incidence and/or prognosis of many of the commoner clinical diseases. The incidence figures, many of which are derived from the Registrar-General's statistics for England and Wales, are designed to act as a general guide and it should not be implied that these are necessarily universally applicable in all geographical areas. The figures for results are approximately the average of reported series.

It is hoped that this method of presenting the subject of pathology will prove to be of value to undergraduate students studying for their final examinations and to postgraduate students preparing for higher qualifications in medical and surgical specialities. It is for these groups that this book has been primarily designed.

After some hesitation we decided not in include references but a list of books for additional reading is appended in many of which lists of references are to be found for the benefit of those seeking further information.

A. D. Thomson
R. E. Cotton

Acknowledgments to First Edition

We would like to thank Professor R. W. Scarff and our other colleagues in the Bland-Sutton Institute of Pathology and in the Middlesex Hospital for the benefit of their helpful advice and criticism on many points. Dr Stephen Jones earns our special gratitude for preparing the diagrams in which he was assisted by Mr W. Turney of the Middlesex Hospital Photographic Department, Dr Robert Jennings of Northwestern University, Chicago, kindly gave considerable assistance with some of the sections, to him also we are greatly indebted. Our thanks are also due to Miss Margaret Smith, Miss Christine De'Antiquis and Miss Julia Mackrill who typed the manuscript and to Mr L. T. Morton who prepared the index. Finally, the unfailing courtesy, good humour and kind cooperation of Mr Per Saugman of Blackwell Scientific Publications was of considerable assistance in the preparation of this book.

Books for Additional Reading
and Reference

Robbins SL, Cotran RS. *Pathologic Basis of Disease*, 2nd ed. Saunders, Philadelphia.

Anderson WAD, Kissane JM. *Pathology*, 7th ed. CV Mosby, St Louis.

Pomerance Ariela, Davies MJ. *Pathology of the Heart*, Blackwell Scientific Publications, Oxford.

Spencer H. *Pathology of the Lung*, 3rd ed. Pergamon, Oxford.

Morson BC, Dawson IMP. *Gastrointestinal Pathology*, 2nd ed. Blackwell, Oxford.

MacSween RNM, Anthony PP, Scheuer PJ. *Pathology of the Liver*, Churchill Livingstone, Edinburgh.

Walter JB, Israel MS. *General Pathology*, 5th ed. Churchill Livingstone, Edinburgh.

Ashley DJB. *Evans' Histological Appearance of Tumours*, 3rd ed. Churchill Livingstone, Edinburgh.

Symmers WStC, ed. *Systemic Pathology*, 2nd ed, Vols. 1–6. Churchill Livingstone, Edinburgh.

Harrison CV, Weinbren K. *Recent Advances in Histopathology*, No. 9. Churchill Livingstone, Edinburgh.

Anthony PP, MacSween RNM. *Recent Advances in Histopathology*, Nos 10 & 11. Churchill Livingstone, Edinburgh.

Fox H, Langley FA. *Tumours of the Ovary*. Heinemann, London.

Blaustein A, ed. *Pathology of the Female Genital Tract*, 2nd ed. Springer-Verlag, New York, Berlin.

International Histological Classification of Tumours, Nos. 1–23. World Health Organisation, Geneva.

Risdon RA, Turner DR. *Atlas of Renal Pathology*. M.T.P. Press, Lancaster.

Holborow EJ, Reeves WG, eds. *Immunology in Medicine*. Academic Press, London.

Taussig MJ. *Processes in Pathology*. Blackwell Scientific Publications, Oxford.

Chanarin I, Brozovic M, Tidmarsh E. *Blood and its Diseases*, 2nd ed. Churchill Livingstone, Edinburgh.

Hirsh J, Brain E. *Haemostasis and Thrombosis – a conceptual approach*. Churchill Livingstone, Edinburgh.

GENERAL PATHOLOGY

Chapter 1
Introduction

Definition

Pathology is the study of disease and disease processes. The abnormalities in the body as a whole, in organs, tissues, cells and in body fluids, are manifestations of these disease processes and, by examination of such altered material, information regarding the basic nature of the disease may be obtained. Pathology is therefore the study upon which the practice of medicine is based.

Just as there are marked variations in clinical signs and symptoms with any particular disease, so the pathological changes may differ in individual cases, but in the majority a broadly constant pattern emerges of gross anatomical, histological, cytological and biochemical changes induced by the disease. Information collected over many years by such studies has led to the establishment of aetiological factors, incidence, complications, results and behaviour, so that a prediction of the clinical course of many diseases may be accurately provided, following pathological examination of suitable tissues or material.

Causes of disease

Although the precise aetiology of many diseases is not exactly known, most illnesses can frequently be placed into a broad type or category, and it is often of assistance to think of any disease as falling within one of the following groups.

CONGENITAL

Inherited or familial
A genetic abnormality inherited from one or both parents and transmitted to the child (see p. 16).

Congenital
An abnormality present from birth, although it may not be manifest at that time. The abnormality does not have a genetic basis and these diseases are acquired *in utero*.

ACQUIRED

Injury
Injury to the body tissues by physical causes, e.g. trauma, heat, cold, ultraviolet light, irradiation, etc., and chemical causes, e.g. organic and inorganic chemical substances.

Inflammations
A large group including all infections due to bacteria, viruses, parasites, worms and fungi. This group is subdivided into two main categories.

NON-SPECIFIC
Acute.
Subacute.
Chronic.

Where the tissue reaction is not diagnostically

3

characteristic of the aetiology, even if known, e.g. pyogenic infections.

SPECIFIC
Acute.
Chronic.

Where the aetiological agent produces some characteristic histological feature diagnostic of the condition, e.g. specific granulomas, fungi and parasites.

Mechanical
This includes all diseases resulting from mechanical factors, e.g. obstructive pulmonary collapse, hydronephrosis, intussusception, intestinal obstruction, etc.

Metabolic
This group includes those diseases causing metabolic disturbance due to starvation or deprivation of specific nutritional substances, e.g. vitamins, as well as diseases due to intrinsic metabolic abnormalities, e.g. gout.

Circulatory
A large group which encompasses all diseases of the heart, blood vessels and blood together with abnormalities of the circulation, e.g. congestion, oedema, thrombosis and infarction.

Endocrine
Diseases caused by imperfect function of the endocrine glands resulting in diabetes mellitus, thyrotoxicosis, hyperparathyroidism and Addison's disease, etc.

Degenerations and infiltrations
Disease processes in which there are retrogressive changes in the body cells manifest by alteration of the cytoplasm or nucleus. The examples vary from reversible and trivial cloudy swelling, to irreversible and sinister cell necrosis.

Tumours
Benign neoplasms and primary and secondary malignant tumours.

Other varieties
It must be admitted that some diseases overlap in this classification whilst other defy classification into any group. Some of these latter diseases are now known to be, or are presumed to be, of immunological pathogenesis, whilst others may be of psychiatric origin and are beyond the scope of this book, as the pathology in most remains obscure. Others are of completely unknown nature and in the present state of knowledge must be regarded as 'idiopathic', e.g. ulcerative colitis.

Chapter 2
Cell Structure and Function

Under the light microscope, cells are seen to be composed of an outer limiting membrane, cytoplasm and a nucleus. It is known from biochemical studies that complex reactions take place within the cell, but not precisely where or how. Electron microscopy shows that the cytoplasm contains not only 'cell sap' but also specialized structures – the organelles. Cell fractionation techniques have enabled biochemists to determine the functions of these structures.

Cell components

Ultrastructural features are represented in Fig. 1.

MEMBRANE

STRUCTURE

From chemical analysis the membranes are known to be composed of a lipid–protein complex. High resolution electron microscopy shows them to be arranged as two electron dense laminae with a central electron-lucent zone. The precise detail of the structure is unknown, but the model which best explains the chemical nature, electron microscopic appearance and function, is that of Singer and Nicolson. This is that the membrane is formed of two layers of lipid molecules with their hydrophilic ends on the outer aspect and their hydrophobic chains towards the centre. The protein component is arranged as globules linked by hydrophobic bonds to the lipid. Some proteins are placed across the whole width of the membrane having expression on both sides, others only being exposed on one side, or the other.

FUNCTIONS

Transport
The cell membrane is the barrier between the cell

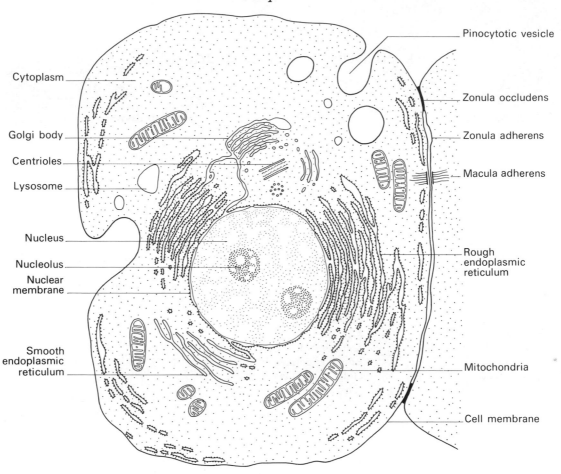

Cytoplasm

Golgi body

Centrioles

Lysosome

Nucleus

Nucleolus

Nuclear
membrane

Smooth
endoplasmic
reticulum

Pinocytotic vesicle

Zonula occludens

Zonula adherens

Macula adherens

Rough
endoplasmic
reticulum

Mitochondria

Cell membrane

Fig. 1. The cell: diagram of ultrastructural features.

interior and the outside. Substances must cross it to gain access to, or to leave, the cell. They can do this by the following methods.

DIFFUSION

This is a passive process involving small ions and water, and is dependent upon concentration gradients.

SODIUM PUMP

To maintain the high concentration of potassium within the cell and the relatively low concentration of sodium, sodium is actively excluded in exchange for potassium by the 'sodium pump' which requires energy.

ACTIVE TRANSPORT

Raw materials for metabolism such as amino acids and glucose are transported into the cell against a concentration gradient. This process is also energy dependent.

BULK TRANSFER

Larger quantities of substances can be transferred into the cell by invaginations of membrane being nipped off into the cytoplasm to form vacuoles. When these contain fluids the process is known as *pinocytosis* – cell drinking – and when there is solid matter – *phagocytosis* – cell eating.

Similarly secretory or excretory vacuoles can fuse

with the cell membrane and discharge their contents. This is called *exocytosis*.

Surface receptors

The membrane proteins probably act as receptors for substances in active transport, e.g. amino acids or groups of amino acids, and may act as receptors for hormones, etc. They also have a role as cell surface antigens.

JUNCTIONS

Cells do not function in isolation. To form organs and maintain structure there must be communication.

Junctional complexes

These are formed of three types of junction.

ZONULA OCCLUDENS

This is where the outer laminae of two adjacent cell membranes appear to fuse.

ZONULA ADHERENS

Here there is an electron-lucent gap between two adjacent membranes. It is thought to contain a substance which acts as a cell glue.

MACULA ADHERENS – OR DESMOSOME

Especially seen in epidermal cells. Tonofilaments converge on the membranes on each side of the junction. They do not cross the junction.

Gap junctions

A fourth type of junction is seen particularly between cells transferring electrical impulses. The two membranes are separated by an electron-lucent gap containing structures which pass from one cell to the other.

NUCLEUS

NUCLEAR MEMBRANE

This is composed of two membranes, each having the same ultrastructure as the cell membrane, separated by a space – the *perinuclear cistern*. At intervals there are nuclear pores at the edges of which the inner and outer membranes join. There is thought to be a single membrane across each pore.

The outer membrane is studded with ribosomes and is continuous with the endoplasmic reticulum.

CHROMATIN

The chromatin, in the human, comprises 46 chromosomes (22 pairs of autosomes and one pair of sex chromosomes). These are only visible during cell division. At other times the chromatin is present as follows:

HETEROCHROMATIN

This is densely staining, inactive chromosomal material such as occupies most of a lymphocyte nucleus.

EUCHROMATIN

More lightly staining, active chromosomal material such as may be seen in plasma cell nuclei.

SEX CHROMATIN

Also known as 'Barr bodies'. Seen particularly in buccal smears, close to the nuclear membrane in cells possessing more than one X chromosome. This heterochromatin represents the inactivated X chromosome. Normal females have one Barr body per cell, normal males have no sex chromatin (see p. 11).

NUCLEOLUS

There may be one or several of these structures per nucleus. They have a granular network – *the nucleolonema*, enclosing spaces – the *pars amorpha*. They are thought to be the site of RNA production and are more numerous in cells which are metabolically active.

CYTOPLASM

CYTOPLASMIC SAP

Owing to the 'sodium pump' there is a relatively high concentration of potassium and a relatively low concentration of sodium in intracellular fluid as compared to extracellular fluid. Also amino acids and other chemicals are in higher concentration due to active transport.

CYTOPLASMIC DNA

The presence of DNA in the cytoplasm in single-celled organisms is well established, e.g. the resistance transfer factor of bacteria, which may be a bacteriophage, contains DNA. Cytoplasmic DNA is also postulated to be present in human cells.

ORGANELLES

Mitochondria

These oval bodies have two membranes. The outer is smooth, the inner is formed into plates and septae called *cristae*. Mitochondria contain DNA and can divide by transverse fission; it has been suggested that they have evolved from intracellular symbionts. They are the powerhouses of the cell. The matrix contains the enzymes of the Kreb's cycle and the electron transport chain enzymes are lined up on the cristae. The energy generated in the mitochondria is stored in the high energy bonds of A.T.P. In actively metabolizing cells, requiring much energy, the mitochondria are large and have numerous cristae. In inactive cells they are small and have few cristae.

Smooth endoplasmic reticulum (S.E.R.)

Within the cytoplasm are complexes of intercommunicating tubes and cisterns called the endoplasmic reticulum which is in continuity with the perinuclear cistern. Some of these channels have ribosomes attached to the outer surface (rough endoplasmic reticulum, R.E.R.) and some do not (smooth endoplasmic reticulum, S.E.R.). S.E.R. is the site of steroid metabolism, glycogen synthesis in the liver and drug detoxification. Increase in S.E.R. can be induced in liver cells by drug administration.

Rough endoplasmic reticulum (R.E.R.)

This is the form of endoplasmic reticulum with attached ribosomes. Protein synthesis takes place along the ribosomes and R.E.R. is abundant in cells making proteins for 'export', e.g. plasma cells. Ribosomes are made of R.N.A. and when R.E.R. is present in large amounts, the R.N.A. can be seen by staining the cells with pyronin.

Golgi apparatus

Adjacent to the nucleus, this structure is composed of a stack of curved cisterns and appears, when well formed, as a clear zone in the cytoplasm on light microscopy. Here the proteins, enzymes, etc., produced by the cell are modified and packaged. The modification may be a combination with carbohydrate to form glycoproteins, aggregation into other forms of complex molecule, or sulphation. Vacuoles containing the finished product are pinched off from the surface of the Golgi apparatus. These vacuoles may be secretory or contain peroxide – *peroxisomes* – or lytic enzymes – *lysosomes*.

Lysosomes

As stated above, lysosomes are released from the Golgi apparatus as vacuoles containing lytic enzymes. These enzymes function at low pH and have the following two main properties.

DIGESTION OF PHAGOCYTOSED MATERIAL

Phagocytic vacuoles which may contain foreign material (heterophagosomes) or effete cell components (autophagosomes) fuse with lysosomes to form *secondary lysosomes*. Within these vacuoles the lysosomal enzymes act upon the phagocytosed material converting it into soluble substances which may be released into the cytoplasmic sap to take part in cell metabolism. Sometimes the process is not complete and indigestible material remains. These particles are known as 'residual bodies' and are seen under the light microscope as 'wear and tear' pigment.

AUTOLYSIS

After cell damage, the number of autophagosomes increases, the damaged material being digested by fusion with lysosomes. If there is sufficient injury to cause cell death, the lysosomal membranes rupture and total autolysis of the cell ensues. This is important in necrosis and post-mortem autolysis.

Centrioles

Close to the nucleus, partly surrounded by the Golgi apparatus there are at least two centrioles. These are formed of nine evenly spaced triplets of microtubules surrounding two central microtubules. Pairs of centrioles are placed at right angles to each other. The first phase of cell division is preceded by reduplication of the centrioles which later migrate to the opposite poles of the cell, forming the spindle.

Flagellae and cilia are composed of a similar arrangement of microtubules, but in some cases they have an outer ring of nine doublets of microtubules rather than triplets.

Cell division

MITOSIS

This involves duplication of the chromosomes and their division into two equal parts to form two identical daughter cells.

Before division the chromosomes replicate, the centrioles divide and begin to move to the poles of the cell and the spindle starts to form.

Prophase
The nuclear membrane breaks down and the condensed and coiled chromosomes become visible. Connections are established between the chromosomal centromeres and the poles formed by the centrioles.

Metaphase
The chromosomes move to the centre of the cell and line up along the equatorial plate.

Anaphase
The duplicated chromosomes split apart, identical material moving towards the poles.

Telophase
The chromosomes uncoil and the nuclear membranes of each new cell are formed. The cell membranes become complete and divide the cytoplasm.

Interphase
This is the period between divisions and is entered as soon as telophase is complete.

MEIOSIS

Meiosis is the division which occurs in germ cells to produce four daughter cells, each with the haploid number of chromosomes (23). The first meiotic division is the reduction division. The second is like mitosis.

1st meiotic division

PROPHASE
This is divided into five stages.

Leptotene
The chromosomes become visible, are thin and delicate.

Zygotene
Each chromosome lies beside its opposite number to form a *bivalent*. One is maternally derived, one paternally derived.

Pachytene
The chromosomes become condensed, so thicker and shorter.

Diplotene
The two chromosomes of the bivalent separate slightly and 'chiasmata' can be seen. These are foci where the arms of the chromosomes appear to link. They commonly break where they cross and immediately reassemble with 'crossing over' of some maternal genetic material to paternal chromosomes and vice versa.

Diakinesis
Further condensation of the chromosomes takes place.

METAPHASE
The chromosomes become arranged along the 'equatorial plate'.

ANAPHASE
Each chromosome bivalent separates and one chromosome moves to each pole of the cell.

TELOPHASE
The formation of two daughter cells becomes complete each having only 23 chromosomes.

2nd meiotic division
In the male the haploid cells almost immediately undergo the second meiotic division (like mitosis). In the female, mitosis follows only if fertilization occurs.

Chapter 3
Medical Genetics – Chromosome Abnormalities

Introduction

Cells of different tissues and organs vary in appearance and degree of specialization but basically they are composed of cytoplasm and nucleus. Within the latter are the *chromosomes*, deeply staining thread-like bodies of varying size and shape. The units of heredity (the *genes*) are arranged in a linear fashion along each chromosome. They are submicroscopic segments of the DNA molecule, occupying a precise position or *locus* and determining inherited characters. The total complement of genes of an individual is known as the *genotype*; the *phenotype* is the expression of those genes as physical and mental traits.

The chromosome number

The nucleus of every cell except the germ cells contains the *diploid* number of 22 pairs of *autosomes* and one pair of *sex chromosomes*, XY in males and XX in females, making a total of 46. Each somatic cell reproduces by *mitotic division* into two daughter cells which exactly resemble the parent cell and contain 46 chromosomes. During the first *meiotic division* of *gametogenesis*, one chromosome from each pair passes into each of the two daughter (or germ) cells thus giving rise to the *haploid* number of 22 autosomes and one sex chromosome which in the oocyte is always X but in the spermatocyte may be X or Y. Fertilization of the *ovum*, by nuclear fusion of the ova and the sperm, reconstitutes the diploid number of 46 chromosomes, the sex chromosome patterns being XY or XX depending on whether the ovum was fertilized by a Y-bearing sperm or an X-bearing sperm.

In dividing cells the chromosomes are seen to be split longitudinally into two *chromatids* except at a single point, the *centromere*, which divides the chromosome into two arms (the long and short arms).

Identification of human chromosomes

Individual chromosomes may be distinguished by several criteria:
(*a*) The total length of the chromosome.
(*b*) The position of the centromere. Those which have the centromere situated at approximately the middle of their length are termed metacentric; those with the centromere towards one end are submetacentric and those with the centromere near the end are acrocentric.
(*c*) The presence of *satellites* (small chromatin masses) attached by narrow stalks to the short arms of all acrocentric chromosomes except the Y chromosome.
(*d*) Special banding techniques.

With the above criteria, the autosomes can be arranged into seven groups of similar morphology numbered A to G, and also in descending order of size (1–22). This systematic arrangement is known as the *karyotype* (Fig. 2 below).

Sex chromatin

There is a difference in the somatic nuclei of males and females. Normal female cells have a distinctive mass, the *sex chromatin*, lying against the inner surface of the nuclear membrane. This mass is absent in normal males. The polymorphonuclear leucocyte in females is also distinctive, having an accessory nuclear lobule (the drumstick).

Only one X chromosome is active in female cells and any others present are inactive and are represented as the *sex chromatin mass*. The number of sex chromatin masses is usually one less than the number of sex chromosomes. Thus a patient with a

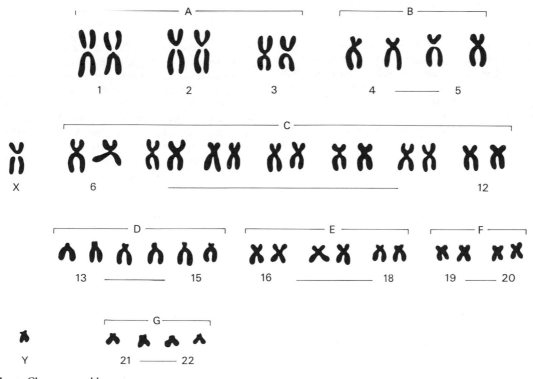

Fig. 2. Chromosomal karyotype.

sex chromosome constitution of XXX has 2 chromatin masses. Epithelium scraped from the inner surface of the cheek provides easily accessible cells for the determination of sex chromatin status.

Chromosome abnormalities

Chromosomal aberrations in man are either alteration in the chromosome number or structural alterations in individual chromosomes. Abnormalities of number are commoner than abnormalities of structure.

ABNORMALITIES OF CHROMOSOME NUMBER

ANEUPLOIDY

A chromosome number is *aneuploid* if it is not an exact multiple of the haploid (23) number, e.g. 45 or 47. The presence of three instead of the usual pair of chromosomes is known as *trisomy* of which the best known example is G trisomy (mongolism or Down's syndrome) where the extra small acrocentric chromosome is considered to be number 21. Two other important trisomic syndromes have been described with typical phenotypes – trisomy 13 producing Patau's syndrome and trisomy 18, Edwards' syndrome.

If one chromosome is missing, the individual is *monosomic* for that particular chromosome. The only example of monosomy in man compatible with life is Turner's syndrome in which only one X chromosome (XO) is present.

Origin of aneuploidy
Trisomy and monosomy is attributed to an error – *non-disjunction*, in either the first or second cell division of meiosis, in which two homologous chromosomes fail to separate, both chromosomes of that pair enter one daughter cell nucleus. The one cell will have 24 chromosomes and the other 22. On their fertilization by a normal germ cell the zygotes formed will have 47 and 45 chromosomes respectively, the former being trisomic and the latter monosomic for that particular chromosome. Non-disjunction can also occur during mitotic cell division.

POLYPLOIDY

A chromosome number is *polyploid* if it is a multiple of the basic haploid (23) number other than the normal diploid (46) number, e.g. 69 or 92. This is occasionally seen in the chromosomes of neoplastic tissue and in some aborted foetuses.

Origin of polyploidy
An error in the formation of the spindle mechanism during meiosis, after the chromosome material has duplicated and before the completion of cell division, results in polyploidy.

ABNORMALITIES OF CHROMOSOME STRUCTURE

Abnormalities can arise as a consequence of the breakage of chromosomes. The common types of structural abnormalities encountered are deletion, ring formation, translocation (interchange), duplication, inversion and isochromosomes.

Deletion
A deletion is the loss of a segment of a chromosome and may be terminal or involve the loss of a segment between two breaks. The deleted chromosome participates in subsequent cell division only if the centromere is present and the small chromosome segment without a centromere is usually lost. Although uncommon, distinctive phenotypes due to deletions have been described. A partial or a complete deletion of a number 5 chromosome is associated with the syndrome known as 'cri du chat', and a condition characterized by multiple congenital abnormalities has been described associated with a partial deletion of other chromosomes, notably 13, 18 and 21.

The *ring chromosome* is a special type of deletion in which both terminal fragments of a chromosome are lost and the broken ends of the chromosome unite.

Translocation (interchange)
A translocation (or interchange) is the result of exchange of a segment from one chromosome to a non-homologous chromosome following breakage of these chromosomes. A number of instances of Down's syndrome are due to translocation between chromosomes 21, 14 and 15 or between chromosomes 21 and 22. Mothers of these individuals are

phenotypically normal but have a karyotype of 45 chromosomes with only one 21 and a composite 15/21. As a result of the translocation, segregation of the chromosomes during meiosis is disturbed and a translocation carrier can produce four types of gametes.

Duplication
A duplication is the inclusion of an extra segment of the chromosome within a chromosome.

Inversion
An inversion follows the detachment of a segment of a chromosome with recombination within the chromosome in an inverted position. Inversions cannot be detected at present, in preparations of human chromosomes, unless they involve the centromere.

Isochromosomes
Isochromosomes are produced when division at the centromere takes place at right angles to the long axis of the chromosome instead of parallel to it. The result is two chromosomes, one composed of two short arms and the other of two long arms. It is partly a duplication and partly a deletion.

CHROMOSOMAL MOSAICS AND CHIMERAS

Mosaicism is the presence in the same individual of two kinds of chromosome constitution derived from a single zygote. Some patients with Down's syndrome are mosaics and have tissues with 46 and 47 chromosomes. Several patients with Turner's syndrome have XO and XX cell lines.

In a chimera there is also more than one kind of chromosome constitution but derived from more than one zygote.

Aetiology of chromosome abnormalities

Chromosome abnormalities may be considered as mutations for they are analogous to point mutations affecting single genes. The aetiology of major abnormalities of chromosomes remains obscure but several factors may be important.

Radiation
Ionization radiations are a possible cause of *non-disjunction* and experimentally can produce chromosome deletions and genetic mutations.

Virus infections
For example, measles can produce fragmentation of chromosomes.

Late maternal age
It is a major factor in the incidence of Down's syndrome which is more frequent in older than younger women. Non-disjunction is thought to occur more frequently in older mothers.

Clinical conditions due to chromosomal abnormalities

There are several well-recognized clinical conditions due to numerical and structural abnormalities of the autosomes and of the sex chromosomes.

AUTOSOMAL ABNORMALITIES

Examples of autosomal abnormalities are as follows.

Down's syndrome
This is the commonest autosomal anomaly, occurring about 1 in 700 live births and characterized by mental retardation, a typical facies with slanted, widespread eyes, epicanthic folds, short neck and flattened occiput, broad flat hands with short incurving fifth digits and abnormal dermatoglyphic patterns (single palmar crease and distal triradius in the palms). Associated anomalies – ventricular and atrial septal defects, oesophageal atresia, tracheo-oesophageal fistulae and duodenal atresia, may also occur.

Most cases of mongolism are associated with an extra chromosome from the G group, the affected individual being conventionally considered trisomic for chromosome 21 with a total chromosome complement of 47. Occasionally the condition may result from a reciprocal translocation of a chromosome of 13–15 (D) group and a chromosome of the 21 and 22 (G) group or a translocation between individual chromosomes of 21–22 (G) group.

Trisomy 18 – Edwards' syndrome

The important clinical features are mental retardation, failure to thrive, micrognathia, low-set ears, a characteristically clenched fist with overlapping fingers, 'rocker-bottom' deformity of the feet and a high proportion of arches in the fingerprints. Affected infants are trisomic for a chromosome of group E (probably number 18) with a chromosome complement of 47. Few cases survive longer than 6 months.

Trisomy 13 – Patau's syndrome

The 13 trisomy, which is less frequent than other trisomies, has karyotype of 47 chromosomes with trisomy for one of the chromosomes in the 13–15 group. The usual features are defects of the central nervous system, mental retardation, cleft palate, harelip, cataracts, polydactyly and anophthalmia.

'Cri du chat' syndrome

One of the most commonly found conditions due to a partial or a complete deletion of the short arms of chromosome number 5. Affected infants have a characteristic high-pitched cry like the mewing of a cat, mental retardation, micrognathia, hypertelorism and low-set ears.

SEX CHROMOSOME ABNORMALITIES

Examples of sex chromosome abnormalities are:

Turner's syndrome – ovarian dysgenesis or monosomy X

Turner's syndrome which occurs about 1 in 2500 female births has three characteristics – sexual infantilism, short stature and congenital anomalies.

SEXUAL INFANTILISM
Manifested by primary amenorrhoea; lack of breast development with widely spaced nipples; scanty sexual hair; infantile external genitalia, uterus and Fallopian tubes; 'streak' gonads which have no ovarian follicles (see p. 432).

SHORT STATURE
Patients rarely attain a height greater than 152 cm.

CONGENITAL ANOMALIES
Webbing of neck; congenital lymphoedema of extremities; frequently coarctation of the aorta and horseshoe kidneys.

Most affected females are chromatin-negative with 45 chromosomes and a single X sex chromosome (45/XO pattern), but there is a small subgroup of mosaics with one of the following patterns: XO/XX, XO/XY, or XO/XYY.

Some cases of ovarian dysgenesis are chromatin-positive. These patients are either mosaics with normal chromosomes (XO/XX, XO/XXX or XO/XX/XXX) or due to deletion or isochromosome formation of the X.

Multiple X syndromes in women

The triplo-X syndrome, which occurs about 1 in every 1000 female births, is characterized by mild mental subnormality, and slightly underdeveloped secondary sex characters with secondary amenorrhoea. The usual karyotype is 47 with trisomy of X chromosome (47/XXX) but occasionally the chromosome number is 48 with four X sex chromosomes (48/XXXX).

Klinefelter's syndrome

The main features of this chromosomal anomaly in males are:
1 *Small azoospermic testes* with sclerosing tubular degeneration, absence of elastic tissue and hyperplasia of interstitial cells.
2 *Bilateral gynaecomastia*, eunuchoid build, sparse sexual hair and beard growth, and high urinary gonadotrophins with low 17-ketosteroid excretion.
3 *Mild intellectual subnormality*. Most affected men are chromatin-positive and have 47 chromosomes with a sex chromosome complement of XXY. Occasionally patients may have XXXY or XXXXY karyotypes and a few may be mosaics XXY/XX, XXY/XY (see p. 409).

The YY syndrome

Individuals with this syndrome may have a mild mental defect with violent and aggressive behaviour and are usually taller than 183 cm. They have XYY karyotypes and occasionally XYYY, XXYY or XXXYY.

CHROMOSOMAL ABNORMALITIES AND ABORTION

About 20 per cent of abortions which occur spontaneously in the first 3 months of pregnancy are due to chromosomal abnormalities in the foetus. Many of these early abortuses are triploids, XO or 21 trisomies.

CHROMOSOMAL ANOMALY AND LEUKAEMIA

A characteristic anomaly – the Philadelphia chromosome (Ph′) is found in the leucocytes of some patients with chronic granulocytic leukaemia. This chromosome marker appears to be a deleted chromosome number 21 (see Fig. 2 on p. 11).

Chapter 4
Medical Genetics – Inherited Disorders

Patterns of inheritance

The patterns within families of single gene inherited diseases are determined by whether the mutant gene is located on one of the autosomes or on the X chromosome; by whether the gene is present in single dosage (*heterozygous*) or in double dosage (*homozygous*); and by whether the trait is *dominant* or *recessive*.

AUTOSOMAL DOMINANT INHERITANCE

Generally rare and usually less severe than autosomal recessive conditions. The abnormal gene is located on one of a pair of autosomes.

Features
1   Trait appears in every generation unless it has arisen as a fresh mutation.
2   Affected persons transmit the trait to half their children.
3   Males and females equally affected.
4   Unaffected persons cannot transmit the condition to their children.

Examples of diseases due to dominant inheritance
Achondroplasia, brachydactyly (short fingers), Huntingdon's chorea, Marfan's syndrome, familial polyposis, multiple neurofibromatosis and tuberose sclerosis.

Variability in autosomal dominant inheritance
Dominant conditions may show a wide variability in severity or *expressivity*. The expression may range from mild to severe. When the disease is extremely mild clinically it is referred to as *forme fruste*. The clinical expression of the mutant dominant gene may be so reduced that the condi-

tion cannot be detected and in such cases is said to be *non-penetrant* and in a pedigree would appear to '*skip a generation*'.

AUTOSOMAL RECESSIVE INHERITANCE

A disease due to autosomal recessive inheritance is expressed only in a person who receives the recessive gene from both his parents and so is homozygous for it.

Features
1　Condition appears also in one-quarter of brothers and sisters.
2　Parents and offspring are clinically normal.
3　Males and females equally affected.
4　Parents of affected individuals often consanguineous.

Examples of diseases due to recessive inheritance
Many inborn errors of metabolism, e.g. phenylketonuria, homocystinuria and alcaptonuria; cystic fibrosis, Morquio's disease and congenital adrenal hyperplasia.

SEX-LINKED INHERITANCE

Sex-linked genes may be X-linked or Y-linked. The only condition due to Y-linked gene is the 'hairy' ear trait transmitted only from male to male, *Holandric inheritance*. X-linked genes have more clinical significance and may be recessive or dominant.

X-LINKED RECESSIVE INHERITANCE

The inherited disease is expressed by all males who have the gene and only by females who are homozygous.

Features
1　Females only rarely affected.
2　If the condition is lethal as in Duchenne type of muscular dystrophy transmission is always through carrier females.

3　Half of the sons of carriers are affected and half of their daughters are carriers.
4　Never male to-male transmission.

Examples of diseases due to X-linked recessive inheritance
Severe Duchenne type of progressive muscular dystrophy, classical haemophilia, Christmas disease and colour blindness.

X-LINKED DOMINANT INHERITANCE

Features
1　Affected men transmit the condition to all their daughters and to none of their sons.
2　Affected women who are heterozygous pass the trait to half their sons and to half their daughters.
3　Affected homozygous females produce only affected children.

Examples of diseases due to X-linked dominant inheritance
Vitamin D-resistant rickets.

SEX-LIMITED TRAITS

A trait which is sex-limited appears in only one sex. Baldness is sex-limited, appearing usually in males.

MULTIFACTORIAL OR POLYGENIC INHERITANCE

Many common diseases and anomalies which are not inherited in a dominant or recessive manner nevertheless show some evidence of a measure of genetic inheritance. The disease may be the result of several genes having an additive effect or produced by an interaction of genetic and environmental factors. The incidence of such conditions among relatives is higher than in the general population.

Examples of diseases due to multifactorial inheritance
Pyloric stenosis, hare lip with or without cleft palate and congenital dislocation of the hip.

Examples of inherited metabolic disorders

DISORDERS OF CARBOHYDRATE METABOLISM

Maturity onset diabetes mellitus

HEREDITY

The usual pattern of inheritance described suggests the participation of a single recessive trait with incomplete penetrance but this evidence is not conclusive (see also p. 634).

Galactosaemia

NATURE

A familial disorder of galactose metabolism.

INHERITANCE

By a single autosomal recessive gene.

AETIOLOGY

This has been shown to be due to a deficiency of galactose-1-phosphate uridyl transferase. The deficiency can be demonstrated in erythrocytes of patients and partially detected in the heterozygous carriers of the disease (see Fig. 3).

CLINICAL MANIFESTATIONS

These characteristically appear in early infancy and include:

1 Nutritional failure with vomiting, diarrhoea and loss of weight.
2 Hepatosplenomegaly.
3 Cataracts.
4 Mental retardation.

LABORATORY FINDINGS

1 Elevation of blood galactose.
2 Galactosaemia, albuminuria, amino-aciduria.
3 Deficient erythrocyte galactose-1-phosphate uridyl transferase.

TREATMENT

If untreated the condition is usually fatal, but improvement and prevention of clinical manifestations may be produced by removal of galactose from the diet.

Glycogen storage disease

NATURE

A collection of distinct diseases resulting from primary abnormalities of glycogen metabolism and resulting in the accumulation of glycogen in the tissues. The clinical picture varies with the enzyme deficiency (see Fig. 4).

INHERITANCE

Each defect inherited by single autosomal recessive gene.

DISORDERS OF AMINO ACID METABOLISM

Phenylketonuria

NATURE

Metabolic disorder caused by deficiency (demonstrable in liver and kidney) of enzyme phenylalanine hydroxylase resulting in accumulation of phenylalanine and its abnormal metabolites.

		Enzyme
1	Galactose + ATP $\longrightarrow$ Galactose-1-phosphate + ADP	Galactokinase
2	Galactose-1-phosphate + UDP glucose $\rightleftharpoons$ UDP galactose + glucose-1-phosphate	Galactose-1-phosphate uridyl transferase
3	UDP galactose $\rightleftharpoons$ UDP glucose	UDP galactose-4-epimerase
4	UTP + glucose-1-phosphate $\rightleftharpoons$ UDP glucose + pyrophosphate	UDP glucose phosphorylase

Fig. 3. Principal chemical pathways involved in galactose to glucose conversion.

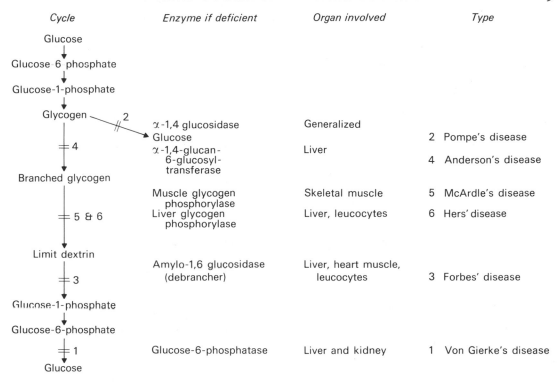

Fig. 4. Principal chemical pathways involved in glycogen metabolism showing site of enzyme deficiencies causing glycogen storage types 1–6.

INHERITANCE
Autosomal recessive in which the heterozygote state can be detected through an elevation of serum phenylalanine following a test load. Chemical defect shown at point 1 in Fig. 5.

CLINICAL MANIFESTATIONS
These include severe mental retardation, convulsions, eczematous skin lesions and deficiency of pigmentation in skin and hair.

TREATMENT
The condition can be improved by low phenylalanine diet and may be largely prevented if treatment is started early in life.

Alcaptonuria

NATURE
One of the original four inborn errors of metabolism described by Garrod in 1908.

INHERITANCE
Autosomal recessive.

AETIOLOGY
Deficiency of enzyme homogentisic acid oxidase prevents breakdown of homogentisic acid and causes its accumulation in serum and excretion in the urine (see Fig. 5 on p. 20).

CLINICAL FEATURES
Homogentisic aciduria, ochronosis (pigmentation of cartilage and other connective tissues), arthritis in later years (see p. 117).

Albinism

NATURE
Inherited disorder of melanin metabolism resulting in decrease or absence of pigment in skin, hair and eyes, possibly due to defective tyrosinase (see also p. 118).

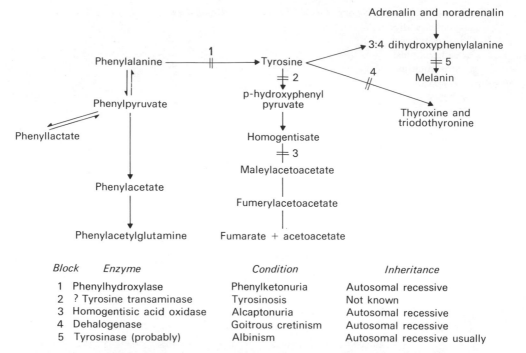

Fig. 5. Principal pathways in phenylalanine and tyrosine metabolism and the blocks causing the conditions described. Modified from Harris H. (1959), *Human Biochemical Genetics*, Cambridge.

CLINICAL MANIFESTATIONS AND INHERITANCE
These are of three types:
1 Oculocutaneous albinism – usually autosomal recessive.
2 Ocular albinism – X-linked recessive.
3 Localized cutaneous albinism – autosomal dominant, sometimes associated with deaf-mutism.

Familial goitre
See p. 308.

See p. 308.

DISORDERS OF LIPID METABOLISM

NATURE
Abnormal increases in the plasma concentrations of various lipid components have been described and some attempts made to classify them according to the disturbed lipid component. The classification, causes and genetic characteristics remain inadequately established but a simplified classification follows.

Familial hypertriglyceridaemia
Characterized by excessive chylomicrons in plasma, waxy skin, visible lipaemia of retina, eruptive xanthomata and in childhood, spasms of abdominal pain, hepatosplenomegaly.

Treatment is usually aimed at prevention of abdominal pain in childhood by low fat diet.

The condition is inherited as an autosomal recessive characteristic.

Familial hypercholesterolaemia
Familial disorder characterized by raised plasma cholesterol and in many patients associated with xanthoma tuberosum and tendinosum.

There is an increased risk of ischaemic heart disease and, in some cases, of aortic stenosis.

INHERITANCE
The disorder is frequently familial and is inherited as an autosomal dominant characteristic with incomplete expression in the heterozygote.

TREATMENT

For heterozygotes a diet low in cholesterol with substitution of polyunsaturated fats may be effective in lowering cholesterol levels. In some ion exchange resins such as cholestyramine it may be necessary to achieve normal serum cholesterol levels. Satisfactory treatment of homozygotes is extremely difficult.

Hypertriglyceridaemia with hypercholesterolaemia

Characterized by abnormally high plasma concentrations of both cholesterol and triglycerides, probably a heterogeneous group of disorders.

Xanthomata may appear and there is an increased risk of peripheral vascular and ischaemic heart disease in affected patients, but negligible amongst relatives.

Abnormal glucose tolerance often found.

Inheritance is probably multifactorial with genetic and environmental factors playing a part.

The condition may be improved by a low carbohydrate diet. Secondary hyperlipaemia may be caused by:

Physiological post-prandial state.
Pregnancy.
Hypothyroidism.
Obstructive jaundice.
Biliary cirrhosis.
Glomerulonephritis.
Nephrotic syndrome.
Diabetes.

Metachromatic leucodystrophy

See p. 610.

Lipid storage diseases

See p. 113.

Chapter 5
Inflammation – Local Manifestations

Definition

Manifestations
  Local
  General

Local manifestations
Macroscopical
Microscopical
  Vessel constriction
  Vessel dilatation
  Vessel permeability
  Exudation
  Haemoconcentration
  Margination of leucocytes
  Emigration of white cells
  Chemotaxis
  Phagocytosis
  Macrophage activity
Components
  Vascular
  Cellular
  Exudate

Local factors

VASCULAR
Chemical mediators
Nerve connections

CELLULAR

Blood-borne
Polymorphs
  Neutrophils
  Eosinophils
  Basophils and mast cells
Lymphocytes and plasma
cells
Monocytes

From tissues
Histiocytes (macrophages)
Fibroblasts
Giant cells

Cells in types of inflammation
Acute
Subacute
Chronic

EXUDATE
Arteriolar dilatation
Vascular permeability

Chemical mediators
Amines
Kinins
Proteases
Cleavage products of
complement
Prostaglandins
Slow reacting substance of
anaphylaxis
Summary

Macroscopical varieties
Serous
Fibrinous
Sero-fibrinous
Haemorrhagic
Suppurative (purulent)
  Ulcer
  Empyema
  Abscess
Catarrhal
Gangrenous
Phlegmonous
Membranous
Cellulitis

Definition

Response of living tissues to injury, resulting in an exudate.

Manifestations

These are:
1 Local.
2 General.

Local manifestations

Regardless of the exciting cause, the basic local

inflammatory response is almost always similar in type.

Macroscopical
There is heat, pain, swelling and redness with a variable loss of function.

Microscopical
The following is the usual sequence of events:
1 Momentary arteriolar constriction.
2 Dilatation of arterioles, capillaries and venules.
3 Increased permeability of vessel walls.
4 Exudation of a protein-rich inflammatory fluid – *exudate*.
5 Haemoconcentration due to fluid loss into tis-

sues but intravascular retention of most of the red cells.

6 Margination of the leucocytes which leave the *axial stream*, pass into the *plasmatic zone* and pavement the endothelial surface.

7 Emigration of white cells and diapedesis of red cells through the vessel walls.

8 Chemotaxis of polymorphonuclear leucocytes (polymorphs).

9 Phagocytosis of organisms by the polymorphs.

10 Appearance of phagocytic histiocytes – macrophages.

Components

Thus, at the local site, there are three basic components.

VASCULAR

With increased but relatively static blood flow in the area – *rubor and calor*.

CELLULAR

Increased cells in the area, mainly derived from the blood, permitting phagocytosis and local antibody increase – *tumor*.

EXUDATE

The protein-rich inflammatory exudate containing fibrinogen and producing oedema – *tumor*, and *dolor* due to stimulation of nerve endings.

Local factors

These components will now be described in greater detail.

VASCULAR

Chemical mediators

Injury evokes the triple response by liberation of chemical mediators which act directly on arterioles, capillaries and venules causing dilatation and increased permeability. Initial vasoconstriction is probably due to direct mechanical stimulation of the capillaries.

Nerve connections

The vascular response may be modified by cutting the sensory nerves and so blocking the axon reflex. This axon reflex causes the 'flare' of the triple response by arteriolar dilatation. Inflammation can occur in denervated tissues but, if the autonomic system is damaged and the local vessels constricted, there is more tissue destruction. A similar effect is produced by injecting adrenalin just before, or with, the injuring agent.

CELLULAR

Different aetiological agents cause variation in the number and types of cells found at the local site of inflammation. The cells present may include any of the following.

BLOOD-BORNE

Polymorphonuclear leucocytes

NEUTROPHILS

The first and most numerous cells seen in acute inflammation. They are motile, amoeboid, actively phagocytic and respond to chemotaxis (see p. 446).

EOSINOPHILS

Emigrate in significant numbers from the blood stream in the later and healing stages. Large numbers are frequently associated with parasitic infestations and allergic conditions (see p. 446).

BASOPHILS AND MAST CELLS

Granules in cytoplasm contain histamine, slow-reacting substance of anaphylaxis (SRS-A), eosinophil – chemotactic factor of anaphylaxis (ECF-A) and platelet activating factor. The cells appear degranulated after release of these substances. They are associated with immunologically mediated disease (see p. 101).

Lymphocytes and plasma cells

Main function is in cellular and humoral immunity (see p. 89). They do not reach inflammatory areas in the early stages, but later play an important part, especially in chronic inflammation and granulomatous diseases, e.g. tuberculosis, syphilis.

Monocytes

Phagocytic cells present in the blood in small numbers which appear in the inflammatory exudate shortly after the initial phases of the reaction. They are motile and exhibit a weak chemotactic response (see p. 446).

FROM TISSUES

Histiocytes or macrophages
These cells are similar in appearance and function to blood monocytes. They are actively phagocytic and motile.

Fibroblasts
Young fibrous tissue cells appearing in the healing stage. They synthesize collagen.

Giant cells
Large multinucleate cells formed by the fusion of histiocytes. There are several types but the most commonly encountered in inflammation are the foreign body and Langhans' types. The foreign body type is a large cell with multiple nuclei arranged centrally; the Langhans' giant cell is of a similar size but is frequently oval and has a peripheral distribution of the nuclei which show a 'horseshoe' arrangement. They are actively phagocytic and ingest foreign particles too large for macrophages to engulf.

Some of the giant cells found in pathological conditions are illustrated in Fig. 6.

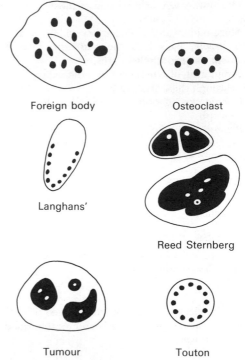

Foreign body   Osteoclast

Langhans'

Reed Sternberg

Tumour   Touton

Fig. 6. Types of giant cells.

CELLS IN TYPES OF INFLAMMATION

The characteristic cells are as follows.

Acute
Polymorphs, except for typhoid fever when mononuclear cells predominate.

Subacute
Polymorphs, plasma cells and lymphocytes.

Chronic
Lymphocytes, plasma cells and fibroblasts. Monocytes and macrophages are present in varying numbers in all infections.

EXUDATE

The main factors are as follows.

Arteriolar dilatation
This increases blood flow and pressure in capil-laries. When pressure exceeds the osmotic pressure of plasma protein, fluid will pass into tissue spaces.

Vascular permeability
Chemical mediators of inflammation increase vascular permeability to plasma proteins, thus decreasing the intravascular osmotic pressure.

CHEMICAL MEDIATORS

The best established mediators include the following.

Amines
Histamine is active in man to produce vasodilatation and increased vascular permeability: 5-Hydroxytryptamine (5-HT, serotonin) although a mediator in the rat and mouse is probably not important in man.

Kinins
Bradykinin and kallidin, formed from plasma pre-

cursors, increase vascular permeability, produce vasodilatation and pain.

Proteases

These substances are released from neutrophils and have many properties including increased vascular permeability, releasing histamine, they are chemotactic for monocytes, cleave C_3 and C_5, activate kinins and immobilize neutrophils. Some are pyrogens.

Cleavage products of complement

C_{3a} and C_{5a} cause histamine release from mast cells. They are chemotactic agents, as is C_{567}.

Prostaglandins

Released from neutrophils during phagocytosis and from platelets. PGE_1 and PGE_2 produce vascular permeability, vasodilatation and pain. Some prostaglandins potentiate the action of kinins, others have a protective effect.

Slow-reacting substance of anaphylaxis – SRS-A

Increases vascular permeability after some delay. Produces bronchospasm.

Summary

The number of substances which have been proposed as mediators in the acute inflammatory response is large and increasing. Their interactions are uncertain. The probable sequence of events is that histamine and the kinins are important initially. Their action is modified by prostaglandins, proteases and cleavage products of complement. SRS-A is important in the later phases.

Macroscopical varieties of acute inflammation

Variations in the proportions of the cellular, vascular and exudative components in any inflammation may result in the following descriptive varieties of acute inflammation.

Serous

Serous exudate of protein-rich fluid (3 g/dl or more) with relative density of 1.020 or above. This type of inflammatory response occurs on serous membranes, e.g. pleurisy with effusion, peritonitis, pericarditis and synovial effusions. It should not be confused with the transudates of renal or cardiac failure which have a low relative density and a protein content of 0.3 g/dl or less.

Fibrinous

An exudate containing exuberant amounts of fibrin forming shaggy strands. Found typically in 'bread and butter' pericarditis, on pleural and peritoneal surfaces and filling the alveoli in lobar pneumonia.

Sero-fibrinous

Frequently, serous and fibrinous varieties are combined to give a serous effusion containing profuse fibrinous strands.

Haemorrhagic

This type shows all the signs of acute inflammation with small or large areas of red cell extravasation due to extensive vascular damage. It is seen in very virulent or fulminating infections: in the obstructed appendix; in the gall bladder with *Clostridium perfringens* infection; in the lungs with viral or haemolytic streptococcal infection; as a generalized manifestation of meningococcal septicaemia (spotted fever).

Suppurative or purulent

This implies the presence of pus, which consists of tissue breakdown products, polymorphs and organisms, frequently associated with some cholesterol, fibrin and red cells.

ULCER

A local defect or excavation of the surface of an organ produced by shedding or sloughing of the surface tissues due to any cause. It is most frequently seen in the skin and gastro-intestinal tract.

EMPYEMA

A localized collection of pus within a closed cavity which is most commonly found in the pleural space or in the gall bladder.

ABSCESS

A localized collection of pus within the substance of an organ or tissue. It is commonly found in solid organs, e.g. brain, liver, kidney, lungs and bones.

Catarrhal

This refers to a type of inflammation associated with a profuse secretion of watery or mucoid fluid from an epithelial surface. It is especially common in the respiratory tract but also occurs in the intestines.

Gangrenous

In some severe infections, vascular stasis is followed by thrombosis and the tissues become devitalized. The discoloration and necrosis so produced give the characteristic appearances of this type of inflammation. Gangrenous inflammation is seen in some cases of acute appendicitis and cholecystitis and also in infections due to clostridia.

Phlegmonous

Occurs rarely as a spreading oedematous necrosis within a tissue plane and can occur in the neck and abdominal wall. It is also seen in the walls of hollow viscera, e.g. phlegmonous gastritis (see p. 187).

Membranous

The formation of a membrane composed of matted fibrin, mucus and inflammatory cells producing a grey-white membrane on the surface – pseudo-membranous colitis (see p. 205). Epithelium may be included in this sheet and it is then called a 'true' membranous inflammation; the absence of epithelium results in a so-called 'false' membrane and this is the type most usually seen in diphtheria.

Cellulitis

A rapidly spreading inflammation in tissues which is usually due to β-haemolytic streptococci and has a red, slightly raised margin. It is frequently accompanied by red tender streaks visible beneath the skin due to an acute lymphangitis.

Chapter 6
Inflammation – Localization: Results: General Effects

Localization of infection

ORGANISM
Dose
Virulence and type
Invasive properties
Site of entry
Phagocytosis
Chemotherapy

HOST
Blood supply
Site of entry
Fibrin barrier
Vascular blockage
Immunity
Systemic conditions
Steroids

Results of acute inflammation
Resolution
    Complete
    Incomplete

Suppuration
Chronic inflammation
Fibrosis
Spread
Death

OTHER TYPES OF INFLAMMATION
Subacute
Chronic

General manifestations of inflammation
FEVER
Normal heat regulation
    Retention of heat
    Loss of heat
Mechanism
    Increased heat production
    Decreased heat loss
Stages
Results

HYPERPYREXIA
Definition
Causes
Results

CHANGES IN THE BLOOD

White cells
Leucocytosis
    Neutrophils
    Eosinophils
    Lymphocytes
    Monocytes
Leucopenia
Abnormal white cells

Red cells
Toxic depression
Haemolysis
Haemorrhage

CHANGES IN ORGANS
Reactive
    Local
    General
Degenerative
Septicaemia
Pyaemia
Bacteraemia

Localization of infection

The inflammatory reaction is fundamentally a protective mechanism for the body and the noxious agent is much more easily overcome if the reaction is successfully localized. There are certain factors which determine whether the infection will remain localized or spread.

ORGANISM

Dose
The larger the number of organisms or the greater the degree of physico-chemical trauma, the greater is the likelihood of an inflammatory reaction, and if the dose is very high the greater the chance of spread beyond the local area.

Virulence and type of organisms
Avirulent organisms of the commensal type rarely produce much inflammation, whereas virulent pyogenic bacteria frequently do; staphylococci resulting in a localized purulent reaction; streptococci in a spreading reaction with cellulitis; rickettsiae and many viruses produce an haemorrhagic variant. It is usually, however, not possible in most cases to specify the precise organism from the type of tissue reaction.

Invasive properties

The comparatively avirulent commensal organisms tend to remain localized, as do the coagulase-producing staphylococci, whilst the streptokinase (fibrinolysin)-producing organisms, e.g. β-haemolytic streptococci, and the hyaluronidase-producing organisms, e.g. *Clostridium perfringens (C. welchii)*, spread more rapidly. This invasive property, therefore, is usually brought about by substances produced by the organisms including both endo- and exotoxins.

Site of entry

The site of entry of many organisms alters the type of disease produced. Thus, anthrax inoculated into the skin produces a 'malignant pustule' but the same organisms aspirated into the lung results in the sinister pneumonia – *wool sorter's disease*. The neurotropic organism of rabies travels to the brain to produce its fatal effect. A bite from a rabid animal on the face is thus more serious than one on the leg. The incubation period is shorter as is the time in which to achieve effective resistance.

Phagocytosis and digestion

Many organisms exhibit positive chemotaxis to polymorphs and are rapidly phagocytosed by histiocytes but some may remain viable intracellularly and thus be transported to other parts of the body.

Chemotherapeutic sensitivity

In all cases of bacterial infection it is important to know the chemotherapeutic sensitivities of the causal organisms.

HOST

Local blood supply

The more vascular the local area involved, the greater the chance of a rapid and successful inflammatory reaction. Vascular tissues, e.g. skin, usually result in a successful localization of the inflammatory process, whereas avascular structures, e.g. cornea and cartilage, offer little resistance to an invading organism.

Site of entry

The location of infection plays a paramount role in its spread. Dense compact tissues resist infective spread whilst loose tissues, e.g. fat or lung tissue, encourage spread. Infection on the surface of a serous cavity or in a joint space may result in spread of the infection to involve the entire surface.

Fibrin barrier

The formation of fibrin in the tissues from the exudation of plasma fibrinogen has been held to have a filtration effect impeding the spread of bacteria. The fibrin 'net' also aids phagocytosis by providing a surface for the action of neutrophils. Massive fibrin formation occurs in well developed inflammations of severe type and probably a partial barrier effect is produced, but it is modified by bacterial action, e.g. β-haemolytic streptococci – *streptokinase* and pathogenic staphylococci – *coagulase*.

Vascular blockage

Some examples of acute inflammation produce such stagnation of the blood flow and vascular endothelial damage that thrombosis results. This blockage tends to prevent spread of infection, but at the same time leads to increased tissue anoxia and subsequently to necrosis. This by itself will tend to perpetuate and extend the infection, especially when gangrene supervenes.

Immunity

Natural or acquired antibodies markedly modify the resistance of the host to infection. Patients who are immunocompromized, naturally due to recent or previous infection or malignant disease, or artificially due to cytotoxic or immunosuppressive therapy, are much more liable to infection (see p. 375).

Systemic conditions

The general health of the patient is of importance and the young, in a good state of nutrition, are in a better condition to withstand infection than the old or undernourished. In addition, the health of the blood vessels supplying the infected areas has a bearing on the outcome of the inflammatory response. In diabetics, where both the circulation and cell metabolism are abnormal, infections are common.

Steroids

These substances, e.g. hydrocortisone and prednisone, act by impairing the antibody response to an antigen, to suppress many aspects of the inflammatory reaction. The danger of spread of an infection is thus increased.

Results of acute inflammation

The outcome of any acute inflammation depends on the balance between the defence mechanisms of the host, of which the inflammatory reaction is of the greatest importance, and the ability of the noxious agent to overcome these defences. The following may result from an inflammatory response.

Resolution

COMPLETE

Complete resolution may occur with retrogression of the acute inflammatory response and the area return to its previous normal appearance and function. This is the ideal end-result of any inflammatory process.

INCOMPLETE
Resolution may be incomplete and the fibrin of the exudate becomes organized to produce a fibrous scar (see p. 34).

Suppuration
The area of inflammation may suppurate with breakdown of tissue resulting in an abscess, ulcer or empyema. The outcome of this will depend on the site and localization, but after spontaneous or surgical drainage of the pus, the area will be replaced by fibrous tissue to produce a permanent scar (see p. 34).

Chronic inflammation
The agent producing the acute inflammatory reaction may not be combated entirely by the inflammatory response and the acute inflammation will subside to a chronic inflammatory reaction characterized by less intense vascularity and diminished exudation. Chronic inflammation shows:
1   Infiltration   by   chronic   inflammatory cells – lymphocytes and plasma cells
2   Overgrowth of the connective tissue elements – fibroblasts.
3   Increased fibrosis of the inflamed area.

Fibrosis
An area of acute inflammation which does not successfully overcome the initiating agent, will not resolve but will become an area of fibrous scarring.

Spread
If local and general defence mechanisms are overwhelmed by the infecting agent the infection will spread:
1   Locally – involvement of adjacent structures, cellulitis, etc.
2   Lymphatic – lymphangitis and regional lymphadenitis.
3   Blood stream – septicaemia.

Death
A fatal outcome may result when:
1   The local and general defence mechanisms fail in fulminating infections, especially when associated with septicaemia, e.g. meningococcal, or with profound toxaemia, e.g. diphtheria and clostridial infections.
2   Dangerous   locations – infections   in   certain sites, e.g. mediastinum, brain, heart and cervical spine, are associated with a high mortality due to complicating local circumstances.

OTHER TYPES OF INFLAMMATION

Subacute
This is a variety of inflammation intermediate between acute and chronic. It shows some of the manifestations of both types of inflammation with a mixture of increased vascularity and exudation as well as increased fibrosis. The predominant cell is the plasma cell but polymorphs and lymphocytes are also present. The fallopian tube is the classical site and subacute salpingitis shows thickening of the fallopian tube which is extensively infiltrated by plasma cells. Occasionally, a similar picture is seen in appendicitis but elsewhere the term 'subacute inflammation' is ill-defined.

Chronic inflammation
This type of inflammation may be:
1   *Secondary to acute inflammation* – already described, p. 29.
2   *Primarily chronic.* The aetiology of type 2 is usually due to an organism of low grade virulence or due to a longstanding chronic irritation. Common sites where this type of inflammation is encountered are in the kidney, the gall bladder when associated with stone formation, and the bronchial tree. In every instance, a chronically inflamed organ or tissue is paler, firmer and thicker than normal. Microscopically, the area shows a mainly lympho-

cytic cellular infiltration with some plasma cells and a marked fibrous replacement of the area. There is little in the way of a vascular response and significant numbers of polymorphs are only present if there is an acute inflammatory exacerbation superimposed on the chronic condition. The difference, therefore, between the acute and chronic inflammatory reaction may be summarized as a productive connective tissue reaction rather than the vascular and exudative response seen in the acute type of inflammation.

General manifestations of inflammation

The foregoing discussion has detailed the local manifestations of inflammation. The general effects of the inflammatory process vary considerably according to several factors including:
1 The infecting agent.
2 Site of infection.
3 The resistance and immunity of the host.
4 Duration of the infection.
5 Localization of the infection.

FEVER

Fever is a fairly constant accompaniment of any inflammation but it may also occur in infarction, haemorrhage, connective tissue diseases, malignant disease, in reactions to foreign proteins and following involvement of the heat centre by lesions of the brain stem.

Normal heat regulation
This is controlled by the heat regulating centre in the hypothalamus which responds to alterations in the temperature of the circulating blood. Normally, heat production is equalized by heat loss to maintain the normal body temperature.

RETENTION OF HEAT
1 Vasoconstriction, especially of skin vessels.
2 Followed by rigors if vasoconstriction is insufficient.

LOSS OF HEAT
1 Vasodilatation, especially of skin vessels.
2 Followed by sweating if vasodilatation is insufficient.

In disease, the cells in the hypothalamic centre are depressed by circulating pyrogens and the temperature is set at a higher level. Bacterial pyrogens act indirectly causing the release of endogenous pyrogen from neutrophil polymorphs. Some neutrophil proteases liberated during phagocytosis are pyrogens. Further pyrogens are produced by monocytes.

Mechanism of fever

INCREASED HEAT PRODUCTION
1 Increased adrenalin secretion.
2 Increased thyroxine secretion.
3 Rigors.

DECREASED HEAT LOSS
1 Vasoconstriction.
2 Diminished sweating.

Stages of fever
1 *Onset* – heat production greater than heat loss.
2 *Fastigium* – heat production = heat loss, but the temperature is at a higher level.
3 *Defervescence* – heat loss greater than heat production.

Results of pyrexia
1 Metabolism increased by 12.6 per cent for each 1°C of pyrexia.
2 Increased pulmonary ventilation and cardiac output.
3 Excessive protein breakdown with a tendency to ketosis and negative nitrogen balance and with body wasting when the pyrexia is prolonged.
4 Increased 'insensible' fluid loss of water and salt by sweating which may be sufficient to cause sodium depletion and circulatory or renal failure.

HYPERPYREXIA

Definition
A pyrexia in excess of 40.5°C. Above 41°C the centre fails to function.

Causes
1 Severe infections.
2 Excessively hot or humid climates – 'heat stroke'.
3 Brain stem damage, e.g. haemorrhage, tumour or trauma.

4   In susceptible individuals, administration of a general anaesthetic – *malignant hyperpyrexia.*

Results

If prolonged, the condition results in irreversible cell damage, especially in the brain, and death.

CHANGES IN THE BLOOD

(see also pp. 441–450)

WHITE CELLS

Normal count $5-10 \times 10^9/l$.

Leucocytosis

In infections there may be an increase up to 30 000 per μl or more. This is due to release of leucocytes from the peripheral pool and the larger reserves in the marrow and to increased production in the marrow. Stimulating factors both for release and production have been isolated.

NEUTROPHILS
Normal count $2.5-7 \times 10^9/l$. These cells increase in pyogenic infections and in tissue breakdown. This cellular increase is greater when there is intense tissue destruction and suppuration rather than with more extensive but well drained infections.

EOSINOPHILS
Normal count $0.04-0.4 \times 10^9/l$. Eosinophils increase particularly in parasitic infections and allergic states, e.g. asthma.

LYMPHOCYTES
Normal count $2.5-3.5 \times 10^9/l$. Lymphocytes frequently increase in chronic infections, in tuberculosis, in virus infections especially glandular fever, and sometimes in acute infections in children.

MONOCYTES
Normal count $0.13-0.8 \times 10^9/l$. A monocytosis may be found in typhoid fever, influenza, malaria and other chronic inflammatory states.

Leucopenia

This implies a decrease of white cells to below $4.0 \times 10^9/l$. This may occur in typhoid, influenza, many viral infections, malaria and in many haematological disorders.

Abnormal white cells

1   Primitive white cells, e.g. myelocytes and metamyelocytes, may circulate in the peripheral blood in cases with a high leucocytosis and are most commonly seen during infections in infancy.
2   Plasma cells are rarely present in the blood but are sometimes found, especially in severe infections.

RED CELLS

Some degree of anaemia frequently accompanies infections. Generally, the longer and more severe the infection the greater the degree of this anaemia. Some of the factors involved are as follows.

Toxic depression

Some toxic depression of bone-marrow function occurs with all infections but the effects are usually minimal unless the infection is of longstanding, or there is actual involvement of the marrow by the inflammatory process.

Haemolysis

Intravascular destruction of the red cells may occur in malaria or be due to haemolysins produced as exotoxins by bacteria, e.g. β-haemolytic streptococci and *Clostridium perfringens* (*C. welchii*).

Haemorrhage

Repeated haemorrhages will induce anaemia and this may be:
(*a*) From localized areas, e.g. peptic ulcer, typhoid, ulcerative colitis.
(*b*) From a generalized haemorrhagic state, e.g. Weil's disease, yellow fever.

CHANGES IN ORGANS

Reactive

This is mainly manifest as follows.

LOCAL
As part of the inflammatory reaction, e.g. macrophage production.

GENERAL

There is reactive hyperplasia, especially of the regional lymph nodes draining the site of infection, but this may also occur elsewhere, e.g. liver, spleen and bone marrow. This hyperplasia is part of the general defence mechanisms of the body and is linked to the development of immunity.

Degenerative

Degenerative changes are usually the effect of toxic substances (bacterial or tissue metabolites) and produce various degenerative changes in the cells of certain organs particularly the liver, kidneys and heart (see pp. 103–107).

Septicaemia

This is the invasion of the blood stream by actively multiplying organisms.

Pyaemia

This implies the carriage of pyogenic organisms in the blood stream, mostly in clumps, which are subsequently arrested in capillaries in various organs and form metastatic pyaemic abscesses, e.g. in the lungs and kidneys, or in the liver when the portal venous system is involved.

Bacteraemia

This is the appearance in the blood stream of organisms which are not actively multiplying, It is usually a transient phenomenon, but may have serious consequences, e.g. bacteraemia following dental treatment may lead to endocarditis if there are previously damaged valves.

Chapter 7
Repair

Nature

Noxious agents causing inflammatory reactions also cause tissue damage. This may be slight, so that, when the agent is overcome, the cells recover and there is no tissue loss. However, when greater tissue damage occurs cells are destroyed. Dead cells or tissues are rapidly removed from the site by phagocytosis thus leaving a tissue defect, e.g. an ulcer or abscess cavity. In these circumstances, the body does not allow such a defect to remain and by the process of repair makes good the deficiency. Moreover, any breach in continuity of a surface or structure likewise requires repair. This is accomplished by:
1 Regeneration of the parenchymal cells of the organ.
2 Growth of the supporting connective tissues.
   The end result of the repair process will depend largely upon the balance between these two factors.

REPAIR MECHANISMS

PRIMARY UNION – HEALING BY FIRST INTENTION

This occurs at a site where there is only minimal loss of tissue, e.g. a surgical incision.

Stages
1 Exudation of blood into the space between the cut but closely apposed tissues.
2 Coagulation of the fluid with the formation of fibrin strands.
3 Invasion of this coagulum by capillary loops and fibroblasts derived from the marginal tissues.
4 Proliferation of adjacent epithelial cells and migration towards the defect to restore continuity occurs early, initially at the base of the epithelium, beneath the uppermost layer of coagulum.

5 Maturation of the fibroblasts whose fibrils lay down collagen.

6 Progressive maturation of the collagen and decreasing vascularity to result in avascular scar tissue.

SECONDARY UNION – HEALING BY SECOND INTENTION OR BY GRANULATION

This process is similar to that occurring in primary union. However, where there has been loss of tissue such that the edges are separated by a defect, e.g. an ulcer or an abscess cavity, a larger bulk of reparative tissue is required and the process takes longer.

Stages

1 If the cause of the defect is an infection, this has to be successfully overcome by an inflammatory response and the debris removed by macrophages. If traumatic in origin, the defect will be filled with coagulated blood.

2 Repair starts in the floor of the defect with invasion of the surface coagulum by proliferating capillary loops and fibroblasts. Fibroblastic maturation continues towards the surface until the whole area of tissue loss has been made good. This tissue, when viewed tangentially, will be red in colour with a granular surface due to capillary loops – *granulation tissue*.

3 The epithelial cells at a small distance from the edges of the defect proliferate and there is migration over the surface of the granulation tissue, beneath the uppermost coagulum, until the area is covered. Overgrowth is prevented by 'contact inhibition' probably mediated via tissue specific chalones.

4 The vascular granulation tissue matures from the base towards the surface until the entire area is converted into a mass of fibrous tissue. This is red in the early stages but later becomes pale as the scar tissue becomes avascular.

5 Contraction of the wound occurs during healing resulting in a scar which is smaller than the original defect. Contraction of the scar collagen subsequent to healing is a different process and may result in deformity, e.g. cicatrization following extensive burns.

Other features

1 It will be noted that specialized structures in the area, e.g. sweat and sebaceous glands and hair follicles, do not regenerate.

2 The presence of infection retards the growth of granulation tissue and therefore delays healing.

3 The presence of dirt, dead tissue or foreign bodies, e.g. fragments of gauze dressings, produce a foreign body giant cell reaction in the granulation tissue which further delays healing.

4 Where the healing process co-exists with active infection, an exuberant amount of inflammatory vascular granulation tissue may be formed in restoring the tissue continuity – *proud flesh*.

REPAIR BY RESOLUTION

One of the end results of inflammation is resolution. When complete this is the anticipated and desired result in many infections but this can only occur where there is minimal tissue damage. Thus, in spite of the profuse exudate in the lung alveoli in lobar pneumonia, absorption is complete in most instances and the lung tissue returns to structural and functional normality.

REPAIR BY ORGANIZATION

A slightly different method of repair is by organization. This occurs when there is incomplete resolution of inflammation (see p. 29). The unabsorbed fibrin forms a scaffold for fibroblasts and capillary loops to invade the coagulum so that fibrosis subsequently develops in the area. Repair by organization may occur in the lung parenchyma following pneumonia, in the myocardium and heart valves following rheumatic carditis, in the pleura following a fibrinous pleurisy and in many other body tissues which have been the site of inflammation. The importance of this mechanism is that such an area does not return to normal, remaining in a scarred state so that the organ or tissue involved is permanently damaged and may be functionally impaired.

REPAIR BY REGENERATION

Some tissues when damaged show great powers of regeneration. This is especially exemplified by fibrous tissue and by bone in respect of the healing of a fracture. Some parenchymal organs also have considerable powers of regeneration, e.g. liver, thyroid, pancreas, salivary glands and to a lesser extent the kidneys. In general, the epithelial elements can regenerate successfully providing that the connective tissue framework of the organ remains intact.

REGENERATION IN SPECIAL TISSUES

As a general rule it is found that the more specialized a cell or tissue, the less are its powers of regeneration. The reparative properties of tissues may be subdivided into three categories:

1 Will regenerate in most circumstances, e.g. bone, fibrous tissue.

2 Will regenerate in favourable circumstances, e.g. liver, thyroid, kidney tubules.

3 Cannot regenerate, e.g. C.N.S. tissue and striated muscle.

EPITHELIUM

The surface epithelia of the skin, respiratory, alimentary and urogenital tracts, retain their powers of regeneration throughout life and, following injury, repair is rapid and complete.

Glandular epithelium is more variable but there are two relevant factors:

1 If a whole organ or tissue is destroyed no regeneration is possible.

2 If the supporting framework of connective tissue of a parenchymal organ is disrupted the regenerated area will be architecturally abnormal and may also be functionally impaired.

With these exceptions and under ideal circumstances, the liver, thyroid, the exocrine glands of the pancreas and the salivary glands show excellent power of regeneration. The kidney is more limited as the glomeruli cannot regenerate, but the renal tubules have regenerative properties. The hair follicles, sweat and sebaceous glands are readily destroyed and do not regenerate. Specialized glands of the stomach, when destroyed by peptic ulceration, are replaced by more simple glands.

CONNECTIVE TISSUES

Fibrous tissue

Excellent powers of regeneration; collagen forms the basis of all replacement scar tissue.

Bone

Excellent powers of regeneration with complete reformation of the bone following a fracture.

Cartilage

This is replaced by fibrous tissue which may subsequently be converted by metaplasia into fibrocartilage.

Muscle

Striated, cardiac and smooth muscle fibres have virtually no powers of regeneration, although hypertrophy of remaining fibres may occur and restore the functional ability of the tissue.

Mesothelium

These cells regenerate rapidly and completely

Blood vessels

Vascular endothelium regenerates well but destroyed muscle and elastic tissue in the vessel walls do not. However, any new blood vessels formed acquire a musculo-elastic wall around an endothelial lining.

Lymphoid tissue

Cells of the lymphoreticular system have excellent powers of complete regeneration, although in lymph nodes, following prolonged chronic inflammation, fibrous scarring frequently occurs.

Nervous tissue

(*a*) Central nervous system tissue has no capacity for regeneration and is replaced by gliosis.

(*b*) Peripheral nerve tissue shows no regeneration if the cell body is destroyed. If the axon only is damaged regeneration can occur (see p. 619).

Factors influencing repair

Tissue involved

This is obviously of paramount importance, particularly in respect of the powers of regeneration of individual tissues (see above).

Vascularity

An adequate blood supply is essential for both the inflammatory reaction and for the ensuing reparative process. Avascular areas do not heal and this is a noteworthy feature in fractures of certain bones, e.g. neck of femur, ulna and carpal scaphoid, where non-union due to avascular bone necrosis frequently occurs.

Protection

Protective covering prevents further injury and re-infection of the damaged area. Immobilization of the damaged soft tissue or bone also facilitates repair.

Infection

Growth of granulation tissue is retarded by the presence of active general or local infection.

Nutrition

Undernourishment due to any cause, with its associated deficiencies, especially of protein, markedly delays healing.

Vitamins

Vitamin C is essential for healing in respect of the integrity of capillary walls and for the maturation of collagen. In avitaminosis C (scurvy) healing may be totally absent. An adequate supply of vitamin D is also necessary in the repair of fractures. Sufficient intake of other vitamins is also desirable to promote healing at the normal rate.

Age

In general, injured tissues in the young heal more rapidly than those of older subjects. However, this is linked to circulatory and other age-related factors. Fit, healthy old people may heal as well as the young.

Endocrines

Thyroid hormones are necessary for healing and myxoedematous patients may be slow to heal. Corticosteroids (prednisone) retard healing in the manner described on p. 28. Diabetic patients heal poorly, largely as a result of their propensity to infection and to vascular disease.

Temperature

Excessive heat or cold retards the reparative process as both may cause tissue damage and vascular thrombosis (see p. 74).

Size

The amount of tissue destroyed is an important factor, thus the bulk of tissue lost dictates whether the process of repair will be by primary or secondary union. The larger the defect the longer the reparative process will be, the greater the scar tissue formation and the increasing likelihood for a correspondingly greater functional deficit.

Foreign bodies

The presence of foreign material within a wound retards healing by the maintenance of irritation and infection within granulation tissue. In this manner suture material, swabs, dead tissue following inadequate *débridement*, detached clothing and other foreign materials may cause persistence of an open wound.

Sinuses and fistulae

A sinus is a blind tract in the tissues communicating with an epithelial surface, e.g. pilonidal sinus. A fistula is an open track joining two epithelial surfaces, e.g. gut to skin surface, stomach to intestine, rectum to vagina, etc. The presence of either a sinus or a fistula will retard repair and permanent healing cannot occur until their causes are removed.

Irradiation

Tissues which have received irradiation therapy in sufficient dosage may show acute tissue damage and later develop vascular narrowing. Injury to such tissue will be followed by delayed healing (see p. 75).

Sensory nerves

The absence of an adequate sensory nerve supply delays healing. This phenomenon is seen in the indolent ulcers on the hands of patients with syringomyelia and the trophic ulcers on the feet of tabetics. The axon reflex which causes the 'flare' of the triple response will be abolished and if the autonomic supply is damaged there will be local vascular constriction and thus impairment of inflammation and subsequent repair. The precise mechanism, however, remains unknown, hence the ill-defined term 'trophic factors' to cover this aspect, but repetitive and unnoticed trauma to the insensitive part may well be a major factor.

Summary

From this account it will be appreciated that perfect repair of destroyed tissue can only occur in those tissues capable of regeneration. Many specialized cells and organs, once they are damaged, are incapable of reformation so that an area of scar tissue becomes inevitable. However, in some tissues such as fibrous tissue, bone, thyroid and liver, a more favourable outcome can be anticipated.

Chapter 8
Diseases due to Bacteria: Viruses: Rickettsiaceae

Bacterial infections

GENERAL
Non-specific
Specific

TETANUS
Organism
Incidence
Pathogenesis
Appearances
   Local
   Nervous system
Diagnosis
Results

BOTULISM
Nature
Effects
Results

BRUCELLOSIS
Nature
Organisms
Pathogenesis
Appearances
Effects
Diagnosis
Results

PLAGUE
Nature
Mode of infection
Types
   Bubonic
   Pneumonic
   Septicaemic
Microscopical
Results

ANTHRAX
Organism
Types
   Local – malignant pustule
   Pulmonary – wool sorter's disease
Diagnosis
Results

Virus infections

GENERAL
Incidence
Organisms
Structure
Classification
   RNA-containing
   DNA-containing
Effects on host cells
Diagnosis

SMALLPOX – VARIOLA
Nature
Incidence
Lesions
   Skin
   Lungs
   General

CHICKENPOX – VARICELLA
Nature
Lesions
Results

HERPES ZOSTER

MUMPS
Nature
Lesions
   Parotid glands
   Other salivary glands
   Testis
   Pancreas
Results

MEASLES
Nature
Lesions
   Skin
   Mucous membranes
   Lymphoid tissue
   Lung
Results

GERMAN MEASLES – RUBELLA

INFECTIOUS MONONUCLEOSIS – GLANDULAR FEVER
Nature
Lesions
   Lymph nodes
   Spleen
   Liver
   Nervous system
   Blood

Chlamydial diseases
Nature
Diseases in man

PSITTACOSIS

Rickettsial infections

'Q' FEVER

TYPHUS
   Louse-borne – epidemic
   Flea-borne – endemic

SCRUB TYPHUS – TSUTSUGAMUSHI FEVER

ROCKY MOUNTAIN SPOTTED FEVER

Bacterial infections

General

In the foregoing chapters the general pattern of the inflammatory response to injurious agents, including bacteria, has been described. Specific bacteria may modify this response in respect of certain features and so produce clinical and pathological appearances characteristic of a specific disease entity.

Non-specific bacterial infections

Many bacteria evoke focal, suppurative, necrotizing inflammation of a non-specific type and affecting many different sites. These pyogenic organisms include: staphylococci, streptococci, coliforms, the haemophilus group, *B. proteus*. The lesions which they produce are subsequently indicated in the special pathology sections in respect of the various sites involved.

Specific bacterial infections

Many bacterial diseases are more conveniently described in relation to the specific organs or tissues which are maximally involved or clinically predominant.

Gas gangrene – see Gangrene (p. 131).

Cholera, dysentery, enteric fever – see Alimentary Section (p. 198).

Gonorrhoea, granuloma inguinale, soft sore – see Urinary Tract (pp. 392, 406, 405).

Meningococcal Infections – see C.N.S. and Adrenal sections (pp. 601 and 290).

Leptospiral Infections – see Liver (p. 555).

Tuberculosis, syphilis, leprosy – see Specific Granulomas (p. 45).

Diphtheria – see Upper Respiratory Tract (p. 642).

TETANUS

Organism

Clostridium tetani – a gram-positive sporing anaerobe. The spores are extremely resistant and may survive in a dormant state for many years.

Incidence

Infrequent, but still the cause of approximately twenty deaths a year in England and Wales.

Pathogenesis

Contamination of penetrating wounds by spores.

Since the organism is a common commensal of the gut of horses and other animals, most cases are seen in agricultural areas. The development of the vegetative form, exotoxin production and thus of clinical disease may be delayed for weeks or months, but is usually 1–2 weeks.

Appearances

LOCAL
Non-specific inflammation with tissue necrosis in the wound.

NERVOUS SYSTEM
Oedema of motor nerve cells in the spinal cord and medulla with degenerative nuclear changes.

Diagnosis

Recovery of the organism from the wound.

Results

The exotoxin is very powerful and selectively affects the spinal cord and medullary nerve cells with resulting voluntary muscle spasms – 'lock-jaw', and progressive respiratory difficulty which is the usual cause of death. The mortality rate is high.

BOTULISM

Nature

A fortunately rare and very severe food poisoning caused by ingestion of the preformed exotoxin of *Clostridium botulinum*. Foods contaminated include canned and preserved meats, fruit and vegetables.

Effects

Motor paralysis of muscles of the orbit, pharynx, larynx, and of respiration. These effects appear very rapidly, usually within 2–3 hours. The brain may show multiple small vascular thromboses.

Results

Even with prompt administration of antitoxin the mortality is in excess of 50 per cent.

BRUCELLOSIS – UNDULANT FEVER

Nature

A chronic febrile disease of insidious onset and protean clinical manifestations caused by several strains of Brucella.

Organisms
Brucella abortus – cows.
B. melitensis – goats.
B. suis – pigs.

Pathogenesis
Infection is by ingestion of contaminated cow's or goat's milk or close contact with these animals or with pigs. There is cross-infection between animals so that any of the strains may be obtained from a particular animal. After gaining access to the tissues, there is widespread dissemination by the blood stream and invasion of lymphoreticular cells in many organs and tissues.

Appearances
Sites most commonly affected are spleen, lymph nodes, liver and bone marrow. They show small foci of granulomatous inflammation consisting of macrophages and histiocytes surrounded by monocytes, lymphocytes and fibroblasts. Giant cells may be present and the lesions may closely resemble those of tuberculosis, sarcoidosis or even Hodgkin's disease.

Effects
1 Splenomegaly and lymphadenopathy.
2 General effects of varying severity, pursuing a course of weeks or months. The fever is characteristically intermittent with diurnal spikes as high as 40°C, hence *undulant fever*.
3 Anaemia is common.

Diagnosis
1 Isolation of the organism from blood culture – early stages only.
2 Rising titre of serum agglutinins.
3 Brucellin skin test – unreliable and seldom used.

Results
A long course with eventual recovery in all but the 2–5 per cent who die from the disease.

PLAGUE

Nature
A severe infection by *Pasteurella pestis* which is still endemic in some Eastern countries.

Mode of infection
The disease is transmitted to man by fleas from rats which are the principal reservoir of the organisms.

Types

BUBONIC
Extreme matted enlargement of the regional lymph nodes draining the site of the flea-bite. The nodes are haemorrhagic, soft and later necrotic, often involving skin and resulting in sinus formation.

PNEUMONIC
Patchy or confluent areas of haemorrhagic bronchopneumonic consolidation.

SEPTICAEMIC
Blood spread with rapid death and only slight organ changes, although usually early pneumonic and lymph node involvement associated with widespread haemorrhages are seen.

Microscopical
There is a severe exudative response to the numerous organisms present, with fibrin, abundant polymorphs, necrosis and vascular thrombosis. The latter results in haemorrhages and infarcts.

Results
The severity is variable but in untreated pneumonic or septicaemic types, death is almost inevitable. The bubonic type may remain localized, or spread with haemorrhagic necrosis in many organs and tissues – *Black Death*.

ANTHRAX

Organism
Bacillus anthracis – a highly pathogenic grampositive sporing organism. Infection occurs by contact with infected animals or their products – sheep, cattle, horses, pigs.

Types

LOCAL – 'MALIGNANT PUSTULE'
Entry is gained through a skin injury and after a few days a pustule develops with very extensive surrounding and spreading oedema. Satellite vesicles and later pustules are commonly seen as is regional lymphadenopathy, but distant spread is unusual. Histologically, there is an haemorrhagic and necrotic oedematous reaction with relative paucity of polymorphs.

PULMONARY – 'WOOL SORTER'S DISEASE'
Inhaled spores produce a profuse sero-fibrinous and haemorrhagic inflammatory reaction seen macroscopically as extensive consolidation. This is commonly followed by a fatal septicaemia.

Diagnosis
Identification of the organism in the skin lesion or its isolation from the blood.

Results
Untreated, there is a very high mortality rate in the pulmonary type and up to 20 per cent mortality with the malignant pustule.

Virus infections

GENERAL

Incidence
Approximately 1000 deaths were attributable to virus diseases in England and Wales in 1978. The number of non-fatal cases is impossible to estimate but is obviously very large and is attended by a considerable morbidity.

Organisms
1   Filterable particles of variable size (10–400 mμ) and shapes.
2   Capable of multiplication only in the presence of living cells.
3   Variable species specificity.
4   Many have a cell-type specificity or a marked affinity for certain tissues or organs.
5   The inflammatory reaction to their presence is usually characterized by mononuclear cells, cell damage or sometimes cell proliferation, but no suppuration.
6   Many form inclusions in the host cells; in the nuclei – herpes simplex and chicken pox; in the cytoplasm – Negri bodies of rabies; or possibly in both – Guarnieri bodies in smallpox.
7   With the exception of the common cold and herpes simplex, most viral infections are followed by a permanent immunity and antibodies can be demonstrated in the host.

Structure
Viruses contain either deoxyribonucleic acid (DNA) or ribonucleic acid (RNA) but not both, unlike all higher forms of life. The nucleic acid forms a central core surrounded by a protein shell – *capsid*, these forming the *elementary body* or *virion*. The capsid is composed of a specific number of identical sub-units – *capsomers*, arranged regularly to form a compact mass. The capsomer arrangement in different viruses produces their individual morphological appearances mostly of spherical or filamentous form.

Some viruses have outer membranes – *envelopes*, one or more in number and largely lipid in composition, e.g. herpes viruses and arborviruses.

Larger viruses may also contain rudimentary but ineffectual enzyme systems and various carbohydrates, but require host cells for growth.

Classification
More than fifty diseases in man and many more in animals are known to be caused by viruses and many more may be caused by them but confirmatory evidence is lacking.

Originally viruses were classified according to their *tropism* (affinity) for specific tissues, e.g. dermatotropic, neurotropic, visccrotropic, but generalized viraemia is common and the organisms have been shown to adapt to produce changes in their affinity.

More recent classifications are based on the nature of the nucleic acid and morphological factors.

RNA-CONTAINING VIRUSES
(*a*) Picornaviruses – small, no envelope, cubical capsid.
    (i) Enteroviruses – polioviruses.
                  Coxsackie viruses.
                  Echo viruses.
    (ii) Rhinoviruses – common cold viruses.
(*b*) Myxoviruses and Paramyxoviruses – intermediate size, outer envelope, helical capsid, e.g. influenza viruses, measles, rabies, mumps.
(*c*) Reoviruses – rather small, no envelope, cubical capsid. May cause some upper respiratory tract infections.
(*d*) Arborviruses – small, outer envolope, capsid shape uncertain. These are transmitted by an insect vector (arthropod-borne), e.g. mosquitoes and ticks.
    Include epidemic encephalitis, yellow, dengue and sandfly fevers.
(*e*) Arenaviruses – a recently described group of which the most important clinically is the dangerous Lassa fever.

DNA-CONTAINING VIRUSES

(a) Poxviruses – large, complex outer envelope, helical capsid, e.g. smallpox and vaccinia.
(b) Adenoviruses – intermediate size, no envelope, cubical capsid. Important cause of upper respiratory tract infections and kerato-conjuntivitis.
(c) Herpes viruses – large, outer envelope, cubical capsid, e.g. herpes simplex and chickenpox-zoster, cytomegalic inclusion disease.
(d) Papillomaviruses – small, no outer envelope, cubical capsid. Cause infective warts of various types in man and include polyomavirus in animals.

Effects on host cells

Usually produce necrosis of infected cells but may cause cellular proliferation, as with the polyomavirus in animals. In man necrosis is the usual effect. Most effects are acute and protracted illnesses are not a common feature but some viruses may lie latent in infected cells and their multiplication be triggered by a non-specific, physical or chemical stimulus, e.g. herpes simplex and fever.

Diagnosis

1 Morphological identification by electron microscopic appearances.
2 Isolation and identification of the agent by cultivation in living cells.
(a) Animals – rarely used.
(b) Fertile eggs – e.g. influenza, herpes, poxviruses.
(c) Tissue-culture systems of various types – recognition by 'cytopathic' effect seen by phase-contrast microscopy and inhibited by specific neutralizing antibody.
3 Serological tests
(a) Complement fixation tests.
(b) Tests for neutralizing antibody
(c) Haemagglutination inhibition tests.

For the serological tests, 'paired' sera from the acute and convalescent phases are usually employed to detect changes in titre of the antibodies and the diagnosis is thus largely retrospective but still important from the epidemiological viewpoint.

Many of the virus diseases affecting man are more conveniently described in the appropriate special sections.

Virus diseases of the nervous system (poliomyelitis, encephalitis, rabies) – see C.N.S. (p. 605).

Virus diseases of the liver (yellow fever, viral hepatitis) – see liver (p. 551).

Respiratory virus infection (influenza, primary atypical pneumonia) – see lungs (p. 661).

Virus diseases of skin (warts, molluscum contagiosum – see skin (p. 729).

A brief account of some of the remaining important virus diseases follows.

SMALLPOX – VARIOLA

Nature

An acute, highly infective disease of high mortality due to variola virus and characterized by fever and a widespread vesicular, later pustular, skin lesion.

Incidence

Due to international co-operation on an unprecedented scale it is now believed to be extinct.

Lesions

SKIN

The lesion starts as a papule, later becoming a vesicle at about 7 days, and then a pustule which forms a scab. Skin involvement is usually complete in 2 days, commencing 12–14 days after exposure on the face and spreading towards the trunk. Histologically, there is congestion, mononuclear cell infiltration and ballooning of the epithelial cells with Guarnieri inclusion bodies consisting of aggregates of virus particles. Vesicle formation occurs and the epithelial cells die.

LUNGS

In severe cases there is an interstitial pneumonia, usually followed by secondary bacterial infection.

GENERAL

Non-specific lympho-reticular hyperplasia; focal degenerations and haemorrhages in liver, kidney, adrenal and testis, may all be present together with a leucopenia due to marrow depression. The patient is generally severely ill.

CHICKENPOX – VARICELLA

Nature
A mild, common and highly communicable childhood disease caused by the varicella virus. The incubation period is about 14 days.

Lesions
Manifest by a skin lesion starting on the trunk and spreading outwards but appearing in successive crops, remaining discrete and, whilst forming vesicles, not all become pustules. The inclusion bodies and histological appearances of the lesion show minor differences from those of smallpox.

Results
The disease is mild. Only rare fatalities occur from complicating pneumonia, ear infection or encephalitis.

HERPES ZOSTER

The virus is identical to that of chickenpox but localizes in dorsal root or cranial nerve ganglia with resulting skin lesions over the sensory distribution of the affected nerve. The vesicles formed resemble those of chickenpox but there is very considerable pain which may remain for months or years – *postherpetic neuralgia*. There are degenerative changes and a mononuclear cell infiltration of the ganglion cells.

MUMPS

Nature
A contagious viral disease, usually, but not invariably, characterized by parotid swelling. Incubation period is 2–4 weeks (average $2\frac{1}{2}$).

Lesions

PAROTID GLANDS
Bilateral or occasionally unilateral painful swelling, due to interstitial inflammation accompanied by mononuclear cell infiltration and exudation.

OTHER SALIVARY GLANDS
Similar changes are found in 20 per cent of cases in the submandibular and sublingual glands.

TESTIS
Interstitial orchitis occurs in 20 per cent of adult male patients, usually unilateral; similar changes sometimes affect the ovaries.

PANCREAS
Interstitial pancreatitis occurs less commonly and may mimic acute pancreatitis (see p. 631).

Results
The lesions heal fairly rapidly but pressure induced by the inflammation and possibly by direct effect of the virus, may lead to epithelial cell necrosis and replacement fibrosis. In the testis this may cause atrophy and, if bilateral, sterility.

MEASLES

Nature
An acute, highly infectious viral disease transmitted by droplet infection and with an incubation period of 10–14 days.

Lesions

SKIN
A generalized maculo-papular rash which shows congestion and perivascular mononuclear cell infiltration.

MUCOUS MEMBRANES
Koplik's spots on the buccal mucous membrane of similar pathological appearances to the skin rash and a tracheobronchitis which produces very viscid mucus.

LYMPHOID TISSUE
Enlarged throughout the body with hyperplasia of germinal follicles and the presence of characteristic and enormous Warthin–Finkeldey giant cells (see p. 211).

LUNG
In addition to the tracheobronchitis, there may be a mild or moderately severe interstitial pneumonia commonly of giant cell type (see p. 661).

Results
Usually resolves spontaneously but death may occur in the very young or very old. There is, however, a considerable morbidity associated with

secondary bacterial infection, e.g. bronchopneumonia or otitis media, and from collapse and bronchiectasis associated with the viscid mucus.

GERMAN MEASLES – RUBELLA

A very mild infective disease similar to a mild attack of measles. It may be important, however, if acquired in the first 3 months of pregnancy, when it is associated with a high rate of congenital deformities, especially of the heart, eye and ear.

INFECTIOUS MONONUCLEOSIS – GLANDULAR FEVER

Nature
A systemic infection by the Epstein–Barr virus. The disease is of low infectivity and is characterized by fever, lymphadenopathy and blood changes. The course is benign but often prolonged and constitutional symptoms may be severe.

Lesions

LYMPH NODES
Moderately enlarged with hyperplastic follicles which may show atypical features, indistinctness of pattern and the presence of 'glandular fever' cells. The changes may thus be difficult to distinguish from the early stages of a malignant lymphoma (see p. 580).

SPLEEN
Enlarged two or three times and soft, fleshy and haemorrhagic. The lymphoid tissue shows similar atypical hyperplastic features to the lymph nodes.

LIVER
Commonly involved, with changes similar to those of a mild viral hepatitis (see p. 551).

NERVOUS SYSTEM
Focal aggregates of mononuclear cells may be seen in the brain and meninges.

BLOOD
There is a leucocytosis with increase in the mononuclear cells many of which show atypical features characteristic of 'glandular fever cells' (see p. 449). There are heterophile antibodies to sheep's red cells present in the serum to a high dilution – Paul–Bunnell test (see p. 449).

Chlamydial diseases

Nature
A group of diseases caused by infection with organisms which enter cells as 'elementary bodies' 3 nm in diameter, and these enlarge to 'giant bodies' 5 μm in diameter. The giant bodies are subdivided to form bodies about the size of staphylococci (1 μm diam.) which are then condensed to form the elementary bodies. All three types of bodies divide by binary fission.

These *Chlamydia* (Bedsonia) may be grown and identified by injecting fertile eggs or mice.

Diseases in man
Clearly identified diseases in man include: lymphogranuloma venereum (see p. 406), psittacosis and ornithosis, trachoma (see p. 327), inclusion conjunctivitis. Other possible chlamydial infections are cat-scratch disease (see p. 579), Reiter's syndrome and other genital tract infections (see p. 392).

PSITTACOSIS

An infection of psittacine birds (parrot family) which is occasionally transmitted to man to produce an acute interstitial pneumonia, commonly complicated by secondary bacterial infection.

The pneumonia is similar to that produced by influenza but with occasional inclusion bodies visible in the hyperplastic alveolar lining cells (see p. 662). There are also focal necroses of liver and spleen; kidneys, heart and brain are less commonly affected. There is a considerable mortality from this uncommon disease.

Rickettsial infections

Rickettsiaceae are pleomorphic cocco-bacillary intracellular oganisms intermediate in size between bacteria and viruses. They contain both DNA and RNA and multiply by binary fission.

There are two groups:
1 Rickettsiae.
2 Coxiella.

The basic lesion caused by these organisms in man is endothelial cell damage with consequential thromboses, infarcts and ischaemic necroses.

'Q' FEVER

Coxiella burnetii – an acute febrile illness of low mortality and predominantly manifest as a respiratory disease. The lungs show a patchy consolidation due to interstitial inflammation and resemble the appearances of a virus pneumonia. The disease is acquired by inhalation and not through a vector.

TYPHUS

Two types:
(*a*) Louse-borne, human, epidemic – *R. prowazeki*.
(*b*) Flea-borne, murine, endemic – *R. typhi*.
  Both are febrile diseases with a mortality of approximately 20 per cent in the epidemic type and 1–2 per cent in murine typhus. The lesions are widespread in the small blood vessels of many organs. Degenerative changes occur due to occlusion associated with endothelial swelling and a mononuclear inflammatory cell infiltrate. The principal organs affected are brain, skin and heart and the vascular lesions result in multiple haemorrhages in the affected areas.

SCRUB TYPHUS – TSUTSUGAMUSHI FEVER

The clinical and pathological appearances of this mite-transmitted disease are very similar to typhus. Additionally, there is usually a localized area of cutaneous necrosis and ulceration at the site of attachment of the larval mite. Where this lesion is present the mortality of untreated cases is 20–60 per cent.

ROCKY MOUNTAIN SPOTTED FEVER

This is the most common member of a group of diseases all of which closely resemble typhus, are transmitted by ticks and have a very variable mortality. Extensive thrombotic vascular occlusions are commonly seen in the brain, skin, lung and heart.

Chapter 9
Infective Granulomas – Tuberculosis

Having described the general features of non-specific inflammation and some specific infections, it is now necessary to consider a number of different diseases due to infective agents which result in characteristic appearances. These are the specific infective granulomas, so called because:

1 They produce a mass of granulation tissue – a granuloma.
2 Each shows specific histological and cellular features which enable the aetiology of the disease process to be recognized without necessarily isolating the causative organism.

Tuberculosis

Organism
Mycobacterium tuberculosis, a slender acid–alcohol fast rod on Ziehl–Neelsen staining. There are many strains of the organisms but only the human and bovine forms are of importance in human pathology.

Incidence
The mortality due to tuberculosis has decreased dramatically in many countries but is still impor-

tant in many parts of the world, particularly where undernourishment remains a serious problem. In the United Kingdom it is only 50 years since tuberculosis was responsible for 10 per cent of all deaths. Recent figures suggest that the annual new notifications in England and Wales in 1976 were 10 000 of which 7700 were pulmonary and half of these were in the 65–74 age group.

Mode of infection

Apart from the rare 'congenital' cases, tuberculosis is acquired as a result of infection from 'open' cases due to inhalation or ingestion of infected material in the form of droplets, dust, food or milk. Rarely, direct inoculation of infected material may produce the disease – *verruca necrogenica*.

Routes of entry

1   Respiratory tract – inhalation
2   Intestinal tract – ingestion.
3   Skin – inoculation.
4   Placenta – 'congenital'.

Risk of infection

There are many factors which determine whether an individual will develop tuberculosis, including the following.

DOSE AND VIRULENCE OF ORGANISM

No information is available as to the minimum dosage of organisms required, but it is known that some strains are comparatively avirulent.

RESISTANCE OF HOST

The resistance to the infection of the host depends on natural and acquired characteristics. Thus, certain races, e.g. Negroes, are more susceptible than Europeans, but as this is a disease of poverty and dirt, the environmental factors in less well-developed communities are probably more important than any racial susceptibility. Infants are more susceptible than adults but young subjects between the ages of 5 and 15 appear curiously resistant. Malnutrition from any cause and intercurrent disease, e.g. diabetes mellitus, predispose to tuberculosis.

OCCUPATION

The occupation of the patient may be an important factor especially in respect of crowded, poorly ventilated working conditions and in those with industrial pneumoconioses, especially coal miners.

THE BASIC LESION – THE TUBERCLE

Macroscopical

The basic lesion of tuberculosis is the tubercle. This appears as a pin-head-sized white or greyish-coloured minute focus in the tissues and is pathognomic of tuberculosis.

Microscopical

1   A central zone of acellular cheesy necrosis – caseation.
2   Surrounding zone of large, pale, pink-staining cells which are modified histiocytes – epithelioid cells.
3   Langhans' giant cells derived from the fusion of epitheloid cells and with a characteristic peripheral distribution of the nuclei in a 'horse-shoe' arrangement (see Fig. 6 on p. 24).
4   A lymphocytic rim of variable thickness.
5   A peripheral zone of fibroblastic tissue merging with the surrounding structures and increasing in amount with the age of the lesion.
N.B. 1   An avascular structure.
      2   There are no polymorphs.
      3   Z.N. staining reveals *M. tuberculosis*.
These are diagrammatically represented in Fig. 7.

Fate

A tuberculous lesion in the tissues is composed of many such tubercles which amalgamate to form the characteristic tuberculous granuloma. This process may heal or spread the disease.

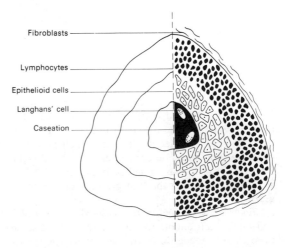

Fig. 7. Diagrammatic representation of a tubercle.

HEAL

Healing is a slow process by progressive fibrosis. The central portions remain caseous for a long time and viable organisms may remain in this apparently inactive and healed lesion. However, reactivation may occur even from calcified or ossified areas to produce further manifestations of the disease at a later date.

SPREAD

The healing process may fail to prevent spread of the tuberculosis.

SPREAD OF TUBERCULOSIS IN THE BODY

Tuberculous infection may spread by the following methods.

Direct spread

Extension of the active lesion occurs with progressive involvement of the adjacent tissues. This can occur in any tissue or organ of the body but is seen especially in the lungs, kidneys and bone, to produce the local clinical manifestations of tuberculosis.

Lymphatic spread

The organisms may pass along the lymphatics and be arrested in the regional lymph nodes or they may be carried to these structures in the epithelioid cells. In the lymph nodes, the organisms produce further tubercles, particularly in the primary type of infection.

Natural passages

The organism may extend to involve and penetrate the walls of natural passages, e.g. bronchus, ureter, vas deferens or gut. Release of infected material into the lumen may result in further spread of the disease.

Blood stream

Organisms may gain entry by:

(*a*) Rupture of a caseous focus into an adjoining blood vessel.

(*b*) Along the lymphatic pathways into the venous system, e.g. via the thoracic duct.

Widespread dissemination by this method leads to the establishment of new tubercles in many organs – miliary tuberculosis, or if more localized, foci occur in one or more organs, e.g. bones, joints, kidney, etc.

ALLERGY, HYPERSENSITIVITY AND IMMUNITY

One of the most complex subjects in tuberculosis hinges around the fact that the reaction on the part of the host differs according to whether it is the first (primary) infection, or whether it is a reactivation or reinfection of a previously infected individual – post-primary or secondary infection. In the primary form, the tissue reaction is a small local focus with a large response in the lymph nodes; in the secondary form, there is a large and localized reaction with minimal lymph nodes changes.

Thus the character of the tissue process is dependent upon whether or not there has been a previous tuberculous infection. In an individual who has not been infected with the disease previously, the organisms at first cause a minimal inflammatory response in the tissues with a mild polymorph reaction during the first 10 days. The polymorphs phagocytose some of the organisms but do not kill them and drain these viable organisms into the regional lymph nodes during the first 24 hours. At approximately the seventh to tenth day of the infection, the tissue reaction dramatically changes when the patient develops an allergy to tuberculoprotein. This will be evident subsequently by a positive Heaf test indicating hypersensitivity to tuberculin. Parallel to this, the tissue reaction changes; the histiocytes become epithelioid cells and caseation occurs at the primary site of infection and in the involved lymph nodes.

It is probable that once this allergic state has developed it is permanent so that in the post-primary form of tuberculosis, the tissues of the body react immediately with epithelioid cells and caseation at the local site of tuberculous invasion, thus preventing early lymphatic spread. Thus, the state of allergy materially modifies the response of the host to tuberculous infection. Does this state produce immunity? A first infection produces a relative degree of resistance associated with the acquisition of hypersensitivity. Subsequent reinfection by tuberculosis will result in an epithelioid cell and caseating reaction at the local area; this probably is a manifestation of hypersensitivity. In addition, the organisms are phagocytosed and may be killed by these epithelioid cells; this positive defence mechanism is an expression of immunity. However, this immunity is only relative and may be insufficiently effective to prevent the establishment of an active tuberculous infection.

PRIMARY TUBERCULOSIS

Nature
This implies the first infection and may occur in the young or in adult life.

Sites

LUNG

This is usually found subpleurally in the mid-zone and is associated with a caseous hilar lymphadenopathy. These two lesions together are the primary complex – the primary focus in the lung is the Ghon focus. Both heal by fibrosis and calcification in almost all cases.

PHARYNX

The primary site is in the lymphoid tissue of the oropharynx, usually the tonsil, with associated caseous enlargement of the regional cervical lymph nodes.

INTESTINES

The site of entry is the lymphoid tissue of the terminal ileum with enlarged and caseous regional mesenteric lymph nodes.

Features
The features of these three examples of primary tuberculosis are:
1 The formation of the primary complex with:
(*a*) A small caseous parenchymal focus.
(*b*) Large caseous regional lymph nodes.
2 The development of a permanent hypersensitivity to tuberculin manifest by a positive Heaf test.
3 Healing by fibrosis, calcification or even ossification usually occurs.
4 The primary infection is usually subclinical and passes unnoticed, except in the cervical region.

Spread
Although most of the primary infections heal, the lack of localizing inflammatory response in the early stages, associated with the late development of allergy, high dosage and high virulence of the organisms, poor host resistance and other factors, may lead to spread of the disease. This is especially likely to occur in adolescents and young adults and produce the following:

DIRECT EXTENSION

Leads to a progressive primary complex, especially in the lung. This is rare (see p. 665).

LYMPHATIC

The regional lymph nodes are already involved but more distant groups may become infected.

NATURAL PASSAGES

For example, tuberculous bronchopneumonia.

BLOOD SPREAD

Miliary tuberculosis, tuberculous meningitis or isolated organ tuberculosis.

The risk of generalized blood dissemination is greater in the previously uninfected patient than in the secondary type of infection, i.e. miliary tuberculosis is more commonly a complication of progressive primary tuberculosis than following the secondary form.

POST-PRIMARY – REINFECTION TUBERCULOSIS

Nature
This implies a reactivation or a reinfection in a patient who has had a previous infection and is already sensitized to tuberculoprotein. Below 40 years of age most cases are believed to be examples of reactivation – *endogenous reinfection* – whereas cases above this age are probably reinfections – *exogenous reinfection*.

Features
The organ changes will be described under their appropriate sections, but the important features are:
1 The lung is the commonest site of involvement.
2 This secondary type of lesion may heal with resulting scarring or may spread:

Spread
Direct
To produce fibrocaseous or caseous pulmonary lesions or pleural involvement.

Lymphatic
Seldom significant in this type.

Natural passages
Via the bronchi to produce bronchopneumonia or

ingestion of infected sputum to result in tuberculous enteritis.

Blood dissemination
To produce either miliary tuberculosis or isolated organ tuberculosis, e.g. urogenital, bone and joint, etc.

These are the common possibilities in the post-primary form of tuberculosis and the histology of the lesions produced in this disease remains characteristically diagnostic in all the affected tissues.

The results of the infection in the various sites will be described under the appropriate organs.

METHODS OF DIAGNOSIS

1 Demonstration or isolation of the organism, e.g. from sputum, urine, etc., by:
(*a*) Smears – Z.N. staining.
(*b*) Culture – e.g. Lowenstein Jensen medium.
(*c*) Guinea-pig inoculation.
2 Biopsy of affected tissues, e.g. lymph nodes, pleura, etc.
3 Skin tests, e.g. Heaf test, skin patch test – positive after the initial stages of the primary infection.

Chapter 10
Infective Granulomas – Sarcoidosis: Leprosy: Syphilis

Sarcoidosis
Nature
Aetiology
Incidence
Age
Macroscopical
Microscopical
Sites
  Skin
  Subcutaneous tissues
  Uveal tract
  Lung
  Spleen
  Salivary glands
  Lymph nodes
  Bones
  Liver
  Other organs
Results
  Resolution
  Fibrosis
  Nephrocalcinosis
  Tuberculosis
  Death
Diagnosis
  Biopsy
  Kveim test
  Blood changes
  Heaf test

Leprosy
Organism
Mode of infection
Tissues involved
Types
  Lepromatous – nodular
    Macroscopical
    Microscopical
  Tuberculoid – anaesthetic –
  maculo-anaesthetic
    Macroscopical
    Microscopical
Diagnosis
  Demonstration of organisms
  Lepromin test
Results

Syphilis
Organism
Types

ACQUIRED
Incidence
Mode of infection
Stages

Primary
  Lesion
  Sites
  Macroscopical
  Microscopical
  Results
  Diagnosis
    Dark ground illumination
    Serology

Secondary
  Manifestations
  Diagnosis
    Demonstration of organism
    Serology
    Results

Tertiary
  Gumma
  Macroscopical
  Microscopical

CHRONIC SYPHILITIC
INTERSTITIAL INFLAMMATION
  Macroscopical
  Microscopical
  Diagnosis
    Serology
    Histology

CONGENITAL

Sarcoidosis

Nature
Although sarcoidosis is not definitely infective, it is placed among the infective granuloma group because of the close similarities between sarcoid and tuberculous lesions.

Aetiology
The cause or causes remain unknown; many aetiological agents have been suggested but none are proven. It has been regarded as an atypical form of tuberculosis; a virus infection; a sensitization manifestation to proteins including pine pollens; an auto-immune disease.

Incidence
An unknown disease restricted to temperate zones of the world.

Age
Sixty-five per cent occur between 20–40 years of age at the time of diagnosis.

50

Macroscopical

The involved tissues in the early stages show multiple white or pale pink sarcoid foci similar to tubercles, which later may become fibrotic.

Microscopical

Each sarcoid granuloma is composed of:

1 A central circular collection of epithelioid cells.
2 Giant cells of the Langhans' or foreign body type.
3 A peripheral narrow zone of lymphocytes.
4 An outer layer of fibrous tissue which may increase with the age of the lesion.

Later:

5 Giant cell inclusions:
(a) Asteroid bodies – star-shaped structures in giant cells.
(b) Schaumann bodies – laminated blue-staining oval bodies.

Later still:

6 Hyaline fibrous tissue may replace the circular sarcoid foci.

N.B. The sarcoid focus shows:

1 No caseation.
2 No *Mycobacterium tuberculosis* on culture, staining or animal inoculation.

Sites of involvement

Sarcoid tissue may be present in one or many tissues or organs to produce protean clinical syndromes.

SKIN

Multiple skin lesions producing Boeck's sarcoidosis or *lupus pernio* – 50 per cent.

SUBCUTANEOUS TISSUES

Erythema nodosum is a frequent manifestation and may be associated with hilar lymphadenopathy.

UVEAL TRACT

Sarcoid involvement of the eye, especially the iris and ciliary body to produce *Heerfordt's syndrome* in 25 per cent of cases.

LUNG

This is the commonest site of clinical involvement – 90 per cent, and may result in a 'miliary' form with a 'snow-storm' radiological appearance. A diffuse infiltration may also occur and this can progress to a *honeycomb lung* (see p. 673).

SPLEEN

Sarcoidosis is a cause of splenomegaly – 13 per cent, resulting in *Stengel–Wolbach's* splenomegaly.

SALIVARY GLANDS

The parotid glands are involved most frequently – 6 per cent, but the submandibular and lacrimal glands may also be affected to produce *Mikulicz's* syndrome (see p. 178).

LYMPH NODES

The lymph nodes are frequently involved at any site – 37 per cent, most commonly in the hilar and cervical groups.

BONES

Bone involvement is unusual except for the phalanges of the feet and hands – 6 per cent, which are demonstrable as radiologically rarefied areas – *osteitis cystica multiplex of Jüngling*.

LIVER

This is probably involved in the majority of cases – 60 per cent, but the diagnosis is dependent on liver biopsy.

OTHER ORGANS

For example, heart, stomach, C.N.S., pituitary and kidneys, all of which are sometimes involved.

N.B. No matter the site involved the histology remains typical of sarcoid. However, it should also be realized that the histological appearances of sarcoid may occur in individuals in reaction to other causes, e.g. skin with injury by silica, lymph nodes draining tumours and in intestine in Crohn's disease. Clinical and histological features must therefore be assessed together.

Results

RESOLUTION

This occurs in the great majority of cases.

FIBROSIS

This is frequently seen in the lymph nodes in the healed stages. It may also occur in other sites:
(a) Lungs – pulmonary fibrosis, honeycomb lung, cor pulmonale.
(b) Eyes – progressive uveal tract fibrosis with blindness.

NEPHROCALCINOSIS

Some cases of sarcoidosis develop a raised serum calcium and this may lead to nephrocalcinosis and subsequently to death from renal failure.

TUBERCULOSIS

A small number of sarcoid patients develop bacteriologically proven tuberculosis with tuberculin test conversion.

DEATH

Due to sarcoid involvement of vital structures on rare occasions, e.g. heart, C.N.S. and the late effects of pulmonary fibrosis.

Diagnosis

BIOPSY

Especially of a lymph node or skin. The histology has to be differentiated from a tuberculous process and, although this is sometimes difficult, the regularity of the epithelioid cell foci and the absence of caseation in the sarcoid lesions are the most certain ways of distinguishing the two conditions.

KVEIM TEST

The intradermal injection of a phenolized preparation of an active sarcoid lymph node. There follows the development of a dermal nodule in approximately 6 weeks and the histology of this lesion shows sarcoid tissue only in those patients with active sarcoidosis.

OTHER LABORATORY TESTS

(a) *Blood count.* This is frequently normal but the E.S.R. may be raised in the active stages and especially with erythema nodosum.

(b) *Serum calcium.* A raised serum calcium occurs in about 5 per cent.

(c) *Alkaline phosphatase.* This is frequently raised and may be due to sarcoid involvement of either the liver or bone.

(d) *Serum proteins.* There is hyperglobulinaemia in about 25 per cent of patients. The main value of this test is in assessing the activity of the disease.

(e) *Electrophoresis.* The serum protein pattern usually shows increased α_2 and γ globulins.

HEAF TEST

This is negative in approximately 50 per cent.

Leprosy

Organism

Mycobacterium leprae, an acid but not alcohol-fast bacillus. The organism is of low virulence and invasiveness and cannot be cultured nor transmitted to animals.

Mode of infection

Not definitely known, but probably due to entry of organisms through abrasions in the skin or mucous membranes followed by lymphatic spread. The incubation period is usually about 3 years. It is probable that the infection is acquired only after prolonged and fairly intimate contact with an infected person.

Tissues involved

Skin, mucous membranes, peripheral nerves.

Types

LEPROMATOUS – NODULAR

Develops in more susceptible individuals.

Macroscopical

Starts with a macular rash which rapidly changes into dermal nodules, particularly on the nose, face, extensor surfaces of the limbs and the mucous membranes of the upper respiratory tract. These may vary from 1 cm in diameter to large disfiguring lesions. Sloughing of the overlying skin is common to produce chronic ulceration. Later there is lymph node and peripheral nerve involvement.

Microscopical

Granulomas composed mainly of large lipid-containing macrophages in which there are very numerous organisms – *lepra cells*. There is an associated mild lymphocytic infiltration.

TUBERCULOID – ANAESTHETIC –
MACULO-ANAESTHETIC

Develops in more resistant hosts.

Macroscopical

Presents as a non-elevated macular skin rash with a nodular hyperaemic border. The lesions vary from discrete areas 1 cm in diameter to large coalescent zones involving the face, trunk and limbs. The local peripheral nerves become involved and the process extends proximally to the larger nerves which become palpable thickened cords.

Microscopical
Localized collections of epithelioid cells surrounded by lymphocytes, plasma cells and scattered giant cells. There is increasing fibrosis as the lesion ages. Organisms are scanty in this type of lesion.

Diagnosis

DEMONSTRATION OF ORGANISMS
(*a*) By biopsy of tissues and staining by modified Z.N. technique.
(*b*) By similar staining of scrapings or washings from ulcerated areas.

LEPROMIN TEST
This skin test is negative in the lepromatous type but positive in the tuberculoid form. As it may also be positive in normal subjects it has only limited clinical application.

Results
A slowly progressive disease with long remissions and recurrent exacerbations. The mortality rate is low but lepromatous cases may die from intercurrent infections. Disfigurement and deformities are considerable. Nerve involvement with anaesthesia is complicated by ulceration, bone decalcification, trophic changes and contractures. This may result in 'claw hands' or even auto-amputation of fingers and toes. The nodular form develops 'leonine facies' due to the lepromatous masses. Ulceration of the mucous membranes of the nose and larynx causes chronic nasal discharge and voice changes.

Syphilis

Organism
Treponema pallidum – a regularly coiled, actively motile, spirochaete about 20 μm in length.

Types
Syphilis may be congenital or acquired.

ACQUIRED SYPHILIS

Incidence
The incidence has considerable geographical variation closely correlated with social factors, promiscuity, etc., and the true frequency in any area is difficult to assess. Effective antibiotic chemotherapy has now markedly decreased the occurrence of late stages.

Mode of infection
The delicate *Treponema pallidum* is rapidly destroyed outside the tissues and almost all cases of syphilis are contracted during close physical contact with an infected person. The organism probably cannot penetrate intact epidermis and gains access through minor abrasions of the surface.

Stages of syphilis
Once the organism has gained access to the tissues of the host, rapid dissemination occurs and the spirochaetes are spread throughout the body, probably within 24 hours of contracting the infection. This spirochaetaemia may be prolonged, lasting for many years and, at any stage, clinical manifestations of the disease may become apparent. The lengthy natural history of the disease is illustrated by the three typical clinical stages.

PRIMARY SYPHILIS

Lesion
The primary lesion is the chancre which develops some 2–6 weeks after infection.

Sites
Usually genital, the penis in the male and the cervix or vulva in the female; the cervical site is frequently missed clinically. Ten per cent have an extra-genital site, e.g. rectum, anus, fingers, breasts or lips.

Macroscopical
A single, painless, indurated ulcer with painless enlargement of the regional lymph nodes.

Microscopical
A predominantly mononuclear cell infiltration with lymphocytes and plasma cells in a fibroblastic granulation tissue. There is thickening of the endothelium and subintimal tissues of the blood vessels which show the characteristic perivascular cuffing of inflammatory cells.

Results
Although the spirochaetes are disseminated

throughout the body at the stage of the primary chancre, the patient appears otherwise perfectly well. The primary chancre heals within 3 months with minimal scarring whether treated or not. In untreated cases it is probable that one-third have a spontaneous cure, one-third never develop clinical lesions but have positive serology, and one-third develop the later syphilitic manifestations.

Diagnosis

DARK GROUND ILLUMINATION
Scrapings of the chancre will reveal the spirochaetes.

SEROLOGY
Wassermann reaction (W.R.), Treponema immobilization test (T.P.I.), Price's precipitin reaction (P.P.R.), Kahn test, Reiter's complement fixation test, etc., are usually positive 4–6 weeks after the development of the chancre, i.e. during the healing stage.

SECONDARY SYPHILIS

The secondary stage with its extremely variable manifestations may become apparent 1–3 months after the primary chancre. However, this stage may remain completely subclinical.

Manifestations
The commoner are:
1   Pyrexia, anorexia, and general malaise.
2   Lymphadenopathy.
3   Skin rashes which tend to be bilateral, copper-coloured and painless. The commonest is maculo-papular in type.
4   Condylomata or venereal warts on the penis or vulva.
5   'Snail-track' ulcers on mucous membranes, e.g. tongue and mouth.
6   Eye changes with retinitis, iritis or iridocyclitis.
7   Alopecia.

Diagnosis

DEMONSTRATION OF THE SPIROCHAETES
This is rarely attempted.

SEROLOGY
Positive W.R., Kahn, etc.

Results
Most of the manifestations of secondary syphilis are transient and tend to disappear whether treated or not.

TERTIARY SYPHILIS

Tertiary manifestations develop in from 3 to 25 years after the primary infection in about one-third of untreated syphilitic patients. The cardiovascular system is involved in the majority of these cases (see p. 244), the C.N.S. in about 10 per cent (see p. 602) whilst the remainder have either solitary gummas or multiple organ involvement. The lesions are as follows.

Gumma

MACROSCOPICAL
Within a solid tissue it forms a localized, firm and rubbery, white or grey mass. In a surface structure it produces an indolent, punched-out ulcer with a 'wash-leather' base.

MICROSCOPICAL
1   Central areas of necrosis with persistence of the ghost outlines of the cell structures – *structured necrosis* (gummatous necrosis). This area is avascular and devoid of inflammatory cells.
2   The necrotic area is enclosed by cellular fibroblastic tissue with more mature collagen merging with the surrounding tissue peripherally.
3   Infiltration of the fibrous area by profuse plasma cells, lymphocytes and scanty giant cells.
4   Endarteritis obliterans of blood vessels with a perivascular cuff of plasma cells and lymphocytes.

Chronic syphilitic interstitial inflammation

MACROSCOPICAL
Diffuse and irregular thickening of the involved structures, e.g. tongue, meninges, aorta and periosteum.

MICROSCOPICAL
1   Diffuse fibroblastic thickening of the tissues.
2   Diffuse infiltration by lymphocytes and plasma cells.
3   Endarteritis obliterans with perivascular cuffing.

4 Multiple minute areas of structured necrosis and scanty giant cells.

Diagnosis

SEROLOGY
The W.R. usually remains positive.

HISTOLOGY
Diagnostic appearances on biopsy.

CONGENITAL SYPHILIS

Congenital syphilis is contracted *in utero* from a syphilitic mother via the placenta. The disease is now less common due to antenatal supervision which normally includes routine serological tests, e.g. V.D.R.L.

The lesions are very protean and may be present at birth or develop in childhood or adolescence, e.g. abnormal-shaped teeth, iridocyclitis or interstitial keratitis.

Chapter 11
Diseases due to Fungi

General

Although significant clinical disease due to infections with fungi are uncommon when compared with bacteria, diseases due to this group of organisms are important and there is considerable evidence to suggest that their incidence is increasing, particularly in patients treated with broad-spectrum antibiotics, corticosteroids or immuno-suppressive drugs. Fungi produce neither exo- nor endotoxins, are only weakly antigenic and are mostly of very limited pathogenicity with little invasive properties. Many of the pathogenic fungi remain limited to the skin surface, e.g. athlete's foot and ringworm, but some produce more serious and generalized diseases which may on occasions prove fatal.

Actinomycosis

Organism
The anaerobic fungus, *Actinomyces israeli*. This organism grows in the tissues in the form of

colonies composed of branching mycelial threads with clubbed ends – *ray fungus*. The colonies appear in pus as *sulphur granules*.

Sites

CERVICO-FACIAL

Accounts for 50 per cent and originates in a site of injury in the jaw, e.g. a tooth socket. The area becomes indurated and the lesion extends by direct spread through adjacent tissues to produce a large, hard, woody mass involving the face, jaw and neck. Softening occurs and multiple sinuses develop, through which the characteristic pus, containing the sulphur granules, exudes.

ABDOMINAL

The abdomen is the site of the disease in 25 per cent and usually presents as an appendicular abscess. This spreads to involve the caecum, intestine, pelvic organs and anterior abdominal wall with multiple sinus formation. The process may also spread in the right paracolic gutter to involve the liver, kidney and vertebral column. The liver may also be involved by blood spread through the portal vein with resulting multiple actinomycotic abscesses. Occasionally, these may spread through the diaphragm into the chest.

PULMONARY

Pulmonary involvement most commonly occurs following aspiration or inhalation of the organisms but rarely may complicate subdiaphragmatic disease. The lower lobes are most commonly involved with characteristic honeycombed abscess formation. Extension may produce empyema, erosion of ribs or vertebrae, pericardial involvement and sinuses in the chest wall. Metastatic abscesses may form in the brain.

ACUTE DISSEMINATED

This is a very rare form, where blood spread produces actinomycosis in many organs.

Macroscopical

The lesions produce a hard indurated swelling of the infected tissues, which, on cross-section, give the appearance of honeycombed abscesses.

Microscopical

The appearances are made specific by the presence of colonies of the fungus, together with a moderate polymorph infiltration and very extensive fibrosis.

Diagnosis

Identification of the organisms in pus or tissue.

Results

Extensive tissue destruction and scarring with rather slow response to antibiotics.

Blastomycosis

EUROPEAN – CRYPTOCOCCOSIS – TORULOSIS

Organism

Cryptococcus neoformans – this is a round or oval organism 5–10 μm diameter which reproduces by budding and has a distinctive and prominent gelatinous capsule.

Geographical distribution

Although described as European, the infection is of world-wide distribution.

Pathogenesis

This is a rare and chronic disease, most commonly seen as a terminal illness in patients with debilitating conditions, e.g. a malignant disease, and in those immunosuppressed.

Sites

SUPERFICIAL

Skin, subcutaneous tissues and joints with the formation of abscesses.

LUNGS

By aspiration or blood dissemination with resulting granulomas.

MENINGES

A meningitis closely resembling that seen in tuberculosis.

Microscopical

The organisms are found in the affected tissues showing a characteristic clear surrounding zone caused by the capsule. There is little inflammatory reaction, particularly in the meninges, although in the lungs, fibrosis and mononuclear cell infiltration create the granulomatous appearance.

Diagnosis
By identification of the organism in C.S.F., sputum, or scrapings of skin lesions.

Results
The disease is resistant to treatment. The meningitic lesion usually proves fatal.

NORTH AMERICAN BLASTOMYCOSIS

Organism
Blastomyces dermatitidis – this is a highly pathogenic round or oval fungus 5–15 μm in diameter which has a characteristically thick and double-contoured wall.

Geographical distribution
The North American continent.

Sites
The fungus enters the body by inhalation or through a skin wound.

SKIN LESIONS
A spreading irregular papule with micro-abscesses in the raised margins.

PULMONARY
Most commonly seen as miliary abscesses throughout the lung. Rarely a solid granulomatous mass forms.

DISSEMINATED
Many organs may be involved, especially bone.

Microscopical
The organisms are present in necrotic zones together with a marked polymorph and lymphocytic inflammatory cell infiltrate.

Diagnosis
By identification of the organism in scrapings from the skin lesions, in sputum or in biopsied tissues.

Results
The disease is extremely resistant to treatment and the skin lesions progressively enlarge. The pulmonary and disseminated forms are commonly, but not invariably, fatal.

Histoplasmosis

Organism
Histoplasma capsulatum. – a small (1–5 μm diameter) budding, oval fungus, with a clear halo caused by a thick capsule.

Geographical distribution
Although most commonly found in the central regions of the U.S.A., cases have been described from many parts of the world.

Sites
A diffuse disease of the lymphoid system which is usually manifest by enlarged spleen, liver and lymph nodes, intestinal ulceration and anaemia.

Microscopical
The organisms are present within macrophages which are the predominant cells of the inflammatory reaction. Central necrosis and giant cell formation may occur.

Diagnosis
1 *Identification of fungi.* In tissues, liver biopsy, bone marrow.
2 *Histoplasmin skin test.*

Results
This is a fatal disease, usually within 1 year of its onset. A mild subclinical form occurs as a transient pulmonary infection which is subsequently demonstrable as calcified foci in lung and regional lymph nodes. These cases also have a positive histoplasmin skin test which serves to differentiate the pulmonary lesions from those of tuberculosis.

Moniliasis – Candidiasis

Organism
Candida albicans – A common inhabitant of skin and the oral cavity, which usually causes superficial infections but occasionally may involve more important organs. Budding, yeast-like forms and long filamentous mycelia penetrating the affected tissues are characteristic.

Geographical distribution
World-wide.

Pathogenesis
The organism is of low virulence and there is usually some predisposing condition which allows its establishment:
1   *Antibiotic therapy*. Very commonly seen after courses of antibiotics particularly when broad-spectrum substances are taken by mouth.
2   *Steroid and immunosuppressive therapy*. There is some evidence to show an increase in the more serious manifestations of disease by this organism in patients who are receiving long courses of corticosteroids or immunosuppressive drugs.
3   *General*. Diabetes, malnutrition, avitaminosis and other generalized metabolic disturbances also predispose.
4   *Venous Lines*. Contamination of central venous feeding or pressure lines by the organism have caused a marked increase in acute systemic moni-liasis.

Sites

SUPERFICIAL
Mouth, vagina, skin creases, e.g. axilla, groin.

OESOPHAGUS
Extension of mouth infection.

LUNGS
Presence of the organism in the sputum does not necessarily mean that it is responsible for the pulmonary disease.

DISSEMINATED
This is rare but blood spread may result in multiple abscesses in many organs.

Macroscopical
There is a white, felted membrane on a red and moist surface – *thrush*. Abscess formation occurs in the lung and in the disseminated form.

Microscopical
The membrane is composed of mycelia with fila-ments penetrating, often deeply, into underlying tissues. There is only a slight inflammatory cell reaction.

Diagnosis
Isolation and identification of the fungus. However, this does not necessarily imply that the monilia is causative of the disease present.

Results
Although only rarely the cause of serious disease, it is commonly rather resistant to treatment once it has become well established in the tissues.

Aspergillosis

Organism
There are many species of Aspergillus but most are contaminants or saprophytes. However, *Aspergillus fumigatus* is associated with disease in man.

Geographical distribution
World-wide.

Lesions

LUNG
This is the commonest form of serious Aspergillus infection. There are two types of disease.

Superficial
An asthmatic type induced by an allergic reaction to the presence of aspergilli in the bronchial tree. The sputum contains the organisms and mycelia may extend for a short distance into the bronchial epithelium.

Granulomatous
Cavitating granulomatous lesions occur occa-sionally, nearly always in patients with chronic bronchitis or previous tuberculosis. The granu-loma may arise due to secondary infection by aspergilli of a pre-existing cavity (abscess or tuber-culosis), or as a result of invasion of previously normal tissues by mycelia with subsequent nec-rosis. These lesions are commonly near the lung surface with bronchopleural fistula formation as a common sequel, spontaneously or following sur-gery.

C.N.S.
May rarely cause meningitis or brain abscesses.

DISSEMINATED
Systemic disease is extremely rare.

EAR AND VAGINA

Superficial infections with aspergilli, particularly in chronic otitis externa and media, are common.

Diagnosis

Aspergillus fumigatus is a commonly occurring saprophyte and therefore cultural isolation from sputum does not necessarily mean the presence of pulmonary aspergillosis. Demonstration of mycelial filaments in smears of sputum or scrapings from superficial lesions is, however, suggestive and evidence of mycelial invasion of epithelial cells is diagnostic.

Coccidioidomycosis

Organism

Coccidioides immitis – a large thick-walled spherule which reproduces by the formation of endospores.

Geographical distribution

Almost entirely confined to South-West United States – San Joaquin fever.

Sites

SKIN

Focal lesions which may be nodular, ulcerated or verrucose, resembling tuberculosis.

LUNG

(*a*) Multiple abscesses.

(*b*) Multiple granulomas resembling tuberculosis.

(*c*) A mild, often subclinical type, with residual calcified lesions.

DISSEMINATED

Occurs very rarely, with involvement of spleen, liver, lymph nodes, bones, C.N.S.

Microscopical

Polymorph infiltration around areas of suppurative necrosis in pulmonary disease with abscess formation.

Epithelioid cell granulomas with central caseation and giant cells in the granulomatous disease.

In both types, the organism is demonstrable lying free within the necrotic areas.

Diagnosis

1 *Demonstration of organism.* In sputum or skin lesions.
2 *Coccidioidin skin test.*

Results

In general the prognosis is good, with fibrous healing and calcification of the lesions but the outlook is grave when the disease becomes generalized. This also is a disease which may mimic pulmonary tuberculosis, but the geographical localization is diagnostically helpful.

Chapter 12
Diseases due to Protozoa

General

Several of the most common and important infectious diseases throughout the world are caused by protozoa, e.g. malaria. Infection with *Entamoeba histolytica* – amoebic dysentery, is more conveniently described in diseases of the alimentary tract (see p. 204). Other important protozoal diseases are outlined below.

Leishmaniasis

Three species of Leishmania infect man, each having a distinctive clinical pattern.

CUTANEOUS LEISHMANIASIS – ORIENTAL SORE

Organism
Leishmania tropica. Round or oval organisms 2 μm diameter with a central nucleus. They are mostly found intracellularly in macrophages.

Geographical distribution
Near, Middle and Far East.

Pathogenesis
Transmitted by the bite of a sand fly from an open case to a new host.

Macroscopical
A papule forms in the area and later a crust of exuded serum and blood appears. The lesion persists for weeks or months before it heals with residual scarring.

Microscopical
Early – macrophages filled with the organism.
Later – released organisms, macrophages and a rim of lymphocytes and plasma cells. Extension to involve the epidermis results in ulceration, a polymorph infiltrate and pseudo-epitheliomatous epidermal hyperplasia.

Diagnosis
Identification of the organisms, in smears from the exudate or in biopsied tissue.

MUCOCUTANEOUS LEISHMANIASIS – ESPUNDIA

Organism
Leishmania braziliensis. This is morphologically indistinguishable from *L. tropica*.

Geographical distribution
Central and South America.

Lesions
Identical to the cutaneous type but with involvement of mucous membranes of the mouth, nose and larynx. Constitutional symptoms may develop.

VISCERAL LEISHMANIASIS – KALA-AZAR

Organism
Leishmania donovani. The organism is of similar appearance to *L. tropica* except for an additional long rod-like structure extending radically from the nucleus and terminating in a blepharoplast.

Geographical distribution
Widely prevalent and endemic in Mediterranean countries, India, Russia, China and parts of Africa.

Pathogenesis
Transmission is by the bite of Phlebotomus sand flies with man as the chief reservoir of infection.

Lesions
The disease is a systemic infection of the lympho-reticular system.

SPLEEN
Grossly enlarged with a thickened capsule, loss of pattern and dark red firm pulp which shows extensive infiltration by phagocytic cells containing large numbers of parasites.

LIVER
Enlarged, often considerably, with distension of the Kupffer cells by the organisms. This may proceed to hepatic cirrhosis.

LYMPH NODES
Generalized lymphadenopathy with parasitic infiltration.

BONE MARROW
Extensively infiltrated by phagocytosed parasites with resulting anaemia and leucopenia.

OTHER ORGANS
Lungs, gastro-intestinal tract, kidneys, skin and pancreas may all show involvement of their lympho-reticular elements.

Diagnosis
1 *Identification of parasite*
(*a*) Tissue biopsy.
(*b*) Bone marrow aspirate.
(*c*) Splenic puncture.
2. *Blood*. Progressive anaemia and leucopenia. The plasma proteins have a low albumin and a high globulin content.
3 *Serological*. A complement fixation test using a fraction of human *Myco tuberculosis* is remarkably specific.

Results
There is a high mortality rate, death usually supervening from intercurrent infection after a clinical course which varies from a few weeks to a few years.

TRYPANOSOMIASIS

Organisms
There are several pathogenic trypanosomes causing disease in man:

Trypanosoma gambiense – Gambian sleeping sickness.

T. rhodesiense – Rhodesian sleeping sickness.

T. cruzi – Chagas' disease (American trypanosomiasis).

All are slender, spindle-shaped, flagellated organisms about 15 μm long and 1–3 μm wide, with a posterior undulating membrane and central nucleus.

Geographical distribution
Central Africa (*T. gambiense* and *T. rhodesiense*); Central and South America (*T. cruzi*).

Mode of infection
The African types are inoculated into man by the bite of a tsetse fly in which the extra-mammalian portion of the life cycle occurs. The vector of the American type is the cone-nosed bug. The inoculated parasites appear in the circulation and subsequently become localized in the tissues.

Lesions
The principal lesions are as follows.

AFRICAN TYPES

Lymph nodes
Enlarged, soft and hyperaemic with gross lymphoreticular hyperplasia. These cells contain the parasites.

Brain
Thickening of the meninges, generalized oedema and scattered haemorrhages in the cerebral substance. There is a meningeal and perivascular inflammatory cell infiltrate with vascular narrowing leading to occlusions and areas of softening.

Other sites
The liver and spleen are sometimes enlarged due to parasitic infestation.

AMERICAN TYPE
Localizes principally in the myocardium within the muscle cells which eventually rupture. There is an accompanying mononuclear cell infiltration. Brain and other organs may also be involved.

Diagnosis
1 *Demonstration of the organism*
(*a*) In the blood.

(*b*) Biopsy of lymph nodes.
2. *C.S.F. Changes* (African types). Increased plasma cells and lymphocytes; raised protein; low sugar and chlorides; occasionally organisms are found.
3 *Complement fixation tests.* Positive in most cases.

Results
The African types present a variable course, as a chronic illness of several years' duration, or as a rapidly fatal process of some months. Most cases show a predominantly neurological picture – *sleeping sickness.*

The American type may show an acute, but rarely fatal, disease, or a chronic slowly progressive clinical course with heart failure.

Toxoplasmosis

Organism
Toxoplasma gondii – an intracellular, round, ovoid or crescent-shaped protozoon with basophilic cytoplasm, prominent nucleus and measuring 5 μm in length by 2·5 μm wide.

Geographical distribution
World-wide and common in all domestic animals, especially dogs, guinea-pigs, mice, rats and pigeons.

Mode of infection
The portal of entry and manner of transfer are obscure. Most of the recognized cases are seen in young infants, who presumably have acquired the infection *in utero* but there are undoubtedly many adults who contract an aysmptomatic form of the disease.

CONGENITAL TOXOPLASMOSIS

Lesions
1 Hydrocephalus.
2 Necrotic or calcified cerebral ganulomas.
3 Bilateral choroidoretinitis.
4 Focal necroses in heart and other viscera.
5 Low-grade fever, skin rash, jaundice and hepatosplenomegaly, may be present.

Diagnosis
1 *Isolation of the organism*
(*a*) From C.S.F.

(*b*) Transmission of the disease to guinea-pigs, mice and fertile eggs.

2 *Serological*

(a) Complement fixation test.

(*b*) Dye test – a rising titre is necessary for diagnosis.

(c) Fluorescent antibody test.

Results

A very variable clinical course; the predominant feature is usually the hydrocephalus which may progress with early death. Alternatively, the disease may 'die out', so that, with suitable surgical procedures, the prognosis may be favourable.

ADULT TOXOPLASMOSIS

Lesions

1 A benign, febrile lymphadenitis of variable severity – this is the most common form.

2 Disseminated infection with cerebral and pulmonary granulomatous lesions – uncommon.

3 Pulmonary infection resembling atypical pneumonia.

4 Choroidoretinitis and uveitis.

Diagnosis

As for the congenital type; the organisms, however, are seldom recoverable. Lymph node biopsy may also be helpful or diagnostic. The slightly enlarged discrete nodes show distortion of the follicular pattern and a rather diffuse infiltration with somewhat foamy histiocytes.

Results

Only in the very rare disseminated form is there danger to life. The disease in mild form may be responsible for some cases of 'P.U.O.' and lymphadenopathy. Moreover, the subclinical or milder types which may occur in pregnant females may explain the existence of the congenital form of the disease by transplacental spread.

Malaria

Incidence

There are still many millions of humans affected

Geographical distribution

World-wide, although most common in tropical and subtropical areas.

Aetiology

Transmission of the malarial parasites by various species of Anopheline mosquitoes.

Parasites

Plasmodium falciparum – causes 'malignant' malaria with continuous fever and brain involvement.

P. vivax ⎫ cause 'benign' malaria with a 'tertian'
P. ovale ⎰ fever.

P. malariae – causes 'benign' malaria with a 'quartan' type of fever.

Malarial life cycle

There are two cycles – in mosquito and in man.

IN MOSQUITO

Sexual cycle – 7–12 days – sporogony.

(a) Female mosquito bites infected man, the natural reservoir of the parasite.

(*b*) The infected blood which contains the female and male gametocytes is ingested into the stomach. These mature and penetration of a female gamete by a male gamete results in a zygote.

(c) The zygote penetrates the wall of the stomach and forms an oocyst.

(*d*) Within the oocyst, sporozoites develop to form a sporocyst.

(e) The sporocyst ruptures into the body cavity with release of sporozoites.

(*f*) The sporozoites migrate to the salivary gland of the mosquito and, following a bite, are introduced to a new host in the saliva.

IN MAN

Asexual cycle—schizogony.

Exo-erythrocytic phase

Seven days

(a) Sporozoites introduced by infected mosquito into the blood stream.

(*b*) These drain into the liver and there develop into merozoites.

(c) The merozoites invade the blood stream and enter erythrocytes.

Erythrocytic phase

Length varies with species – 36–72 hours.

(a) Merozoites in erythrocytes mature into trophozoites.

(*b*) The trophozoites develop into schizonts which divide into numerous merozoites.

(*c*) The erythrocytes rupture with release of merozoites into the blood stream.

(*d*) Some released merozoites penetrate further red cells, the remainder being destroyed by defence mechanisms.

(*e*) After about five such cycles in man, the merozoites change into male and female gametocytes from which a mosquito can be infected and the cycle continued.

Effects

RING FORMS
The trophozoites appear as ring forms in the erythrocytes about 10–14 days after the bite.

PYREXIA
New merozoites are released:

Every 48 hours with *P. vivax* and *ovale* – 'tertian' malaria.

Every 36 hours with *P. falciparum* – 'malignant' malaria.

Every 72 hours with *P. malariae* – 'quartan' malaria.

The bouts of pyrexia coincide with this merozoite release.

ANAEMIA
The destruction of the red cells produces an haemolytic anaemia and pigmentation by haemoglobin derivatives.

LYMPHORETICULAR SYSTEM
Phagocytosis of parasites causes lymphoid hyperplasia resulting in enlargement of spleen, lymph nodes and liver.

SPLENOMEGALY
In the acute stage the spleen is enlarged, soft and haemorrhagic. Microscopically, there is congestion, increased pigmentation and many parasites in the histiocytic cells. In the chronic stage, the spleen is grossly enlarged, firm and deep brown or almost black in colour. Microscopically, there is marked fibrosis with pigmentation due to haematin and also lymphoreticular overgrowth.

LIVER
Shows enlargement and the Kupffer cells are laden with pigment and parasites in the acute stage. The lymph nodes and bone marrow show similar changes.

BRAIN
In 'malignant' malaria of *P. falciparum* there is extreme congestion of the brain and the red cells may plug the cerebral vessels to produce areas of cerebral softening or small white foci of increased gliosis – 'malarial granulomas'.

BLACKWATER FEVER
Is produced by the sudden disruption of red cells releasing haemoglobin in large quantities to result in jaundice, gross haemoglobinuria and often oliguria progressing to acute renal failure.

Results

ACUTE BENIGN MALARIA
A severe febrile illness which, spontaneously or with treatment, subsides, but the patients are liable to repeated exacerbations over the years.

ACUTE MALIGNANT MALARIA
Rapidly progressive with high fever, convulsions and other cerebral manifestations, vascular collapse and death within a few days or weeks if untreated.

CHRONIC MALARIA
This is the usual pattern in native populations who have developed some resistance to the infection. Repeated attacks of benign malaria result in progressive, severe hepatosplenomegaly, chronic anaemia, poor general health and a shortening of the normal life span.

Diagnosis

Readily made by examination of thick blood films at the time of the acute attack or during an exacerbation. Morphological differences in the organisms enable identification of the species of parasite to be made. Malarial antibody studies may be an additional aid.

Chapter 13
Diseases due to Worms

Although disease due to Helminths (worms) are un-common in Western countries, there are many parts of the world, notably Africa and the Middle and Far East, where manifestations with these parasites are very common and result in chronic ill-health with reduction of the normal life span.

Classification

Nematodes
These are worms in the commonly used sense of the word and include round, thread, muscle, hook, blood and Guinea worms.

Cestodes

These are the tapeworms and include the beef, pork and fish tapeworms. Man can be infested with the adult worm or the cystic stage, e.g. hydatid disease.

Trematodes

These are flukes and include several families, of which the most important are the Schistosomata.

Brief descriptions of some of the more important diseases due to these worms follow.

Nematodes

The whole life cycle of nearly all the members of this class of worms occurs without the interposition of an intermediate host.

ROUNDWORM – ASCARIASIS

Parasite

Ascaris lumbricoides – resembles the common earthworm but is cylindrical and pointed at both ends, measuring 15–35 cm in length. The ova are oval with a thick, nodular capsule.

Geographical distribution
World-wide

Life cycle
Cycle complete in 1 months (Fig. 8).

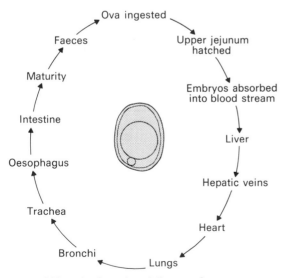

Fig. 8. Life cycle of ascaris and diagram of ovum.

Origin of infection
Water, vegetables and auto-infection.

Effects

INTESTINES
(*a*) Slight inflammatory reaction with eosinophilia.
(*b*) Nutritional deprivation, particularly in children, with growth retardation and weight loss.
(*c*) Occasionally peritonitis or intestinal obstruction.

LUNGS
(*a*) Loeffler's syndrome – eosinophilia associated with an haemorrhagic 'pneumonitis'.
(*b*) Asthmatic symptoms producing asphyxia on rare occasions.

Diagnosis
Recovery of ova or adult worm from the faeces.

THREADWORMS – OXYURIASIS

Parasite
Enterobius vermicularis (Oxyuris vermicularis) – the male is 4 mm in length with a spirally coiled tail; the female is 10 mm long with a pointed tail. The ova are bean-shaped with a thin capsule.

Geographical distribution
World-wide

Life cycle
The fertilized females emerge from the intestine and ova are deposited around the anus. These are transferred to new hosts by faecal contamination or by auto-infection via the fingers to the mouth. The ova mature in the intestines and attach themselves to the mucosa of the caecum, ileum and appendix. The structure of the ovum is illustrated in Fig. 9.

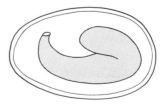

Fig. 9. Threadworm ovum.

Effects

Usually insignificant and are often an incidental finding in appendectomy specimens. Infrequently they may cause an inflammatory reaction with abundant eosinophils or a chronic granulomatous lesion in tissues. Mature worms migrate to the anus and cause intense pruritus, especially at night in children, in whom the scratching results in auto-infection.

Diagnosis

Ova may be collected on a cellophane strip applied to the anal margin at night.

MUSCLE WORM – TRICHINIASIS

Parasite

Trichinella spiralis – 2–6 mm long. A characteristic phase is that of the encysted larvae in voluntary muscles.

Geographical distribution

World-wide but particularly common where improperly cooked meat, particularly pork, is eaten, e.g. in sausages.

Life cycle (Fig. 10)

The chief source for man is the infected pig with in-fection due to ingestion of uncooked or inadequately cooked trichinous pork.

In muscle fibres embryos coil up, become less active and encysted, but in the early stages destroy the affected fibres with an accompanying lymphocytic and eosinophilic infiltration. Later there is scarring and calcification of the fibrous cyst wall 1–2 years after invasion. The worm, however, may remain viable for as long as 10 years.

Effects

These are variable. The stage of muscular invasion is marked by severe muscular pain with fever and dyspnoea if the diaphragm is involved. Myocardial involvement may rarely lead to heart failure and C.N.S. involvement produces fits or an encephalitic clinical picture.

Diagnosis

1   Muscle biopsy with demonstration of the encysted larvae.
2   Precipitin or complement fixation tests.

HOOK WORM – ANCYLOSTOMIASIS

Parasite

Ancylostoma duodenale a small cylindrical worm 10–13 mm long with a large mouth containing two pairs of hook-shaped teeth. The ova are oval and segmented into four to eight cells.

Geographical distribution

Found in all tropical and subtropical countries but particularly India and Ceylon. Infestation is extremely common and is second only to malaria as a world producer of death and chronic ill-health.

Life cycle

Cycle takes 7 weeks to complete (Fig. 11).

Effects

In the intestine, the worm attaches itself to the mucosal villi where there is oedema and an inflammatory reaction which may lead to ulceration or gangrene. The parasite extracts blood at this site so that severe anaemia is common.

Diagnosis

Identification of ova in the faeces.

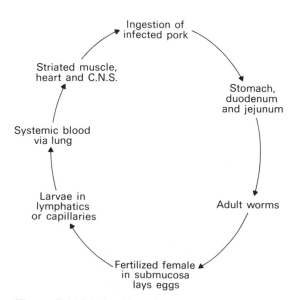

Fig. 10. Trichiniasis – life cycle.

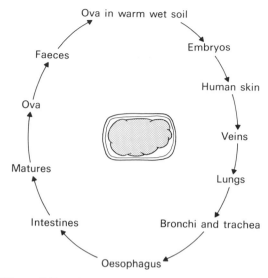

Fig. 11. Life cycle – hook worm.

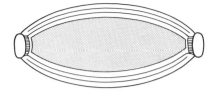

Fig. 12. Whip worm – diagram of ovum.

WHIP WORM – TRICHURIASIS

Parasite
Trichuris trichiura – adult worm is 30–50 mm long with a thin anterior portion, thick posteriorly, and thus resembling a whip. The ova are oval, dark brown and with characteristic protruding knobs at both ends.

Geographical distribution
World-wide but most common in the tropics.

Life cycle
Similar to threadworms (p. 67) The structure of an ovum is illustrated in Fig. 12.

Effects
The adult worm inhabits the caecum and is implanted only very superficially. It causes minimal or no clinical effects.

Diagnosis
Identification of ova in the faeces.

FILARIASIS

Clinical
The common denominator in filarial infections is the involvement of the subcutaneous tissues and lymph nodes producing elephantiasis, mostly affecting the lower limbs and external genitalia.

Parasites
There are several types, the most important being *Wuchereria bancrofti* – a hair-like worm 40–100 mm long found in the thoracic duct, lymphatics and lymph nodes. The motile microfilariae are only 0.3 mm long and 7 μm wide and can thus pass through capillaries. They inhabit the peripheral blood by night.

Geographical distribution
Middle and Far East, Hungary, Turkey, Central and parts of South America, Pacific Islands and Northern Australia.

Life cycle
Takes 12–30 days to complete (Fig. 13).

Effects
Inflammatory reaction around the sites of localization in the lymph nodes and lymphatics. The worms die and often calcify but there is an accompanying granulomatous tissue reaction producing lymphatic obstruction and chronic lymphoedema. The elephantiasis is manifest by subcutaneous fibrosis, hyperkeratosis of the skin and impairment of the blood supply.

Other filariae
1 *Loa loa* – '*Eye-Worm*' – predilection for migrating across the temporal region beneath the corneal epithelium and across the bridge of the nose to the other side.
2 *Onchocerciasis* – *Onchocerca volvulus* affects the upper trunk and upper extremities as fibrous masses containing 'reservoirs' of the parasites. These may subsequently migrate around the tissues of head and neck including the eye, with resulting blindness – 'blinding worm'.

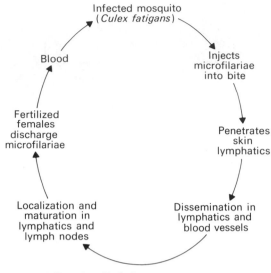

Fig. 13. Life cycle – filariasis.

TAENIA

Parasites

Man is infected by eating the flesh of infected intermediate hosts which contain the cystic stage of the parasite. *T. solium* and *T. saginata* are both long, flat and multisegmented, 304 and 608 cm long respectively; the fish tape worm is even longer – 912 cm. There is a small head whose characteristics vary with the species and 1–3000 hermaphrodite segments which, when mature, are filled with numerous fertilized ova which are subsequently discharged in the faeces. The head is essential for the survival of the whole parasite.

The main distinguishing features are illustrated in Fig. 14

Geographical distribution

World-wide

Life cycle

For example, *T. solium* (Fig. 15).

Effects

1   *Adult worm.* Very variable; there may be minimal gastro-intestinal disturbances or diarrhoea, anorexia, and loss of weight which may be marked and associated with an anaemia which is sometimes

Diagnosis

Filariae may be identified:

1   In blood taken at night – microfilariae seen in Bancroft's filariasis.

2   In blood taken by day – other types.

3   Biopsy of subcutaneous tissues, lymph nodes, etc.

4   Fluorescent antibody testing is additionally helpful.

Cestodes

These are hermaphrodite tape worms which require the interposition of an intermediate host for the completion of their life cycles.

Man is the definitive host of the adult worm of:

Taenia solium – pork tape worm – pig intermediate host.

T. saginata – beef tape worm – cattle intermediate host.

Diphyllobothrium latum – fish tape worm – freshwater fish (perch and pike) and species of Cyclops are intermediate hosts.

Man is the intermediate host of *Taenia echinococcus* (*Echinococcus granulosus*) – hydatid disease; rarely of *Taenia solium* – cysticercosis.

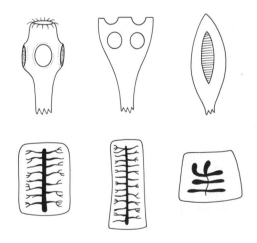

Taenia solium   Taenia saginata   Diphyllobothrium latum

Fig. 14. Diagram of heads and segments of types of tape worms.

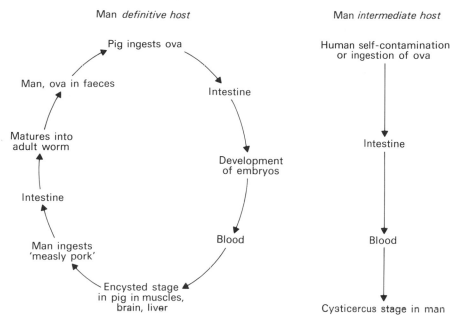

Fig. 15. Life cycle – tape worms.

macrocytic and resembles pernicious anaemia (see p. 482).

2 *Cysticerus stage.* Inflammatory reaction with eosinophils and neutrophil polymorphs followed by a granuloma around the dead encysted parasite which may subsequently calcify. These foci are important in the brain, frequently causing Jacksonian epilepsy.

Diagnosis

1 Isolation of tape worm segments or head in the faeces.

2 Biopsy of the affected area in the cysticercus stage.

HYDATID DISEASE

Infestation of man with the cystic stage of *Echinococcus granulosus.* The adult worm inhabits the intestine of the dog and many other animals and is only 2.5–6 mm long, but the cysts may reach an enormous size, especially in the liver. The disease is described in the liver section (p. 557).

Trematodes

These are flukes with complex life cycles and showing a specialized affinity for tissues of the definitive hosts. All require at least one intermediate host but many require two. The primary intermediate host is always a gastropod or water snail; the second intermediate host may be a mollusc, crustacean, insect, fish or vegetable matter. The most important trematode infestation of man is schistosomiasis.

SCHISTOSOMIASIS – BILHARZIASIS

Parasites

Three species:

Schistosoma haematobium – bladder involvement.

S. mansoni – intestinal and visceral involvement.

S. japonicum – intestinal and visceral involvement.

The male is 11–15 mm long by 1 mm wide with sides curved to form a gynaecophoric canal in which the long filamentous female lies. The adult worms mature in the portal or mesenteric veins and then migrate to the small veins of the bladder, intestines or liver, where ova are deposited. The ova traverse the tissues to the lumen and are excreted in the urine or faeces.

Geographical distribution

S. haematobium – Africa and parts of Middle East, especially Egypt, but also Greece, Cyprus and Portugal.

S. mansoni – Africa, Central and South America, Caribbean.

S. japonicum – Far East, especially China, Japan and Philippines.

In these areas, infestations with the worms are very common – up to 60 per cent of the population.

Life cycle

The cycle in man takes 6 weeks to complete (Fig. 16).

Mode of infection

The cercariae in water have the power of penetrating intact skin. In some countries, flooded rice fields are enriched by human excreta thereby perpetuating the infestation.

Effects

Mainly in three organs:

1 *Liver*. *S. mansoni* and *S. japonicum* – cause fibrosis around the ova with eventual 'pipe-stem' cirrhosis (see p. 558).

2 *Rectum*. Intense acute, followed by chronic, granulomatous inflammation around the worms and ova. Ulceration and necrosis are followed by fibrosis, mucosal hyperplasia with polyp formation and sometimes stricture or carcinoma.

3 *Bladder*. *S. haematobium* – chronic cystitis with fibrosis, mucosal metaplasia, fistula formation and carcinoma (see p. 388).

Diagnosis

1 Identification of ova in urine or faeces.

2 Biopsy of affected tissue.

3 Complement fixation and fluorescent tests are invaluable.

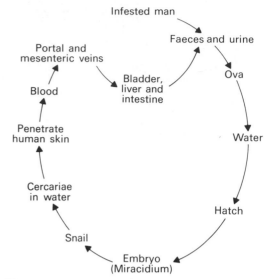

Fig. 16. Life cycle – schistosomiasis.

OTHER TREMATODE INFESTATIONS

Intestinal fluke

Fasciolopsis buski – a common fluke in China, producing diarrhoea and anaemia. The intermediate hosts are a snail and a water plant which is eaten raw in salads.

Liver flukes

(*a*) *Fasciola hepatica* – Causes 'liver-rot' in sheep, goats and cattle. Only rarely parasitic to man in sheep-raising areas.

(*b*) *Chinese liver fluke* – *Clonorchis sinensis* – found in the Far East only.

Both these flukes cause biliary tract inflammation with obstructive jaundice and hepatic abscesses.

Lung fluke

Paragonimus westermani. – limited to the Orient. Two intermediate hosts: the snail, then crayfish and crabs which are eaten by man. The flukes produce focal consolidation, abscess formation and fibrosis of the lungs.

Chapter 14
Special Forms of Injury

Burns
Classification
  Degrees
Microscopical
Practical classification
  Partial thickness
  Full thickness
Causes
  Thermal
  Electrical
  Chemical
  X-rays
Sites
Local effects
Systemic effects

High temperature injuries
Causes
  Endogenous
  Exogenous
Possible mechanisms

Low temperature injuries
Local
  Immersion foot – trench foot
  Frostbite
Systemic

Crush injuries – crush syndrome
Aetiology
Effects
Results

Blast injuries
Aetiology
Results
  Air blast
  Immersion blast

Radiation injuries
Nature

IRRADIATION EFFECTS
Absorption
Intensity
Rate of administration
Latency of effects

TISSUE CHANGES
Radiosensitive
Radioresistant
Radioresponsive

RESULTS

Immediate or early
Local and superficial
Internal

Delayed or late
Radionecrosis
Induced malignancy
Aplastic anaemia
Genetic

Burns

Classification
A time-honoured method is:
1 *First degree*. Erythema of the epidermis only.
2 *Second degree*. Coagulation with vesicle formation in the epidermis.
3 *Third degree*. Destruction of full thickness of the epidermis down to and including the superficial dermis and some accessory organs, e.g. hair follicle destruction.
4 *Fourth degree*. Extension of the burn to the deep fascia or with involvement of muscle, bone, etc.

Microscopical
In all, except the first degree burn, there is coagulation of the proteins, cell death, gross exudation of fluid due to vascular damage and an inflammatory cell infiltration.

Practical classification

PARTIAL THICKNESS
Incorporating first and second degree burns.

FULL THICKNESS
Incorporating third and fourth degree burns.

The practical significance of this classification is that partial thickness burns will heal by regeneration from residual epithelium without significant scarring. Full thickness burns will heal only by granulation and by marginal epithelialization with gross scarring unless excised and skin grafted.

Causes

1 Thermal.
2 Electrical.
3 Chemical.
4 X-rays and other irradiations.

Sites

Although most commonly on the skin surface, similar burns may follow thermal or chemical injuries to the mouth, respiratory and alimentary tracts.

Local effects

1 Loss of epithelium with exposure of a raw and unprotected area.
2 Infection of the burned area due to loss of protective surface.
3 Profuse plasma loss from the burned area due to capillary damage.
4 Loss of function.
5 Pain from exposed nerve endings.
6 Scarring with contactures and sometimes keloid formation.

Systemic effects

1 Shock – see p. 123.
2 Electrolyte disturbances due to plasma and fluid loss.
3 Haemoconcentration.
4 Fall of plasma protein levels.
5 Generalization of infection.
6 Organ changes:
(a) *Liver*. Cloudy swelling and fatty change. Occasionally there are areas of focal necrosis.
(b) *Kidneys*. Tubular degeneration or, with severe burns, acute tubular necrosis (see p. 365).
(c) *Adrenals*. Stress reaction with cortical lipid depletion and sometimes cell necrosis.
(d) *Gut*. Acute ulceration in duodenum or in stomach – 'Curling's ulcer'.
(e) *Brain*. Hyperaemia, oedema and sometimes fat embolism.
(f) *Lungs*. Bronchopneumonia as a complication.

High temperature injuries

Causes

ENDOGENOUS
Fever and hyperpyrexia with damage to vital centres in the brain stem (see p. 30).

EXOGENOUS
(a) *Local*. Burns.
(b) *Systemic*. 'Heat stroke' – general exposure of the body to excessive temperatures may result in circulatory collapse and death, mainly due to fluid loss and electrolyte disturbances. A major factor in the development of heat stroke is the failure of the sweating mechanism whereby heat can no longer be lost in sufficient amounts. It is thus most commonly found in hot and humid climates.

Possible mechanisms

Cell death may be caused by:
1 Denaturation of cell proteins.
2 Inactivation or destruction of cellular enzyme systems.
3 Increased cell metabolism with accumulation of metabolites.

Low temperature injuries

Local

IMMERSION FOOT
'*Trench foot*' exposure to long-continued low but non-freezing temperatures resulting in vascular damage and tissue ischaemia. The part is initially pale and blotchy when cold and, on subsequent warming, becomes oedematous and hyperaemic. Thrombosis and gangrene may follow in severe cases.

FROSTBITE
Exposure to freezing temperatures with the production of ice crystals in the tissues, vascular thrombosis and death of cells. When warmed, the part remains cold and pale and gangrene ensues.

Systemic

With whole body exposure to low temperatures there is skin blanching due to vasoconstriction later followed by hyperaemia due to loss of vasomotor control. Depression of vital centres, particularly in the brain, occurs and is fatal if severe and prolonged at or below a body temperature of approximately 21°C. Controlled hypothermia is occasionally used deliberately to reduce metabolic activity during operations on the heart and brain as this allows greater surgical freedom of action.

Crush injuries – crush syndrome

Aetiology
Prolonged external pressure on tissue particularly a limb, e.g. by fallen masonry, etc.

Effects
Shock with release of myoglobin from the muscles following ischaemic changes in the tissues, which result from pressure occlusion of the blood vessels.

Results
Severe shock with peripheral vascular failure, acute renal tubular necrosis and death from renal failure when severe or prolonged (see p. 365).

Blast injuries

Aetiology
1 Air blast from an explosion producing high pressure followed by low pressure from one direction.
2 Immersion blast in water producing high pressure followed by low pressure from all directions.

Results

AIR BLAST
Direct pressure on the body surface produces collapse of the thorax and rupture of solid viscera with haemorrhage. The compressive wave may enter the lungs and rupture alveoli with laceration and haemorrhage.

IMMERSION BLAST
The high pressure is applied to the body from all sides if the body is erect in the water, but if floating, the force will tend to raise the body unharmed out of the water. In the erect posture, the pressure will compress the abdominal wall with laceration of the diaphragm and solid viscera, or may pass up the anal canal to rupture the intestines. Sudden re-expansion of the abdomen in the ensuing negative pressure phase may result in intestinal rupture.

Radiation injuries

Nature
All types of radiation act in a basically similar fashion on tissues and cells although their powers of tissue penetration vary. Thus alpha and beta particles have little penetrative ability and are absorbed by the superficial tissues of the body, whereas gamma rays, used in therapy, penetrate deeply into the body tissues.

IRRADIATION EFFECTS

The effects of irradiation on tissue cells depend on the following.

Absorption
The greater the absorption of radiation the greater the tissue effect, e.g. gamma rays.

Intensity
The effects of irradiation depend on the intensity of the rays absorbed and the penetrating gamma rays produce the maximal biological results.

Rate of administration
Large doses over a short period of time produce the maximal effects and this results in damage to both normal and abnormal tissues so that a compromise has to be adopted in therapy. Thus a tumour is treated by multiple fields through different ports to concentrate the dosage to the tumour area and minimize the damage to adjacent normal tissues.

Latency of effects
There is a time-lag between absorption and its apparent biological action, varying from a few hours to several weeks.

TISSUE CHANGES

Normal tissues may be subdivided into three groups in respect of their sensitivity to radiation.

Radiosensitive
Cells killed or seriously injured by 2500 rad or less,

e.g. bone marrow, intestinal epithelium, lymphoid tissue and gonadal cells.

Radioresistant

More than 5000 rad necessary to kill or seriously injure the cells, e.g. kidney, liver, pancreas, endocrine glands, mature bone and cartilage, muscle and brain.

Radioresponsive

Intermediate in sensitivity, 2500 to 5000 rad being required for cell death or injury, e.g. skin, blood vessels, elastin and collagen. Growing bone and cartilage are also in this group and thus arrest of bone growth may occur following irradiation in the region of the epiphyseal line.

RESULTS OF IRRADIATION

IMMEDIATE OR EARLY

Local and superficial

Radiation burns. Appear after about 2 weeks. They may be of all degrees and involve the skin surface or deeper tissues. Healing is slow with residual scarring.

Radiation dermatitis. Follows frequent exposure to small doses of irradiation. Atrophy, hyperkeratosis, pigmentation, telangiectasis and splitting of nails with dermal fibrosis, occur secondarily to endarteritis obliterans induced by the irradiation.

Internal

Radionecrosis. Necrosis of abnormal, radiosensitive and other normal tissues occurs in the irradiated area when the dosage is high. There may be extensive tissue destruction and slow healing with scarring.

Storage. Ingested or injected radioactive elements are selectively stored in various tissues, e.g. strontium-90 in bones, iodine-131 in the thyroid and may produce eventual effects, usually of a chronic nature.

DELAYED OR LATE

Radionecrosis

Due to endarteritis obliterans in any affected tissue with:

(a) Chronic ulceration and tissue destruction, e.g. intestinal perforation.

(b) Gross fibrosis, e.g. pulmonary or renal fibrosis, lymphoedema, ureteric obstruction.

(c) Failure to heal due to the combination of these factors, e.g. persistent ulcers or fistulae.

Induced malignancy

Squamous cell and basal cell carcinomas. In areas of irradiated skin.

Leukaemia. Increased incidence of leukaemia in extensively irradiated persons, e.g. Hiroshima and Nagasaki, patients treated for ankylosing spondylitis by X-rays, and occupationally in radiologists.

Bone tumours. With radioactive phosphorus and strontium-90.

Other tumours. May less commonly develop in irradiated organs or tissues. The precise part played by irradiation in the induction of many forms of malignancy remains speculative.

Aplastic anaemia and thrombocytopenia

Although this is mostly an acute depression of bone marrow function it may also follow prolonged exposure to small doses (see p. 454).

Genetic

The possible effects of gonadal irradiation on subsequent progeny is not definitely known but it is possible that mutations could be induced and thus lead to genetic abnormalities in future generations (see p. 13).

Chapter 15
Water: Electrolytes:
Acid-base Balance

Objectives

This aims to be a clinically orientated introduction to water, electrolytes and acid-base balance as seen on the wards through the two standard laboratory requests: *urea and electrolytes* and *blood gases*. The intention is to give an understanding of relevant normal physiology, and to provide simple explanations for some of the problems which arise, and for their treatment.

Sodium and water

NORMAL PHYSIOLOGY

Sodium and its associated anions – mainly chloride and bicarbonate – are by far the largest contributors to the ionic and osmotic content of the extracellular fluid. Sodium and water are therefore considered together, since abnormalities of the two are closely related.

Water makes up about 65 per cent of body weight in men, and about 55 per cent in women.

About two-thirds of the water is intracellular, and some three litres of the extracellular water is in the plasma.

The body contains in the region of 4000 mmol of sodium: 1600 mmol in bone – non-exchangeable, the rest dissolved in the body water.

Cell membranes have an ATP-dependent 'pump' which excludes sodium from the cells and maintains the electrical potential across the membrane. The concentration of sodium in health is approximately 5 mmol/l in intracellular fluid and 140 mmol/l in extracellular fluid.

Most people ingest 80–120 mmol of sodium and 1500–2500 ml of water each day. Insensible water losses in sweat and from the lungs are about 1000 ml, and some 500 ml of water is produced by metabolic oxidative processes. In normal circumstances, therefore, the urine volume will be 1000–2000 ml. If, as is usual, sodium is neither gained nor lost by the body, urine will contain the same amount of sodium as is taken in i.e. 80–120 mmol.

Sodium and water balance is controlled by the kidneys. There is, for all practical purposes, no limit to the amount of water that can be excreted in health. At the other end of the scale, the maximum urine concentration that can be achieved is around 1200–1400 mosm/kg and with the normal solute load that has to be excreted, this means that there is a minimum obligatory urine volume of 400–500 ml/day. Water excretion is controlled by hypothalamic osmoreceptors governing anti-diuretic hormone (ADH) release. ADH acts on the proximal portion of the collecting ducts in the kidney, increasing its permeability to water, which then passes back into the capillaries.

Most of the controlling functions of the kidney are dependent on sodium transport. With a normal glomerular filtration rate of 120 ml/min, and a plasma sodium concentration of 140 mmol/l, some 17 mmol of sodium are filtered every minute and in the region of 25 000 mmol during the course of a day. Less than 0.5 per cent of this appears in the urine, so there is a large margin for increase in sodium excretion. The kidneys are also extremely good at conserving sodium, and normal persons placed on a sodium-free diet reduce their urinary sodium losses to less than 2 mmol/day within 2–3 days. The control of sodium excretion is achieved through intra-renal mechanisms influenced by renin, angiotensin and aldosterone, and probably by other factors.

Under most circumstances, the volume and sodium content of the urine are determined largely by the intakes of water and sodium.

The body normally maintains sodium and water balance by excreting the difference between intake and requirements in the urine, but stress or disease can bring into play more powerful mechanisms than those which produce that result.

Maintenance of circulating volume is the highest priority, and hypovolaemia – or under-perfusion of the kidneys – causes maximal sodium retention, irrespective of the intake of sodium or of water. Hypovolaemia also causes ADH release and reduced water excretion.

There are no normal values for urine volume or electrolyte concentrations, only values that are appropriate or inappropriate for the clinical situation.

DISORDERS OF HYDRATION

Pure deficiencies or excesses of sodium or water are rare, but they are seen in clinical practice. All possible combinations are therefore considered.

Pure water deficiency

CAUSES
1 Insufficient intake:
(a) No water available.
(b) Loss of sensation of thirst, e.g. in cerebral disease.
(c) Unconsciousness with no water supplied.
2 Excess losses:
(a) Hot climate with sweating – some sodium loss too.
(b) Osmotic diuresis – water losses usually greater than those of sodium.
(c) Diabetes insipidus:
Pituitary.
Nephrogenic.

EFFECTS
1 Reduced intracellular and extracellular fluid volume.
2 Concentration of all solutes, including sodium.

TREATMENT
Water replacement, see Hypernatraemia (p. 81).

Water replacement may be achieved orally, by nasogastric tube or intravenously. In the latter case, water itself cannot be given because its hypotonicity in relation to plasma causes haemolysis: 5 per cent w/v glucose is usually used, which is almost isotonic with normal plasma. The glucose is metabolized and the water remains.

Pituitary diabetes insipidus is treated with rehydration and vasopressin (ADH) or the synthetic DDAVP.

Nephrogenic diabetes insipidus can be treated with thiazide diuretics, chlorpropamide and/or increased water intake.

Pure sodium deficiency

CAUSES
1 Deficient intake. Impossible in health in a normal climate.
2 Excess losses:
(a) Sweating in a hot climate.
(b) Intestinal. Loss of sodium and water with replacement, by drinking or intravenous 5 per cent glucose, of the water. For example:
Pyloric stenosis.
Vomiting.
Fistulae.
Diarrhoea.
(c) Renal sodium and water losses with replacement of the water:
Diuretics.
Osmotic diuresis.
Analgesic nephropathy.
Other tubular disorders.

EFFECTS
1 Reduced extracellular fluid volume.
2 Hyponatraemia.

TREATMENT
1 Sodium replacement. Oral or intravenous.
2 Treatment of underlying cause.

Sodium and water deficiency

CAUSES
1 Deficient intake. Impossible in health in a normal climate.
2 Excess losses
(a) Sweating in a hot climate.
(b) Intestinal:
Pyloric stenosis.

Vomiting.
Fistulae.
Diarrhoea.
(c) Renal:
Diuretics.
Tubular disorders.
Osmotic diuresis.
(d) Endocrine. Mineralocorticoid deficiency:
Addison's disease (p. 290).
Sheehan's syndrome (p. 299).

EFFECTS
1 Postural hypotension.
2 Hypotension.
3 Tachycardia.
4 Poor organ perfusion.
5 Poor peripheral perfusion.
6 Reduced skin turgor.
7 Reduced intra-ocular tension.
8 Dry mouth and tongue.

TREATMENT
1 Replacement with (usually) isotonic (0.9 per cent w/v) saline.
2 Review of drug therapy.
3 Treatment of underlying cause.

Pure water excess

CAUSES
1 Excess intake:
(a) Hysterical polydipsia.
(b) Iatrogenic. Only occurs if renal and/or endocrine function disturbed.
2 Reduced excretion:
(a) Any acute illness.
(b) 'Inappropriate ADH syndrome', e.g. in carcinoma of lung (see p. 301).
(c) Drugs, e.g. carbamazepine.

The 'inappropriate ADH syndrome' is rare. The hyponatraemia commonly seen in ill patients is usually due to *appropriate* water retention secondary to hypovolaemia.

EFFECTS
Hyponatraemia.

TREATMENT
Water restriction, see Hyponatraemia, p. 80).
Hypertonic saline. Diuretics (if clinically urgent).

Pure sodium excess

CAUSES
1 Saline emetics.
2 Saline purges.
3 Inappropriate intravenous fluids, e.g. excess hypertonic sodium bicarbonate.

EFFECTS
Hypernatraemia.

TREATMENT
Administration of water, see Hypernatraemia (p. 81).

Sodium and water excess

CAUSES
1 Heart failure.
2 Renal failure – sometimes.
3 Hypoproteinaemia, e.g.:
    Nephrotic syndrome.
    Liver disease.
    Starvation.
    Any severe illness.
4 Drugs, e.g. carbenoxylone.
5 Cushing's syndrome – unusual (see p. 291).
6 Conn's syndrome – unusual (see p. 292).
    This is nearly always due to inability to excrete sodium, with appropriate retention of water to maintain normal osmolality. Sometimes, there is inappropriate water retention in addition – causing *reduced* plasma osmolality.

EFFECTS
1 Oedema.
2 Pulmonary oedema.
3 Hypertension.

TREATMENT
1 Review of drug therapy.
2 Treatment of underlying illness:
(*a*) Heart failure. Digoxin and diuretics.
(*b*) Renal failure. Diuretics. Dialysis.
(*c*) Liver disease. Fluid restriction. Diuretics.
(*d*) Nephrotic syndrome. Diuretics, steroids, intravenous albumin.

DISORDERS OF SODIUM CONCENTRATION

Hyponatraemia
A plasma sodium concentration below the local reference range. It is determined by a change in the relative amounts of sodium and water in the extracellular fluid.

CAUSES
1 *Abnormalities of total amounts of sodium and water.* Low plasma sodium concentrations can occur in all the following circumstances.

Total amount of:

Sodium	Much reduced	Reduced	Normal	Increased
Water	Reduced	Normal	Increased	Much increased

The causes are diagnosed from history and clinical examination.
2 *Abnormalities of sodium distribution.* In ill patients, the sodium pump does not function normally – the 'sick-cell' syndrome – and sodium leaks into the cells. Other ions leak out and osmotic and electrical equilibrium is maintained, resulting in hyponatraemia. The 'sick-cell syndrome' is often wrongly diagnosed. The hyponatraemia is usually due to water overload.
3 *Abnormalities of water distribution.* In severe hyperglycaemia, or when any other osmotically active substance – e.g. mannitol – is present in much greater quantities in the extracellular than intracellular fluid, water is drawn out of the cells to maintain osmotic equilibrium, diluting all substances in the extracellular water. This is diagnosed by measuring plasma osmolality and comparing the actual value with that calculated from the known concentrations of sodium, potassium, urea and glucose. The history is of great importance.
4 *Artefact:* (*a*) 'Drip arm'. This can occur if blood is taken from anywhere in the same arm as an intravenous infusion containing little or no sodium.
(*b*) Hyperlipaemia. Sodium is present in plasma *water*, but measurements are made per litre of whole plasma. Concentrations may therefore appear low if fat, or in rare instances protein, makes up a significant amount of the plasma volume.

EFFECTS

Severe hyponatraemia can cause unconsciousness, fits, or mental changes, e.g. disorientation, confusion.

TREATMENT

Depends on the cause. Not all abnormalities justify treatment.

Successful treatment of abnormalities of total amounts of sodium and water can be achieved if correct assessment of deficiencies or excesses is made.

The 'sick-cell' syndrome may be improved by treatment of the underlying cause and by administration of glucose and insulin if appropriate.

Abnormalities of water distribution due to osmotically active substances in the plasma are treated according to the substance present.

In general, aggressive attempts to change ionic concentrations in plasma rapidly may result in 'disequilibrium syndromes' which themselves cause abnormal behaviour, impaired consciousness or fits, so treatment should proceed as gently as is consistent with safety.

Hypernatraemia

A plasma sodium concentration above the local reference range. As with hyponatraemia, the concentration is determined by changes in the relative amounts of sodium and water in the extracellular fluid.

High sodium concentrations can occur in all the following circumstances.

Total amount of:

Sodium	Reduced	Normal	Increased	Much increased
Water	Much Reduced	Reduced	Normal	Increased

CAUSES

Hypernatraemia is most commonly due to *water depletion* (see p. 78), but may also occur when hypertonic saline purges, emetics or excess hypertonic intravenous fluids are given.

EFFECTS

Impairment of consciousness if severe.

TREATMENT

Administration of water (see p. 79), either to replace the deficit or to facilitate excretion of the sodium load. As with hyponatraemia, treatment should be as gentle as clinical circumstances allow.

Potassium

NORMAL PHYSIOLOGY

Potassium is quantitatively the most important intracellular cation. The body contains about 3000 mmol of potassium, of which 98 per cent is intracellular at a concentration of about 150 mmol/l intracellular water. Although only a very small amount of potassium is in the extracellular fluid, the concentration is very closely maintained in health at between 3.5 and 4.5 mmol/l.

The normal dietary potassium intake is 70–100 mmol/day, and normally the same amount is excreted in the urine. Control of potassium excretion occurs in the distal renal tubule, where it is exchanged in competition with hydrogen ion for sodium. The kidney cannot conserve potassium as effectively as sodium. The minimum concentration in urine is about 15 mmol/l and there is a minimum daily urinary loss of 20–25 mmol, which must therefore be taken in if balance is to be maintained.

In marked distinction to sodium, the concentration in the plasma is not primarily determined by the total amounts of potassium and water in the body, since so little potassium is present in the extracellular fluid. More important are the factors determining the distribution between the intra- and extracellular water. Abnormalities of extracellular potassium concentration are very important clinically because they can arise rapidly with shifts of very small amounts of potassium across cell membranes. Membrane potentials are affected and dangerous cardiac arrhythmias and muscular weakness may occur.

DISORDERS OF POTASSIUM CONCENTRATION

Hypokalaemia

A plasma potassium concentration below the local reference range.

CAUSES

1 *Depletion of potassium*
(a) Intestinal losses:
   Vomiting.

Diarrhoea.
Purgatives.
(*b*) Metabolic alkalosis.
(*c*) Renal tubular acidosis.
(*d*) Diuretics.
(*e*) Osmotic diuresis.
(*f*) Mineralocorticoid excess:
Cushing's syndrome.
Conn's syndrome.
'Ectopic ACTH syndrome', e.g. carcinoma of bronchus (see p. 000) and other tumours.
(*g*) Drugs, e.g. carbenoxylone, liquorice.
2 *Abnormal distribution*
(*a*) Metabolic alkalosis.
(*b*) Treatment of acidosis with bicarbonate.
(*c*) Treatment of hyperkalaemia with insulin.
(*d*) Familial hypokalaemic periodic paralysis.

In many of the causes of metabolic alkalosis, there is potassium depletion due to secondary potassium loss in the urine, and abnormal distribution due to hydrogen ion losses.

EFFECTS
1 Muscle weakness.
2 Cardiac arrhythmias.
3 Cardiac arrest.
4 Renal tubular damage.

TREATMENT
1 Identification and treatment of underlying cause.
2 Potassium replacement in suitable form – usually potassium chloride, if there is a deficiency.

Urgent replacement is necessary if the concentration is below 2.5 mmol/l. Intravenous therapy may be necessary initially. If so, the ECG should be monitored.

Hyperkalaemia
A plasma potassium concentration above the local reference range.

CAUSES
1 *Potassium excess*
(*a*) Renal failure.
(*b*) Potassium-retaining diuretics, e.g. amiloride.
(*c*) Iatrogenic – rapid administration of potassium in intravenous fluids.
2 *Abnormalities of distribution*
(*a*) Some metabolic acidoses.
(*b*) Mineralocorticoid deficiency – adrenal failure.

(*c*) Familial hyperkalaemic periodic paralysis.
(*d*) Crush injury – rapid release from damaged muscle cells.

EFFECTS
1 Muscle weakness.
2 Cardiac arrhythmias.
3 Cardiac arrest.

TREATMENT
1 Rapidly-acting – seconds or minutes.
(*a*) Glucose and insulin intravenously.
(*b*) Bicarbonate intravenously to increase pH.
(*c*) Calcium chloride or gluconate intravenously – does not affect concentration of potassium, but stabilizes cell membranes.
2 Longer term – hours or days.
(*a*) Ion exchange resins orally or rectally.
(*b*) Dialysis:
Peritoneal.
Haemodialysis.
(*c*) Hydrocortisone in replacement doses, if due to adrenal failure.

Treatment is urgent if the concentration is above 6 mmol/l. The ECG should be monitored.

Chloride and bicarbonate

The concentrations of chloride and bicarbonate in the plasma are most useful in the differential diagnosis of metabolic acidosis.

The total concentrations of anions and cations in the plasma are equal and maintain electrical neutrality. The majority of the cationic charges come from sodium (140 mEq/l). The remainder come from potassium (4 mEq/l), calcium (4 mEq/l), magnesium (2 mEq/l). The main anionic charges come from chloride (95–105 mEq/l), bicarbonate (22–28 mEq/l), and protein (15–20 mEq/l). The remainder of the charges are associated with phosphate and other organic compounds.

N.B. The concentrations are given in mEq/l rather than mmol/l because this section deals with ionic charges and not molar concentrations.

Sodium, potassium, chloride and bicarbonate are the electrolytes which are usually measured. If the concentrations of these anions and cations are added, there will usually be a difference in their sums of some 12–15 mEq/l. This is called the *anion gap*, and is really the difference between the ionic concentrations of the unmeasured cations and anions.

$$\text{Anion gap} = [(Na^+) + (K^+)] - [(Cl^-) + (HCO_3^-)].$$

The 'normal range' for the anion gap will vary between laboratories, depending on the analytical methods used for electrolyte measurement.

Metabolic acidoses may be regarded as being of two main types, one associated with an increased anion gap, and the other in which the difference is normal in magnitude. In any metabolic acidosis, the plasma bicarbonate concentration must, by definition, be low. In acidoses due to bicarbonate ion loss or hydrogen ion retention, the concentration of chloride rises to maintain electrical neutrality. The sum of the two ions remains the same, and the anion gap is normal.

In the other type of metabolic acidosis, bicarbonate is replaced by different organic anions, e.g. ketones, lactate, methanol, ethylene glycol, retained unmeasured anions in renal failure, and the chloride concentration remains the same, so the sum of chloride and bicarbonate falls. The anion gap is increased, and this provides an important clue that anions not normally present in significant quantities are responsible, with their associated hydrogen ions partially buffered by bicarbonate, for the acidosis.

Urea

Urea is the major end product of protein metabolism in man. With an average protein intake of 50–80 g/day, about 250–400 mmol of urea (15–25 g) is produced daily in the liver and excreted in the urine. The concentration in the plasma is usually 4–7 mmol/l. Urea is filtered by the glomerulus and passes unchanged down the renal tubule. At low urine flow rates, some urea diffuses passively back into the bloodstream, which makes measurement of endogenous urea clearance a less reliable indicator of glomerular filtration rate than the clearance of creatinine (see below).

Causes of high plasma urea
1 Low glomerular filtration rate:
(*a*) Renal failure (renal and post-renal).
(*b*) Hypovolaemia (pre-renal uraemia).
2 High production (pre-renal uraemia):
(*a*) High protein intake.

(*b*) Metabolic response to injury – general effects on body protein.
(*c*) Resolving haematoma or lysis of injured tissue.
(*d*) Melaena – bacterial action on blood in the bowel releases ammonia, which is absorbed and converted to urea by the liver.

Causes of low plasma urea
1 Low protein intake.
2 Starvation.
3 Liver failure.
4 Overhydration – dilution and 'wash-out'.

Creatinine

Creatinine production results from turnover of muscle protein. It is affected very little by protein intake or injury, and is dependent largely on the total amount of muscle present.

The average production of creatinine is around 10 mmol/day and is higher in men than women. It may be as low as 5 mmol/day in the very frail, or as high as 20 mmol/day in large physically fit men. The concentration of creatinine in the plasma varies in different individuals, but is usually between 80 and 120 μmol/l.

Endogenous creatinine clearance is widely used as a test of renal function. Creatinine is completely filtered at the glomerulus, and is neither secreted into the tubule nor reabsorbed from it. This enables an estimate of glomerular filtration rate to be made.

$$\text{Clearance} = \frac{UV}{P} = \frac{\text{Urine creatinine} \times \text{volume}}{\text{Plasma creatinine}}$$

Many doctors prefer to use repeated measurements of plasma creatinine when following the progress of patients with renal problems. Although creatinine clearance is not difficult to perform and is theoretically a better indicator, as a single measurement, of glomerular function, the plasma concentration alone is perfectly adequate for most purposes, and inaccuracies in urine collection may give misleading results.

Causes of high plasma creatinine
1 Raised production. Fit men with large muscle mass – physiological.
2 Decreased excretion. Renal failure.

Causes of low plasma creatinine
1 Reduced production. Small people – physiological.
2 Starvation – reflects low muscle mass.

Acid-base balance

BACKGROUND

For the optimal working of the body's enzyme systems, the degree of acidity of the intra- and extracellular fluids must be maintained. The intake of hydrogen and other acids or basic ions is variable, but usually some 50–70 mmol of acidic (mainly H^+) ions need to be excreted by the kidney to keep the total hydrogen ion activity (pH) constant. These ions are excreted in the urine largely buffered by phosphate or by the formation of ammonia, with subsequent excretion as ammonium ions.

pH is simply a convenient way of expressing hydrogen ion activity. It is defined as 'the negative logarithm (base 10) of the hydrogen ion activity', expressed in terms of molarity.

The normal hydrogen ion activity in arterial blood is between 36 and 44 nmol/l. The range in venous blood is very variable and measurements of this give little information about the body's acid-base status. 10 nmol/l is equivalent to a pH of 8.0 (conc. $1 \times 10^{-8.0}$ M). 100 nmol/l gives a pH of 7.0 (conc. $1 \times 10^{-7.0}$ M). 36 and 44 nM are equal to pH 7.44 and pH 7.36 respectively. The coincidence of the figures 36 and 44 is mere chance. The range of extracellular pH compatible with survival is about 6.8–7.7. This is a range of hydrogen ion activity of between 160 and 20 nmol/l, so the concentration can change a great deal more than with many other ions, a fact that is often not fully appreciated since pH is still almost universally used as the scale of acidity.

The Henderson–Hasselbach equation
The relationship between pH, bicarbonate and carbonic acid concentrations can be expressed as follows:

$$pH = pK' + Log_{10} \frac{[HCO_3^-]}{[H_2CO_3^-]}.$$

pK' is a mass action constant for all the chemical reaction equilibria and remains fairly constant at 6.1. There are small changes with variations in temperature, but these are not important clinically.

Since a constant proportion of dissolved carbon dioxide is present as $[H_2CO_3]$ and the amount dissolved depends directly on the partial pressure of carbon dioxide in arterial blood (p_aCO_2), the equation may be rewritten for practical use as:

$$pH = 6.1 + Log_{10} \frac{[HCO_3^-] \, (mmol/l)}{p_aCO_2 \, (kPa) \times 0.225}.$$

If two of the variables are measured, the third can be calculated. Most 'blood gas' analysers measure pH and P_aCO_2 and calculate the bicarbonate concentration. Values for the bicarbonate concentration derived in this way are slightly lower than those estimated by direct chemical methods in the laboratory because most chemical methods measure dissolved carbon dioxide as well as 'true' bicarbonate.

There are other problems with these measurements such as variation due to carbon dioxide diffusing out of solution *in vitro*, and the buffering effect of haemoglobin. Correction may be made for the latter, and efforts to compensate for the former include measuring bicarbonate at a fixed P_{CO_2} of 5.3 kPa (40 mmHg) – *standard bicarbonate*, and deriving various different values – *buffer base*, *base excess* etc. These efforts are chemically quite valid, but make very little difference in diagnosing and treating disorders of acid-base balance as seen on the wards. Only the bicarbonate concentration estimated by blood gas analysis will be considered here.

DISTURBANCES OF ACID-BASE BALANCE

Definitions
Metabolic disturbances occur when the primary problem is with the bicarbonate concentration.

Respiratory disturbances occur when the primary problem is with the partial pressure of carbon dioxide.

Disturbances are *compensated* when the arterial blood pH is between 7.36 and 7.44, and *uncompensated* when it is outside these limits.

pK' remains constant, and so maintenance of the pH requires a constant ratio between P_aCO_2 and bicarbonate. In any disturbance, compensation occurs by a change in concentration of the substance not involved in the primary problem, such that the *ratio* is brought back to its original value – although both bicarbonate concentration and p_aCO_2 will usually be outside their normal ranges. As a general rule, the p_aCO_2 and bicarbonate must change in the same direction. A summary of findings in the common disturbances will be found in Fig. 17.

It is important to remember that compensated respiratory acidosis and metabolic alkalosis may give very similar results on blood gas analysis. History and physical examination are most important and will usually dispel any confusion.

METABOLIC DISTURBANCES

Metabolic acidosis

The primary change is a fall in bicarbonate. Compensation is achieved by hyperventilation to reduce the P_aCO_2.

CAUSES
1 Normal anion gap – hyperchloraemic:
(*a*) Loss of intestinal secretions:
  Biliary fistulae.
  Pancreatic fistulae.
  Diarrhoea.
(*b*) Renal tubular acidosis.
(*c*) Ureterocolostomy.
(*d*) Excess intake of acid – rare.
2 High anion gap:
(*a*) Renal failure – failure of hydrogen ion excretion by the kidneys, but other cations retained as well.

(*b*) Diabetic ketoacidosis.
(*c*) Lactic acidosis.
(*d*) Poisons, e.g. methanol, ethylene glycol.

TREATMENT
1 Treatment of underlying cause.
2 Replacement of deficits with bicarbonate or an anionic compound converted to bicarbonate, e.g. citrate, lactate, if appropriate.

Metabolic alkalosis

The primary change is a rise in bicarbonate. Compensation occurs to some extent by hypoventilation, but the process is often not very efficient.

CAUSES
1 Excess ingestion of alkali – milk-alkali syndrome.
2 Excess loss of acid:
  Vomiting.
  Pyloric stenosis.
3 Hypokalaemia – when not caused by bicarbonate loss or hydrogen ion retention:
  Diuretics.
  'Ectopic ACTH syndrome'.
  Conn's syndrome.
  Drugs, e.g. carbenoxylone.

If due to hypokalaemia, the urine may be paradoxically acid despite a severe alkalosis.

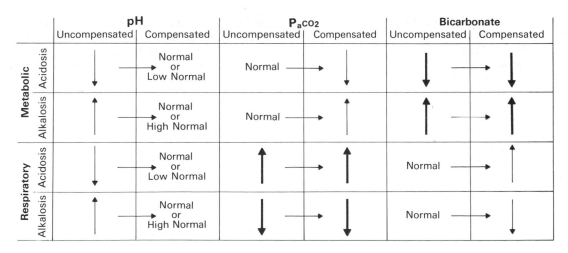

Fig. 17. Summary of common acid-base disturbances. The primary changes are marked in thick arrows.

TREATMENT
1　Review of drug therapy: N.B. self medication.
2　Replacement of Na^+, Cl^- and K^+ (they may all contribute to the problem).
3　Rarely, dilute sterile HCl or NH_4Cl intravenously if urgent.

RESPIRATORY DISTURBANCES

Respiratory acidosis
The primary change is a rise in P_aCO_2. Compensation occurs by renal retention of bicarbonate.

CAUSES
1　Excess production – rare. High metabolic rate with very high carbohydrate intake can raise the R.Q. above 1.0. However, carbon dioxide production above normal is only a problem when alveolar ventilatory ability is already compromised.
2　Reduced excretion:
(*a*)　Failure of alveolar ventilation:
　　　Bronchial asthma – late.
　　　Chronic obstructive airways disease.
　　　Pain.
　　　Respiratory depressants.
(*b*)　Hypoventilation during mechanical ventilation.

TREATMENT
1　Review of energy intake.
2　Review of drug therapy.
3　Treatment of chronic obstructive airways disease.
4　Alteration of mechanical ventilation.

Respiratory alkalosis
The primary change is a fall in P_aCO_2. Compensation occurs by production of an alkaline urine to reduce plasma bicarbonate concentration.

CAUSES
Hyperventilation:
(*a*)　Hysterical.
(*b*)　Hyperventilation during mechanical ventilation.

(*c*)　Anoxia.
(*d*)　Bronchial asthma – early.
(*e*)　Cerebral disease.
(*f*)　Salicylate – direct effect on respiratory centre.

TREATMENT
1　Treatment of underlying cause.
2　Alteration of mechanical ventilation.

MIXED DISTURBANCES

These are not uncommon. The component parts of the total disturbance may act in the same, or opposite directions on the blood pH, P_aCO_2 and bicarbonate. Measurement of *blood gases* is therefore essential if a problem of this type is suspected.

Examples

RESPIRATORY ALKALOSIS AND METABOLIC ACIDOSIS
Occurs with salicylate poisoning. There is an initial respiratory alkalosis, due to a direct stimulation of respiration, followed by a metabolic (lactic and salicylic) acidosis. In both cases, there will be a reduction in the bicarbonate, so the pH should be measured to find out which abnormality predominates.

RESPIRATORY AND METABOLIC ACIDOSIS
Seen in severely ill patients, and usually representing ventilatory and circulatory failure. Inadequate ventilation, either due to weakness, pulmonary problems or mechanical underventilation, causes carbon dioxide retention. Poor circulation and hypoxia leads to lactic acidosis and failure of the kidney to excrete hydrogen ion. These disturbances tend to change the bicarbonate concentration in opposite directions and its level may therefore be within the normal range. The unwary may not realize that this does not preclude a severe mixed acidosis and fail to make the diagnosis. Again, in all cases of doubt, the arterial pH and P_{CO_2} should be measured.

Chapter 16
Basic Immunology

The immune response

The protection or exemption (immune = exempt) which follows the successful outcome of an infectious disease has been known for many centuries.

'Immunity', and hence immunology, grew from considerations of defence against life-threatening infection and early observations confirmed the view that 'bugs were bad' and the host response essentially 'good'. Subsequently, several lines of evidence suggested that this was not always the case. The classical descriptions of anaphylaxis, serum sickness and delayed hypersensitivity to tuberculin all demonstrated the potential for host damage which could be brought about during an immunological response to foreign material. Von Pirquet embraced both good and ill effects within his concept of 'altered reactivity' although the term *allergy* which he ascribed to this has generally fallen into misuse and the term *immunity* is now used in its stead whether it implies protection alone or includes some element of immunopathology.

Cardinal features
The adaptive immune response displays several features which distinguish it from other forms of biological reactivity. It readily divides into two sequential processes: 'recognition' and 'defence'.

Complex recognition processes occur in many biological systems. The immune system represents a remarkable specialization of this innate cellular attribute, and is one in which the diversity of recognition is immense.

SPECIFICITY
The recognition ability of the immune system is sharply focused in mammalian organisms. Any minor modification in the chemical make-up of a particular antigen results in a significant change in its recognition by an animal that has been immunized with the unaltered material. Important clinical examples of the specificity of the immune response are the ability to distinguish between identical and non-identical tissue grafts and the use of blood group antibodies (isohaemagglutinins) in the forensic analysis of blood stains.

DIVERSITY
The attribute of specificity implies that many different responses will be necessary to cope with the total demands made upon the immunological system. This is indeed the case and the immune system contains millions of potential reactivities. The molecular diversity is partly heritable and partly due to variability which arises as the immune system matures.

MEMORY

When an individual antigen 'selects' the specific cell clone which shows specificity for it, it also stimulates a quantitative expansion of that reactive cell population as well as inducing qualitative changes in the nature of the reacting products. This 'heightening' of the specific response confers a state of *memory* upon the responding organism so that a secondary encounter takes place with greater speed and efficiency.

DEFENCE

Although the recognition event is sometimes associated with inhibition or inactivation of foreign material this tends to be the exception and it is usually only after the recognition process has triggered various effector mechanisms that the processes of defence are marshalled. These involve various cells, e.g. macrophages, polymorphs (neutrophils, eosinophils, basophils) and mast cells and molecular systems, e.g. inflammatory amines, complement, kinins, lysosomal enzymes and lymphokines (see p. 94). A considerable degree of amplification takes place during the effector response such that, in molecular terms, the initial encounter of one antigen with one recognition unit (be it cell or antibody) generates the production of large numbers of effector molecules. These defence or effector systems are non-specific in their function and rely entirely upon the recognition moiety of the immune response for their aim. Fig. 18 lists each of the components of the immune response according to their specific or non-specific characteristics.

Recognition	Defence
specific	non-specific
Antibody molecules	Macrophages
B lymphocytes	Polymorphonuclear cells
T lymphocytes	Mast cells
	Histamine, SRS-A
	Complement
	Kinins
	Lysosomal enzymes
	Lymphokines

Fig. 18. Components of the immune response.

Analogous systems

It is important not to attribute an immunological basis to every response to foreign material. In favism, a haemolytic episode may follow the ingestion of a wide variety of different drugs and other substances. Yet it was not until glucose-6-phosphate dehydrogenase deficiency was identified (see p. 493) that an immunological basis was discarded. Likewise, the asthmatic episodes induced in susceptible subjects by aspirin and other analgesic substances has often been thought to be immunologically mediated. The poor degree of chemical specificity in both these instances is most unlike an immunological event and in the latter case the disorder is now thought to be one of prostaglandin metabolism.

The nature of antigenic material

An *antigen* is a substance capable of inducing a specific change in the responsiveness of a whole organism. This may operate in positive or negative directions. An antigen capable of inducing a positive immunological response is often referred to as an *immunogen* whereas a substance which can induce a state of specific *un*responsiveness is called a *tolerogen*. Tolerance is rarely described in man although much animal work has demonstrated that such a condition can be readily induced by varying the dose or chemical form of a substance which is otherwise immunogenic. There are, nevertheless, important implications for autoimmune and malignant disease where the presence or absence of tolerogenic stimuli may be of especial importance.

The smallest recognizable unit contained within an antigen is often referred to as a *hapten*. This is synonymous with an *epitope* or *antigenic determinant*. A hapten is not capable of inducing an immunological response when present in a free and unconjugated form although it is able to combine specifically with the recognition unit, be it a specific cell or antibody. Haptenic material only becomes *immunogenic* when it is complexed with a 'carrier' molecule. The latter can be almost any molecule of larger size and is often a protein. Most drugs and many other smaller molecules (i.e. of mol. wt less than 1000) are too small to be immunogenic in their own right and only become so after complexing with blood or tissue proteins.

DEGREES OF FOREIGNNESS

When foreign tissue or protein is inoculated into man or experimental animals, the degree of responsiveness relates to the difference in genetic background between donor and recipient. Two parallel but synonymous sets of terms are in common use, e.g. homograft and allograft (see Fig. 19). However, the suffix *-geneic* tends to be used to describe tissues or cells (e.g. xenogeneic) whereas those words with the suffix *-ologous* are more often used for sera (e.g. heterologous).

The lymphoid system

Paul Ehrlich proposed in his 'side-chain theory' of immunity that the protective serum factors or antibodies were the product of a cell which was itself reactive with antigen. The identity of the 'immunocompetent' cell remained a mystery until the immunological properties of the lymphocyte were identified. The lymphocyte was shown to have a key role in graft rejection as well as antibody formation and recirculation of this cell through the lymph as well as the blood was shown to be an important part of its normal physiology.

Lymphocyte development
Although different varieties of lymphocyte exist, it is clear that they are all derived from stem cells present in adult bone marrow. In earlier development stem cells are found in yolk sac and liver. The lymphoid cells that leave bone marrow (or its precursor equivalent) are immature and in the case of the T lymphocyte there is an obligatory requirement for processing in the thymus before it acquires all the characteristics of a functionally mature cell. The epithelial component of the thymus secretes a trophic hormone – *thymopoietin* (also called *thymosin*).

The key role of the thymus has been confirmed by experiments involving neo-natal thymectomy in animals as well as evidence from several rare but well documented forms of thymic aplasia in man in which T-cell development is impaired. In birds, B lymphocyte differentiation only takes place in the micro-environment of the Bursa of Fabricius which develops from the hind-gut. Chemical or surgical bursectomy induces a severe antibody deficiency syndrome. An intensive search for a 'bursa-equivalent' in mammals has not been successful and it looks as if B lymphocytes continue to differentiate in, and after leaving, the marrow without passing through any other tissue micro-environment although the existence of a trophic hormone has not been excluded. These initial sites of lymphoid differentiation are known as *primary lymphoid organs* and such development is entirely independent of antigenic stimulation. Both major populations of lymphocytes then migrate into *secondary lymphoid organs* such as the lymph nodes, spleen and gut-associated lymphoid tissue and it is here that further proliferation and development occurs in response to antigenic stimulation (see Fig. 22, p. 94).

T and B lymphocytes

The B lymphocyte population consists of those lymphocytes which, following antigenic stimulation, further differentiate and divide to form the antibody secreting plasma cells. B lymphocytes have readily detectable antibody on their surface. This antibody is characteristic for an individual cell or clone of cells and is the receptor by which such cells recognize antigen. The thymus-processed or T lymphocytes, on the other hand, do not contain readily detectable surface immunoglobulin and although they too become stimulated when they meet specific antigen they give rise to further T

Relationship	Terms	
Genetically identical i.e. from same organism, identical twin or member of an inbred strain	Autologous Isologous	} Syngeneic
Genetically non-identical member of same species	Homologous	Allogeneic
Different species	Heterologous	Xenogeneic

Fig. 19. Terms used to describe the antigenic relationship of biological material.

lymphocytes following cell division. T and B lymphocytes can be distinguished in many other ways, some of which are listed in Fig. 20. T lymphocytes subserve classical cell-mediated immune responses and have an important role in 'delayed hypersensitivity' reactions including graft rejection (see p. 375).

Blood lymphocytes consist of c. 10 per cent B cells and c. 70 per cent T cells. The remaining 20 per cent or so of cells are often referred to as 'null' cells. Peripheral blood lymphocytes represent only a small fraction of the total lymphocyte pool and the large majority reside in secondary lymphoid organs. B lymphocytes are found in the lymphoid follicles and medulla of lymph nodes and in the follicles of the spleen whereas T lymphocytes occur in the paracortical zone of the lymph nodes and in the area between follicles in the spleen (see also p. 578).

The major route of entry of lymphocytes into the lymph node is directly from the vascular circulation via the post-capillary venules (P.C.V.'s). These specialized vessels contain tall endothelial cells and are situated at the cortico-medullary junction (see p. 579). A few lymphocytes arrive via afferent lymphatics and a smaller percentage arise by cell division within the node itself. Both T and B cells show complex traffic routes through secondary lymphoid organs and come into intimate contact with each other particularly during the acute phase of an immunological response when the structural and functional state of these organs undergoes considerable change. Both kinds of cell recirculate through blood and lymph.

Lymphocyte interaction

The compartmentation of the lymphoid system into T- and B-cell functions is not complete and there is mutual interaction in the elaboration of most immunological responses. Certain T lymphocytes (and macrophages) co-operate with B lymphocytes to enable them to proliferate in response to antigen and produce specific antibody. This sub-population of T cells are known as *helper* cells and there are also T *suppressor* cells which regulate the proliferative response of B cells. Failure of these cells to regulate the immune response may be an important cause of auto-immune disease.

The phagocytic cell system

Phagocytic cells are widely distributed. They include blood monocytes, Kupffer cells lining the liver sinusoids, alveolar macrophages in the lung, and tissue macrophages (or histiocytes) present throughout the body. The particular importance of the mononuclear phagocyte or monocyte (both in blood and tissues) is emphasized in the term *mononuclear phagocyte system* which replaces the earlier designations of 'reticulo-endothelial system' or 'lymphoreticular system'. It assists the lymphoid system in its non-specific handling of foreign and particulate material which may then be processed by the lymphoid system itself. Many of its cells can acquire specificity by virtue of their ability to take up cytophilic or opsonizing antibody which then enhances the phagocytosis of specific antigen.

	T cells	B cells
Rosette formation	Sheep red blood cells	Mouse red blood cells
Other surface chemistry	T-cell glycoproteins	Surface Ig (detectable by immunofluorescence) Fc receptor C3 receptor
Mitogen reactivity	Phytohaemagglutinin Concanavalin A	Poke-weed mitogen

Fig. 20. Human T and B lymphocyte markers.

Immunoglobulins

The three main varieties of immunoglobulin are now known as IgG, IgM and IgA (previously defined electrophoretically as γG, γM and β_2A). The remaining two classes of antibody, IgD and IgE, were discovered following identification of myeloma proteins which did not type with reagents for the other known classes.

An intriguing feature of the immunoglobulin molecule is its ability to perform two quite separate biological functions:

1 To complex specifically with antigen.
2 To activate various mediator systems, e.g. complement.

Immunoglobulin molecules consist of two 'heavy' and two 'light' polypeptide chains joined by disulphide bridges. Two antigen-combining sites are present at one end of the molecule each composed jointly of one end of a light chain and the corresponding end of a heavy chain. This portion of the molecule (which can be split off by proteolytic enzymes) is known as the Fab portion. The Fc portion is that part of the molecule which triggers the various effector systems and is variable from class to class.

IgG is the most plentiful antibody in the circulation (Fig. 21) and is also detectable in the extra-vascular compartment. The much larger IgM molecule is mostly restricted to the circulation and is the predominant antibody of the primary response to antigen. IgA is most plentifully found in the secretions of mucosal epithelia where it has an important protective role. The function of IgD is still largely obscure. IgE is present in least amount of all in peripheral blood although it does have a high affinity for tissue mast cells and triggers their degranulation on contact with specific antigen.

The attainment of adult serum levels of immunoglobulins is a slow process and for the first 3 months of life the newborn infant relies almost entirely upon IgG antibody acquired transplacentally during gestation.

Antibody molecules can themselves be antigenic and 'anti-globulins' can be raised against them in other species. They are frequently used as reagents for the specific detection and quantitation of immunoglobulin molecules. Sometimes they develop spontaneously, e.g. rheumatoid factor (see p. 286) (which is an antibody reactive with IgG) and these antiglobulins may show specificity for localized areas where heritable differences or *allotypes* occur. Parts of the antigen-combining site itself can be recognized as foreign, the resultant antibody then reacting with the individual chemistry – or *idiotype* – of the immunizing molecule.

Antigen – antibody combination

The formation of a complex between specific antigen and specific antibody may, of itself, produce some degree of inactivation or inhibition of the antigen, e.g. if it is an exotoxin, a mobile flagellum or a virus seeking a host cell receptor. However, most of the significant effector events which follow antigen–antibody combination are due to the antibody mediated triggering of the various mediator systems which give rise to immunological damage, e.g. amine release, complement fixation, phagocytosis and macrophage activation.

DETECTION OF ANTIGEN – ANTIBODY INTERACTION

Both primary and secondary phenomena are exploited in the laboratory to analyse both antigen and antibody. *Immunoprecipitation* – usually performed in transparent gels such as agar – relies on

Class	Mean serum concentration (mg/100 ml)	Complement activation	Phagocyte binding	Mast cell binding	Mucosal secretion	Placental transfer
IgG	1000	+	+	−	−	+
IgA	250	+*	−	−	+	−
IgM	100	+	−	−	−	−
IgD	3	−	−	−	−	−
IgE	0.1	−	−	+	−	−

Fig. 21. Properties of the five classes of immunoglobulins. (* This effect is mediated by the alternative pathway.)

the formation of large complexes which form a precipitate. Antibodies which do not readily form precipitates can be demonstrated by using other methods such as *haemagglutination* (where the antigen is located on the surface of a red cell), *immunofluorescence* (where the combinational event is observed by the use of fluorescein-labelled antibody) and *complement fixation methods* (where the combinational event is detected by virtue of a secondary consumption of complement). Other biological systems can be used for the detection of IgE antibodies although radioactive methods are often used to give greater sensitivity.

Antibody synthesis

The immunoglobulin found on the surface of a B lymphocyte is usually confined to one class and a single antigen specificity. Plasma cells which arise from it secrete antibody of the same specificity but the class of antibody may vary from that originally found on the surface of the B cell. This switch (e.g. IgM to IgG) takes place during the process of B cell stimulation and requires the presence of co-operating T lymphocytes. The mature plasma cell synthesizes and secretes about 2000 antibody molecules per hour during its short life of several days. Most antibody responses are polyclonal in nature, the total antibody produced arising from a number of different antibody producing clones of cells. In some circumstances a single clone of cells synthesizes an inordinate amount of antibody. This is described as a monoclonal response and is typically found in myelomatosis and macroglobulinaemia (see p. 470). These are important conditions to diagnose and distinguish and here the technique of immuno-electrophoresis is necessary to confirm that a 'compact band' seen on conventional protein electrophoresis is due to the presence of monoclonal antibody.

The light chains of antibody molecules can be of two types, κ (Kappa) and λ (Lambda) and both light chains of any one antibody molecule are of the same chemical type. Thus, antibody molecules which represent the product of a single clone of antibody forming cells share the same heavy and light chain type and the same antigen specificity. The normal slight excess of light-chain production is exaggerated in monoclonal disorders giving rise to excess free light chains in the urine – also called *Bence-Jones proteinuria* (see p. 471). The trigger for monoclonal proliferation in man is still obscure. An antigenic stimulus is likely to be involved at some stage although a second and less specific stimulus may be necessary to give rise to uncontrolled growth and antibody production.

Mediator systems

Figure 18, p. 88 has distinguished those components of the immunological system which are specifically involved in its recognition function from the various non-specific mediator systems which generate the inflammatory process. The relationship between these two is one of subtle triggering such that their inflammatory potential is only realized at the site of a specific immunological event. This may occur either in the fluid phase of various tissue fluids or on the surface of mediator cells. The triggering events that follow the combination of antigen with specific T lymphocytes are less clearly understood.

Histamine and slow-reacting substance of anaphylaxis (SRS-A)

The granules of mast cells and basophils contain histamine and SRS-A in addition to other substances such as heparin. Both kinds of cell have a receptor on their surface with a high avidity for the Fc fragment of IgE molecules. The cross-linking of two adjacent and specific IgE molecules by antigen causes the cell to discharge most of its mediator-containing granules by a process of exocytosis. The cell is not lysed and can regenerate its mediator discharging potential within a short period of time. Mast cells predominantly occur on the adventitial surface of small blood vessels as well as within smooth muscle. The chief effect of these two mediators is to increase capillary permeability and to cause the contraction of smooth muscle (see p. 25). Physiologically, the local increase in capillary permeability can be seen as a means of enhancing extra-vascular immunity by allowing the egress of significant quantities of serum proteins and inflammatory cells so that other mechanisms of immune elimination can proceed in the extra-vascular compartment. Clinically, smooth muscle contraction is important in disorders such as bronchial asthma (see p. 647).

Mast cell degranulation is also caused by products of the complement activation pathway. IgE-mediated release can be blocked by sodium cromoglycate although this does not prevent antigen–antibody combination at the cell surface. This effect is peculiar to the mast cell and does not prevent mediator release by basophils.

The complement system

This complex system of proteins is of paramount importance in the intra-vascular compartment although it can also operate in other tissue environments, e.g. synovial fluid and C.S.F. It functions as an enzyme cascade and shows several similarities with the coagulation sequence. There are nine numerically identified proteins which function in the sequence 142356789; the events of major biological importance occurring at the C3 stage. The pathway commencing at C1 is known as the *classical* pathway in contrast to the *alternative* pathway which has a separate route of entry at the C3 stage.

The classical pathway is triggered when a sub-component of C1 (C1q) reacts with the complexed Fc fragments of IgG or IgM antibody. Alterations within the C1 complex generate an active enzyme –C1 esterase–which is then able to activate both C4 and C2 to produce a C3 convertase–C42. C1 esterase is under the control of a C1 esterase inhibitor and patients who lack this enzyme are prone to recurrent inflammatory episodes–a condition known as *hereditary angio-oedema*.

The alternative pathway involves C3b and properdin as well as factors B and D which by interaction form the C3 convertase designated C3bBbP. Various agents enhance the activity of this feedback loop including complexed IgA and various cell wall lipopolysaccharides, e.g. endotoxin and zymosan, and *nephritic factor* causes increased C3 consumption by a similar mechanism.

The activation of C3 gives rise to several active fragments. Fluid phase C3a is chemotactic for neutrophil polymorphs and causes release of histamine and SRS-A from mast cells. C3b is bound at the site of complex formation and mediates the phenomenon of 'immune adherence' to neutrophil polymorphs and macrophages. Thus increased capillary permeability, chemotactic attraction of phagocytic cells and their adherence at the site of complement fixation are all brought about by activities generated at the C3 stage.

The terminal stages of the complement sequence are necessary for lysis of the 'target' cell upon which complement activation has taken place, e.g. an invading bacterium or an incompatible red blood cell. Deficiencies of the classical pathway prior to C3 are not associated with an increased incidence of infection and deficiencies in the later components

are not associated with obvious disease. C3 deficiency on the other hand is complicated by severe and recurrent infections. This emphasizes the critical importance of C3 activation in defence against pathogenic organisms.

Coagulation and kinins

Factor XII or Hageman factor which initiates the intrinsic coagulation pathway (see p. 519) also activates the kinin-forming pathway. The coagulation sequence is often involved locally during complement activation and has an augmenting role in various immunopathological situations.

Bradykinin is the most potent mammalian vasodilator and in conjunction with the fibrinolytic action of plasmin has a role in the re-establishment of vascular patency following activation of the coagulation and complement pathways. The first component in the pathway is prekallikrein which is converted to kallikrein by Hageman factor. Kallikrein then acts on kininogens to form the active kinin molecules. These give rise to increased capillary permeability, dilatation of peripheral arterioles, a chemotactic effect on leucocytes and the production of pain at the site of release. Kallikrein conversion is inhibited by the C1 esterase inhibitor as well as other protease inhibitors, e.g. α_2 macroglobulin. Following generation, kinins are broken down by kininases.

Hageman factor also converts plasminogen to plasmin and plasmin is able to activate C1 esterase. The inordinate activation of C1 and kallikrein are of importance in the production of symptoms – in hereditary angio-oedema where there is a deficiency of the C1 esterase inhibitor. The kinin system is also of importance in the pathogenesis of gram-negative septicaemia where factor XII activation follows endothelial cell damage by endotoxin with activation of kallikrein, a fall in kininogen and the production of free kinins. Endotoxinaemia is also associated with complement activation and disseminated intravascular coagulation (see p. 531).

Lysosomal enzymes

The involvement of phagocytic cells in immunological responses is associated with the release of lysosomal enzymes from their granules. These enzymes fall into four main groups: hydrolases, neutral serine proteinases, metallo-proteinases and microbicidal elements such as myeloperoxidase, lysozyme and lactoferrin. Their release adds a further amplifying dimension to the original im-

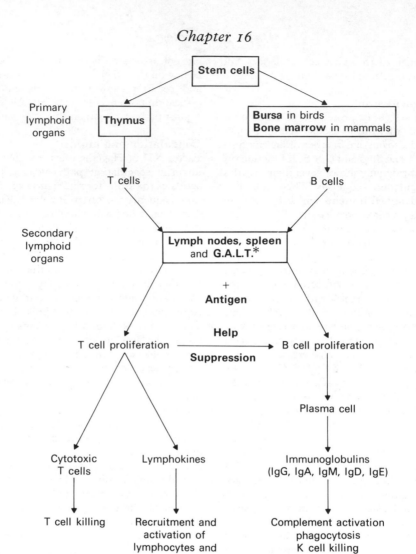

* Gut-associated lymphoid tissue.

Fig. 22. An overall view of the immune system.

munological event and they have an important role in digesting and breaking down foreign material. Deficiency of such materials, e.g. myeloperoxidase is associated with abnormal defence against infection.

Prostaglandins
These ubiquitous substances are becoming increasingly implicated in immunological events. They are capable of producing most of the cardinal features of inflammation although their ability to induce

oedema may be due to a reduced threshold for the permeability effect of kinins. Certain analogues are chemotactic for polymorphonuclear leucocytes.

Lymphokines
These are soluble factors released from the cytoplasm of T lymphocytes during the synthetic phase following antigen or mitogen stimulation. Lymphokine material may also be produced by B lymphocytes although its role in normal immune processes is uncertain. These factors are able to

attract other cells to the site of antigen recognition by T cells (chemotactic factors); are able to retain such cells at the site of inflammation (migration inhibition factors) and can stimulate other cells to become activated (mitogenic factors). The chemical nature of most of these factors is still in doubt although it is known that they are of small molecular weight (20–50 000) and are unlike immunoglobulins in structure.

Membrane effects

Most of the above mediator systems function extra-cellularly. However, there is evidence that cell damage can occur following the direct apposition of lymphocyte and other effector cell membranes with the 'target' cell. This is unlikely to involve any of the above mediator systems and may be an important mechanism for eliminating and destroying foreign cellular material. Macrophages, polymorphonuclear leucocytes, K cells and lymphocytes may all act in this manner.

Modulating effects

Each mediator system has considerable potential for amplifying and extending the initial immunological event. This implies that inhibitory factors are important in controlling these systems and preventing them from inordinate activity. As well as specifically identifiable inhibitory molecules which act at various key points in each sequence, many of the effector events, and particularly those involving cell function, are under humoral control via adrenergic and cholinergic systems. Their effect is mediated intra-cellularly by various cyclic nucleotides (e.g. cAMP, cGMP) and considerable inhibition or augmentation of processes such as mast cell degranulation, phagocytosis and lymphocyte stimulation can be shown to take place when the intracellular levels of these substances are significantly disturbed.

An overall view

The various components of the immune system are linked together in Fig. 22 to provide an overall picture of their sequential role in the reaction to specific antigen. The immune system can be divided horizontally into:

1 Antigen-independent differentiation of specific clones of mature T or B lymphocytes.

2 Antigen-dependent expansion of specific clones with further differentiation of the T and B lymphocyte pathways.

3 The combination of specific antigen with the mature immune system.

4 The consequences of such combination and triggering of various effector mechanisms.

A vertical division can be made into T and B cell compartments of the immune system and although these two compartments have important physiological interactions with each other their capability for independent function is evidenced by the behaviour of animals and human beings that fail to develop T or B cells. Other more localized defects, e.g. complement deficiencies, help to demonstrate the importance of individual components in the successful function of the whole system.

Immunodeficiency disorders	Phagocyte abnormalities
Stem cell deficiency	Neutropenia
T cell deficiency	Defects of motility
B cell deficiency and hypo-γ-globulinaemia	Intra-cellular defects
	Complement deficiencies
	Secondary or acquired immunodeficiency

Immunodeficiency disorders

Many of the severe forms of immunodeficiency are fortunately rare but localized defects are relatively common and any patient who is prone to recurrent, atypical or unexplained infections should be screened for an underlying immunodeficiency disorder. This should include an assessment of immunoglobulins, complement, T and B lymphocytes and phagocytic cells.

Stem cell deficiency

Severe combined immunodeficiency (SCID) is caused by an absence of lymphocyte precursor cells and thus both T and B cell compartments are deficient. Such cases present in the first few weeks or months of life with several bacterial, fungal or viral infections often of an opportunistic kind, e.g. with *Candida*, *Pneumocystis*, etc. One form is associated with the lack of an intra-cellular enzyme, adenosine deaminase and is inherited as an autosomal recessive. Children with SCID usually die in early life unless given a histocompatible marrow transplant.

T cell deficiency

If the thymus is absent or hypoplastic then T cell differentiation is impaired. Such patients are especially prone to infection with fungi and viruses. The DiGeorge and Nezelof syndromes are examples of this and although B cells and immunoglobulins may be present in normal amounts, antibody responses are often impaired. The DiGeorge syndrome is associated with other abnormalities of development of the third and fourth branchial arches, e.g.

hypoparathyroidism and abnormalities of the great vessels. Thymus grafting is usually successful in correcting the immunological abnormality. The administration of thymic hormone or transfer factor has also been shown to improve the T cell defect.

Minor forms of T cell abnormality are more common and have been described in such diverse conditions as chronic muco-cutaneous candidiasis, recurrent herpes simplex infection, leprosy (see p. 52) and Down's syndrome (see p. 13). In the first two examples the defect has been localized to an inability of T lymphocytes to produce the appropriate lymphokines.

B cell deficiency and hypo-γ-globulinaemia

In its classical form levels of all five classes of immunoglobulins are low and infections – mostly bacterial and of the upper and lower respiratory tract – start becoming a problem during the first year of life. In the congenital X-linked variety, B lymphocytes form less than 0.5 per cent of the total lymphocyte count. Some patients do possess circulating B lymphocytes and in this more variable form, in which the clinical onset may not occur until adult life, the defect appears to be one of plasma cell differentiation from the B lymphocyte. Here the antibody deficiency is usually less severe and one or more classes, e.g. IgM, may be spared. Nevertheless, all such patients are prone to repeated infection and bronchiectasis is common. Patients often have chronic steatorrhoea which may be associated with *Giardia* infection. A polyarthritis is common. Each of these clinical disturbances are greatly improved by the administration of intramuscular γ-globulin in association with appropriate anti-microbial therapy.

Partial forms of antibody defect are relatively common. Isolated IgA deficiency occurs in about 1 in 700 of the population and is associated with an increased incidence of auto-immune and atopic diseases.

Phagocyte abnormalities

NEUTROPENIA

Severe infections occur when the neutrophil count falls to less than 500 cells/mm^3. In the dominant familial variety the count is usually toward 1000 cells/mm^3 and many affected individuals are asymptomatic. With cyclical neutropenia the count may transiently fall as low as 50 cells/mm^3 and prophylactic antibiotics may help to prevent infection.

DEFECTS OF MOTILITY

A number of defects in the motile response of phagocytic cells to chemotactic stimuli have been described and the random mobility of these cells can also be abnormal. The failure of polymorphonuclear leucocytes to localize at inflammatory sites causes an increased incidence and severity of bacterial and fungal infections.

INTRA-CELLULAR DEFECTS

Chronic granulomatous disease is the most closely studied example in which repeated infection occurs with catalase-positive organisms, e.g. staphylococci and fungi. The polymorphs phagocytose normally but cannot kill because of an enzyme abnormality which prevents the synthesis of bactericidal peroxide. Catalase-negative organisms can make their own peroxide and are killed normally.

This inherited condition is usually confined to the male sex and presents in early life with recurrent boils, cellulitis, suppurating lymph nodes, intermittent fever and visceral abscesses. Some milder cases reach adult life and are relatively symptom-free.

In vitro testing using the stimulated nitroblue tetrazolium (NBT) test shows that less than 10 per cent of an affected patient's neutrophils are able to reduce the dye. This test is also able to detect the carrier state in the mothers of affected patients.

Complement deficiencies

Defects have now been identified in most of the individual complement components of the classical pathway. Their discovery has confirmed the paramount importance of the C3 stage of the complement sequence, for marked deficiency of this substance is associated with recurrent and severe bacterial infections. In contrast, deficiencies of the earlier or later components are not associated with life-threatening infection although there is accumulating evidence of an increased incidence of other immunological disorders, e.g. systemic lupus, and Henoch–Schönlein purpura, in patients who lack early components, e.g. C2.

Deficiency of the C1 esterase *inhibitor* is associated with hereditary angioedema. The intercurrent activation of C1 in the absence of this inhibitor causes the development of acute episodes of tissue oedema which can involve the subglottic region and intestinal tract, sometimes with fatal results. Drug treatment is helpful in preventing attacks.

Secondary or acquired immunodeficiency

Immunodeficiency most often occurs as a sequel to other diseases or their treatment. Patients with malignant disease develop secondary forms of immunodeficiency as in chronic lymphatic leukaemia and Hodgkin's disease and complicating infection may be a problem. The use of powerful cytotoxic and 'immunosuppressive' agents has brought with it a steady toll of immunodeficiency and this is most evident in those patients receiving drugs to suppress graft rejection (see p. 375) and auto-immune disease. Splenectomy is associated with an increased risk of serious infection with pneumococci, meningococci and *Haemophilus influenzae*.

Chapter 18
Immunopathological Mechanisms in Disease

Hetero-immune responses

It has been known for many years that much of the tissue damage seen in post-primary tuberculosis is a consequence of the host response to the tubercle bacillus. The majority of patients with hepatitis B infection have detectable antigen in the blood, followed by antibody, and make a spontaneous recovery. Uraemic patients on dialysis may harbour the antigen for long periods without showing any ill effect, whereas the serum of those individuals who develop fulminating hepatitis usually contains both antigen and antibody simultaneously and antigen–antibody complexes can be demonstrated in the liver.

Lymphocytic choriomeningitis virus infection in mice clearly demonstrates the importance of host factors in determining the natural history of infectious disease. If animals are inoculated with virus in adult life they develop an acute encephalitis and die within 6–8 days. Animals inoculated during the neonatal period (when they are immunologically immature) become life-long carriers of the virus with low levels of antibody present in the circulation. A similar carrier state can be induced in adult animals by giving cyclophosphamide 3 days after virus inoculation. However, the administration of normal syngeneic (see p. 89) lymphocytes to carrier animals causes acute encephalitis and death within a few days. It is clear that few infectious diseases occur without the amplified and elaborate immune response involving host tissue in some way and such damage is designated *hetero-immune* (Fig. 23). Thus it is of little profit to try and classify responses into those that are entirely protective (to which the term 'immune' is sometimes restricted) and those where pathological features are striking (sometimes called 'allergic'). The object of any immunization programme is to reduce the latter to a minimum although sometimes the untoward effects prove insurmountable, e.g. immunization against respiratory syncitial virus infection.

Many other kinds of foreign material can induce hetero-immune responses, e.g. pollens, danders, drugs and foreign tissues and therapeutic manipulation (e.g 'desensitization' or 'enhancement' – see below) can successfully modify the response.

Auto-immune responses

A number of human diseases are characterized by an immune response which is primarily directed against one or more components of host tissue (Fig. 23). Although the potential for host damage is obvious, here too, this often extends away from the primary target to involve antigenically irrelevant tissue, e.g. renal damage in systemic lupus.

The tissue damage is caused by one or more of the established mechanisms described below. The aetiology, or trigger, for the development of auto-immune disease is less clearly understood but there are several possible ways in which it can arise.

RELEASE OF SEQUESTERED ANTIGEN

If foreign tissue is introduced into an animal before it is immunologically mature then it may be accepted as 'self'. In this situation the adult animal does not respond even when challenged with

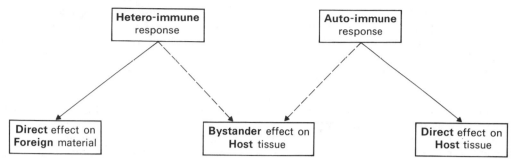

Fig. 23. Hetero-immune and auto-immune responses.

further doses of similar material. Normal body constituents exist, e.g. the lens protein of the eye, which do not come into contact with the immunological recognition system during its development. If such constituents are released during adult life, because of trauma, irradiation or other kinds of injury, then an immune response is likely to follow. This is the suggested basis for sympathetic ophthalmia (see p. 335) and may underlie other more common auto-immune disorders.

BYPASSING T CELL TOLERANCE VIA A 'CARRIER EFFECT'

Experiments in which an artificial state of specific unresponsiveness (or 'tolerance') to foreign antigen has been achieved in adult life have demonstrated that both T and B lymphocytes can be involved. However, T cells are rendered tolerant with much greater ease than B lymphocytes and the discovery of self-reactive B cells in normal individuals suggests that T cell tolerance may be the most crucial physiological requirement. T cell help is necessary before B cells can produce significant amounts of auto-antibody. T cells will only co-operate in this way if they recognize a complementary part of antigenic material – designated the *carrier* – which is intimately associated with the *hapten* – recognized by the B cell.

Thus if foreign material bearing 'carrier' determinants (against which the host has responsive T cells) happens to complex covalently with host tissue (against which the host has reactive B cells) then T cell help is available and a potent anti-self response will ensue.

Experimentally there are many examples of this mechanism whereas few are proven in the human situation. Nevertheless, there is evidence that the red cell antibodies which develop against the I antigen following infection with *Mycoplasma pneu-*

moniae are induced by a combination of the mycoplasma organism with host red cells. The same may also apply to the anti-red cell antibodies with Rhesus specificity which may appear during treatment with the hypotensive agent α-methyl dopa.

The fact that budding viruses often incorporate host cell material and that virus antigens are often expressed on the surface of host cells suggests that this mechanism may apply to the initiation of auto-immune disease during virus infection. The appearance of smooth muscle antibodies during infection with viruses, e.g. hepatitis B, EBV and cytomegalovirus, may be a sequel to the combination of virus material with myofibrillar components of host cells.

This mode of auto-immunization can only explain the production of self-reactive antibody and does not provide an explanation for T cell responses against self.

SPONTANEOUS APPEARANCE OF SELF-REACTIVE T CELLS

Most forms of spontaneously occurring auto-immune disease show an increasing incidence with age. This could reflect a gradual failure of the normal mechanisms which suppress self-reactive T cells. Animals rendered T-cell depleted have been shown to develop an increased incidence of auto-immune disorders. Evidence from the New Zealand hybrid mice (NZB/NZW) demonstrates a correlation between failure of suppressor cell activity and the severity of the lupus-like disease to which they are prone. It is possible that certain viruses may disturb the balance between helper and suppressor lymphocytes.

Alternatively, somatic mutation may give rise to *de novo* generation of 'forbidden clones' of self-reactive cells.

Genetic basis

An increasing body of evidence suggests that there are important constitutional factors which affect the development of immunological disease of both hetero-immune and auto-immune varieties. The severity of disease induced by LCM virus varies with the genetic strain of mouse and its histocompatibility antigens. Several infections in man that are associated with a significant immunopathological component, e.g. leprosy, are linked to HLA type. The familial proneness to organ-specific auto-immune disease is also closely linked to HLA and other disorders, e.g. systemic lupus, rheumatoid arthritis, Sjögren's disease, Goodpasture's syndrome, multiple sclerosis, dermatitis herpetiformis and coeliac disease, also show significant associations with particular phenotypes.

In addition to the four HLA loci (A, B, C and D) the region of chromosome six which bears the major histocompatibility complex also contains genes coding for individual complement components (e.g. C2, C4 and factor B), glycoproteins on phagocyte cell surfaces and other genes controlling immune responsiveness analogous to the Ir genes in

mice. However, the exact mechanism(s) of disease association in man have yet to be clarified. Thus both the 'seed' e.g. virus or chemical, as well as the 'soil', i.e. genetic background of the host, are important determinants of the hetero-immune and auto-immune disorders.

Mechanisms of immunological damage

Whether an immunopathological process is hetero-immune or auto-immune, there are a limited number of mechanisms by which host or foreign tissue can be damaged and inflamed (Fig. 24). These are now described in turn with, in each case, a comparison being drawn between their physiological basis and their – often more striking – pathological effects.

REAGINIC

Here the initiator is reaginic antibody of class IgE which induces the release of mediators (see p. 92) from mast cells and basophils following its combination with specific antigen. There is also evidence that the IgG$_4$ subclass may trigger a similar release of mediators from these cells in certain

	Initiator	Mediators	Clinical examples	
			Hetero-immune	Auto-immune
Reaginic	Reaginic antibody (IgE or possibly IgG$_4$)	Histamine, SRS-A, etc.	Extrinsic asthma Allergic rhinitis	
Membrane-reactive	Antibody (IgG, IgM or IgA) with specificity for membrane-bound antigen	Complement, polymorphs and their lysosomal enzymes	Incompatible blood transfusion	Haemolytic anaemia Pemphigus Goodpasture's syndrome
Immune-complex	Cell-free antigen–antibody complexes	Complement, polymorphs and their lysosomal enzymes	Serum sickness Allergic alveolitis Glomerulonephritis	Systemic lupus Rheumatoid arthritis
Cell-mediated (including K cells)	T lymphocytes and other mononuclear cells	Soluble factors + membrane effects	Graft rejection Contact dermatitis Tuberculin reaction	Thyroiditis Chronic hepatitis

Fig. 24. Mechanisms of immunological damage with examples.

circumstances. The inflammatory mediators are histamine and SRS-A. Their release may be important in controlling the release of colloid and cells from the vascular compartment into local extravascular sites, but when such mediator release takes place to an inordinate degree it can give rise to a variety of clinical disorders often categorized as *atopic*, including extrinsic asthma, allergic rhinitis and eczema. At least one form of gastro-intestinal allergy to dietary proteins, e.g. those found in cows' milk, is mediated in this way and the rare but potentially fatal condition of *acute anaphylaxis* is a reaginic event provoked by foreign antigen.

Atopic disorders are usually characterized by an elevation in the serum IgE level in association with tissue and blood eosinophilia. This mechanism of damage can be effectively blocked by the administration of sodium cromoglycate which blocks the cellular events subsequent to the combination of antigen with cell-bound reaginic antibody.

MEMBRANE-REACTIVE

In this instance the antigens involved are an intrinsic part of a cell or basement membrane. Damage is induced following the combination of specific antibody of class IgG or IgM, and possibly IgA, which then fixes complement on the surface of the cell or basement membrane. The damage may be caused by membrane lysis due to activation of the entire complement sequence or may follow the activation of lysosome-containing cells, e.g. neutrophils and macrophages, following their attraction and adherence by intermediate components of the complement pathway (see p. 93). These events enhance the phagocytic potential of these cells as well as their release of lysosomal enzymes. Physiologically, such a mechanism is important in the prompt inactivation and elimination of foreign material including bacteria and extra-cellular viruses. A similar mechanism obtains when host cells are involved in auto-immune disease, e.g. Goodpasture's syndrome – characterized by the presence of anti-glomerular basement membrane antibody (see p. 361); pemphigus, characterized by antibody against the intercellular substance of epidermis (see p. 723), and auto-immune haemolytic anaemia – where red cell destruction is brought about by the presence of red cell antibodies (see p. 505).

IMMUNE-COMPLEX

Here both antigen and antibody occur in soluble form. When they meet in the circulation or following diffusion through tissues they may fix complement causing inflammatory damage as well as activating phagocytic cells and their lysosomal enzymes. The prompt formation of antigen–antibody complexes is probably an important part of the 'sensitization' process whereby the antigen-dependent expansion of clones of specifically reactive cells is achieved in normal circumstances. Complex formation is often necessary for the localization and elimination of foreign antigen and in some instances this alone, without recourse to other effector mechanisms, is capable of inhibiting the pathogenic behaviour of living organisms and their products.

In most instances immune complexes are cleared rapidly and efficiently without the production of significant host damage. However, if there is a liberal and persistent source of antigen or the antibody is of poor quality, then complexes may persist in the circulation or in particular tissues with immunopathological consequences. Local tissue damage may be intense as in extrinsic allergic alveolitis (see p. 671) glomerulonephritis (see p. 359) or rheumatoid synovitis (see p. 286) and persistent presence of complexes in the circulation is usually associated with their deposition in blood vessels throughout the body. The particular pattern of localization of circulating complexes is determined by many factors including their size, antigen-antibody ratio, the class of antibody involved and its ability to fix complement, the vascular status of a particular organ and any local release of permeability factors, e.g. histamine, SRS-A and lymphokines, as well as prior trauma to a local site.

'Immune-complex disease' can occur in many situations, e.g. following the injection of foreign sera and the administration of certain drugs, e.g. penicillin and streptomycin, as well as in various kinds of auto-immune disease, e.g. systemic lupus erythematosus, where the circulating complex contains nuclear antigens in combination with antibody (see p. 281).

CELL-MEDIATED

In this instance the immunological event takes place independently of antibody, the primary event being one of combination of antigen with the specific receptor of a T cell. This results in stimulation of the lymphocyte with the synthesis and secretion of inflammatory lymphokines (see above) and the involvement of macrophages. This mechanism is normally of paramount importance in the defence against intra-cellular parasites, e.g. certain viruses, which may express antigenic material on the surface of the parasitized cell. Various immuno-pathological states result from such a mechanism including contact dermatitis, graft rejection (see p. 375) and the post-primary response to tuberculosis (see p. 665). The longer time course of cell-mediated reactions gave rise to the description *delayed hypersensitivity* in contrast to the more 'immediate' reaginic, membrane-reactive and immune-complex mechanisms.

K or 'killer' cells are morphologically indistinguishable from lymphocytes but have a receptor for the Fc region of IgG antibody and are able to lyse 'target' cells coated with specific antibody. These cells do not bear B or T cell markers and have to be in intimate contact with antibody coated target cells before damage takes place. The physiological role of this mechanism is still debated but it is likely that this mechanism is effective in defence against infection in extra-vascular sites where antibody concentrations may be comparatively low and where complement is not always present in sufficient quantity to permit a membrane-reactive mechanism of damage to take place. There is evidence for this mechanism having a role in the damage which occurs in auto-immune thyroiditis (see p. 306) and some forms of chronic hepatitis.

The different mechanisms of immunological damage are summarized in Fig. 24. It is not uncommon for more than one mechanism to co-exist in a particular disease or pathological state. Consideration of the mechanism(s) involved in a particular condition has important implications for therapy as well as aetiology and pathogenesis. The amplification potential of each of these effector mechanisms is enormous and emphasizes the need for important inhibitory and control mechanisms to contain the inflammatory process and maintain physiological homeostasis.

Chapter 19
Degenerations: Infiltrations: Necrosis

Nature

The degenerations and infiltrations imply alterations in the morphology of cells produced by:

1 Accumulation of metabolites or other substances in a cell damaged by preceding injury – *degeneration*.

2 The overloading of a previously normal cell by materials which are abnormal in either type or quantity – *infiltration*.

The changes in the cells in both degeneration and infiltration may appear similar and are indicative of cell derangement short of actual death of that cell. Most of the changes are reversible if the initiating cause is removed but, if prolonged or if of severe degree, cell death will result – *necrosis*.

Water disturbances

Water may pass across the cell membrane by passive diffusion, dependent upon concentration gradients. Under normal conditions the osmotic pressure of the intracellular fluid (due to potassium, magnesium, phosphate and protein) is the same as that of the extracellular fluid (due to sodium, chloride and bicarbonate). The osmotic pressure of the intracellular fluid is maintained by the sodium pump. If this fails, the pressure rises and the cell swells as water enters.

Cloudy swelling
Frequently an artefactual change due to autolytic changes in the cells after death or poor fixation. When seen in life:

CAUSES
1 *Infections.* Any febrile illness.
2 *Physico-chemical injuries.* Direct toxic effect.
3 *Nutritional.* Either local as in ischaemia, or general associated with anaemia, anoxia or malnutrition.

SITES
Any cell, but especially the parenchymal cells of the liver, kidney and heart.

APPEARANCES
The cells are slightly swollen and show a hazy and granular cytoplasm. Under the electron microscope there is swelling of the tubules of the rough endoplasmic reticulum (see p. 8) and loss of their ribosomes. The mitochondria may be slightly swollen. Any reduction in ATP production is a factor in the accumulation of further water due to malfunction of the energy-dependent 'sodium pump'.

RESULTS
This is the earliest detectable degenerative change of a cell and is completely reversible. The clinical and pathological significances are disputed.

Hydropic degeneration

Characterized by further water accumulation in the cell. This may be due to more marked mitochondrial damage, cessation of ATP production and failure of the 'sodium pump' leading to increased osmotic pressure within the cell. Alterations in the permeability of the cell membrane to other substances can be produced by toxic agents.

CAUSES
1   *Severe water and electrolyte disturbances*. Especially potassium depletion.
2   *Physico-chemical agents*, e.g. burns, scalds, chloroform and carbon tetrachloride.
3   *Infective conditions*.
4   *Following cloudy swelling*. If prolonged.

SITES
Liver cells and the convoluted tubules of the kidney.

APPEARANCES
Vacuoles appear in the cytoplasm, these may coalesce to form one large vacuole. Ultrastructurally the rough endoplasmic reticulum shows dilatation and large cisterns. Mitochondria are swollen with loss of cristae.

RESULTS
The condition is reversible but is an indication of severe damage and may proceed to death of the cell if the causative factors are maintained.

Protein disturbances

Protein from the diet is split into amino acids which, after absorption, are reconstituted to form tissue protein. The 'normal' appearances of nuclear and cytoplasmic proteins in fixed and stained sections vary according to the techniques employed, but, under standard conditions, the distortions so produced are minimal. Alterations from this 'normal' appearance are seen in the degenerations and infiltrations.

Hyaline change and protein accumulation

The term 'hyaline' describes a pink-staining homogeneous glassy appearance of the cytoplasmic protein of the cell and is not always due to a degeneration, it may be a protein accumulation.

CAUSES
1   Excess reabsorption of protein as in renal tubular cells where protein has leaked through damaged glomeruli.
2   Russell bodies. Accumulations of immunoglobulin in plasma cells.
3   Alcoholic hyaline in liver cells (Mallory's hyaline) see p. 550). Probably broken down fibrils of rough endoplasmic reticulum.
4   Inclusion bodies in viral infections (see p. 40).
5   Collagenization with maturation. Seen in collagen fibres themselves, blood vessel walls, chronically inflamed lymph nodes and in slowly growing benign tumours, e.g. fibroids.
6   Fibrinoid. A special form of protein accumulation, called fibrinoid due to its resemblance to precipitated fibrin. It is found in blood vessel walls and connective tissue and contains plasma proteins including fibrin, albumin, globulins – particularly immunoglobulins and complement. It is associated with immunological damage and increased vascular permeability and often is accompanied by necrosis within the vessel wall or connective tissue.

Myxoid and mucoid degeneration

Mucopolysaccharides are widespread in the body as secretions of epithelial cells and as the ground substance of connective tissues and cartilage. They are conjugates of carbohydrate and protein. Excessive accumulation of this material is described as myxoid degeneration and is readily demonstrated by periodic acid–Schiff (P.A.S.) staining. The term 'mucoid degeneration' is applied to the production of large amounts of mucinous secretion by cells.

CONNECTIVE TISSUES

The formation of 'myxomatous' tissue which looks like Wharton's jelly and is histologically composed of stellate-shaped cells in a mucoid matrix. It occurs in many connective tissues but especially in fibrous tissue and is seen in collagen diseases, in blood vessels, especially medionecrosis of the aorta, and in many connective tissue tumours.

EPITHELIUM

Excessive production of epithelial mucin is associated with degeneration of the cells in catarrhal inflammation. Excessive mucus production in tumours may occur in 'colloid' cancers, mucinous cystadenoma of the ovary and in 'pleomorphic' adenomas of salivary glands.

Carbohydrate disturbances

All carbohydrates in the diet are broken down by enzymes and absorbed from the intestinal tract as monosaccharides. In the liver they are converted to glucose which may be:

1 Immediately oxidized for energy.
2 Converted and stored as muscle glycogen.
3 Converted and stored in the liver as glycogen with subsequent release as glucose by glycogenolysis when necessary.

Glucose may also be formed from protein by gluconeogenesis under the control of the hormones of the pituitary, thyroid, pancreas and adrenal cortex. The storage of glucose as glycogen is under the influence of insulin and the hyperglycaemia of diabetes mellitus is usually due to insulin deficiency. Liver disease, by impairing glycogen storage, may have the same effect. In hyperglycaemia, more glucose is delivered to the renal tubular epithelium than these cells can reabsorb, thus leading to glycosuria. Glycogen, the storage form of glucose, is recognized in fresh tissues by Best's carmine stain (red) or P.A.S. (rose-violet). Glycogen is normally found in the liver, kidney, heart and polymorphs.

Glycogen infiltration

This is an excessive amount of intracellular glycogen.

CAUSES

Diabetes mellitus
Present in the tissues in excess due to hyperglycae-

mia and especially prominent in renal and liver epithelium. The cells are distended and show nuclear ballooning or clear cytoplasmic vacuoles of glycogen.

Tumours
Some tumour cells are rich in glycogen, e.g. seminoma, renal carcinoma, squamous cell carcinoma and chondroma.

Glycogen storage disease
See p. 112.

Fat disturbances

Nature
'Fatty change' in cells concerns neutral fats, the glycerides of palmitic, stearic and oleic acids. Dietary fat is absorbed from the intestines, transported to the liver and thence utilized for:

1 Immediate energy requirements.
2 As an essential component of all tissue cells.
3 Storage in fat depots.

There is a continuous turnover of body fat via the blood stream due to its utilization and replacement in the tissues. In health, neutral fat can be readily demonstrated in adipose tissues – fat depots. Histological sections are prepared by the frozen section technique and Sudan or Oil Red O staining will reveal the red-staining fat. Healthy parenchymal tissues, e.g. heart, liver and kidney, show no demonstrable fat when stained by this method.

OBESITY

In obesity, whether due to over-eating or endocrine disturbances, there is an excess of fat of normal composition in the fat depots, e.g. buttocks, breasts, anterior abdominal wall, subcutaneous tissues, perinephric tissues and epicardium, but there is no demonstrable intracellular fat in the heart, liver or kidney cells. Thus obesity is totally different from fatty change.

FATTY CHANGE – FATTY DEGENERATION AND INFILTRATION – STEATOSIS

Nature
This implies the presence of demonstrable fat

within parenchymal cells, especially those of the liver, kidney and heart.

Historical
The original concept was of two types of 'fatty change'.

FATTY INFILTRATION
A single globule of fat distending the cytoplasm of the cell and displacing the nucleus to one side. It was postulated that this was 'transport fat' derived from the fat depots and carried by the blood stream; it was further surmised that the parenchymal cells could not deal with the excessive amounts of fat carried to them in the blood stream but were otherwise normal.

FATTY DEGENERATION
The presence of multiple small droplets of fat within the cytoplasm of the cell without nuclear displacement. This was regarded as evidence of cell degeneration with unmasking of previously un-stainable fat – *fat phanerosis*, such fat being entirely derived from within the affected cells. The presence of some nuclear degenerative changes supported the view that this was a primary degenerative change in the cell.

It was then shown experimentally that all demonstrable fat within a cell was dervived from the fat depots. Thus, it was postulated the 'degenerative' type of fatty change was due to the inability of a previously damaged cell to metabolize a normal amount of fat transported to it. Fat, therefore, accumulated within the cytoplasm.

Present view
The current views still lack complete clarity but the following is a possible compromise harmonizing the various opinions:
1 The presence of stainable fat in a parenchymal cell is indicative of damage to that cell.
2 This fat is derived from the fat depots via the blood stream.
3 The cell nuclei may show degenerative changes or appear normal.
4 The fat may be in the form of multiple small droplets or in a single globule.

Thus, all 'fatty change' is fatty infiltration by transport fat accumulating in a damaged parenchymal cell.

Causes
Any cause of cell damage including:
1 *Infection.* Bacterial, viral or their products.
2 *Physico-chemical*, e.g. chloroform, carbon tetrachloride, phosphorus, etc.
3 *Anoxia*, e.g. chronic passive venous congestion, anaemia.
4 *Nutritional factors*, e.g. lack of dietary factors, especially choline, and methionine, in alcoholics and in pregnancy.

The aetiological factors are further discussed in the liver section (see p. 548).

Sites
Parenchymal cells, especially those of the heart, liver and kidney.

Macroscopical
The organs show pallor and on cross-section may impart a 'greasy' feel, especially in the liver. The heart may show the 'tabby cat' or 'thrush breast' appearance whilst the kidney usually shows linear pale streaks due to the fat in the renal tubules.

Microscopical
The presence of stainable fat within the cell cytoplasm as a single globule or in multiple minute droplets. The nuclei may or may not show histological evidence of degenerative changes. Initially the excess fat is found in the endoplasmic reticulum, golgi apparatus and within vacuoles – 'liposomes'. With increased accumulation, large amounts of fat are found free in the cytoplasm.

Results
'Fatty change' is a reversible process and if the cause is removed the cells usually return to normal. However, long-continued fatty change with evidence of nuclear degeneration eventually proves irreversible and progresses to necrosis or fibrous replacement.

Necrosis

Definition
Necrosis is cell death.

Causes
Any factor causing cell damage including:
1 *Ischaemia.* Deprivation of oxygen or other metabolic necessities.

2 *Infective*. e.g. bacterial, viral, etc.

3 *Physico-chemical*. Direct action, e.g. heat, X-rays, acids, etc.

Appearances

Morphological changes indicative of cell death are produced by enzymes of extra- or intracellular origin. It thus follows that some time must elapse before modification of cell structure becomes visible. Sudden death with immediate fixation, i.e. an operative specimen, prevents enzyme action and so no histological changes of necrosis are seen.

NUCLEAR CHANGES

Enzymic breakdown of DNA into acidic subunits increases staining with basic dyes including haematoxylin. The chromatin thus looks darker and condensed – *pyknosis*. The nuclear membrane then ruptures and the chromatin fragments into small, darkly staining aggregates – *karyorrhexis*. The disappearance of nuclear material indicates *karyolysis*. An analogy may be seen here with the normal maturation of an adult red cell from the nucleated normoblast via the reticulocyte.

CYTOPLASMIC CHANGES

The cytoplasm passes through variable degenerative changes which may include cloudy swelling, hydropic, fatty or hyaline degeneration as previously described. The nuclear changes of death of the cell are occurring *pari passu* and the cell terminates as an anuclear ghost, the cytoplasm forming an amorphous, granular, opaque mass, the organelles having undergone autolysis (see p. 8).

Types

There are two basic types of necrosis:

COAGULATIVE NECROSIS

This type of necrosis is due to denaturation of the cellular protein to result in a firm mass of necrotic cells whose outlines may persist for days or even weeks before becoming dissolved and removed by enzymic lysis. This type of necrosis is commonly seen following deprivation of the blood supply, e.g. in infarcts.

COLLIQUATIVE NECROSIS

In contrast to the firm coagulative necrosis, colliquative necrosis implies the rapid liquefaction of dead cells. This occurs particularly in the central nervous system where the liquefaction is due to the breakdown of myelin and results in cerebral softening, e.g. following vascular occlusion.

Other types of necrosis

FAT NECROSIS

This is of two types:

(a) *Traumatic*. Produced by traumatic rupture of fat cells. The free fat evokes a tissue reaction resulting in a fibroblastic area of scar tissue and a firm nodule which may mimic a tumour (see p. 223).

(b) *Enzymic*. This occurs when the neutral fats are split by lipases into fatty acids and glycerol. The fatty acids saponify with alkalis to form chalky white precipitates. This is seen in the peritoneal fat in acute pancreatitis, in which condition enzymes, including lipase, escape into the tissues (see p. 631).

MUSCLE NECROSIS

In striated muscle in severe infections, e.g. typhoid, the striations disappear as do the nuclei. The appearances resemble hyalinization (see above), but this is in fact necrosis. It is traditionally known as 'Zenker's degeneration'.

CASEATION

This is the descriptive term reserved for the characteristic friable, cheesy, amorphous material in the centre of a tuberculous lesion. The appearances are due to a mixture of degenerative tissue protein and fat, the latter being derived from the lipid capsule of the organism.

GUMMATOUS

This is the 'structured necrosis' of the tertiary syphilitic lesion in which the ghostly outlines of the cells of the affected organ are still faintly preserved.

SUPPURATIVE

A special form of liquefaction necrosis is the production of pus due to the presence of proteolytic enzymes in organisms and polymorphs.

FIBRINOID

Necrosis associated with the accumulation of fibrinoid (see above) seen in connective tissue and blood vessel walls.

GANGRENE

This is necrosis of tissue in bulk, commonly with added putrefaction and is considered on p. 130.

Chapter 20
Amyloid Disease

Nature

Amyloidosis is a disease process in which there is extra-cellular deposition of a fibrillary protein in the tissues. The term was applied by Virchow because this waxy hyaline substance stains dark brown with iodine.

Classification

Numerous classifications have been devised, based on the staining reactions, organ distribution, association with connective tissue fibres and relationship with underlying conditions. None is entirely satisfactory but the latter is the most widely used.

Primary amyloid
Amyloid deposition may occur in the absence of any associated factors. There are two subgroups:

LOCALIZED
Localized deposits, forming tumour-like nodules, may occur, either single or multiple in several organs, notably larynx, lung, bladder and subcutaneous tissue.

GENERALIZED
A diagnosis of primary amyloidosis is only made after exclusion of all possible associated conditions. In some cases Bence-Jones proteinuria may be found, and this suggests an overlap with the plasma cell dyscrasias (see p. 471).

Secondary
Previously, secondary amyloid occurred mainly in relation to tertiary syphilis, pulmonary tuberculosis and chronic suppuration such as osteomyelitis and bronchiectasis. Now it is more commonly associated with rheumatoid arthritis and chronic urinary tract infection in paraplegics.

Genetic
Amyloid can be genetically determined. A number of hereditofamilial syndromes have been described, e.g. polyneuropathy in Portugal, nephropathy in familial Mediterranean fever.

Senile
Amyloid is commonly found in the brain and heart of elderly people, the frequency increasing with age. Clinical effects are not usual.

Tumours
Systemic amyloidosis may complicate some tumours, e.g. myelomatosis, Hodgkin's disease, renal carcinoma. Local amyloid deposition has been described mainly in endocrine neoplasms, e.g. medullary carcinoma of thyroid (see p. 315).

Distribution

The previous belief that primary and secondary amyloidosis could be distinguished in part by the organ distribution is erroneous. Systemic amyloidosis may affect any organ, those most commonly involved being kidney, spleen, liver, gastrointestinal tract, skeletal muscles and heart.

Organ changes

The amorphous amyloid material is deposited mainly in the walls of small blood vessels and in the interstitial tissues. There may be atrophy and replacement of adjacent parenchymal cells, e.g.:

1 *Kidney*. Deposition of amyloid in glomerular tufts, arterioles and basement membranes of tubules to produce enlarged pale kidneys. Renal involvement often leads to the nephrotic syndrome or progressive chronic renal failure (see p. 374).

2 *Liver*. Deposition of amyloid in the walls of the sinusoids and in arterioles. Liver cell atrophy may occur and the liver becomes large, pale, firm and waxy.

3 *Spleen*. The pattern may be either:

(*a*) Focal. Amyloid is deposited in the arterioles of the white pulp, replacing the Malpighian bodies and resembling *sago* granules on section.

(*b*) Diffuse. Amyloid is deposited in the walls of the sinusoids, causing diffuse involvement of the red pulp and the spleen becomes enlarged, firm and waxy.

Nature

Staining reactions

1 *Iodine*. Mahogany brown colour when poured onto affected tissues.

2 *Congo red*. The most reliable histological stain. The dye is soluble in amyloid and stains it a rose-pink colour. Greater specificity is achieved using polarizing microscopy, when characteristic green birefrigence is exhibited.

3 *Methyl violet*. Amyloid stains metachromatically in histological sections.

4 *Thioflavine T*. When stained with this fluorochrome and examined in ultraviolet light, a characteristic greenish fluorescence is seen.

Structure

The early view that amyloid was composed of glycoprotein and polysaccharide has now been disproved; it is a fibrillar protein.

High resolution electron microscopy has shown that both experimental animal and human amyloid has a fibrillary structure arranged either at random or in parallel bundles and a molecular weight ranging from 5000 to 18 000.

Chemical analysis has been hampered by the insolubility of amyloid, but modern immunochemical methods have shown that it is composed of polypeptide chains. In primary amyloid these are whole or fragmented immunoglobulin light chains, but secondary amyloid is probably not derived from immunoglobulins.

It is likely that amyloid is, in fact, a heterogenous spectrum of proteins rather than homogenous.

Pathogenesis

There is strong evidence that systemic amyloidosis has an immunological basis. Primary amyloid is known to be composed of immunoglobulin light chains and the condition may be a form of plasma cell dyscrasia. Secondary amyloid usually follows prolonged immunological stimulation as in chronic infections or rheumatoid arthritis. The precise mechanism for the laying down of amyloid is unknown.

Clinical effects

In both primary and secondary amyloidosis there is a progressive increase in the deposition of amyloid material. The clinical effects depend on which organ is the most severely affected. Hepatosplenomegaly is usual although liver failure is rare. The nephrotic syndrome may occur, and heart failure may follow significant cardiac involvement. Rarer clinical syndromes include hypo-adrenalism and neuropathies. Death usually occurs from renal or cardiac failure.

Diagnosis

The systemic Congo red test is no longer used because of anaphylactic reactions reported in some subjects.

The best diagnostic method is tissue biopsy. The sites most commonly investigated are random rectal biopsy with renal or liver biopsy when there is clinical evidence of involvement of these organs.

Prognosis

The outlook in systemic amyloidosis is very poor, and there is no effective treatment. Trials of cytotoxic and immunosuppressive agents are being undertaken but have not yet been evaluated.

Senile amyloid is usually an incidental finding at autopsy, and has no systemic effects.

Chapter 21
Metabolic Disorders of Proteins: Carbohydrates: Lipids

Metabolic disorders of protein

GOUT

Purine metabolism
Purines are derived from breakdown of nucleoproteins. The end-products of purine metabolism are uric acid and urea.

Nature
A common disease, predominantly in males over 50 years who frequently have a family history of gout, although occasionally the gouty manifestations may be symptomatic of other diseases (see below). The deposition of urates in the tissues is usually associated with an increased serum uric acid level – in excess of 0.40 mmol/l in males and 0.35 mmol/l in females.

Aetiology
The increased serum uric level is due to one or both of the following mechanisms:

1 Increased uric acid production:
(a) In 'idiopathic' gout this is probably due to an inborn metabolic defect leading to increased endogenous synthesis.
(b) May also occur in excessive nuclear breakdown associated with extensive areas of necrosis, e.g. infarcts, or in leukaemia, polycythaemia, and other myeloproliferative disorders. These result in 'symptomatic' gout (see p. 458).
2 Decreased uric acid excretion. This is usually associated with renal damage or renal failure and an increased blood urea.

Macroscopical
There may be a diffuse infiltration, but more typically there are hard, localized nodules composed of white, chalky material – *tophi*. These tophi are found in:
1 Soft tissue around the joints, e.g. big toe, sometimes extending into bone (see p. 710).
2 Ear cartilages.

3 Subcutaneous tissue and bursae.

4 In the heart and kidneys, but rarely to any significant degree.

Microscopical

A tophus consists of collections of crystalline sodium biurate surrounded by a fibroblastic inflammatory reaction containing foreign body giant cells. Similar but not identical appearances may be caused by the pyrophosphate crystals of *pseudogout*.

Results

The disease usually runs a chronic course with acute and painful exacerbations of the joint lesions and long intervening periods of remission. Hypertension and renal disease may be associated, but the gout is probably only rarely causative. Treatment with allopurinol and related substances may maintain a lowered uric acid blood level, prevent acute episodes and relieve symptoms.

Metabolic disorders of carbohydrate

DIABETES MELLITUS

Although diabetes is principally a disorder of carbohydrate metabolism due to a relative or an absolute insulin insufficiency, fat and protein metabolism are also severely affected. This extremely common disease accounting for over 4000 deaths in England and Wales annually is discussed in the section on pancreatic diseases (see p. 633).

GLYCOGEN STORAGE DISEASES

Nature

Rare abnormalities of glycogen metabolism resulting in the progressive accumulation of glycogen in the tissues of young subjects.

Aetiology

At least nine forms have now been identified, each associated with a different enzyme deficiency, e.g. Type I – Von Gierke's Disease – absence of glucose-6-phosphatase. The inheritance is rare recessive (see p. 18).

Sites

Liver, kidney, heart and skeletal muscles.

Macroscopical

Enlarged, pale, firm organs, with clinical hepatomegaly or cardiomegaly.

Microscopical

Cytoplasmic vacuoles of glycogen are present in hepatocytes, renal tubular epithelium and myocardial fibres. Some enzyme defects can be demonstrated histochemically.

Results

Premature death due to heart failure or intercurrent infection.

Lipid disturbances

Nature

Lipids are a group of fatty substances which includes cholesterol and its esters. Cholesterol is deposited in the tissues in two forms, in foam cells and as crystals which are doubly refractile on polarization. Lipids within foam cells require special histological staining techniques for identification of their chemical composition.

RAISED BLOOD CHOLESTEROL

Causes

Obesity, pregnancy, obstructive jaundice, primary biliary cirrhosis, glomerulonephritis, myxoedema and primary familial cholesterolaemia.

Results

There is deposition of cholesterol in various tissues, e.g. subcutaneous tissues – *xanthelasma* (see p. 326), blood vessels – *atheroma* (see pp. 258–259).

INCREASED LOCAL LIPID

The local deposition of cholesterol is found in many conditions, including the following.

Cholesterosis of the gall bladder

Pale flecks due to collections of foam cells in the submucosa (see p. 572).

Degenerations

(*a*) Epithelial. Wherever epithelial degeneration occurs.

(b) Connective tissue. In connective tissue tumours especially neurofibromas and meningiomas, and in atheromatous lesions (p. 258).

(c) Abscesses and haematomas. In the wall of any chronic abscess or haematoma.

CRYSTALLINE CHOLESTEROL

(a) Cholesterol 'solitaire' stone in the gall bladder.

(b) In any degenerating or inflammatory tissue.

(c) In cysts with fluid contents, e.g. branchial and dermoid cysts, hydrocoele, etc.

Histologically, these appear as rhomboid crystals in frozen sections, but otherwise as linear clefts in the tissues frequently surrounded by foreign body giant cells.

LIPID STORAGE DISEASES – LIPOIDOSES

Nature
These form a rare group of diseases of unknown causation, all of which show accumulation of lipid substances of differing chemical composition.

GAUCHER'S DISEASE

A congenital, familial disease with autosomal recessive inheritance in which there is an accumulation of glucocerebrosides in the cytoplasm of cells in the lymphoreticular system.

Sites
Spleen, bone marrow, liver, lymph nodes and brain, with enlargement of spleen and liver.

Microscopical
The Gaucher cell is large (20–100 μm) with a central hyperchromatic nucleus, and pale irregularly striated cytoplasm. The striae are strongly PAS positive.

Results
There are two types:

(a) *Acute neuropathic (infantile)*. Appears within the first year of life and is rapidly progressive with death within 6 months. Cerebral involvement is usually prominent.

(b) *Chronic adult*. This is the commonest form, and unlike the acute neuropathic type has a predilection for Jews. It appears usually before the age of 30 years with hepatosplenomegaly and anaemia which is slowly progressive over a period of 10 years or more.

NIEMANN – PICK DISEASE

A severe congenital familial disease, with autosomal recessive inheritance, due to the accumulation of cholesterol and sphingomyelin in the cells of the lymphoreticular system.

Sites
Spleen, liver, lymph nodes and bone marrow.

Microscopical
Collections of foam cells containing lipid droplets which are sudanophilic and PAS positive. The cells are large, but usually smaller than the Gaucher cell.

Results
Usually presents in infancy and is rapidly progressive with death before the age of 3 years.

HAND–SCHÜLLER–CHRISTIAN DISEASE

This condition is part of a wider disease entity of Histiocytosis X and is described on p. 691.

TAY–SACHS DISEASE–AMAUROTIC FAMILIAL IDIOCY

This disease of ganglioside deposition in cerebral tissues is described on p. 611.

Chapter 22
Calcification : Pigmentation

Calcification
Physiological
Damaged tissues
Stone formation
Metastatic calcification
    Causes
    Sites
    Mechanisms
Congenital calcinosis

Heterotopic bone formation
Nature
Secondary to calcification
Myositis ossificans

Pigmentation

EXOGENOUS
Metals
Coarse particles
Soluble substances
Fungi

ENDOGENOUS

Haemoglobin derivatives
Haematin
Haemosiderin
Haematoidin (bilirubin)

Porphyrins
    Congenital porphyria
    Acute idiopathic porphyria
    Drug porphyria

Melanin
Nature
Increased pigment
Decreased pigment

Lipochromes

Calcification

This may occur in many sites, some of the more common examples being illustrated in Fig. 25 on p. 115.

Physiological
Deposits of calcium occur in costal cartilages, larynx, tracheal rings, pineal body, etc., with increasing frequency with advancing age. This is believed to represent a physiological manifestation associated with ageing processes. Indeed, calcification is frequently seen in placental tissues, especially when parturition is delayed.

In damaged tissues
Calcium salts show an affinity for degenerate material and scar tissues. Thus, calcification occurs in caseous material, fibrous tissue of the heart valves pericardium, pleura, surrounding worms, ii tumours of many types, e.g. fibroids, and in the media of the arteries in old age and in atheroma at any age.

Stone formation
Calcium salts are incorporated in many calculi in the urinary tract, pancreas, salivary glands, biliary tract, etc. (see pp. 371, 570).

Metastatic calcification
This is calcification occurring in previously normal tissues due to an excess of ionized calcium in the blood and tissue fluids, usually following excessive mobilization from the skeleton.

CAUSES
The main causes are:
1 Hyperparathyroidism – primary or secondary (see p. 316).
2 Hypervitaminosis D.
3 Tumour-associated products causing hypercalcaemia (see p. 159).

SITES
Kidney, stomach, lung and especially urinary calculi.

MECHANISMS
These are extremely complex and are the subject of much debate. There are obvious interrelationships between calcium, phosphate, vitamin D, parathor-

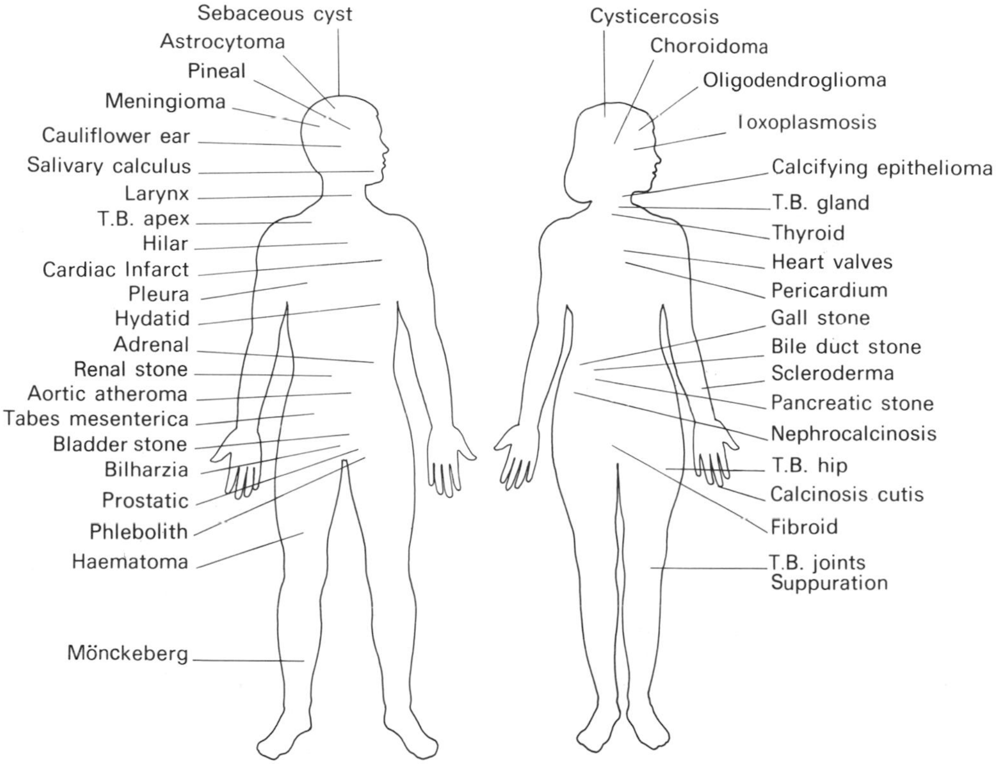
Sebaceous cyst
Astrocytoma
Pineal
Meningioma
Cauliflower ear
Salivary calculus
Larynx
T.B. apex
Hilar
Cardiac Infarct
Pleura
Hydatid
Adrenal
Renal stone
Aortic atheroma
Tabes mesenterica
Bladder stone
Bilharzia
Prostatic
Phlebolith
Haematoma
Mönckeberg
Cysticercosis
Choroidoma
Oligodendroglioma
Toxoplasmosis
Calcifying epithelioma
T.B. gland
Thyroid
Heart valves
Pericardium
Gall stone
Bile duct stone
Scleroderma
Pancreatic stone
Nephrocalcinosis
T.B. hip
Calcinosis cutis
Fibroid
T.B. joints
Suppuration

Fig. 25. Sites of calcification.

mone, calcitonin, phosphatase. Some of these are discussed on pp. 692–697.

Congenital calcinosis

A very rare condition in which there is deposition of calcium salts in the skin, subcutaneous tissues, muscles and tendons but without any detectable abnormality of blood calcium levels. The cause is not known.

Heterotopic bone formation

Nature

This implies bone formation outside the skeletal system. It is uncommon but may occur.

Secondary to any form of calcification

Osteoblasts lay down osteoid tissue in the calcium to produce bone, e.g. Mönckeberg's medial sclerosis, old haematomas, pleural thickening, tuberculous scars, etc.

Myositis ossificans

This occurs in two forms:

(*a*) Traumatic myositis ossificans. Following trauma, the muscle is replaced by fibrous tissue which is subsequently ossified. One of the more common sites is at the adductor insertion in the thigh – 'Rider's bone'. The osteoblasts may arise by metaplasia from fibroblasts in extra-osseous sites.

(*b*) Myositis ossificans progressiva. A very rare disorder affecting young males whereby muscles, tendons and ligaments progressively ossify. The aetiology is completely unknown.

Pigmentation

EXOGENOUS PIGMENTATION

Pigmentation may follow injection, inhalation or absorption from the gut of a large number of coloured foreign materials. These may be distributed in the body via the lymphatics or blood stream. This group includes the following.

Metals

Silver, lead, bismuth or gold acquired accidentally from water supplies or occupations, e.g. workers in precious metals, or following prolonged therapeutic administration. Lead poisoning results in 'blue lines', whilst silver is deposited in the skin as an albuminate which imparts a permanent grey discoloration.

Coarse particles

Inhalation of carbon, iron ore, silica and asbestos dust result in pigmentation of the lungs associated with the pneumoconioses (see p. 668). A common form of pigmentation is due to the injection of coarse particles into the skin in tattooing.

Coloured soluble substances

A slight yellow discoloration of the skin may follow the ingestion of some soluble substances; this may be carotene in individuals who eat a surfeit of carrots, or chemical substances, e.g. some antimalarial drugs.

Fungi

Some fungi cause local pigmentation at the diseased site, e.g. monilia – white, aspergilli – black or dark brown.

ENDOGENOUS PIGMENTATION

Pigmentation may be due to endogenous substances and these include blood derivatives, e.g. haemoglobin, bile and porphyrins, as well as melanin and the lipochromes.

HAEMOGLOBIN DERIVATIVES

Pigmentation of tissues is frequently due to one of the many breakdown products of haemoglobin. This may be schematically represented as shown in Fig. 26.

Haematin

Haematin appears in the tissues as a dark brown pigment but the Prussian blue reaction for iron is negative as the iron is 'bound'. Haematin is the

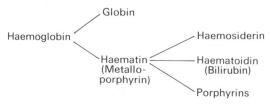

Fig. 26. Haemoglobin derivatives.

pigment found in malaria in Blackwater fever and its also occurs in the kidneys in acute haemolytic states, e.g. following an incompatible blood transfusion (see p. 365).

Haemosiderin

Appears in the tissues as a brown, granular pigment which gives a positive Prussian blue reaction as the iron is 'free'. This pigment is found within cells in excess in:

(*a*) Trauma – producing local haemorrhage or bruising.

(*b*) Prolonged and excessive therapeutic iron administration.

(*c*) Repeated blood transfusions usually involving several hundred units over a prolonged period of time – *haemosiderosis.*

(*d*) Haemochromatosis (see pp. 562 – 563).

(*e*) Excessive blood destruction – in haemolytic anaemias from any cause.

(*f*) In cardiac failure – in 'heart failure cells' in brown induration of lungs.

(*g*) In the 'siderotic nodules' in the spleen associated with splenomegaly and hepatic cirrhosis (see p. 737).

Haematoidin or bilirubin

These are probably identical substances which occur as yellow-brown granules or crystals and do not contain iron. They are present in areas of local haemorrhage and bilirubin is the pigment responsible for jaundice. The mechanism of its formation and its role in jaundice are described in the liver section (see p. 575).

Porphyrins

The haematoporphyrins are the respiratory pigments of the blood. These iron-free porphyrins are normally present in minute quantities in the plasma and in the urine where they are excreted as coproporphyrins. In the condition of porphyria there is an excretion of many milligrams per day, due to inborn errors of porphyrin metabolism.

CONGENITAL PORPHYRIA

The disease may not become manifest until several years after birth. It is associated with a Burgundy-red colour of the urine which develops on standing due to excessive urinary excretion of porphyrins. A red-brown discoloration is also found in the teeth and bones. In addition skin lesions, including photosensitivity (*hydroa aestivale*) may be manifest and this dermatological condition may result in gross scarring and deformity (see p. 722).

ACUTE IDIOPATHIC PORPHYRIA

This is also an inherited disease and occurs especially in females, who present with abdominal colic, vomiting and a dark-coloured urine. Later, skin involvement, neuritis, paralysis and mental symptoms may develop.

DRUG PORPHYRIA

Similar signs and symptoms may occur in patients following administration of certain drugs, e.g. phosphorus, lead, sulphonamides, barbiturates, alcohol and arsenicals. It is probable, however, that these substances merely precipitate the clinical manifestations of the previously undetected inborn metabolic defect.

MELANIN PIGMENTATION

Nature

Melanin is a dark brown pigment which is normally found in the skin, the choroid of the eye, the adrenal cortex, in the substantia nigra and in the meninges. In the skin, the pigment is produced by melanoblasts which are situated in the basal layer. Some authorities regard these cells as of ectodermal origin whilst others regard them as being derived from nerve end-organs (neuroectoderm) followed by migration into the epidermis. Melanin is a granular protein-containing pigment formed:

$$\text{Tyrosine} \xrightarrow{\text{Tyrosinase}} \text{Phenylalanine} \xrightarrow{\text{Melaninogenase}} \text{Melanin}$$

Some of the melanoblasts show no visible pigment but all are DOPA positive. This implies the

ability of these cells to convert dihydroxyphenylalanine (DOPA) into melanin and indicates the presence within these cells of melaninogenase. Melanophores are also pigmented cells but are only phagocytes which transport the pigment and are all DOPA negative. The metabolism of melanin is influenced by a hormone from the pituitary (melanin-stimulating hormone, MSH).

Increased melanin pigmentation

Occurs in many conditions including:

1 *Sunlight*. To produce the normal 'sun-tan' or freckles.
2 *Heat*. As in furnace workers.
3 *Irradiation*.
4 *Pregnancy*. Producing 'chloasma' of pregnancy.
5 *Addison's disease* (see p. 290).
6 *Haemochromatosis*. The pigment is a mixture of haemosiderin and haemofuscin as well as melanin (see pp. 562 – 563).
7 *Melanosis coli*. Producing an asymptomatic brown or black discoloration of the large bowel. This may be due to the local conversion of proteins into melanin and is associated with constipation and sometimes with anthracene purgatives.
8 *Ochronosis*. This is a rare inborn error of metabolism whereby homogentisic acid, which is a breakdown product of tyrosine and phenylalanine, is excreted but accumulates in cartilage to produce the ochre-discoloration of both articular and intervertebral disc cartilages. The urine also develops a dark colour on standing – *alcaptonuria* (see p. 19), due to the presence of homogentisic acid and similar pigment may be present in the renal tubules.
9 *Benign naevus*. A tumour-like lesion of DOPA positive 'naevus cells' (see p. 733).
10 *Malignant melanoma*. A malignant tumour of melanoblasts (see p. 734).
11 *Neurofibromatosis*. Von Recklinghausen's disease is associated with '*café-au-lait*' spots (see p. 620).

Decreased melanin pigmentation

May be due to:

1 *Congenital*:

(*a*) *Complete*. Total absence of melanin pigment, an autosomal recessive trait – *albinos*.

(*b*) *Localized.* A patchy depigmentation with absence of melanin occurs in vitiligo or leucoderma. Piebaldism and white forelock is an autosomal dominant disorder and localized eye lesions with absence of pigment are sex-linked recessive. Albinos with ocular defects and deaf-mutism are irregular dominants.

2 *Acquired.* Loss of melanin frequently occurs following skin injury so that depigmentation is associated with any extensive scar formation, e.g. leprosy, burns, granulomas, scleroderma, etc.

LIPOCHROMES

Lipochrome is a yellow fat-soluble pigment which is normally present in the adrenal cortex, in ganglion cells, testes and luteal cells. Lipochrome occurs in excess as pathological pigmentation in brown atrophy of the heart. In this condition, the heart is both smaller and browner than normal and the lipochrome is visible microscopically in the paranuclear areas of the myocardial fibres – 'wear and tear' granules (see p. 238).

Chapter 23
Circulatory Disorders – Congestion: Oedema: Shock

Congestion

Nature
Congestion or hyperaemia is an increase in the amount of blood in the tissues.

ACTIVE CONGESTION

This is dilatation of arterioles and capillaries occurring in exercise and in inflammation.

PASSIVE VENOUS CONGESTION

This is venous stasis and may be acute or chronic, local or general

Acute passive venous congestion
Organs or tissues are deep red and engorged with blood. Extravasation of blood to produce haemorrhages may also occur.

LOCAL
Due to sudden obstruction of the venous return, e.g. venous thrombosis, strangulation at a hernial site, torsion of a vascular pedicle, volvulus, etc. The sudden mechanical occlusion prevents the return of venous blood; the more resistant arterial walls remain patent and blood continues to enter the area thus producing the hyperaemia. Eventually, the tissue tension is so elevated that the arterial supply becomes occluded and necrosis follows.

GENERAL
Generalized acute hyperaemia occurs with acute heart failure and asphyxia, causing raised venous pressure and overdistension of the viscera.

Chronic passive venous congestion

LOCAL
Caused by prolonged gradual obstruction of veins with or without thrombosis. The causes include enlarged lymph nodes, tumours and other masses

compressing veins. Thus, mediastinal tumours and retrosternal goitres may cause vena caval obstruction and likewise cirrhosis of the liver produces chronic passive venous congestion confined to the portal circulation, with oesophageal varices, splenomegaly and visceral hyperaemia.

GENERAL

Generalized chronic passive venous congestion occurs in chronic cardiac failure when the venous return is impeded – congestive heart failure from any cause.

Organ changes

When congestion is mild, the organ changes are restricted to hyperaemia. In more severe or prolonged cases, the stasis of blood results in tissue anoxia and consequently parenchymal cell degeneration. There is frequently evidence of fibrous replacement of the anoxic tissues with haemorrhages due both to the anoxia and the raised venous pressure. Oedema is also an accompanying feature in many cases (see p. 122).

1   *Lungs*. This is the most commonly seen in chronic left ventricular failure and in mitral valve obstruction. In both circumstances there is gross hyperaemia and stagnant anoxia in the vessels of the oedematous alveolar walls. Red blood cells and fluid escape into the alveoli and later there is fibrous thickening of the alveolar walls. The red cells are phagocytosed by histiocytes to produce the haemosiderin-containing 'heart-failure' cells. The lung thus becomes firm, brown and fibrous – *brown induration*.

2   *Liver*. Rapid congestion of the liver occurs in right heart failure as there are no valves between the hepatic veins and the right atrium.

Early. The central vein of each liver lobule shows extreme dilatation and the central portions of the sinusoids are congested to produce the deeply congested liver which drips blood on section.

Later. The ensuing anoxia produces centrilobular liver cell damage. The peripheral portion of the lobule around the portal tracts remains normal with an intermediate zone of fatty change due to interference with cell metabolism. The result is a deeply congested and mottled liver – 'nutmeg' liver.

Late. If the congestion is unrelieved, there is necrosis of the anoxic central zones with replacement fibrosis – 'cardiac cirrhosis' (see p. 565).

3   *Spleen*. In the early stages, the spleen is slightly enlarged due to engorgement. Later, especially with portal vein obstruction, e.g. hepatic cirrhosis, the spleen is grossly enlarged with increased fibrosis of the walls of the sinusoids and excessive haemosiderin pigmentation. This is produced by the same mechanism as in the lung and is sometimes known as 'brown induration' of the spleen. On occasions, firm white or brown plaques are present in the splenic pulp. These '*siderotic nodules*' are composed of localized collections of haemosiderin surrounded by fibrous tissue.

4   *Kidneys*. Slightly enlarged, tense and deep red in colour with an exaggerated cortico-medullary differentiation. The glomeruli may be visible as small red haemorrhagic dots on the cut surface. Microscopically, the glomeruli are extremely engorged and the tubules may show anoxic degenerative changes.

5   *Other organs*. The intestines, stomach and other abdominal viscera show engorgement with blood. The limbs, especially the legs, are over-filled with blood and are frequently oedematous.

Results of prolonged venous congestion

1   Enlargement due to engorgement.
2   Stagnant anoxia with parenchymal cell degeneration and increased fibrosis.
3   Oedema.

Oedema

Nature

Oedema is the excessive accumulation of extracellular fluid in the tissues. It may be in the form of a transudate (r.d. less than 1.021), or an exudate (r.d. more than 1.020).

Normal tissue fluid

Factors involved in the formation and removal of normal tissue fluid are schematically represented in Fig. 28.

The extracellular fluid has a total volume of 10–11 litre. This is the *milieu interne* of Claude Bernard and is the fluid which bathes all the cells of the body and through which all cell metabolites pass. The fluid is never static, being in constant exchange with the intracellular fluid and with the blood.

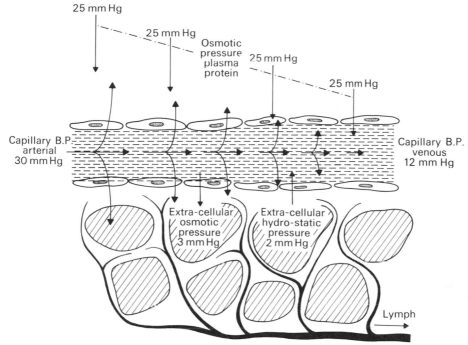

Fig. 28. Diagram of capillary to show factors involved in tissue fluid formation.

Factors involved in the formation and removal of tissue fluid

CAPILLARY BLOOD PRESSURE
The hydrostatic pressure of the capillary blood is approximately 25–30 mmHg at the arterial end and only 7–12 mmHg at the venous end. This results in a net outflow of fluid into the tissues at the arterial end, but a net inflow into the vessels at the venous end.

CAPILLARY PERMEABILITY
An, intact, healthy endothelium acts as a semi-permeable membrane, allowing the free passage of electrolytes but opposing the passage of proteins. If the permeability is increased, e.g. in inflammation, protein may pass through the vessel wall.

OSMOTIC PRESSURE OF BLOOD
This is largely maintained by the contained plasma proteins, particularly albumin, which exert a pressure of approximately 25 mmHg attracting fluid back into the blood, especially at the venous end.

OSMOTIC PRESSURE OF EXTRACELLULAR FLUID
Extracellular fluid contains 4–6 g/l of protein, mainly albumin, which exerts an osmotic pressue of 2–3 mmHg to attract fluid from the blood. The electrolyte contents of plasma and extracellular fluid are normally in equilibrium.

HYDROSTATIC PRESSURE OF EXTRACELLULAR FLUID
The elastic properties of tissue produce a slightly positive pressure which varies between 1 and 2 mmHg, and deters the escape of fluid from the blood. The tissue tension at different sites varies according to the tissue components. Thus, subcutaneous and other loose tissues show a greater degree of oedema than firm collagen or other compact tissues.

LYMPHATIC DRAINAGE
Lymphatic vessels normally remove any excess of extracellular fluid.

These six factors, working in conjunction, ensure

a constant circulation of extracellular fluid. In oedema, one or more of these factors become deranged to result in the pathological excess of extracellular fluid.

Causes of oedema

INCREASED HYDROSTATIC PRESSURE
Increased venous pressure will force fluid out of the blood vessels into the extracellular spaces:
(a) *Systemic.* Cardiac failure results in increased venous pressure. This is not the only factor, however, as tissue anoxia is also produced and causes vascular dilatation and increased permeability thus increasing the amount of extracellular fluid.
(b) *Local.* Mechanical obstruction to venous drainage, e.g. gravid uterus pressing on pelvic veins causing leg oedema, venous thrombosis, varicose veins, etc.

DECREASED OSMOTIC PRESSURE OF THE BLOOD
Oedema usually occurs when the plasma proteins fall below 40 g/l.

Causes of protein decrease
(a) *Inadequate intake*, e.g. starvation oedema, malabsorption syndrome, etc.
(b) *Excessive output*, e.g. renal disease with albuminuria, especially in the nephrotic syndrome; outpouring of protein in severe burns; recurrent ascites.
(c) *Underproduction*, e.g. severe liver disease with deficient protein synthesis, etc.

INCREASED CAPILLARY PERMEABILITY
Increased vascular permeability allows an excess of fluid and plasma proteins to pass into the tissues.

Causes
(a) *Systemic.* Bacterial products and some chemicals may produce generalized oedema. This is the type seen in anaphylaxis. Probably the most common cause is the anoxia associated with cardiac failure.
(b) *Local.* Local injury to blood vessels by burns, chemicals and infections results in vascular damage with increased permeability and a resulting inflammatory exudate. In *angioneurotic oedema*, a local hypersensitivity reaction to an antigen produces a transient but often severe local oedema by increasing capillary permeability. A common site for this to occur is the glottis.

INCREASED OSMOTIC PRESSURE OF THE EXTRACELLULAR FLUID
Excess of sodium ions in the extracellular fluid retains water and therefore produces oedema. This factor is operative in cardiac failure and in any condition impairing the excretion of sodium, e.g. renal failure, excess secretion of adrenal glucocorticoids and mineralocorticoids and also with an excessive dietary intake of sodium.

LYMPHATIC OBSTRUCTION
Obstruction to the lymphatics may prevent the drainage of tissue fluids and if persistent may lead to *lymphoedema* – a brawny, non-pitting oedema with subsequent overgrowth of the connective tissue and thickening of the skin. When severe this is *elephantiasis* (see p. 278).

Causes
1　*Congenital.* Milroy's disease (see p. 278)
2　*Parasitic*, e.g. filarial infection (see p. 69).
3　*Scarring*, e.g. fibrosis following infection – lymphogranuloma venereum, or following irradiation (see p. 76).
4　*Surgery.* Following removal of inguinal or axillary lymph nodes, e.g. for carcinoma of breast.
5　*Malignant disease.* Lymphatic blockage by tumour cells.

Clinical types
The two most commonly encountered clinical types of generalized oedema are those associated with cardiac failure and renal disease.
1　*Cardiac oedema.* The chief factors are:
(a) Increased hydrostatic pressure in the veins.
(b) Stagnant anoxia with increased vascular permeability.
(c) Sodium ion retention with increased osmotic pressure of the extracellular fluid.
2　*Renal oedema.* The factors involved vary with renal diseases but include:
(a) Decreased plasma proteins and thus decreased plasma osmotic pressure due to albuminuria, e.g. nephrotic syndrome.
(b) Increased osmotic pressure of extracellular fluid due to electrolyte disturbance, e.g. acute renal failure.
(c) Increased capillary permeability – believed to

be a factor in the oedema of acute glomerulonephritis.

(*d*) Oedema due to cardiac failure may be superimposed, particularly when there is associated
hypertension secondary to the renal disease.

Effects

The effects of oedema of the tissues depend largely
on the site of accumulation of the fluid. Little
functional disturbance is occasioned by mild subcutaneous oedema but cerebral oedema leads to
raised intracranial tension, coma and even death
when severe. In pulmonary oedema, there is displacement of air by the fluid in the alveoli thereby
impeding gaseous exchange; thus dyspnoea and
cyanosis frequently result.

Shock

Nature

A clinical state resulting from reduction of the
effective circulating blood volume.

Pathogenesis

The precise cause or causes of the severe reduction
of circulating blood volume are not always obvious,
but commonly one or more of the following factors
are involved:

1   *Blood loss*. Severe external or internal haemorrhage is a self-evident cause and will result in a rapid
reduction of circulating blood volume – haemorrhagic shock.

2   *Capillary bed dilatation*. Pooling of large quantities of blood in the capillary bed can lead to
diminished circulating blood volume. The exact
mechanism by which this is produced is unknown
but it is postulated that after initial vasoconstriction
in response to catecholamine release, the precapill-
ary vessels become refractory and dilate. The
post-capillary venules remain constricted and pooling occurs. Dilatation of pre-capillary arterioles

also happens in the presence of metabolic acidosis.

3   *Neurogenic*. It has been suggested that nervous
pathways may be involved in the production of the
initial and transient phase of shock – *primary shock*.
Certainly some individuals faint at the thought of
venesection, or at the site of blood. Alterations of
vasomotor tone with resulting redistribution of
blood mediated by nervous mechanisms may well
operate in the longer-lasting true clinical shock.

4   *Cardiogenic*. Also known as central shock, this is
seen in acute cardiac failure especially following
myocardial infarction and is due to 'pump failure'.

5   *Plasma and fluid loss*. Severe local plasma loss
occurs into the area of extensive burns and other
injuries and a more generalized fluid loss occurs
with increased capillary permeability. This is seen
in anaphylaxis (see p. 101), in the shock associated
with peritonitis and severe systemic acute infections including endotoxic shock. Copious vomiting,
salt loss, severe water deprivation and diarrhoea
will also cause shock by haemoconcentration and
reduction of the blood volume.

Effects

These vary according to the severity and duration
of the condition.

In general the condition leads to hypotension and
reduction of blood flow to vital organs, which thus
become anoxic and may show:

1   *Brain*. Loss of consciousness may be followed
by permanent structural damage due to anoxic
oedema, raised intracranial tension and degeneration of neurones with cerebral softening.

2   *Kidneys*. Acute tubular necrosis with anuria (see
p. 365).

3   *Adrenals*. 'Adrenal exhaustion' may occur with
cortical lipid depletion.

4   *Liver*. Fatty change of variable degree.

5   *Heart*. Fatty change, usually minimal.

6   *Lungs*. Extremely variable, but usually congested.

Chapter 24
Circulatory Disorders – Thrombosis: Embolism

Thrombosis

Definition
The formation of a solid mass–thrombus, from the constituents of the blood within the vascular system during life.

Normal coagulation mechanisms
These are described on p. 523.

POST-MORTEM CLOT

This is merely the clotting of the blood which occurs after death. The clot is shiny, elastic, non-adherent and takes the shape of the vessel in which it lies. It is usually composed of two layers; an upper of clotted plasma – *chicken fat*; a lower layer of sedimented red cells – *redcurrant jelly*. This post-mortem clot is not a true thrombus as it is not formed during life.

ANTE-MORTEM THROMBUS

Macroscopical
A fully formed thrombus is a laminated structure which is firm, often friable, has a rough or granular

external surface and may be loosely or firmly adherent to its site or origin on the vessel wall. The laminated appearance – *lines of Zahn* – is due to successive waves of platelet disposition and thrombus formation.

Microscopical

The first change visible microscopically on the endothelial surface in thrombus formation is the deposition and disintegration of platelets which appear as pink-staining homogeneous material. The presence of damaged platelets leads to accumulation of various clotting factors and initiates fibrin deposition. Red and white cells are trapped in the fibrin meshes, followed by further deposition of aggregated platelets. Successive layers of platelets and thrombus produce the laminated structure of the thrombus.

Types

PLATELET THROMBUS
Composed almost entirely of platelets. Forms the initial phase of a coralline thrombus (see below), and also endocardial vegetations, e.g. rheumatic, infective endocarditis (see p. 246).

CORALLINE THROMBUS
The typical laminated thrombus, which may become *occlusive*, e.g. coronary artery, deep vein of leg.

PROPAGATING THROMBUS
Progressive extension proximally of thrombus following thrombotic occlusion in the venous system.

MURAL THROMBUS
A thrombus adherent to one aspect of the wall of a large vessel or chamber of the heart but which does not completely obliterate the lumen, e.g. thrombus overlying a myocardial infarction.

BALL THROMBUS
An unattached spherical thrombus within the cavity of the atrium too large to pass through the valve orifice and which may thus cause intermittent valvular obstruction (see p. 251).

SEPTIC THROMBUS
A thrombus may form as a result of infection or a previously bland thrombus may subsequently become secondarily infected (see p. 277).

Predisposing factors

CHANGES IN VESSEL WALL
Any factor or disease which disturbs the smooth integrity of the vessel wall and its endothelial surface predisposes to platelet deposition.
(a) *Damage to wall.* Trauma, infection, external pressure.
(b) *Disease of vessel.* Atheroma, polyarteritis nodosa.

CHANGES IN BLOOD FLOW
(a) *General.* Stasis is the most important factor, e.g. venous stasis in leg veins in congestive heart failure, or dehydration.
(b) *Local.* Stasis may again be important, e.g. in leg veins post-operatively.

Local turbulence produced by distortion of the vascular lumen from narrowing or dilatation, predisposes to thrombus formation, e.g. rigid valves, walls of aneurysms.

CHANGES IN COMPOSITION OF BLOOD
(a) *Platelets.* Following surgery, childbirth or severe haemorrhage, the platelets may be transiently increased in number, and clotting is thereby promoted. A raised platelet count may be persistent in polycythaemia rubra vera, and prolonged for a considerable time after splenectomy.
(b) *Polycythaemia.* Apart from the raised platelet count, the blood is more viscous, flow may be reduced and red cell clumping occurs.
(c) *Plasma proteins.* In conditions such as macroglobulinaemia increased viscosity promotes stasis and thrombosis (see p. 471).

Fate of thrombus

ORGANIZATION
A thrombus becomes organized by fibroblasts and capillaries growing in at the point of attachment. The fibrous area so produced may later calcify to form a phlebolith or be recanalized by multiple narrow endothelial-lined channels to restore the continuity of the blood flow. In arteries, this recanalization seldom leads to any significant re-establishment of the circulation.

DETACHMENT
A portion of the friable thrombus may become detached and form an embolus. This may occur in

any situation but most commonly complicates a mural thrombus of the ventricle following cardiac infarction, from the atrial appendage associated with fibrillation, and from leg vein thrombosis to produce pulmonary infarcts. Detachment commonly results from propagation of thrombus when the advancing end reaches the junction with a larger vein.

INFECTION
Infected thrombus becomes softened by proteolytic ferments and portions may become detached to produce:
(a) Septic infarction.
(b) Pyaemic abscesses.
(c) Other embolic phenomena, e.g. mycotic aneurysms, Osler's nodes.

Embolism

Definition
Embolism is the impaction in some part of the vascular system of any undissolved material brought there by the blood stream. This definition therefore includes many types of emboli of varying composition, the commonest being a thrombus.

THROMBUS

Venous thrombosis

SITES
(a) Leg veins.
(b) Pelvic veins. Prostatic plexus, uterine, vesical or pelvic vessels.
(c) Intracranial venous sinuses. Rare

RESULTS
Dislodgement results in an embolus being transported towards the heart thence through the right site of the heart to:
1 Occlude pulmonary vessels:
(a) 'Saddle embolus' obstructing the bifurcation.
(b) Occlude main pulmonary trunks.
(c) Occlude smaller pulmonary arteries.
2 Paradoxical embolus. By passing through a patent foramen ovale into the left side of the heart and thus to the systemic arteries. This is very rare.

Arterial thrombosis

SITES
(a) *Heart*. Vegetations on mitral and aortic valve cusps; mural thrombus on ventricular wall following cardiac infarction; thrombosis in atrial appendages or on the left atrial wall in mitral stenosis and atrial fibrillation.
(b) *Arteries*. Thrombus superimposed on arterial disease, particularly atheroma.

RESULTS
Detachment of the thrombus to lodge in branches of systemic arteries in the brain, kidney, spleen, etc., or to obstruct the aortic bifurcation – 'saddle embolus', or more distally in the limb vessels.

FAT EMBOLISM

Nature
Globules of fat (and more rarely bone marrow) circulating in the blood stream with subsequent impaction.

Causes
1 *Fractures*. Nearly all cases are due to fractures through long bones containing fatty marrow, especially the femur and tibia.
2 *Burns*. Occurs when extensive burns involve subcutaneous fat.

Clinical
Pulmonary involvement leads to dyspnoea and rarely, if severe, to death. The most important effect of systemic fat embolism is cerebral involvement. Signs of cerebral irritation may ensue 24–48 hours after injury, and in severe cases coma is followed by death.

Diagnosis
This may sometimes be confirmed by examination of urine and sputum for fat globules, but the tests are unreliable.

Organ changes
The changes are seldom very obvious and fat stains on frozen section material are usually necessary to demonstrate the fat emboli in the small vessels of the affected organ:
1 *Brain*. Multiple petechial haemorrhages diffusely scattered throughout the cerebral substance.

The fat globules are able to traverse the pulmonary capillaries by moulding of their shape and thus particles of 15 μm or more may gain access to the systemic circulation.

2 *Lungs*. These are heavy, occasionally show petechial haemorrhages or may appear normal. However, some are detectably greasy on palpation of the cut surface.

3 *Kidneys*. Usually appear macroscopically normal.

Pathogenesis

The mechanisms is not fully understood. It seems clear that mechanical entry of fatty tissue into the venous system is of greatest importance, but occasionally the degree of trauma appears inadequate to account for the severity of the lesion. It has been proposed that fat emboli may in fact be composed of aggregated chylomicrons derived from circulating blood lipids, but experimental evidence does not support this. It has also been suggested that the effects of fat embolism are due more to the toxic effect on vascular endothelium of fatty acids than to simple ischaemia.

Results

It is probable that minor degrees of fat embolism occur in most fractures of long bones but only rarely is this clinically apparent. The mortality rate of clinically symptomatic cases is high, particularly when cerebral signs develop.

GASEOUS EMBOLISM

Air

AETIOLOGY

Air bubbles in the blood act as non-compressible physical masses which may coalesce and produce obstruction or result in the production of a frothy non-expulsive mass in the chambers of the heart, thus impeding the circulation. It seems probable that more than 100 ml of gas must be introduced into the circulation before detectable effects occur. Significant quantities of gas may gain entry from:

1 Incision of large neck veins due to surgery or suicidal cut throat.

2 Intravenous therapy using grossly faulty apparatus or technique.

3 Procedures involving injection of air or gas, e.g. pneumoperitoneum, pneumothorax, insufflation of fallopian tubes, presacral oxygen insufflation, etc.

4 Separation of the placenta during labour when the uterine contractions raise the intra-uterine pressure, especially when the foetal head is enagaged.

5 Chest injuries involving lung and chest wall when air may be absorbed into the blood stream during the negative pressure phase of respiration.

6 In cerebral surgery through open veins or venous sinuses.

ORGAN CHANGES

At post-mortem, numerous blood vessels are filled with bubbles of gas and affected organs, particularly the brain, may show petechial haemorrhages. In order to establish the diagnosis the body must be opened under water when bubbles will escape from the incised blood vessels and the heart.

Nitrogen – Caisson disease

AETIOLOGY

Decompression sickness or Caisson disease occurs in those working in increased atmospheric pressure, e.g. divers and underwater construction workers. At high pressure there is increased solution of atmospheric gases in the blood. If the return towards lower pressure is too rapid, dissolved oxygen, carbon dioxide and nitrogen come out of solution as bubbles of gas. The oxygen and carbon dioxide are rapidly reabsorbed, but the inert nitrogen remains in the tissues with a particular affinity for fat, e.g. subcutaneous tissue, nervous system.

RESULTS

Gas bubbles in the bones and joints produce '*the bends*'. Those in the brain produce mental disturbances and even coma, whilst bubbles in the lung vessels result in '*the chokes*'. Infarction of the ends of long bones may occur, with destruction of articular surfaces, and involvement of the spinal cord leads to paraplegia. The condition can be relieved by placing the patient in a decompression chamber with subsequent slow decompression to allow time for reabsorption of the nitrogen to occur.

AMNIOTIC EMBOLISM

Nature

This occurs during labour due to the entry of

amniotic fluid into the circulation with subsequent lung involvement. This may give rise to three different manifestations.

Types

1 Patients develop sudden respiratory distress during the first stage of labour. They may die immediately or survive for a few hours, whilst others develop severe shock which may be successfully treated. At post-mortem the pulmonary vessels are found to be plugged by keratin and lanugo from the amniotic fluid.

2 Other patients develop multiple intravascular capillary thromboses. This is due to the sudden release of amniotic fluid, with its high content of thromboplastins, into the maternal circulation and thus initiating intravascular clotting.

3 A few patients develop depletion of blood fibrinogen with resulting bleeding tendencies which may prove fatal (see p. 531).

Pathogenesis

During labour the engagement of the foetal head in the lower uterine segment acts as the 'cork'. With uterine contractions creating a high pressure in the uterus, the amniotic fluid is forced into the blood stream via open maternal placental sinuses.

TUMOUR EMBOLISM

In some instances of blood-borne tumour metastases, the tumour fragments may be sufficiently large to cause manifestations on impaction. This may occur with renal carcinoma growing along the renal vein into the inferior vena cava and with bronchial carcinoma in the pulmonary vessels. Compared with the high incidence of metastases by single cells or small groups of cells, this is extremely uncommon.

TISSUE FRAGMENTS

Fragments of necrotic tissue, e.g. atheroma, liver following liver biopsy or trauma, may become dislodged and produce emboli.

PARASITES

Clumps of parasites may circulate in the blood stream and produce embolic manifestations, e.g. cerebral malaria (see p. 65).

INFECTED EMBOLI

These may arise from infected thrombus or from vegetations in infective endocarditis to result in infarction and infection at the site of impaction.

EFFECTS OF EMBOLISM

The effects of emboli depend on many factors particularly:
(a) Site of origin – arteries or veins.
(b) Site of impaction.
(c) Collateral circulation.
(d) Infection – aseptic (bland) or septic.

Sudden Death

This may be due to:
(a) Pulmonary embolism.
(b) Cerebral embolism (see p. 599).
(c) Coronary embolism – a very rare cause of coronary occlusion.

PULMONARY EMBOLISM
This is the most common and most important.

Incidence
It is estimated that about 0.5 per cent of all hospital admissions die from pulmonary embolism and that this accounts for between 5 and 10 per cent of all post-operative deaths.

Predisposing factor
Venous thrombosis, especially in the legs.

Macroscopical
Occlusion of one or both pulmonary vessels by embolic thrombus having the dimensions of the vein of origin. The lungs frequently show no abnormalities but may reveal some congestion and oedema or be dry and bloodless. Areas of recent infarction may be present due to previous small emboli.

Nil

No clinical or pathological manifestations may be apparent if the embolus lodges and blocks a small vessel where the collateral blood supply maintains an adequate nutrition of the affected tissues, e.g. skeletal muscles, intestines, etc.

Infarction

Embolic occlusion of the vessel supplying a part or whole of an organ will, in the absence of adequate collateral circulation, result in death of the affected tissue – *infarction* (see p. 131).

Obstruction to a limb artery

If the brachial or femoral artery is blocked, the limb becomes cold, pale, numb and weak with absent distal pulsations. If the collateral blood supply is adequate and the blood vessels are healthy, sufficient circulation will develop to restore the limb to clinical normality. If the blood supply remains inadequate, death of the limb will occur – *gangrene*.

Chapter 25
Circulatory Disorders – Gangrene: Infarction

Gangrene

Definition
Death of tissue in bulk, often with putrefaction.

Types

DRY GANGRENE
Death of a part, usually a limb, due to ischaemia in the absence of gross oedema or infection. The limb mummifies and there is a line of demarcation due to an inflammatory reaction at the junction of the living and dead tissues. This is the appearance which usually follows a gradual arterial occlusion.

MOIST GANGRENE
The swollen putrefying part, organ, or limb which follows arterial, or sometimes venous, occlusion complicated by an infection, frequently by saprophytic organisms. This is commonly seen in strangulation of the intestine but may result in a limb infection of a previously dry gangrene.

Causes

VASCULAR
(a) *Vessel disease*, e.g. atheroma, aneurysm, arterial and venous thrombosis, connective tissue diseases, etc.
(b) *Vascular spasm*, e.g. Raynaud's phenomenon, ergot poisoning.
(c) *External pressure*, e.g. tumour, cervical rib, bandage, tourniquet, plaster, haematoma, ligature, torsion of pedicle, strangulation.
(d) *Embolism*.

TRAUMATIC
For example, crushing injuries with deprivation of blood supply, bed sores, etc.

PHYSIO-CHEMICAL
For example, heat, cold, acids, alkalis, X-rays, etc.

INFECTIVE
For example, acute pyogenic (carbuncle); severe infection with vascular thrombosis (gangrenous appendix); clostridial infection (gas gangrene).

NERVOUS DISEASES
For example, syringomyelia and tabes dorsalis associated with sensory nerve loss – 'trophic ulcers'.

Effects

LOCAL

(*a*) Necrosis of tissues, often accompanied by pain.

(*b*) Ulceration.

(*c*) Infection and suppuration.

(*d*) Functional loss.

(*e*) Perforation of hollow viscera, e.g. gangrenous intestine with peritonitis.

GENERAL

Absorption of products of tissue breakdown and infection causing serious systemic effects from which death may ensue.

GAS GANGRENE

Aetiology

Anaerobic spore-bearing clostridia, especially *Clostridia perfringens* (*welchii*), *C. novyi* (*oedematiens*), *C. septicum* and *C. sporogenes*.

Predisposing factors

Compound fractures, penetrating and other injuries where there is impairment of the blood supply or inadequate *débridement* of devitalized tissue encouraging the establishment of the infection. The presence of blood clot, dead tissue, foreign bodies and implanted dirt predispose to the anoxic conditions necessary for multiplication of the clostridia.

Macroscopical

The area is painful, rapidly enlarging and exudes a foul-smelling sero-sanguinous discharge. The tissue passes through stages of discolouration and crepitus, due to gas formation.

Microscopical

The connective tissue and muscles are oedematous and necrotic with a non-specific inflammatory reaction and gas production. There is lysis of red cells and destruction of blood vessels with areas of thrombosis. Numerous gram-positive organisms are present but usually there is a paucity of inflammatory cells.

Pathogenesis

The clinical condition of gas gangrene is produced by a variety of bacterial enzymes and toxins. These include saccharolytic and proteolytic enzymes, fibrinolysin, hyaluronidase, haemolysins and lecithinase which is the α-toxin. These ferments break down the infected tissues and produce further anaerobic areas enhancing progressive spread.

Results

Unless dramatically treated, the infection spreads rapidly and the disease becomes generalized with gas production in the viscera, including the liver and spleen, following blood dissemination. The haemolysins are absorbed, resulting in systemic haemolysis with staining of the vascular endothelium and producing a rapid fall in the Hb level. There is a profound toxaemia and death rapidly follows this generalization.

Infarction

Definition

An area of ischaemic necrosis produced by deprivation of the blood supply. This is usually induced by embolism or thrombosis.

Predisposing factors

Infarction only occurs in areas where, following blockage of a vessel, there is inadequate collateral circulation to maintain the life of the tissues. Thus many organs of rich vascularity are only rarely the site of infarcts, e.g. skin, thyroid, liver. It is, therefore, in tissues with so-called 'end-arteries' that infarction most commonly occurs.

Types

1 *Aseptic.*

2 *Septic.*

Each of these may be:

(*a*) Pale or anaemic, e.g. kidney, spleen, heart, brain.

(*b*) Red or haemorrhagic, e.g. lung, intestine.

This is an unsatisfactory descriptive subdivision as the colour of the infarct is dependent only on the amount of blood which passes into the area of tissue death. All infarcts are red initially, but in solid organs rapid tissue coagulation allows fewer red cells to enter the area and they therefore appear paler at an earlier stage than in less solid organs.

Macroscopical

Infarcts involve the periphery of a solid organ to

produce a wedge-shaped area having the base on the capsular aspect and the apex at the site of vascular obstruction. The surface is slightly raised above the surrounding tissues. Following vascular occlusion, the blood pressure in the ischaemic area falls, but the adjacent viable tissues have a normal blood pressure so that, in the early stages, there is a suffusion of red cells from the adjacent living tissues into the dead area. Where there is a serosal surface, a fibrinous exudate frequently forms and there is also an hyperaemic zone, due to an inflammatory response, at the junction of the living and dead tissues.

Microscopical

In all tissues except the C.N.S., the cells of an infarct undergo coagulative necrosis. In the first few hours, the infarct is stuffed with blood, but after 24 hours the cell cytoplasm becomes coagulated and granular and the nuclei show *pyknosis* and *karyorrhexis*. In addition, there will be a variable number of red cells present, intact in the early stages, but showing lysis from about 24 hours onwards. Later still, haemosiderin will be visible. At the margin there is a vascular inflammatory reaction which gradually extends into the infarcted area.

Fate of infarcts

Very small infarcts may become softened and subsequently be absorbed. The usual end result is the phagocytic removal of the dead tissue followed by organization of the area by repair tissues which grow in from the margins. Finally, there remains a pale depressed scar at the site of the infarct.

Organ changes

1 *Renal infarct*. A pale, wedge-shaped area involving mainly the cortex and usually sharply demarcated by an hyperaemic zone. There is a separate renal capsular blood supply so that the capsule and the immediate subcapsular tissues remain healthy and usually there is no pain.

2 *Splenic infarct*. This may occasionally be red but is usually pale and there is involvement of the capsule with production of pain and a fibrinous exudate on the peritoneal surface. Splenic infarcts, like normal splenic tissue, frequently soften due to autolysis after death and thus aseptic infarcts may be difficult to differentiate from septic infarcts on macroscopic appearances alone.

3 *Cardiac infarct*. If the thrombotic obstruction produces sudden death there may be no detectable abnormality in the myocardium. Later, acute myocardial infarction appears as a pale yellow area of soft muscle – *myomalacia cordis*, with red foci. If the endocardium is involved, there may be mural thrombus deposition and if the pericardium is affected, a fibrinous pericarditis (see p. 233).

4 *Liver infarct*. Infarction is rare due to the dual blood supply from both portal and hepatic vessels. Infarction does occur when there is some predisposing disturbance of this blood supply, e.g. tumours, and the infarct may be red or anaemic.

5 *Lung infarct*. This is the most common site of infarction in spite of a dual blood supply from the pulmonary and bronchial arteries. A pulmonary infarct shows the classical red appearance with a pyramidal shape and pleural involvement which produces pleural pain (see p. 649).

6 *Intestinal infarct*. This may be due to venous occlusion, e.g. in torsion, volvulus or strangulation, or to arterial occlusion by thrombus or embolus. It is haemorrhagic in type as venous occlusion produces gross congestion and oedema due to over-filling of the affected portion of the gut by arterial blood, followed by stagnant anoxia and tissue death. Occlusion of a mesenteric artery results in a fall of pressure, reflux of portal venous blood, congestion, stagnation and anoxia with tissue death (see p. 195).

7 *C.N.S. infarct*. This is the underlying pathology of many cases of hemiplegia and is very common.

(a) *Cerebral softening*. This is due to cerebral artery occlusion by thrombosis or embolism or to ischaemia caused by occlusive disease of the carotid or vertebral vessels in the neck. There results an area of colliquative necrosis visible as cerebral softening. The myelin is phagocytosed by microglia which become laden with fatty material – 'compound granular corpuscles'. Later, the neuroglia of the surrounding tissue proliferate – *gliosis*, to enclose a cystic cavity containing yellow fluid – 'apoplectic cyst' (see p. 599).

(b) *Spinal cord*. Similar changes occur, resulting in partial or complete transection of the cord.

(c) *Central artery of the retina*. Thrombotic or embolic obstruction of the central artery produces a haemorrhage at the macula, necrosis of the retina and blindness.

SEPTIC INFARCTION

Causes
Septic infarction is due to:
(*a*) An infected embolus.
(*b*) Secondary infection of an established infarct.

Macroscopical
The basic changes are those of an aseptic infarct but the infection results in liquefaction of the necrotic area and abscess formation.

Microscopical
There is nuclear and cytoplasmic death of the tissue with the additional features of a pyogenic inflammation within the infarcted tissues.

Chapter 26
Abnormalities of Cell Growth

Aplasia – Agenesis

Definition
Aplasia or agenesis is the failure of development of a tissue or an organ.

Aetiology
A developmental abnormality, presumably occurring early in intra-uterine life.

Organs
Aplastic organs are either totally absent or are represented by a small mass of fibrous or fatty tissue containing a few rudimentary cells. The commoner clinical examples occur in paired organs, e.g. adrenal, kidney and lungs, with no immediate clinical effect. When such tissues as the pituitary and aorta are aplastic, however, the lesion is incompatible with life.

Hypoplasia

Definition
Hypoplasia is the failure of organs to develop to full size.

Aetiology
A developmental abnormality less severe than aplasia.

134

Organs

Rudimentary organs are found which are smaller than normal and lack their full complement of cells. Function may therefore be reduced and hypoplasia usually affects the same paired and unpaired organs as aplasia.

Atrophy

Definition

Atrophy implies an acquired change in a previously normal tissue and is the subsequent decrease in the size of an organ or tissue. The reduction in size may be due to a decrease in the number or the size of individual cells, or both.

Types

PHYSIOLOGICAL

Atrophy occurs in many tissues as a normal manifestation, e.g. the thymus gland and lymphoid tissue following puberty, the ovaries at the menopause and most tissues with increasing age.

NUTRITIONAL

Inadequate or abnormal dietary intake will lead to wasting, e.g. in starvation.

VASCULAR

Vascular disease producing ischaemia leads to loss of tissue cells.

DISUSE

Disuse atrophy occurs in a paralysed limb, in the muscles in rheumatoid arthritis or in any other tissue where functional activity is reduced.

PRESSURE

Prolonged pressure produces atrophy, e.g. aneurysm of aorta on the sternum or spine, corsets pressing ribs into the liver and 'cough furrows' on the liver surface. This probably mediates through vascular insufficiency due to the pressure.

INFECTIONS

In prolonged infectious diseases, particularly those associated with toxaemia, alterations of metabolism and depletion of nutritional reserves predispose to atrophy, e.g. tuberculosis, etc.

ENDOCRINE

Involution of breast and the uterus at the menopause and many endocrine organs in hypopituitarism, due to loss of trophic hormones.

METABOLIC

Severe uncontrolled generalized metabolic disturbances may cause severe wasting and organ atrophy, e.g. diabetes mellitus, thyrotoxicosis, malabsorption syndrome, etc.

MALIGNANT DISEASE

Association with the 'cachexia' of malignant disease (see p. 159).

Macroscopical

The affected tissues or organs are smaller than normal but usually retain their normal shape.

Microscopical

There are fewer cells than normal and these cells are smaller than normal. The tissue may, however, appear more cellular due to the diminished amount of cytoplasm surrounding the remaining nuclei.

Nature

The differing types already listed are based on clinical varieties but the basic aetiology is a deprivation of blood supply or nutritional requirements to the tissue with resultant atrophy.

Hypertrophy and hyperplasia

Definition

Hypertrophy. An increase in the size of the tissues due to an increase in individual cell size.
Hyperplasia. An increase in the size of the tissues due to increase in total cell numbers.

Frequently these two changes occur simultaneously in the tissues but hypertrophy occurs alone in those tissues which are incapable of regeneration, e.g. cardiac muscle.

Types

The main factors are work load or endocrine stimulation, giving rise to the following types:

ENDOCRINE

For example, breast in lactation; many organs in acromegaly.

COMPENSATORY
The kidney, when the other kidney is hypoplastic or has been removed; the fibula following destruction of the tibia, etc.

FUNCTIONAL
For example, the left ventricular myocardium in hypertension or aortic stenosis; the athletic individual with muscular hypertrophy in response to exercise; the bladder wall following prostatic obstruction, etc.

REPLACEMENT
As part of the repair process, e.g. healing of a liver defect by regeneration.

REACTIVE
For example, reactive hyperplasia of the lymphoid tissue and bone marrow in response to infection or anaemia.

NEOPLASTIC
Tumours are formed as a result of localized areas of increase in cell numbers. Although characteristically this neoplasia is uncontrolled hyperplasia with no physiological function, the borderline between neoplasia and hyperplasia is not always sharply defined.

Metaplasia

Definition
Metaplasia is the change from one type of cell to another. It is usually reversible and is most commonly seen as a change from more specialized to less specialized cells, e.g. columnar or transitional cell types to squamous epithelium.

EPITHELIAL METAPLASIA

Aetiology
Prolonged irritation or chronic infection, e.g. calculi in urinary or biliary tracts, bronchiectasis.

Sites
Endocervix, gall bladder, urinary bladder, renal pelvis, respiratory tract, stomach, small and large intestine.

Changes
The original mucosa, usually columnar or transitional, changes to squamous epithelium. In the stomach there is a change from the specialized acid or enzyme-secreting epithelium to a colonic and only mucus-secreting type – 'intestinal metaplasia', (see p. 190).

CONNECTIVE TISSUE METAPLASIA

Aetiology
Most commonly found in association with repair processes.

Changes
Fibroblasts retain their mesenchymal ability to change into other connective tissue cells, e.g. osteoblasts. Thus fibrous tissue may metaplase to bone, or to fibrocartilage as in replacement of a removed semilunar cartilage in the knee.

Results of metaplasia

The squamous epithelium resulting from the metaplasia may undergo malignant change, e.g. squamous cell carcinomas of bronchus, renal pelvis and gall bladder, but the metaplasia may be reversible if its cause is removed.

Dysplasia

Definition
Dysplasia is an alteration in the size, shape and orientation of epithelial cells.

Aetiology
Commonly associated with chronic irritation or inflammation but sometimes occurs with no apparent cause.

Sites
Epithelium of cervix (see p. 420), skin, oesophagus, endometrium, etc.

Changes
Instead of the orderly pattern of squamous epithelium with a basal cell layer, prickle cell layer and horn cells in a regular sequence, or the regimented orderly columns of columnar epithelium, the cells

become disorderly showing disruption of the normal progression of cell layers and with variation in size, shape and staining of the individual cells. These cells may increase in number with thickening of the epithelium and, in squamous epithelium, the basal cells frequently show a marked increase in their number. In addition, mitotic activity is increased and mitotic figures may appear abnormal. Some features of maturation, however, remain.

Results

This is usually a reversible change and, particularly if the chronic irritation or inflammation is successfully treated, the epithelium can return to normal. The changes may, however, persist and ultimately progress to malignancy.

Neoplasia – tumours

Definition

There are many definitions of neoplasia:
1 An autonomous parasite.
2 A new growth arising from pre-existing tissue, independent of the needs of the organism and subserving no useful physiological function.
3 'A tumour is an abnormal mass of tissue, the growth of which exceeds and is unco-ordinated with that of normal tissues, and persists in the same excessive manner after cessation of the stimuli which evoked the change' (Willis).

CLASSIFICATION

There is no uniformity of opinion regarding the best method of tumour classification. A complete form lists every known type of tumour and becomes a catalogue, whilst the shorter methods are inevitably incomplete. The following compromise is adopted and is based on the tissue of origin.

Connective tissue
(*a*) *Benign*. Lipoma, chondroma, osteoma, etc.
(*b*) *Malignant*. Liposarcoma, chondrosarcoma, osteosarcoma.

Epithelium
(*a*) *Benign*. Papilloma, adenoma.
(*b*) *Malignant*. Carcinoma.

Lymphoid tissue
(*a*) *Benign*. Benign lymphoid lesions.
(*b*) *Malignant*. Malignant lymphoma.

Naevus cells
(*a*) *Benign*. Benign pigmented naevus.
(*b*) *Malignant*. Malignant melanoma.

Nervous system
Meningioma, glioma, neuroblastoma, etc.

Teratomas and embryonal tumours
(*a*) *Benign*. Benign teratoma, e.g. ovarian dermoid.
(*b*) *Malignant*. Malignant teratoma, Wilms' tumour (nephroblastoma).

Endothelium
(*a*) *Benign*. Haemangioma, lymphangioma.
(*b*) *Malignant*. Haemangiosarcoma.

Chapter 27
Tumours – Comparisons Between Benign and Malignant Tumours

Structure
 Benign
 Malignant
Mode of growth
 Benign
 Malignant
Rate of growth
 Benign
 Malignant
Continuation of growth
 Benign
 Malignant
Metastases
 Benign
 Malignant
Clinical results
 Benign
 Malignant

**Characteristics of
 malignancy**
Invasion of tissue
Evidence of atypical structure
 Differentiated
 Undifferentiated
Evidence of rapid growth
Evidence of irregular cell growth
Atypical blood vessels
Metastases

**Spread of malignant
 tumours**
Direct spread
 Expansion
 Invasion
Lymphatic spread
Blood spread
Implantation
 Natural
 Induced
Transcoelomic spread
 Peritoneum
 Pleura
 Pericardium

This section indicates only the major differences between benign and malignant tumours. These generalizations are sometimes subject to uncommon exceptions which will be specified subsequently in the appropriate sections.

Structure

BENIGN
Attain a high degree of structural differentiation and thus closely resemble their tissue of origin. A lipoma therefore looks like fat and a colonic adenoma is readily recognizable as being of glandular tissue origin.

MALIGNANT
There are varying degrees of imperfect differentiation, varying from the well-differentiated tumour, e.g. keratin-forming squamous cell carcinoma, through all stages of dedifferentiation to the anaplastic tumour.

Mode of growth

BENIGN
Grows by expansion with compression of adjacent tissues which form a capsule.

MALIGNANT
Grows by expansion but extends by invasion. The tumour cells are not confined by a capsule and infiltrate between the adjacent tissue cells which they destroy.

Rate of growth

BENIGN
Usually slowly growing and showing an increased number of mitoses but these are of normal appearance.

MALIGNANT
Frequently rapidly growing, usually with numerous and abnormal mitotic figures.

Continuation of growth

BENIGN

Usually continue to grow slowly. However, growth may stop after a variable period of time or spontaneous regression may occur, e.g. thyroid adenoma, fibroids of uterus and some meningiomas.

MALIGNANT

Continue to grow, if untreated, until death occurs and only very rarely does spontaneous regression occur.

Metastases

BENIGN

Never metastasize; if this occurs, the diagnosis is incorrect.

MALIGNANT

Almost all malignant tumours will eventually metastasize if left untreated, although some tumours, e.g. basal cell carcinomas and adamantinomas, are predominantly of local malignancy only and thus only rarely metastasize.

Clinical results

RENIGN

Benign tumours are harmless except:

By virtue of position, e.g. brain, mediastinum, etc., thus interfering with the function of vital structures.

By incidental complications, e.g. torsion, haemorrhage, ulceration, infection, intussusception.

By hormone production, e.g. pituitary, pancreatic, adrenal and parathyroid adenomas.

By subsequent malignant change, e.g. intestinal polypi, naevi, chondroma, etc.

MALIGNANT

These may result in similar manifestations as above but also kill by virtue of their invasiveness and their ability to metastasize.

Characteristics of malignancy

Invasion of tissue

The presence of invasion is indicative of malignancy (see p. 140).

Evidence of atypical structure

(a) *Differentiated tumours.* These, imperfectly but recognizably, reproduce adult tissue, e.g. glandular tubules in adenocarcinoma, keratin in squamous cell carcinoma, etc., through varying grades of dedifferentiation to:

(b) *Undifferentiated tumours.* These have no resemblance to adult tissues, e.g. anaplastic carcinoma or spindle-cell sarcoma.

Histological grading of the malignancy of a tumour relies mainly on the degree of differentiation observed.

Evidence of rapid growth

The presence of many mitotic figures indicates rapid cell division and therefore rapid tissue growth. An increased mitotic rate does not necessarily indicate that malignant change has occurred in a tissue, although it is a strong pointer, particularly if abnormal mitotic figures are seen.

Evidence of irregular cell growth

The tumour cells show abnormal features indicative of irregular growth. These histological features include hyperchromatism of nuclei, irregularity of size, shape and staining of the cells, increase of nuclear:cytoplasmic ratio, giant or bilobed nuclei, tumour giant cells (see Fig. 6 on p. 24), prominent and large nucleoli and abnormal mitotic figures, e.g. triradiate mitoses.

Atypical blood vessels

All tumours require a blood supply which is additional to the normal vascularity of the area, but in malignant tumours the actual blood vessels may show structural abnormalities with deficiency of their wall or endothelial lining. In very rapidly growing sarcomas, the tumour cells may line the vascular channels so that neoplastic cells are in direct contact with the blood stream. Rapidly growing tumours commonly outstrip their blood supply, resulting in necrosis, most marked in the centre.

Metastases

A metastasis is a secondary deposit of tumour derived from the primary neoplasm but separate from its primary site of origin.

Spread of malignant tumours

The basic behaviour of a particularly malignant

tumour depends largely upon its ability to invade and metastasize. The methods of spread are as follows.

Direct spread

EXPANSION

As a result of cell proliferation, the tumour increases in bulk and expands to compress the adjacent tissues which may then react to form an apparent capsule, e.g. renal carcinoma. This capsule, is, however, incomplete due to the associated tumour cell infiltration.

INVASION

Direct infiltration in continuity by the proliferating tumour cells occurs between the cells of the adjacent tissue. Considerable variation in resistance to this invasion is shown by different tissues. Thus, direct spread occurs more rapidly through loose connective tissues and along tissue planes than in compact structures such as bone, cartilage or fascia. As a result the shape of a tumour may be moulded at points of contact with these relatively resistant tissues. No tissues, however, are inviolate from invasion and the local infiltration results eventually in destruction of the adjacent tissue and in fixation of the tumour to other structures in the area.

Lymphatic spread

Small groups of tumour cells infiltrating tissue spaces gain access to the lymphatic vessels and are carried as tumour emboli within the lumen to the regional lymph nodes draining the site of origin of the tumour, where they may be arrested. The tumour cells are first visible in the peripheral sinus of the lymph node where they form separate tumours. Eventually the lymph nodes may become solid with tumour and the lymph flow ceases, or the lymphatic vessels be permeated by solid cords of tumour. In these circumstances, flow of lymph may be reversed and retrograde spread of tumour cells may result, e.g. '*peau d'orange*' of the breast, lymphoedema, etc. Further lymphatic spread of tumour may result from invasion of efferent lymphatics from the lymph nodes and thus other and more distant groups of nodes become invaded. Eventually, cells may enter the thoracic duct or other major lymph channels and so reach the blood stream.

Blood spread

Bloodstream invasion occurs as a result of:

(*a*) Invasion of a blood vessel within the tumour itself, especially when the vessel wall is defective.

(*b*) Invasion of a vein by direct extension of the tumour, or by erosion of a vessel from a lymph node metastasis.

(*c*) Via the lymphatic system into the blood stream.

If the systemic venous system is involved, the lungs are the commonest site of blood-borne metastases, but if the portal venous radicles are invaded, the tumour usually metastasizes to the liver. However, following blood stream invasion, tumour deposits may form in any organ of the body. There is a considerable variation from one type of malignant tumour to another in the distribution of their metastases. As a generalization, the liver, lungs, bone and brain are the most common sites and yet metastases are only rarely found in the spleen and muscles and are uncommon in the kidneys. Thus, the volume of the blood supplied to an organ cannot be the only consideration. Furthermore, some tumours have a predilection for certain sites, e.g. prostate to bone and lung to adrenal, which are not readily explicable. A further point of note is that numerous cells gain access to the blood stream yet this may result in few, solitary or even no metastatic tumour masses. No acceptable explanation can as yet be offered for these phenomena, but obviously tumour cell characteristics and host tissue resistance factors must be both involved in the subsequent fate of blood-borne tumour cells.

Implantation

The tumour may spread as a result of implantation of viable tumour cells in a tissue distant from the primary tumour but occurring without lymphatic or blood invasion. This may occur by:

NATURAL IMPLANTATION

Tumours on the surface of a hollow structure exfoliate and the viable cells, carried in the contents within the lumen, implant elsewhere, e.g. carcinoma of renal pelvis to bladder, carcinoma of bladder to urethra, carcinoma of bowel to implant into a *fistula-in-ano*, medulloblastoma with 'seedlings' in the spinal subarachnoid space.

INDUCED IMPLANTATION

As a result of surgical intervention, viable tumour cells may 'contaminate' the wound at the time of operation and there become established, grow and produce clinical recurrence at a later date. This can occur as tumour nodules in the scar of a mastectomy, at the site of anastomosis following resection for intestinal carcinomas and at any other site where raw or granulating areas form a suitable 'soil' for tumour cell implantation.

Transcoelomic spread

The occurrence of separate nodules of tumour as a result of spread across a body cavity.

PERITONEUM

Carcinomatosis peritonei frequently follows a primary tumour of the stomach, ovary or intestine which has invaded the serosal coat.

PLEURA

Multiple tumour nodules on the visceral and parietal pleura are frequently due to spread from a primary or secondary lung tumour.

PERICARDIUM

This is uncommon except when the pericardium is invaded by a carcinoma of the bronchus, or tumour has invaded the mediastinal lymph nodes.

In each case, the serous cavity lining becomes studded with tumour nodules and there is frequently a reactive exudate containing malignant cells.

Chapter 28
Benign and Malignant Epithelial Tumours

Benign epithelial tumours

SURFACE EPITHELIUM –
PAPILLOMA
Nature
Squamous cell papilloma
    Sites
    Microscopical
Transitional cell papilloma
    Sites
    Microscopical

GLANDULAR EPITHELIUM –
ADENOMA OR PAPILLOMA
Nature
Adenoma
    Sites
    Microscopical
Cystadenoma
    Sites
    Microscopical
Papilloma
    Sites
    Microscopical

Papillary cystadenoma
    Sites
    Microscopical

**Malignant epithelial
tumours**
Nature
Features
Squamous cell carcinoma
    Sites
    Macroscopical
    Microscopical
Transitional cell carcinoma
    Sites
    Macroscopical
    Microscopical
Adenocarcinoma
    Nature
    Sites
    Macroscopical

Microscopical
    Tubular adenocarcinoma
    Papillary adenocarcinoma
    Papillary cystadeno-
        carcinoma
    Mucoid carcinoma
    Clear cell carcinoma
Carcinoid tumours and
APUDomas
    Nature
    Distribution
    Microscopical
    Function
    Behaviour
Basal cell carcinoma –
rodent ulcer
    Sites
    Macroscopical
    Microscopical
Mucous gland tumours
Choriocarcinoma
    Nature
    Sites
    Microscopical

Benign epithelial tumours

TUMOURS OF SURFACE
EPITHELIUM – PAPILLOMA

Nature
A papilloma is a simple epithelial tumour which
projects from an epithelial surface and is covered by
squamous, transitional or columnar epithelium,
according to its tissue of origin.

Squamous cell papilloma

SITES
Common skin tumours but they can arise from any
other squamous-covered surface, e.g. tongue,
larynx, etc.

MICROSCOPICAL
There is regular overgrowth of the squamous
epithelium in the form of papillary fronds, frequently with hyperkeratosis. The basement membrane remains intact.

Transitional cell papilloma

SITES
Arise anywhere within the urinary tract. They are
often multiple and usually have a narrow pedicle
and long villous processes.

MICROSCOPICAL
The transitional epithelium is papillary and the
fronds have a delicate connective tissue core in
which there are thin-walled blood vessels. They

commonly produce haematuria and frequently recur after removal. Differentiation from transitional cell carcinoma may be impracticable, and clinically all transitional cell papillomas are regarded as malignant growths (see p. 389).

TUMOURS OF GLANDULAR EPITHELIUM – ADENOMA OR PAPILLOMA

Nature
These are benign tumours derived from glandular columnar cell epithelium. In general adenomas reproduce the tubular structure of the parent tissue, whilst papillomas take on a fronded finger-like appearance.

Adenoma

SITES
Arise from any glandular structure and are most commonly found in the intestine, pituitary, pancreas, parathyroid, salivary gland and thyroid.

MICROSCOPICAL
The tumour tissue consists of well differentiated tubular or acinar structures which reproduce with variable exactitude the glandular tissue of origin so that it may be difficult to distinguish in some cases between the tumour and normal tissue. Adenomas do not form ducts, so that, if secretion continues, areas of cystic dilatation may result – *cystadenoma*.

Cystadenoma

SITES
These are most commonly found in the ovary but also occur in the breast, thyroid, pancreas, etc.

MICROSCOPICAL
An adenoma in which there develops single or multiple cysts.

Papilloma

SITES
May arise from the surface of any glandular epithelium, but are found mainly in small and large intestine, breast and thyroid.

MICROSCOPICAL
The fronded papillary tumour is covered by thickened but benign columnar or cuboidal epithelium. They are frequently multiple, especially in the colon – villous adenoma, and breast – intraduct papilloma.

Papillary cystadenoma

SITES
Found commonly in the ovary and in other sites of cystadenomas.

MICROSCOPICAL
The cyst contains a papillary tumour covered by columnar or cuboidal epithelium. Malignant change not uncommonly occurs with the formation of a papillary cystadenocarcinoma (see p. 144).

Malignant epithelial tumours

Nature
A malignant epithelial tumour is a carcinoma. This may arise from squamous, transitional or columnar epithelium, from an epithelial surface or from glandular tissue. Most carcinomas have the following pathological features in common:

Features
(*a*) Occur mostly over the age of 50 years.
(*b*) Growth is generally less rapid than in sarcomas.
(*c*) Spread is predominantly by local and lymphatic invasion in early stages with blood dissemination as a later manifestation.
(*d*) The stroma is fibrous and commonly abundant, separating groups or columns of the malignant epithelial cells.

Squamous cell carcinoma

SITES
Occur in situations normally covered by squamous epithelium but they also arise in areas of metaplasia of transitional epithelium, e.g. urinary tract, or metaplasia of columnar epithelium, e.g. bronchus.

MACROSCOPICAL
They may be nodular, papillary, diffusely infiltrative or ulcerative. The ulcers characteristically show induration due to local infiltration, with raised, rolled, nodular, everted edges.

MICROSCOPICAL
The commonest type is a keratinizing squamous

cell carcinoma which invades the underlying tissue in the form of 'cell nests' composed of central laminated keratin surrounded by prickle cells and an outer layer of basal cells. Depending upon the degree of differentiation, i.e. the amount of keratin and maturity of the tumour cells, four grades of malignancy are recognized; grade I being the fully keratinizing tumour of low grade malignancy and grade IV the non-keratinizing undifferentiated form of high grade malignancy, grades II and III being intermediate in differentiation and malignancy.

There are two variants of squamous cell carcinoma – 'transitional cell' and 'lymphoepithelioma'. They are both rare, occur mostly in the upper respiratory tract and pharynx and are described on p. 122.

Transitional cell carcinoma

SITES
They occur in any part of the urinary transitional epithelium – 'urothelium' – but are most frequent in the bladder.

MACROSCOPICAL
They form papillary, nodular, diffuse or ulcerated tumours and are frequently multiple.

MICROSCOPICAL
Formed by atypical transitional epithelial cells showing varying loss of polarity, and an increased mitotic rate. Three grades of differentiation are recognized, based on nuclear appearances and cytological regularity: grade I – well differentiated; grade II – moderately differentiated; grade III – poorly differentiated. In some cases squamous metaplasia occurs (see p. 339).

Adenocarcinoma

NATURE
This term is applied to tumours which form glandular structures and arise from glandular organs.

SITES
This is the commonest type of malignant tumour and arises from any columnar epithelial surface or from glandular tissue. The common sites include the breast, stomach, intestines, kidneys, uterus, thyroid, pancreas.

MACROSCOPICAL
They produce polypoid, papillary, fungating, nodular, diffusely infiltrating, stenosing, ulcerating or mucoid tumours at the site of origin.

MICROSCOPICAL
The appearances within the group of carcinomas are very variable and include the following descriptive types:

Tubular adenocarcinoma.
This is the commonest form of carcinoma and is the malignant counterpart of the benign adenoma. There is invasion of tissues by malignant, atypical, columnar epithelium forming atypical and irregular glandular structures. These tumours may be graded into degrees of malignancy by their degree of histological differentiation. The criteria are the size, uniformity and staining of the cells, their mitotic activity and the amount of tubule formation. The well-differentiated low-grade tumours are composed of comparatively regular and uniform cells with scanty mitoses and well-marked tubule formation. There are all grades of dedifferentiation with increasing cellular atypicality, lessening degree of tubule formation and greater numbers of mitoses with increasing malignancy. In this manner, the tumours are graded into: grade I – well differentiated; grade II – moderately differentiated; and grade III – poorly differentiated (anaplastic).

Papillary adenocarcinoma
This is the malignant counterpart of the benign columnar cell papilloma, from which it may arise. There is irregular hyperplasia with reduplication of the surface epithelium covering the fronds and invasion of the stroma of the stalk or the underlying tissues with penetration of the basement membrane.

Papillary cystadenocarcinoma.
Formed as a result of malignant change in a papillary cystadenoma to form a mixture of papillary and more solid areas with evidence of invasion of the adjacent tissues (see p. 433).

Mucoid carcinoma
These have a gelatinous or mucoid appearance due to the presence of abundant mucoid material produced by the epithelial cells of the tumour. They are seen most commonly in the gastro-intestinal tract or in the breast.

Clear cell carcinoma

These tumours are composed of sheets and cords of cells with clear, often granular cytoplasm due to the presence of glycogen and lipid. The most common sites are kidney and adrenal.

Carcinoid tumours and APUDomas

NATURE

Tumours which arise from cells of the *neuro-endocrine system* which is widespread throughout the body. The cells contain neurosecretory granules at electron microscopy level and can be identified by immunohistochemical methods as producing one or more hormones.

Originally considered to be of neural crest origin this concept has recently had to be widened.

The term APUD cell was originally created to indicate a function of 'amine-polypeptide-uptake-decarboxylation', but again the original concept has required extension beyond that aspect.

DISTRIBUTION

Anterior pituitary, thyroid (C cell), islets of Langerhans, stomach, small intestine, appendix and lung (Kultschitzsky cell), carotid body, skin, adrenal medulla, urogenital tract, etc.

MICROSCOPICAL

Some of these tumours have a classical 'carcinoid' appearance with ribbons, columns and acini of small regular cells with eosinophilic cytoplasm and usually little pleomorphism or mitotic activity. They are argyrophilic but not always argentaffinic and can be shown by immuno-peroxidase methods with specific antisera, to contain hormonal polypeptides.

Other tumours have an 'endocrine' appearance without the characteristic carcinoid pattern.

FUNCTION

The list of substances produced by cells of the diffuse endocrine system and their tumours grows almost daily. Some will be identified in specific sites (see p. 159).

BEHAVIOUR

Biological behaviour is unpredictable and histological appearances may belie both the natural history and functional activity.

The appendicular carcinoid (see p. 213) is benign and inactive but the small intestinal equivalent produces large amounts of 5-hydroxytryptamine and in advanced cases the carcinoid syndrome (see p. 247). It also metastasizes frequently but is slow growing.

Only rarely are these tumours very aggressive.

Basal cell carcinoma – rodent ulcer

SITES

These occur especially on exposed parts and particularly on the face in the region of the eyelids, nose and cheek. However, they may occur anywhere on the skin surface and are sometimes multiple.

MACROSCOPICAL

Slowly growing but potentially destructive and invasive tumours showing an irregular, slightly raised, pearly appearance and a central scab covering an ulcer with irregular margins.

MICROSCOPICAL

The tumour is usually composed of solid nests of darkly staining basal type cells with a characteristic outer palisaded layer. They are now thought to arise from immature skin appendage epithelium rather than the basal layer of the epidermis, and at least seven histological variants are described, e.g. keratotic, cystic, adenoid, morphoea-like. They are thus related to other types of skin appendage tumour (p. 732).

Mucous gland tumours

Uncommon tumours arising from any mucous gland but most frequently in the parotid and other salivary glands. The characteristics of this group of tumours of variable behaviour are described in the salivary gland section (see p. 179).

Choriocarcinoma

NATURE

This is a unique tumour in that it is not derived from the host tissues but from the trophoblastic tissue of a parasite (foetus).

SITES

Occur in the uterus and at ectopic placental sites. Trophoblastic tissue may also be present in malignant teratomas, e.g. testicular, ovarian.

MICROSCOPICAL

These rapidly growing, haemorrhagic tumours are composed of malignant cyto- and syncytiotrophoblast and do not form chorionic villi. They invade extensively into the myometrium with early spread into blood vessels giving rise to disseminated metastases (see p. 430).

Chapter 29
Benign and Malignant Tumours of
Connective Tissue

Benign

Fibroma
Many of the benign fibroblastic proliferations previously called fibromas have now been reclassified under the heading 'fibromatosis' (see below). However, localized benign fibromatous tumours do occasionally occur notably in the ovary and the breast.

Myxoma

SITES
Fascial planes, subcutaneous tissues and intermuscular septa. Also found as a specific entity in the left atrium (see p. 251).

MACROSCOPICAL
These encapsulated tumours have a soft, mucoid or gelatinous appearance.

MICROSCOPICAL
The tumour is composed of stellate cells in a connective tissue mucoid matrix. The majority of myxomas are fibroblastic proliferations particularly of nerve origin, showing extensive myxomatous degeneration.

Lipoma

SITES
Slowly growing very common, encapsulated, yellow tumours occurring anywhere in the subcutaneous tissues but especially on the back of the neck, the shoulders and the buttocks. They also occur in the subperiosteal, intestinal submucosal and retroperitoneal tissues. Very occasionally, particularly in the retroperitoneal tissues, malignant change to liposarcoma may occur. There is also a localized or diffuse lipomatous condition with painful fatty masses in female subjects – *adiposis dolorosa* (Dercum's disease).

MACROSCOPICAL
Encapsulated, lobulated, soft, yellow and fatty tumours.

MICROSCOPICAL
Formed by adult adipose tissue divided into lobules by fibrous septa. The fibrous tissue may be excessive and the tumour is then called a *fibrolipoma*. Areas of fat necrosis are frequently found due to either infection or trauma.

Hibernoma

A rare variant is the hibernoma, a brown tumour composed of finely vacuolated fat cells of foetal type and reminiscent of the hibernating gland of bears and certain other mammals.

Chondroma

Lobulated, glistening, semi-translucent tumours formed by mature cartilage and most frequently found in the metacarpals and at the ends of long bones. There are two types, ecchondromas which are frequently associated with diaphyseal aclasia and enchondromas which are most commonly situated in the bones of the hands (see p. 700).

Osteoma

The term osteoma embraces a miscellaneous group of lesions, some of which are simply congenital cartilage-capped exostoses (see p. 699). The rare ivory osteoma of the skull and the commoner osteoid osteoma are probably true benign neoplasms.

Leiomyoma

SITES
Leiomyomas can occur wherever there is smooth muscle but are especially common in the subcutaneous tissues arising from the media of blood vessels or from the arrectores pilorum muscles. They also occur in the ovary, kidney and gastrointestinal tract. The uterine 'fibroid' is probably the commonest benign tumour of humans and is a mixture of smooth muscle and fibrous tissue – *fibromyoma* or *fibroleiomyoma* (see p. 416).

MACROSCOPICAL
Circular, pale, whorled, encapsulated tumours, frequently multiple.

MICROSCOPICAL
Comparatively acellular tumours composed of myofibrils with blunt-ended nuclei and arranged in a whorled pattern.

Rhabdomyoma

This is a very rare lesion of developmental origin which can occur in skeletal muscle, in the heart or in other organs associated with tuberose sclerosis (see p. 593). Histologically, there is a benign overgrowth of striated or cardiac muscle fibres.

Neurofibroma

This includes both neurofibromas and Schwannomas, both of which arise from the connective tissues of peripheral and cranial nerves. They form firm swellings on the nerves and are composed of fibrous tissue from the perineural tissues or from Schwann cells. They are more fully described in the peripheral nerve section (p. 620).

Fibromatoses

Nature
The term fibromatosis has been applied to a wide variety of dysplastic lesions of connective tissue which do not have the features of an inflammatory response nor of unequivocal malignancy. Some of these conditions are unquestionably benign and others possess locally aggressive properties and may infiltrate muscle and fat. None metastasizes. They are grouped together because of the similarities in histological appearance, and to distinguish them from fibrosarcoma, which carries a more

sinister prognosis. They can be considered in two main groups.

Types

CONGENITAL AND JUVENILE

Included in the group are *fibromatosis colli* affecting the sternomastoid muscle and causing congenital torticollis, *infantile and juvenile fibromatosis* which may be nodular or diffuse, in subcutaneous tissue or skeletal muscle, and which may recur if excision is incomplete, and *calcifying juvenile aponeurotic fibroma*, which is also liable to recur if incompletely excised.

MISCELLANEOUS

Palmar and plantar fibromatosis

Palmar fibromatosis – Dupytren's contracture – and its plantar equivalent are the commonest fibromatoses. Men are affected more commonly than women (ratio 7:1). The process presents with one or more nodules in the ulnar part of the palm. With time the nodules flatten and contractures evolve. Histologically the lesion is composed of cellular proliferating fibroblasts. It may recur if excision is incomplete.

Musculo-aponeurotic fibromatosis – Desmoid tumour

Typically these occur in the rectus sheath and the majority of cases are women, usually parous. They also occur in association with other muscle sheets, in particular the neck, shoulder and upper limbs. The tumour nodules vary in size, have an ill-defined outline, and may infiltrate muscle. They are composed of proliferating fibroblasts arranged in a whorled pattern. Recurrence is usual if excision is incomplete.

Generalized multifocal fibromatosis

In rare cases, nodules of fibromatosis occur at several sites in the body, usually in subcutaneous tissue, but occasionally in muscle.

OTHER FIBROBLASTIC PROLIFERATIONS

Apart from the fibromatoses, a miscellaneous collection of lesions are composed in the main of proliferating connective tissue. Some are thought to be reactive or inflammatory, e.g. keloids, nodular fasciitis, proliferative myositis, retroperitoneal fibrosis, whilst others are of doubtful neoplastic origin, e.g. dermatofibroma (benign histiocytoma), non-osteogenic fibroma of bone.

Malignant connective tissue tumours

SARCOMAS

Nature

A malignant tumour arising from mesodermal connective tissue is a sarcoma.

N.B. A glioma, although arising from neuroglial connective tissues, is not a sarcoma as it is derived from ectoderm. Sarcomas have certain features in common.

Clinical

(a) Frequently affect the young age groups.
(b) Rapid growth to form a large tumour.
(c) Early and widespread blood dissemination due to imperfectly formed blood vessels within the tumour.
(d) May arise from previously benign tumours, e.g. chondrosarcoma from chondroma.
(e) May arise from a growth disorder, e.g. osteitis deformans – osteosarcoma, neurofibromatosis – neurofibrosarcoma.

Histological

(a) The tumour cells are usually discrete.
(b) There is evidence of all the histological features of malignancy including marked cellularity, numerous mitoses, tumour giant cells, hyperchromatism of the nuclei, areas of haemorrhage and necrosis.
(c) There are areas of stromal differentiation, e.g. the cells form cartilage or bone or fibrous tissue and it is this recognizable differentiation which enables recognition of the type and gives the prefix to the sarcoma, e.g. chondrosarcoma.
(d) New blood vessels are formed in excess within the tumour tissue and these are frequently ill-formed so that tumour cells are in direct contact with the blood.
(e) Some sarcomas show no diagnostic differentiation and are composed of masses of spindle-shaped cells. It may thus be impossible to say from which tissue this *spindle cell sarcoma* has arisen.

Fibrosarcoma

SITES
The common sites are fascial planes between the muscles of the limbs, retroperitoneal and subcutaneous tissues, within bones and from the periosteum.

MACROSCOPICAL
Large, firm and pale pseudo-encapsulated infiltrating masses.

MICROSCOPICAL
Composed of malignant fibroblastic tissue with varying degrees of cellularity and collagen formation.

Myxosarcoma
This is usually a fibrosarcoma in which extensive myxomatous degeneration has occurred. The tumours arise from the same sites as fibrosarcomas and behave in a similar manner.

Liposarcoma

SITES
A rare tumour which may arise from a pre-existing lipoma, especially in the retroperitoneal tissues.

MACROSCOPICAL
Forms a soft and yellow or myxoid non-encapsulated fatty tumour.

MICROSCOPICAL
Composed of atypical fat cells of embryonic type. This tumour has to be differentiated from a fibrosarcoma invading adipose tissue, a far more frequent occurrence. A differentiated myxoid variant is not uncommon.

Chondrosarcoma
This tumour is related to bones where it forms a large, lobulated, glistening mass. It is composed of atypical cartilage cells with evidence of irregular growth and is further considered on p. 700.

Osteosarcoma
The osteosarcoma is a highly malignant tumour of osteoblasts occurring in young persons and presenting as a large irregular, destructive, bone mass. Variable amounts of bone or osteoid tissue are produced by the tumour cells and the appearances are described in the bone tumour section (p. 699).

Leiomyosarcoma

SITES
The common sites are uterus and intestines where they probably arise in pre-existing leiomyomas.

MACROSCOPICAL
Soft, pale and non-encapsulated tumours which are commonly necrotic when large, e.g. in the uterus.

MICROSCOPICAL
Spindle-shaped cells with pink-staining cytoplasm, resembling smooth muscle cells but showing cellularity, mitotic activity and atypicality indicative of malignancy.

Rhabdomyosarcoma

NATURE
These extremely rare tumours may arise from skeletal muscles, but also occur in the urogenital tract, nasopharynx and subcutaneous tissue. Three varieties are recognized, adult pleomorphic, embryonal alveolar and embryonal botryoid.

MACROSCOPICAL
They form large, bulky, pale and necrotic invasive tumours.

MICROSCOPICAL
The essential feature is the presence of irregular malignant cells with large hyperchromatic nuclei and abundant pink cytoplasm – 'Strap cells'. Cross striations are visible in the cytoplasm. These striations must be present in the actual neoplastic cells and should not be confused with the altered appearances of skeletal muscle invaded by another type of sarcoma.

Neurofibrosarcoma
These arise from pre-existing neurofibromas and Schwannomas. They occur most commonly in cases of neurofibromatosis and result in rapid enlargement of the pre-existing tumour. Histologically, there is evidence of increased cellularity, atypicality and invasiveness (see p. 620).

Synovial sarcoma

SITES

Arise in relation to the synovial membranes of large joints especially the hip, knee and ankle.

MACROSCOPICAL

Large, pale, firm tumours which show a distinct tendency to grow away from the joint of origin and invade the adjacent soft tissues and bone.

MICROSCOPICAL

The essential biphasic feature is the cleft-like spaces lined by epithelial-like, synovial type cells, with a stroma that varies from fibroblastic to spindle cell in type (see p. 712).

Mesothelioma – pleura and peritoneum

NATURE

These are very rare neoplasms derived from the mesothelial lining cells of the pleural or peritoneum. The majority of cases are associated with inhalation of asbestos fibres, usually from industrial exposure (see p. 670).

MACROSCOPICAL

The pleura or peritoneum is grossly thickened and densely bound to adjacent structures. The tumour tissue is hard and pale, and usually diffuse. Care must be taken to exclude a primary elsewhere, as diffuse metastatic tumours may mimic a mesothelioma.

MICROSCOPICAL

A tumour is composed of a mixture of malignant stromal spindle cells and clefts lined by cuboidal mesothelial lining cells. In one variant there is a marked papillary pattern, and in another the spindle cell element predominates.

Undifferentiated (spindle-cell) sarcoma

This is the histologically descriptive name given to any sarcoma composed exclusively of spindle-shaped cells and having no diagnostic stroma, i.e. no cartilage, bone, fibrous tissue, etc. This descriptive type implies lack of differentiation, and the tumour may arise from any connective tissue. It exhibits rapid growth, frequently with early blood-borne dissemination and thus carries a grave prognosis.

Chapter 30
Other Tumours

Tumours of lymphoreticular system

BENIGN LYMPHOID LESIONS

Nodular infiltrations of lymphoid cells occur in several organs, forming tumour-like masses, e.g. 'lymphocytoma cutis' in the skin, 'benign lymphoid polyp' in the rectum. They are rare. Microscopically the lesions are composed of mature lymphoid tissue, occasionally forming follicles with germinal centres.

MALIGNANT LYMPHOMA

There are two main types with subgroups, as follows.

Hodgkin's disease
A tumour composed of multicellular infiltrate consisting of large atypical mononuclear cells, giant cells (Reed–Sternberg cells), lymphocytes, plasma cells and eosinophils set in a variable fibrous stroma (see p. 581).

Non-Hodgkin's lymphoma

FOLLICULAR
These tumours are derived from follicle centre lymphoid cells and have a well-defined follicular or nodular pattern. The overall prognosis is good, but progression to a diffuse type of lymphocytic lymphoma may occur, with a consequent worsening of the prognosis (see p. 582).

DIFFUSE

In these lymphomas the lymph node is replaced by sheets of tumour cells with no attempt at formation of a follicular or nodular pattern. They are further subdivided as follows.

Lymphocytic

There are two variants, small cell and large cell types. The small cell type, which is the homologue of chronic lymphatic leukaemia (C.L.L) is composed of cells closely resembling normal small lymphocytes and carries a relatively good prognosis. The large cell type is composed of large lymphoid cells (lymphoblasts) and has a relatively poor prognosis (see p. 582).

Histiocytic

Rare tumours, derived from cells of the macrophage system sometimes known as 'Malignant histiocytosis' (see p. 583).

Undifferentiated

Although the cytological detail of these tumours does not permit a more precise typing, more specialized techniques suggest that most are lymphoid in origin. They are of extremely poor prognosis (see p. 582).

Burkitt's lymphoma

A particular variety of undifferentiated lymphoma occurring most commonly in Africa and with a predilection for mandible, maxilla, soft tissues, retroperitoneum, testis and ovary. Some patients respond dramatically to cytotoxic therapy (see p. 583).

These are the main types of malignant lymphoma. Other rarer varieties include *Mycosis fungoides*, Sézary syndrome and immunoblastic sarcoma. In addition there are the following closely related tumours.

Myeloma

A tumour composed of neoplastic plasma cells, producing abnormal immunoglobulins, and forming deposits mainly in skeletal tissues (see p. 470).

Leukaemia

Malignant proliferations of myeloid, lymphatic or monocytic cells, which clinically behave as acute or chronic forms (see p. 462).

Tumours of naevus cells

Nature

A group of melanin-containing tumours derived from pigment-forming cells (melanocytes). Most authorities now agree that these cells are derived from the neural crest (i.e. neuro-ectoderm), and migrate to the basal layer of the skin in early intra-uterine life.

Benign pigmented naevus

A naevus or mole implies a benign pigmented tumour derived from melanocytes and containing 'naevus cells'. Many of the lesions are of developmental origin and are present in the form of moles in variable numbers in the skin of every individual. In one variety the proliferating naevus cells are confined to the epidermo-dermal junction – the 'junctional naevus'. In adults this must be distinguished from pre-malignant change. The commonest variety is the 'intradermal naevus' in which the naevus cells are entirely within the dermis.

Malignant melanoma

NATURE

This is the malignant counterpart of the benign naevus, and is thus a malignant tumour of melanocytes (see p. 117).

SITES

The commonest site of origin is the skin, especially of the head and neck, but they may also arise from the choroid, meninges and conjunctiva.

MACROSCOPICAL

A variably pigmented, rapidly growing, often ulcerated and bleeding lesion of the skin, commonly with a history of deepening or irregular pigmentation.

MICROSCOPICAL

The tumour is composed of pleomorphic, malignant, melanin-containing cells invading the underlying tissues and the overlying epidermis and frequently showing junctional activity at the margins. Sometimes the tumour cells show no melanin pigment – *amelanotic melanoma* – although the tumour cells are still DOPA positive (see p. 117).

Tumours of the central nervous system

This is a complex group of tumours derived from the tissues within the central nervous system. The details of this group are given in the C.N.S. section (pp. 623–628) and include:

(a) From meninges. Meningioma (see p. 627).
(b) From neuroglia. The glioma group which includes astrocytoma, oligodendroglioma, medulloblastoma and ependymoma (see p. 624).
(c) From nerve cells. Neuroblastoma, neurocytoma (see pp. 295 and 626).
(d) From microglia (lymphoreticular cells). Lymphoma (see p. 626).

Developmental tumours

Embryonal tumours

These are uncommon tumours which usually occur in early childhood and may be present at birth. Very rarely cases occur in adult life, presumably because the lesion has remained latent. The tumours are composed of primitive structures normally found in the organ of origin, unlike the teratomas which contain a wide assortment of body tissues (see below). They are usually highly malignant. Examples are as follows.

NEUROBLASTOMA
This tumour arises almost invariably from the adrenal medulla or one of the sympathetic ganglia. It is composed of tightly packed nests of darkly staining round cells, sometimes having a rosette-like pattern. Primitive nerve fibres may be recognized (see p. 295).

NEPHROBLASTOMA (WILM'S TUMOUR)
This is composed of embryonic tubules, sometimes admixed with primitive glomerular structures, and set in a spindle-cell stroma in which striated muscle fibres may be visible (see p. 378).

RETINOBLASTOMA
This tumour has a definite hereditary incidence. It is also composed of small darkly staining cells, with a rosette appearance (see p. 342).

Teratomas – benign and malignant

NATURE
These are tumours consisting of multiple tissues foreign to the part from which they arise – *heterotopia*. They are thought to arise from totipotential germ cells which have escaped the influence of the 'primary organizer' during early embryonic development. They remain as 'rests' with slow growth, or malignant change may supervene. They are most common in early adult life, but may occur at any age.

SITES
Teratomas occur in the ovaries, testes, retroperitoneal tissues, anterior mediastinum, sacrococcygeal region and base of the skull, in approximate order of frequency.

MACROSCOPICAL
The benign teratoma is usually cystic with solid areas and frequently contains recognizable hair, sebaceous material, teeth or bone. The malignant teratoma is usually solid but may be partially cystic.

MICROSCOPICAL
The benign teratoma (e.g. ovarian), is typically represented by a squamous cyst in which there is an elevated nodule containing hair follicles, sebaceous glands, muscle, cartilage, bone, respiratory epithelium, brain tissue or any other tissue. All these tissues show mature differentiation.

The histological appearances of the malignant teratoma are very variable. There may be recognizable 'organoid' structures as in the benign teratoma but, in addition, there are features of malignancy in one or more of the tissue elements, with varying dedifferentiation. Some malignant teratomas are composed entirely of undifferentiated malignant elements.

Hamartomas
These are tumour-like malformations in which the tissues of a particular part of the body are arranged in an irregular, haphazard manner. They are not true neoplasms and can be distinguished from teratomas (a) because the tissues they contain are not foreign to the part and (b) the lesion itself has no tendency to excessive growth. However, tumours may subsequently develop in hamartomas. Examples of hamartomas are angiomata, chondroid harmartoma of lung, solitary exostosis (osteochon-

droma). Some authorities believe that pigmented naevi are also hamartomas.

Tumours of endothelium

Haemangioma

TYPES
These include many different types, e.g. capillary, cavernous, sclerosing and glomangioma. The capillary type is formed by multiple small capillary blood vessels and the cavernous variety by larger endothelial-lined vascular spaces. Many of these are not true tumours but are congenital harmartomatous malformations of the blood vessels (see p. 278).

SITES
(a) *Skin*. Form de Morgan spots, spider naevi, mulberry naevi and port-wine stains.
(b) *Muscles*. Present as vascular tumours in any muscle but especially in thigh, calf, biceps, triceps and sternomastoid.
(c) *Bones*. Usually cavernous in type and commonly seen in vertebrae and skull (see p. 718).
(d) *C.N.S.* Capillary or cavernous lesions can occur anywhere in the brain but particularly in the cerebellum (see p. 627).
(e) *Viscera*. Cavernous haemangiomas are frequently found in the liver or other viscera. When sited in the pyramid of a kidney or in the intestinal mucosa they may cause clinical bleeding (see p. 377).

SYNDROMES
(a) *Hereditary multiple telangiectasia*. Multiple angiomas of skin and mucous membranes resulting in haemorrhages (see p. 516).
(b) *Kast's syndrome*. Angiomas of skin associated with dyschondroplasia of bone (see p. 683).
(c) *Lindau's syndrome*. Angiomas of retina and cerebellum associated with tumours or cysts in visceral sites (see p. 341).
(d) *Sturge–Weber syndrome*. Angioma of face and of the underlying cerebrum.

Lymphangioma

These are all of congenital origin and their structure is similar to haemangiomas in that they are lined by endothelium but they contain lymph and not blood.

TYPES
(a) *Capillary lymphangioma*. Occurs mainly on the lips, cheeks and tongue; the enlargement results in *macrocheilia* or *macroglossia* (see p. 168).
(b) *Cavernous lymphangioma*. Occurs especially in the spleen and results in splenomegaly (see p. 738).
(c) *Cystic*. A thin-walled multilocular cystic mass usually in the neck – *cystic hygroma*.

Haemangiosarcoma

NATURE
A rare and highly malignant tumour of vascular endothelium.

SITES
Any site where haemangiomas are found. Although rare tumours, they are found in the subcutaneous tissues, nose, bones, brain, breast and viscera.

MACROSCOPICAL
Rapidly enlarging, highly vascular and frequently pulsating, red-blue or dusky coloured tumours.

MICROSCOPICAL
The tumour is vasoformative with atypical vascular spaces of irregular size and shape produced by the proliferating malignant endothelial cells.

Lymphangiosarcoma

NATURE
A very rare malignant tumour of lymphatic endothelium.

SITES
The most acceptable examples have arisen in pre-existing and long-standing lymphoedema, e.g. following radical mastectomy for carcinoma of breast.

MACROSCOPICAL
The brawny arm increases in size and contains an area of increased hardness and swelling.

MICROSCOPICAL
The tumour area shows marked atypicality of the lymphatic endothelium in which there are multiple lymph-containing spaces and channels of variable size, formed by the atypical and proliferating malignant lymphatic endothelium.

Chapter 31
Tumours – Predisposing Factors: Effects

Contributory and predisposing factors

INTRINSIC FACTORS
Racial
Genetic
Sex
Age
Benign tumours

EXTRINSIC FACTORS
Chronic irritation
  Physical
    Burns
    Chronic skin ulcers
    Leukoplakia
    Calculi

Chemical
  Skin
  Lung, pleura, nasopharynx
  Urinary tract
  Inflammatory
  Irradiation
Hormonal
Nutritional
Infective agents

Carcinogenesis – theoretical considerations

Effects of tumours
Obstruction
Irritation of serous membranes
Destruction of tissue
Infection
Malignant 'cachexia'
Fever
Anaemia
Hormonal effects
  Appropriate
  Inappropriate
Other tumour products
  Oncofoetal
  Enzymes
  Macromolecules
Tumour markers
Neurological disturbances

Contributory and predisposing factors

The basic cause (or causes) of tumour formation and human carcinogenesis are unknown. There are, however, a number of types and sites of tumours where contributory or predisposing causes are known and which throw some light on the possible factors involved in neoplasia in general.

INTRINSIC FACTORS

Racial
Whilst all races are susceptible to malignant disease, there is considerable geographical variation in organ incidence. For example, liver tumours are uncommon in Europe, but are extremely common in Bantus, and carcinoma of the breast occurs more frequently in the United States and Europe than in Japan. However, virtually all such geographical variations are due to environmental and other extrinsic factors, and there is little evidence to suggest that innate racial differences exist.

Genetic
A definite genetic predisposition has been established with some uncommon tumours, e.g. dominant inheritance in retinoblastoma, polyposis coli; familial occurrence in multiple endocrine adenoma syndrome. Less definite genetic relationships exist for most of the more common tumours, but a number of 'cancer families' have been described.

Sex
There is considerable variation in sex incidence of different tumours, e.g. carcinomas of the bronchus, tongue and lip are predominantly diseases of males.

Age
In general the prevalence of tumours increases with age. Carcinomas are commonest over 50 years, some sarcomas occur in young persons whilst rare embryonal tumours, e.g. nephroblastoma, neuroblastoma, occur only in childhood.

Benign tumours
Many malignant tumours arise in pre-existing

benign neoplasms. Sometimes the risk of this change is slight but definite, e.g. sarcomatous change in fibroids, development of malignant melanoma in a naevus, but on occasions the change occurs so frequently as to constitute a considerable hazard and justifies immediate removal of the benign lesion, e.g. neoplastic polyps of the gastro-intestinal tract, papillomas of nasal sinuses.

EXTRINSIC FACTORS

These are environmental or occupational factors which over many years may result in malignant disease. Many are local and operate at specific sites or on individual organs or tissues. Where these factors are established as pre-cancerous influences they are discussed in the relative special sections. Some general inferences can, however, be made.

Chronic irritation
This may be in the form of physical, chemical or inflammatory agents including irradiation. The irritation is commonly of very longstanding and there is usually an intermediate phase showing metaplasia or dysplasia.

PHYSICAL
(a) Burns. Repetitive burns on the lips of clay pipe smokers predispose to carcinoma at this site.
(b) Marjolin's ulcer. Carcinoma may arise in the scars of burns, sinuses, lupus vulgaris, varicose (gravitational) ulcers.
(c) Leukoplakia. The development of leukoplakia is often associated with chronic irritation by physical agents and frequently progresses to malignancy, e.g. tongue, lip.
(d) Calculi. Chronic irritation by calculi in the biliary and urinary tract may result in squamous metaplasia and subsequently lead to the development of carcinoma.

CHEMICAL
There are many known chemical carcinogens which, on repeated application, may give rise to tumours. Thus, certain occupations predispose to carcinoma at particular sites after prolonged exposure to such agents.
(a) Skin.
Chimney sweep's cancer of the scrotum due to coal-tar derivatives.
Mule spinner's cancer due to lubricating oil.

Shale oil cancers due to paraffin hydrocarbons.
Arsenic. Prolonged administration produces an arsenical dermatitis and sometimes a squamous cell carcinoma develops in these lesions.
(b) Lung, pleura and nasopharynx.
Cigarette smoking. The risk of bronchial carcinoma is twenty times greater in heavy smokers than in non-smokers (see p. 675).
Haematite workers. Haematite lung (see p. 670).
Asbestos workers. Asbestosis (see p. 670) mesothelioma.
Nickel and chromium workers (see p. 675).
(c) Urinary tract. Aniline dye workers have a high incidence of bladder carcinoma due to the presence in their urine of β-naphthylamine (see p. 388).

INFLAMMATORY
Chronic low-grade inflammation alone, or as a concomitant of calculi and other physical agents, may bring about metaplastic changes in epithelium and be pre-cancerous, e.g. schistosomiasis of the urinary tract (see p. 388), ulcerative colitis of long standing (see p. 203), chronic gastric ulcer (see p. 189).

IRRADIATION
Various types of radiation may lead to malignancy (see p. 76). Excessive exposure to sunlight (ultra-violet rays), especially in fair-skinned persons may result in basal cell or squamous carcinoma (see p. 731). An increased incidence of skin cancer was noted in the pioneers of radiology. Lung cancer occurs in the Schneeberg and Joachimsthal miners, due to exposure to radon. Survivors of the Japanese atom bomb explosions have an increased incidence of leukaemia. These factors, and several others, point to an important carcinogenic effect of irradiation.

Hormonal
Cancers in certain 'target organs', particularly carcinomas of the breast and prostate, are so profoundly influenced in growth and behaviour by hormones that they are sometimes classified as 'hormone dependent'. This applies, however, to their behaviour once established and does not necessarily signify that the hormonal factors are causative in their development. There is now evidence to suggest that some cancers may arise following hormonal stimulation, e.g. carcinoma of endometrium in menopausal women receiving hor-

mone replacement therapy, carcinoma of the breast associated with mammary dysplasia.

Nutritional
It is now well established that the marked geographical variation in the incidence of liver cancer is mostly due to the high rate of cirrhosis of nutritional origin in Bantus and other African and Eastern races. A further example of nutritional influence is the development of post-cricoid carcinoma in females with longstanding iron deficiency.

Infective agents
Most of the evidence ascribing a carcinogenic effect to infective agents is derived from experimental animal work. There are numerous examples of the unequivocal induction of malignant tumours by oncogenic viruses in a variety of animals, e.g. chicken sarcoma, mouse leukaemia, mouse mammary tumour, although other types of agent have been implicated. In the human the evidence is more circumstantial. There is a clear association between Burkitt's lymphoma and EB virus, a herpes virus which is the causative agent of infectious mononucleosis. However, proof that the virus induces the neoplastic change is lacking – it may simply be a passenger in the tumour cells. Women with carcinoma of the cervix have a higher incidence of antibodies to herpes simplex virus type 2 than normal women, but again conclusive proof of causation is lacking. Some epidemiological evidence suggests that Hodgkin's disease may occur in epidemic clusters, but no significant agent has been isolated from tumour tissue.

Carcinogenesis – theoretical considerations

Although the basic cause of most tumours remains unknown, the associations described above, together with evidence from experimental studies, provide greater insight into the process of carcinogenesis. In most cases prolonged stimulation by the carcinogenic agents is required, and tumours may take up to 20 years to develop. These may be a reversible intermediate pre-malignant stage in the process, e.g. cervical epithelial dysplasia. In some tumours this constitutes a 'field change' from which the tumours arises, often as multiples lesions, e.g. urothelial carcinoma. From work on experimental animal tumours, e.g. skin cancers in rabbits induced by the application of croton oil to areas pre-treated with hydrocarbons, arose the concept of tumour *initiation* and *promotion*. This two-stage concept has now been replaced by the recognition that most tumours have a multifactorial basis. For example, although heavy cigarette smoking is a very strong risk factor, not all heavy smokers develop bronchial carcinoma suggesting that other factors, genetic or environmental, also play a part. Recent evidence that patients receiving immunosuppressive therapy, e.g. for renal transplants, have a higher incidence of malignant tumours particularly lymphoma suggests that a defect in the immune surveillance mechanism may be an important factor in carcinogenesis. Immunological factors, and the role of viral infection are obvious targets for further basic research into carcinogenetic mechanisms.

Effects of tumours

These are space-occupying lesions and inevitably produce some distortion of surrounding tissues. The general and local effects are extremely variable from site to site but include the following.

Obstruction
May be caused in a hollow viscus by tumours in the lumen, arising from the wall or pressing on the wall from outside. This may be at the primary site of the lesion or due to metastases, e.g.:

Intestine – intestinal obstruction or intussusception.
Biliary tract – obstructive jaundice, e.g. by carcinoma of pancreas, lymph nodes in the porta hepatis, intrahepatic duct obstruction by blood-borne metastases.
Urinary tract – hydronephrosis.
Bronchus – pulmonary collapse.
Portal vein – ascites and varices.
Mediastinum – vena caval syndromes.

Irritation of serous membranes
Deposits of tumour on serous membranes result in the formation of an inflammatory exudate of high protein content which is frequently bloodstained, e.g. malignant ascites.

Destruction of tissue
Progressive destruction and replacement of tissue may produce functional loss, perforation, fistulous communications or haemorrhage.

Infection

Infection is almost inevitable in surface tumours and is very common at other sites.

Malignant 'cachexia'

There is frequently progressive weakness and loss of weight in malignant disease. It was formerly stated that tumours produced 'toxic' substances which induced this cachexia. It is probable, however, that the wasting of malignant disease only occurs in those cases where there is direct interference with nutrition, or complications such as recurrent haemorrhage, ulceration, bacterial infection, pain and insomnia. There is often, however, some relationship between the degree of cachexia and the total mass of the tumour.

Fever

Pyrexia is a frequent accompaniment of malignant disease and is usually due to infection. However, certain tumours, notably Ewing's tumour of bone, tumours in the hypothalamic region and carcinomas of kidney and adrenal, often produce pyrexia in the absence of infection. The causation in these circumstances is uncertain.

Anaemia

Progressive anaemia is frequently found. This may be due to prolonged malnutrition, recurrent blood loss, or longstanding infection producing marrow depression. Multiple secondary deposits in the bone marrow may result in leuco-erythroblastic anaemia, whilst progressive destruction of the stomach by carcinoma may lead to vitamin B_{12} deficiency. The anaemia associated with malignant disease may thus be hypochromic microcytic, normochromic, or macrocytic. Not uncommonly more than one factor is involved and a mixed picture results.

Hormonal effects

These can be divided into two categories.

APPROPRIATE

Tumours of endocrine tissues secreting their own hormones, e.g.:

Ovary – granulosa cell tumours – feminizing; androblastoma – feminizing or masculinizing.
Adrenal – Cushing's syndrome
Pituitary – adenomas may be functionally active to produce acromegaly, or growth in the restricted space of the pituitary fossa may compress the gland and ultimately lead to hypopituitarism.
Parathyroid – metastatic calcification, particularly renal; osteitis fibrosa cystica.

INAPPROPRIATE

Tumours of endocrine and non-endocrine origin secreting hormones not normally associated with that issue, e.g.:

Lung – oat cell carcinomas may secrete polypeptide hormones with parathormone, ACTH or ADH-like activity (see p. 676).
Hydatidiform mole – may secrete a specific thyrotropic hormone causing hyperthyroidism.

Other tumour products

In addition to hormonal secretion, a wide variety of other substances may be produced by tumours, e.g.:

(a) Oncofoetal products and other 'antigens'.
Carcinoembryonic antigen (CEA) – gastrointestinal tumours.
Alpha fetoprotein (AFP) – hepatocellular carcinoma, germ cell tumours.
Pregnancy associated proteins (HCG) – breast carcinoma, teratoma of testis.
(b) Enzymes.
Phosphatases – prostatic carcinoma, hepatocellular carcinoma.
(c) Other macromolecules.
Casein and lactalbumin.
Paraproteins – malignant myeloma, lymphoma.
Polyamines – by many tumours particularly those of the neuroendocrine system (see p. 145).

Tumour markers

These are all *tumour-derived* markers produced either by the epithelial cells of the tumour or by stromal cells.

Additionally there are *tumour-associated* markers which may be produced by cells of uninvolved organs as a secondary effect from tumour cells, e.g. hydroxyproline released by bone infiltrated by osteolytic metastases.

These substances may be useful in the diagnosis and monitoring of certain types of malignant disease, e.g. CEA levels as indicators of recurrence of colonic carcinoma, HCG levels in germ cell tumours and in choriocarcinoma, AFP titre in diagnosis of hepatocellular carcinoma.

Furthermore they may often explain some of the systemic effects of malignant disease including cachexia and hypercalcaemia in the absence of raised parathormone levels.

Neurological disturbances

Myopathy or neuropathy, usually of peripheral or cranial nerves, may complicate some cases of malignant disease, e.g. carcinoma of bronchus. In such cases, tumour cells are rarely found in the affected site and this appears to be a 'metabolic' effect from a tumour which is sometimes remarkably small and occult.

Chapter 32
Exfoliative Cytology

Definition

The study of cells detached spontaneously or artificially from the surface of an organ or membrane.

Introduction

Most tissues are constantly changing due to removal or shedding of effete old cells and replacement by newly formed and generally more active cells. There is thus a turnover of cells in many organs whose speed varies from tissue to tissue (see p. 35). Epithelial cells are amongst the most active in this respect and as many epithelia line accessible orifices and cavities the most mature surface cells are shed or exfoliated into the lumen or on to the surface. Examination of such cells may give valuable information and has the advantage of causing no discomfort to the patient as they are readily collected or detached.

When malignant disease arises from or ulcerates through such an epithelial surface it usually casts off cells which manifest the increased rapidity and atypicality of neoplastic growth (see p. 139).

Historical

Dudgeon and Bamforth in London pioneered this work but a big impetus came from the prolonged studies and modified staining techniques of Papanicolaou. In recent years the scope of the subject has widened very considerably to include not only cancer screening and diagnosis but hormonal effects and histochemical and genetic studies.

Female genital tract

Usually confined to examination of exfoliated cells from the cervix, uterus and vagina. Of less practical importance are cells from endometrium, ovaries and vulva.

Techniques

AYRE SCRAPING OF CERVIX
A specially shaped spatula made so that a rounded prolongation which fits the external os is rotated through a full circle. This removes mucus and the surface cells from the squamo-columnar junctional area at which site most carcinomas of the cervix arise (see p. 420). Rapid spreading on slides and

immediate wet fixation is followed by staining by the Papanicolaou method.

VAGINAL ASPIRATE
The pool of mucus and cells exfoliated from the vaginal, cervix, and endometrium is aspirated into a pipette from the posterior fornix and smeared, fixed and stained as above.

Results

CANCER DETECTION
(*a*) *Carcinoma of cervix* (see also p. 420). The Ayre scrape gives a positive yield of over 90 per cent on first examination. Vaginal aspirate is less satisfactory with a false negative rate of about 25 per cent.

By this technique, presymptomatic diagnosis of dysplasias, preinvasive (*in situ*) carcinoma and very early (micro or occult) invasive carcinoma may be readily established. Results with florid invasive carcinomas are less reliable due to contamination with eyrthrocytes and necrosis of tumour cells.

It is now clearly established that cytology can detect the whole range of epithelial abnormalities of the cervix from mild dysplasia onwards and that this spans on average 20 or more years, 10 years or so from the stage of preinvasive (*in situ*) carcinoma. Population screening should commence with risk, starting when regular sexual activity is established and particularly from 25 years onwards. Conservative methods of treatment now allow earlier intervention in the natural history of the disease. The cytology positive yield in asymptomatic persons is of the order of 1 per cent.

(*b*) *Carcinoma body of uterus.* Only about 25 per cent of cases are cytologically diagnosed by the cervical scrape but a rather higher but still unsatisfactory yield is obtained from examination of the vaginal pool aspirate. The test, however, gives too many false negatives to be a reliable screening procedure.

(*c*) *Other genital tract tumours.* Occasional positive results are achieved in ovarian or tubal carcinomas and in chorion carcinoma and uterine sarcoma.

HORMONAL ABNORMALITIES
Epithelial cells of the female genital tract are profoundly influenced by hormonal activity resulting in morphological and staining variations due to these effects, particularly in respect of oestrogens and progestogens. Thus the cellular appearances change during the phases of normal and abnormal menstrual cycles, and in pregnant, menopausal and post-menopausal patients. Vaginal cells are more sensitive to these influences than cervical cells and hormonal studies are best conducted on vaginal pool specimens. Prediction of hormonal background of menstrual disorders may be accurately achieved.

TRICHOMONAL AND MONILIAL INFECTIONS
Cervical smears have demonstrated the great frequency of unsuspected infections of these aetiologies, particularly the former. Cytological examination is the most reliable method of demonstration of trichomonads.

Urinary tract

Tumour cells of renal, bladder and urethral carcinomas may be detected on cytological examination of urinary deposits. Regular urinary examinations of persons at risk occupationally from chemically induced carcinogenesis (especially aniline dye and synthetic rubber industries) should be carried out to produce pre-symptomatic diagnosis. The technique is particularly useful in the diagnosis and management of *in situ carcinoma* of the bladder (see p. 389). Prostatic massage or fine needle aspirate smears may also be useful diagnostic adjuncts.

Alimentary tract

Mouth

SEX CHROMATIN
Cytological examination of scrapings of buccal mucosa is the most reliable method of study of nuclear sex chromatin, e.g. in suspected Klinefelter's syndrome (see p. 409). The presence of the Barr body denotes the presence of XX sex chromatin and female nuclear sex.

ATYPICAL AND MALIGNANT CELLS
Several conditions affecting the buccal mucosa are premalignant including leukoplakia and lichen planus. Scrapings of such lesions may yield positive malignant criteria before clinical evidence of malignant change. Clinically suspicious lesions may yield confirmatory positive smears.

Stomach

Gastric washings, with suitable preparation and concentration, may provide confirmatory evidence of clinically suspected gastric carcinoma even when radiological evidence is lacking. In the rare condition of *surface cancer of the stomach*, other investigations are commonly normal but the technique has only limited application.

Large intestine

Although theoretically cytological techniques can be applied to detection of colonic carcinoma, faecal contamination complicates the examination. Fluorescent screening techniques dependent on high concentrations of DNA in nuclei of malignant cells may prove to be of some diagnostic significance.

Respiratory tract

Cytological examination of sputum in cases of suspected carcinoma of the lung is an important ancillary diagnostic investigation but is of little value as a screening procedure. Three good specimens of sputum, and not saliva, preferably consecutive early morning samples, should be examined and any purulent or blood-stained flecks selected for examination. Some 60–80 per cent of bronchial carcinomas will exfoliate malignant cells which can be detected in sputum.

Pleural and peritoneal aspirates

Ascites and pleural effusions are common complications of abdominal and thoracic malignant disease. Examination of aspirated material is usually performed by cytological examination of stained smears of the centrifuged deposits together with histological examination of sections of any clot which may form associated with the high protein content of the exudates. However, mesothelial cells, shed from the surface of these membranes in most inflammatory conditions and in infarction, may mimic malignant cells to such a degree as to make interpretation difficult, even for the highly experienced. The techniques are, however, effective diagnostic adjuncts and appearances may be pathognomonic and save unnecessary diagnostic laparotomies or thoracotomies.

Cyst contents

Cysts may be aspirated and contents examined for the type of content and the presence of malignant cells. In practice this is usually reserved for cysts in the breast and ovary and results require expert evaluation.

C.S.F.

Primary and secondary brain tumours may involve the lining of the ventricular system or theca and exfoliated cells become detectable on examination of the C.S.F.

This occurs occasionally in secondary tumours and in medulloblastoma and ependymomas which tend to spread by 'seeding' via the C.S.F. (see p. 626).

Blood

Although occasionally circulating malignant cells can be demonstrated in blood samples, this is now known to be an infrequent occurrence of little or no diagnostic importance.

Fine needle tumour aspirates

Parenchymal or lymph nodal tumours in sites accessible from the skin surface may be successfully aspirated by fine needles and the stained, smeared, aspirate yield diagnostic malignant cells. Breast, prostatic and lymph node lesions are particularly appropriate for this technique.

SPECIAL PATHOLOGY

Chapter 33
Alimentary System –
Mouth: Lips: Tongue: Gums

Congenital
Hare lip
Cleft palate
Stomal abnormalities
Jaw abnormalities

Lip
Infections
Tumours
Carcinoma of lip
  Age
  Sex
  Sites
  Predisposing factors
  Macroscopical
  Microscopical
  Spread
  Prognosis

Oral inflammations
Vincent's infection – trench
  mouth
Herpetic stomatitis
Aphthous stomatitis
Moniliasis
Tuberculosis
Actinomycosis
Cancrum oris

Syphilis
  Primary
  Secondary
  Tertiary
    Leukoplakia
    Gumma
    Interstitial
  Congenital

**Miscellaneous mouth
  lesions**

Infections
Blood diseases
Vitamin deficiency diseases
Pigmentations
Leukoplakia
  Nature
  Age
  Sites
  Aetiology
  Macroscopical
  Microscopical
  Results
Carcinoma of tongue
  Incidence
  Age
  Sex
  Sites
  Predisposing factors
  Macroscopical
  Microscopical
  Spread
  Prognosis

Carcinoma of floor of mouth,
  cheek, palate
  Age
  Sex
  Predisposing factors
  Structure
  Prognosis
Carcinoma of pharynx and
  tonsil
  Types
  Squamous cell carcinoma
  'Transitional cell' carcinoma
  Lymphoepithelioma
  Spread
  Prognosis

Gums
Inflammation
Pyorrhoea
Swellings
  Epilepsy therapy
  Scurvy
  Epulis
    Myeloid
    Fibrous
    Haemangeiomatous
    'Myoblastoma'

Congenital

Hare lip
An abnormality due to failure of fusion of the nasal and maxillary processes which form the upper lip and maxilla. There may be only a slight indentation in the outer part of the middle third of the upper lip, or a fissure may extend to the anterior nares. The condition may be unilateral or bilateral.

There are genetic and environmental factors in the aetiology: risks to children are 1 in 30 with one affected parent.

Cleft palate

This may be associated with hare lip and is also of variable degree. It may affect both the hard and soft palates in complete cases. The fissure then forms a direct communication between mouth and nose and requires urgent operative closure to avoid inhalation of food into the respiratory tract.

Stomal abnormalities

Lip development may extend too far towards the midline – *microstomia*, or conversely, a failure of development – *macrostomia*, shows as a fissure extending towards the ear. The lips may be the site of a congenital lymphangeioma – *macrocheilia*.

Jaw abnormalities

These are rare but include absence of the jaw – *agnathia*; underdevelopment of the mandible or maxilla – *micrognathia*; failure of formation of the condyle.

Lip

Infections

The lip usually involved secondarily from infections of the oral cavity (see below).

Tumours

Benign tumours, e.g. haemangeioma, lymphangioma, fibroma, squamous cell papilloma, rarely occur in the lip. Benign non-neoplastic retention mucous gland cysts are common.

Carcinoma of lip

AGE
This tumour is very rare in the young and usually occurs in the 50–70 age group.

SEX
M:F 20:1.

SITES
The lower lip is involved in 90 per cent of cases.

PREDISPOSING FACTORS
In many cases there is no definite predisposing factor but one or more of the following may be operative:
1 *Leukoplakia.*
2 *Betel chewers.*

3 *Clay pipe smoking.* The main factor is repetitive thermal injury. This raises the incidence in women who smoke pipes.
4 *Sunlight.* Actinic carcinoma – outdoor workers, e.g. sailors, farmers, fishermen and fair-skinned people in sunny climates, have an increased incidence.
5 *Tar.* The repeated contact with tar in fish net menders.

MACROSCOPICAL
The tumour may be nodular, papillary, fissured or ulcerated and approximately 50 per cent of the patients have cervical or submandibular lymph node metastases at the time of diagnosis.

MICROSCOPICAL
Squamous cell carcinomas usually with well marked keratin formation.

SPREAD
Direct spread to adjacent structures, e.g. gum and bone; lymphatic spread to the submandibular and cervical lymph nodes. Blood spread to many organs may occur but is a late manifestation.

PROGNOSIS
Thirty per cent 5-year survival for upper lip tumours. Fifty per cent 5-year survival for lower lip tumours.

Inflammations of the oral cavity

Vincent's infection – trench mouth

NATURE
An ulcerating infection, maximal on the gums around the teeth. It does not occur in edentulous mouths.

AETIOLOGY
The organisms are Vincent's spirochaetes and fusiform bacilli, which are frequently present as commensals in normal mouths. The factors leading to their pathogenicity remain unknown but a symbiotic effect of the two organisms is apparent.

MACROSCOPICAL
Widespread, irregular, painful ulceration with slough formation, involving the gum margins and

resulting, in untreated cases, in progressive destruction of gum tissues.

MICROSCOPICAL

There is an acute, non-specific necrotizing inflammation in which there are pus cells and the causative spirochaetes and fusiform bacilli.

RESULTS

The condition rapidly clears with antibiotic therapy but repeated relapses are common.

Herpetic stomatitis

AETIOLOGY

The virus of herpes simplex.

PATHOGENESIS

The lesions are very commonly associated with infections of the upper respiratory tract and pneumonia. It is believed that the virus is present in a dormant state in the squamous cells of many individuals and is activated by febrile illnesses.

MACROSCOPICAL

Multiple, small, clear, discrete vesicles on the lips, gums and oral mucosa, which after 24 hours rupture to form shallow ulcers. These become encrusted and are frequently secondarily infected.

MICROSCOPICAL

Intra-epidermal vesicle formation with swelling and enlargement of the squamous cell in some of which nuclear inclusions may be seen.

RESULTS

The virus may rarely cause vesicle formation on the cornea which heals with scarring. An encephalitis also occasionally occurs (see p. 607).

Aphthous stomatitis

AETIOLOGY

Unknown.

MACROSCOPICAL

Multiple, small, painful, shallow ulcers on the tip of the tongue, floor or elsewhere in the mouth.

MICROSCOPICAL

Inflammatory ulceration which is non-specific.

RESULTS

Often resistant to treatment, these ulcers pursue a chronic course but have no significant sequelae.

Oral moniliasis

AETIOLOGY

The disease is due to *Candida albicans*, but the precise pathogenesis remains obscure. Many cases occur in children but, when adults are infected, they are frequently debilitated or the condition follows antibiotic, immunosuppresive or steroid administration.

MACROSCOPICAL

Multiple white patches on the mucosal surfaces, particularly the tonsils, which leave a bleeding surface on scraping –*thrush*.

MICROSCOPICAL

There is an acute inflammatory reaction with the yeasts visible on direct examination or on culture.

RESULTS

This usually remains a superficial infection which is commonly difficult to eradicate. Spread to the oesophagus or respiratory tract rarely occurs (see p. 59).

Tuberculosis

A rare buccal manifestion due to infection from a tuberculous pulmonary focus. A tuberculous ulcer may be present on the lip, tongue or tonsil and produces a painful, watery, irregular ulcer with slightly undermined edges. Biopsy is the usual method of diagnosis, but when suspected, smears and cultural methods may demonstrate the organisms.

Actinomycosis

INCIDENCE

Cervico-facial actinomycosis accounts for at least 50 per cent of all cases of infection by *Actinomyces israeli*.

MACROSCOPICAL

The mouth or jaw, commonly a tooth socket, is the primary site, with direct extension to involve the skin surface. This becomes red-blue in colour with multiple hard nodules and marked surrounding very firm induration. Multiple sinuses of face, mouth, jaw or neck develop, from which the pathognomonic 'sulphur granules' may be expressed.

MICROSCOPICAL

An intense polymorph infiltration around colonies of the fungus, surrounded by dense fibrosis.

RESULTS

From this cervico-facial site the process may remain localized, spread to the lungs, or become disseminated by the blood stream (see p. 57). Local deformity is usually marked unless treated by appropriate antibiotics.

Cancrum oris

AETIOLOGY

A rare gangrenous condition of the mouth, usually in children in whom it is preceded by a debilatating illness or malnutrition. The organisms involved are the normal commensals of the area and sometimes additionally anaerobic streptococci which have a synergistic effect.

MACROSCOPICAL

The process starts on the oral mucous membrane and rapidly penetrates the skin of the face producing discoloured, sloughing areas of gangrene.

MICROSCOPICAL

There is extensive tissue necrosis with only a sparse inflammatory cell response.

RESULTS

Extensive deformity of the mouth which is rapidly progressive and may prove fatal in untreated cases.

Syphilis

PRIMARY

A chancre may occur on the lip, tongue, or even tonsil.

SECONDARY

Linear superficial ulcers with irregular margins occur on the mucous membranes – 'snail track' ulcers.

TERTIARY

Three lesions of tertiary syphilis may affect the tongue:

1 *Leukoplakia* (see p. 171).
2 *Gumma.* A typical punched-out ulcer with a wash-leather slough in the base, most common on the dorsum of the tongue.
3 *Chronic interstitial inflammation.* The tongue may be hard and involved by a diffuse syphilitic inflammatory granulomatous reaction.

CONGENITAL

Rhagades at the angle of the mouth or occasionally a gumma.

Miscellaneous lesions in the mouth

INFECTIONS
(a) *Measles.* Koplik's spots on the buccal mucosa (see p. 42).
(b) *Chickenpox.* Small vesicles or a papular eruption (see p. 42).
(c) *Diphtheria.* A grey-coloured membrane on the mucosa of the oropharynx (see p. 642).
(d) *Scarlet fever.* 'Strawberry tongue' with prominence of papillae, is associated with this infection by erythrogenic strains of β-haemolytic streptococci.

BLOOD DISEASES
(a) *Iron deficiency anaemia.* Atrophic glossitis with a smooth pale tongue – Plummer-Vinson syndrome (see p. 476).
(b) *Pernicious anaemia.* Smooth red tongue with pallor of mucous membranes (see p. 482).
(c) *Leukaemia.* The lymphoid tissue of the oropharynx may enlarge or ulcerate, especially in acute leukaemia. Hyperplastic ulcerative gum lesions may be a presenting feature of the disease (see p. 463).
(d) *Agranulocytosis.* Pharyngeal ulceration is a common feature (see p. 452).
(e) *Infectious mononucleosis.* Pharyngeal ulceration with the membrane mimicking diphtheria is frequent in the 'anginose' type (see p. 449).
(f) *Polycythaemia.* Reddish-blue discoloration of the tongue.
(g) *Osler's familial telangiectasia.* Multiple small spider-like vascular dilatations of mucosal blood vessels (see p. 516).
(h) *Thrombocytopenic purpura.* Multiple petechial haemorrhages of skin and mucosae (see p. 517).

VITAMIN DEFICIENCY DISEASES
(a) *Vitamin B complex* – angular cheilosis.
Nicotinic acid – angular cheilosis and a red beefy tongue with atrophy of papillae.
Riboflavine – atrophic glossitis, angular cheilosis and gingivo-stomatitis.
(b) *Vitamin C.* Gingivitis, with swollen haemorrhagic gums and loose teeth, occurs in scurvy (see p. 693).

PIGMENTATIONS
(a) *Metals.* Prolonged industrial or therapeutic exposure to metals may produce pigmentation and gingivitis.
Arsenic – black line.
Bismuth – black line.
Lead – blue-grey line.
Mercury – grey-violet line.
Silver – grey line.
(b) *Addison's disease.* Patches of brown-black melanotic pigmentation of the buccal mucosa.
(c) *Haemochromatosis.* Bronze colour.
(d) *Peutz–Jegher's syndrome.* Mouth and lip melanin pigmentation associated with congenital polyposis of the intestinal tract.

Leukoplakia

NATURE
Hyperplasia of the squamous epithelium with hyperkeratosis producing raised white plaques. Related conditions also occur on the vulva (p. 424) and in the larynx (p. 643).

AGE
Rare under 30, the majority occur at about 50 years of age.

SITES
The most common site is the tongue, but the lips, gums, cheeks and floor of mouth may also be involved.

AETIOLOGY
A small percentage are syphilitic in origin, but otherwise the aetiology is obscure. Dental sepsis, pipe smoking, trauma from teeth and dental plates, electrical currents from fillings of dissimilar metals, vitamin A deficiency and hormonal factors, may all be contributory.

MACROSCOPICAL
The process starts as an area of surface thickening which is white and raised. At a later stage, multiple foci may coalesce to form a large area which becomes rough, white and fissured – 'coat of white paint'. Carcinoma may subsequently develop, usually in one of the fissures.

MICROSCOPICAL
The white appearance is due to surface keratin and hyperplasia of the prickle and basal cell layers to form atypical thickened rete pegs which extend downwards into the underlying tissues. There is also increased fibrosis and a lymphocyte and plasma cell infiltrate in the dermis.

RESULTS
Leukoplakia should be regarded as pre-cancerous since carcinoma will ultimately develop in approximately 30 per cent of cases. The time interval, however, is very variable.

Carcinoma of tongue

INCIDENCE
Tumours of the mouth, including tongue, lip and pharynx, account for about 2 per cent of malignant tumours.

AGE
Average 55 years of age.

SEX
M:F 9:1.

SITES
Sixty-five per cent arise on the lateral borders of the tongue; approximately 70 per cent on the anterior two-thirds.

PREDISPOSING FACTORS
Leukoplakia predisposes to tongue cancer and is present in many cases. Betel chewers have a high incidence and the Plummer–Vinson syndrome predisposes in women.

MACROSCOPICAL
The tumours may be papillary, nodular, diffuse, fissured or ulcerated, with an area of leukoplakia frequently visible at the periphery.

MICROSCOPICAL
Usually a keratinizing squamous cell carcinoma but poorly differentiated types, including lympho-epithelioma, do occur, especially in the posterior third (see below).

SPREAD
Direct spread through the tongue results in fixation to adjacent structures, e.g. floor of mouth. Approximately 50 per cent of patients have evidence of lymph node metastases in the cervical glands when first diagnosed and, at death, 40 per cent have evidence of blood-borne metastases in lungs, liver or other viscera.

PROGNOSIS
This is poor; tumours of the anterior two-thirds have a 5-year survival of 20 per cent; of the posterior third 12 per cent. Most of the long term survivors are stage 1 cases, i.e. growth restricted to the tongue.

Carcinoma of floor of mouth, cheek, palate

AGE
Average age is about 60 years.

SEX
M:F 9:1.

PREDISPOSING FACTORS
As for tongue (see above).

STRUCTURE
The tumours are keratinizing squamous cell carcinomas; only rarely are they undifferentiated.

PROGNOSIS
Five-year survival figures are:
   Floor of mouth – 17 per cent.
   Cheek – 14 per cent.
   Palate – 14 per cent.

Carcinoma of pharynx and tonsil

TYPES
The commonest tumours are keratizing squamous cell carcinomas, but in addition in this region there are undifferentiated types.

'TRANSITIONAL CELL' CARCINOMA
Composed of sheets and strands of undifferentiated epithelial cells with a palisade arrangement at the periphery mimicking to some extent the true transitional epithelial tumours seen in the urinary tract. There are no prickle cells and keratin formation is not seen.

LYMPHOEPITHELIOMA
A tumour in which there are sheets of undifferentiated tumour cells intermingled with a diffuse lymphocytic infiltrate. These tumours present at a younger age (30–40), usually with enlarged regional lymph nodes. The primary lesion in the nasopharynx or tonsil is usually very small and readily missed clinically. They are extremely radiosensitive tumours but are rarely radiocurable.

It is probable that keratinizing squamous cell carcinoma, 'transitional cell' carcinoma and lympho-epithelioma are all examples of varying degrees of dedifferentiation and all should be regarded as variants of squamous cell tumours.

SPREAD
Direct spread plays an important part at this site due to the close proximity of the base of the skull which is invaded at an early stage. The tumours frequently, therefore, cause cranial nerve palsies. Lymphatic and blood dissemination occur early, consequently the prognosis is poor.

PROGNOSIS
Pharynx and tonsil – 10 per cent 5-year survival.

Gums

Inflammation
Any of the inflammatory processes described on p. 168 may involve the gums. In addition there is the condition of pyorrhoea.

Pyorrhoea

NATURE
A progressive inflammatory gingivitis involving the periodontal tissues, resulting in bone destruction, loss of the tooth-bearing tissues and eventual loss of teeth.

AETIOLOGY
Frequently occurs over 30 years of age and may be associated with other types of inflammatory lesions elsewhere in the oral cavity. However, it is more

common as a primary process and in such cases the aetiology remains obscure, although nutritional and endocrine factors may be contributory.

MACROSCOPICAL

Starts as a gingivitis which then involves the gingival sulcus to produce a periodontal pocket. Suppuration occurs in the pocket and destroys the gum margin. Underlying bone is also destroyed resulting in exposure of the tooth roots and loss of tooth-holding tissues. Eventually the tooth is loossened and falls out.

MICROSCOPICAL

There is a non-specific suppurative infection of the soft tissues of the gum and the underlying bone with osteoclastic bone resorption. Organisms isolated are usually the normal mouth commensals.

Swellings

EPILEPSY THERAPY

Swelling of the gums occurs in many epileptic patients treated by diphenylhydantoin sodium.

SCURVY

Vitamin C deficiency with spongy scorbutic gums.

EPULIS

Localized swellings of the gum which are of different histological types:

(a) *Myeloid or giant cell epulis.* A squamous-covered nodule of cellular fibroblastic tissue containing many giant cells. These are of foreign body type and are smaller than osteoclasts. The lesion is reactive.

(b) *Fibrous epulis.* A squamous-covered nodule of benign, but often vascular, fibrous tissue.

(c) *Haemangiomatous epulis.* This squamous-covered nodule is composed of extremely vascular tissue and commonly arises during pregnancy – 'pregnancy tumour'. Sometimes there is ulceration of the epithelium with an inflammatory reaction and the nodule is then called 'granuloma pyogenicum'.

(d) *'Myoblastoma' epulis.* A rare epulis composed of pink-staining granular cells which form small lumps in children. The tumours may occur on the tongue, gum or elsewhere in the body. They are frequently associated with thickening of the overlying squamous epithelium. The 'myoblasts' are of uncertain origin, but are probably histiocytes or fibroblasts and not of muscular origin. The lesions are benign and excision is curative.

Chapter 34
Alimentary System – Jaw: Salivary Glands

Jaw

NORMAL TOOTH DEVELOPMENT

A tooth is derived from two germ layers:
1 The ectodermal dental lamina derived from oral squamous epithelium forms a downgrowth to produce the bell-shaped enamel organ (see Fig. 28). The enamel organ has an inner layer of cells which form the enamel – ameloblasts. The remainder of the organ, including the stellate reticulum forming the bulk of the structure, does not form enamel but

persists as the sheath of Hertwig in the periodontal membrane around the fully formed tooth. Small epithelial foci may persist as the rests of Malassez. In addition, the cells of the dental lamina may not completely disappear but may remain as the epithelial islands of Serres.

2 The mesodermal dental papilla forms the dentine, cementum and pulp of the tooth (see Fig. 28).

TUMOURS OF DENTAL TISSUES

Due to inductive changes exerted by dental tissues on each other, this is a very complex group. Many of the lesions are not true tumours in the neoplastic sense but are developmental anomalies or overgrowths. The term odontogenic tumours is used here in its broadest sense. Many are very rare and incompletely documented in respect of natural history but the W.H.O. classification is, at present, the most logical, in that it groups the various lesions according to their structural characteristics.

Lesions consisting of odontogenic epithelium
AMELOBLASTOMA – ADAMANTINOMA
This relatively common true tumour accounts for 1 per cent of all oral tumours; average age 33 years and 80 per cent in the mandible. There is wide geographical variability in incidence which is much greater in Africans. The tumour is slowly growing, may reach a very large size and is commonly polycystic. There is a very common association with an unerupted tooth and it is widely believed that the tumour may arise in a pre-existing dentigerous cyst. Histological appearances are of epidermal epithelial cells resembling ameloblasts surrounding a central core of stellate reticulum which forms microcysts due to degeneration. Histogenetically, the tumour almost certainly arises from the enamel organ. Whilst largely expansile in growth, local invasion can occur but metastasis is exceptionally rare. Recurrence after curettage is frequent but permanent cure is usually achieved by formal resection.

ADENOMATOID ODONTOGENIC TUMOUR
A variably cystic/solid, benign, truly neoplastic tumour mostly in young persons in the second or third decade and with an epithelial-like glandular histological appearance which probably represents abortive attempts to form enamel organs.

CALCIFYING EPITHELIAL TUMOUR – PINDBORG TUMOUR
A potentially recurrent, locally destructive true tumour, consisting of sheets of polyhedral epithelial cells of epidermal characteristics in an eosino-

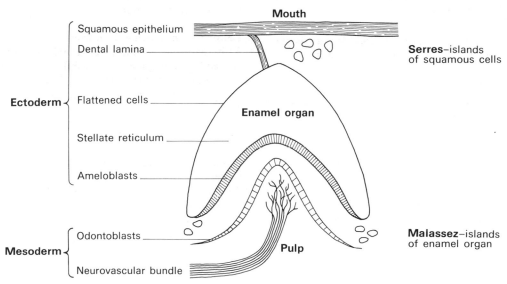

Fig. 28. Development of a tooth.

philic matrix which stains as amyloid and in which extensive calcium deposition occurs in a concentric manner. The lesions usually contain an unerupted tooth, present at an average age of 42 years and probably develop from the reduced enamel epithelium of this associated tooth.

CALCIFYING ODONTOGENIC CYST

A benign intraosseous or gingival cystic lesion showing histological similarity to ameloblastoma but with characteristic keratinous ghost cells and masses with accompanying foreign body giant cells and focal calcification.

Lesions consisting of odontogenic epithelium and mesenchyme

AMELOBLASTIC FIBROMA AND AMELOBLASTIC SARCOMA

The fibroma is a soft solid mass expanding bone but non-invasive. Ameloblastic-like epithelium is embedded in an abundant fibroblastic stroma resembling the dental papilla. In the rare sarcoma this stroma shows frank malignant appearances.

Lesions consisting of odontogenic epithelium and calcified dental tissues

ODONTO-AMELOBLASTOMA

A mixture of odontogenic epithelium with mature enamel and dentine.

Lesions consisting of calcified dental tissues but without odontogenic epithelium

COMPLEX ODONTOME

A tumour-like mass of enamel, dentine and cementum deposited in an irregular manner.

COMPOUND ODONTOME

More highly organized, the enamel and dentine forming recognizable tooth-like structures.

DENS INVAGINATUS

A developmental malformation in which an invagination of enamel is formed in a tooth.

ENAMELOMA

A malformation consisting of ectopic deposits of enamel on a tooth.

DENTINOMA

A tumour-like lesion composed of dentine.

CEMENTOMA

A fibrous lesion containing cementum.

Lesions consisting of odontogenic mesenchyme

FIBROMA AND MYXOMA

These resemble similarly named lesions elsewhere in the body.

Non-neoplastic cysts

DENTAL CYST

Whereas some simple squamous-lined cysts are of developmental origin, most follow epithelialization of an apical abscess or granuloma.

DENTIGEROUS CYST

An epithelial-lined cyst around an unerupted tooth and which may be associated with development of ameloblastoma or of a calcifying epithelial tumour.

INFLAMMATIONS

Both acute and chronic osteomyelitis may occur in the jaw bones, in the mandible usually associated with tooth infection, and in the maxilla with either tooth or sinus infection.

Leontiasis osseum – 'lion face'

This deformity of the maxilla and nose may be caused by a low grade chronic inflammation of the bone or by fibrous dysplasia, although Paget's disease of bone may produce an identical clinical picture. Also see leprosy p. 53.

TUMOURS OF THE JAW

Tumours of the jaw are infrequent but, in addition to the tumours of dental tissues mentioned above, the following types may be found:
1 *Skeletal tissues*
   (*a*) *Bone tumours*
      Osteoma
      Osteosarcoma
   (*b*) *Cartilaginous tumours*
      Chondroma
      Chondrosarcoma

(c) *Giant cell lesions*
   Giant cell variants
   Reparative granuloma.
2 *Soft tissues within bone*
   (a) *Fibrous tissue*
      Fibroma
      Ossifying fibroma
      Fibrosarcoma
   (b) *Blood vessels*
      Haemangeioma
      Angiosarcoma
   (c) *Nerve tissue*
      Neurofibroma
      Neurofibrosarcoma
   (d) *Marrow cells*
      Myeloma
      Ewing's tumour
      *Lymphoma

Thus, any tumour which is encountered elsewhere in the skeleton may occur in the jaws and detailed descriptions will be avoided, except where they are pertinent to the jaw lesion (see pp. 698–706).

Skeletal tissues

BONY TUMOURS
The osteoma is usually of the ivory type and the osteosarcoma is frequently associated with Paget's disease of bone.

CARTILAGINOUS TUMOURS
Chondromas occur in the lower jaw but are rare. Chondrosarcoma may also be associated with Paget's disease.

GIANT CELL LESIONS
It was formerly stated that giant cell tumours frequently arose in the jaw. This true tumour entity is in fact an extreme rarity in the jaw bones, but 'giant cell variants', all of which are benign, are common. A giant cell epulis has to be distinguished from the true osteoclastoma and there is also the condition of *'reparative granuloma'*. This is a destructive osteolytic lesion in the jaws of young adults consisting of a cellular fibroblastic stroma in which there are red cells, some foam cells and giant cells which simulate osteoclasts but which are phagocytic. This lesion, which mimics a giant cell tumour, is probably a reactive process and is benign. Other giant cell variants may occur in the jaw and are considered on p. 703.

Soft tissues

FIBROUS TUMOURS
Fibromas, many of which show ossification, are common in the jaw and various names have been attached to the lesions. They form radiotranslucent swellings with a mottled appearance due to new bone formation. Histologically, they are composed of fibrous tissue in the pure fibroma, with osteoid tissue or bone in the ossifying fibromas. Some authorities have disputed a true tumorous nature and regard them all as variants of fibrous dysplasia (see p. 689).

BLOOD VESSELS
Haemangioma and its malignant counterpart, angiosarcoma are rare in the jaw.

NERVE TISSUE
The inferior dental nerve is incorporated within the mandibular canal and from this nerve, neurofibromas or neurofibrosarcomas may arise

MARROW CELLS
The jaw may occasionally be the site of involvement by malignant marrow cell tumours, e.g. myeloma, lymphoma and Ewing's tumour (see p. 704).

Salivary glands

Introduction
Mucous glands are widespread throughout the upper alimentary and respiratory tracts. Large aggregations occur in the major salivary glands – parotid, submandibular and sublingual; minor collections are numerous in the mouth, palate, lip, cheek, nose, larynx, pharynx, whilst the trachea and major bronchi and the lacrimal glands contain similar mucous glands.

Whilst most attention is usually focused on the major salivary glands, diseases affecting these organs commonly produce similar changes in any mucous gland at any site.

Congenital
Congenital abnormalities are rare, but include atresias and anomalies of the ducts. Occasionally, one or more glands may be absent.

INFLAMMATIONS – SIALOADENITIS

Non-specific

ACUTE SUPPURATIVE

This usually occurs in debilitated individuals, particularly children. The exact pathogenesis is obscure but there seems little doubt that the pyogenic organisms gain access to the glands via the duct from the mouth. In severe cases, frank suppuration with abscess formation may occur with destruction of the gland.

CHRONIC

This is usually associated with duct calculi but occasionally can arise *de novo* as a low grade chronic inflammatory process of obscure pathogenesis. The involved gland is firm and may be swollen and there is fibrosis and a chronic inflammatory cell infiltration with loss of epithelium. The condition may mimic a tumour, from which clinical differentiation may be difficult.

Specific

MUMPS

The diffuse interstitial parotid inflammation in mumps is usually bilateral but occasionally unilateral. In 20 per cent, the submandibular and other salivary glands are involved (see p. 42).

GRANULOMATOUS

Tuberculosis or actinomycosis may rarely involve salivary glands. Salivary gland involvement by sarcoidosis is rather more frequent.

CYTOMEGALIC INCLUSION DISEASE

Nature. A rare disease of infancy and childhood characterized by the presence of inclusion bodies in the nucleus and cytoplasm of the epithelial cells of salivary glands, renal tubules, septal cells of the lungs and less commonly in other sites. Infection may also become established at any age group in patients receiving immunosuppressive therapy.

Aetiology. The cytomegalovirus.

Appearances. The affected cells, particularly in the salivary glands, are grossly swollen and contain large inclusion bodies in the nucleus and cytoplasm.

Effects. The clinical pattern and course are extremely variable, the usual manifestations being of a blood dyscrasia and hepatomegaly. When the salivary glands only are affected, the disease is of no significance, but when of widespread distribution, death may result.

SIALOLITHIASIS

Stone formation in the duct results in acute or chronic sialoadenitis with eventual atrophy of the salivary gland acini. The submandibular duct is the most common site. The pathogenesis of the calculi is obscure.

BENIGN LYMPHOEPITHELIAL LESION

Nature

Salivary gland enlargement characterized histologically by atrophy of glandular parenchyma and lymphocytic infiltration with epimyothelial islands replacing the intralobular ducts.

The term largely replaces Mikulicz's and Sjögren's syndromes, in which affected glands are usually enlarged (bilateral in Mikulicz's syndrome) and there are associated connective tissue diseases in over half the patients who present with dry mouth and conjunctivae (Sjögren's syndrome).

Pathogenesis

The high incidence of hypergammaglobulinaemia, positive rheumatoid factor in 90 per cent and frequently positive anti-nuclear factor together with a specific anti-salivary duct antibody in many cases indicates an immunological disorder.

Incidence

Largely in the middle aged with a female preponderance.

Macroscopical

Affected glands are painless and have usually progressively enlarged. One or more parotid, submandibular and lacrimal glands are most typically involved. The lesion may be diffuse or discretely nodular with a rubbery whitish cut surface and retention of the normal lobular pattern.

Microscopical

Glandular atrophy, lymphocytic infiltration usually without follicle formation and duct proliferation forming the epimyothelial islands.

Course

Slowly progressive benign course with a slight risk of development of malignant change to lymphoma or, rarely, carcinoma.

CYSTS

Non-neoplastic cysts of retention type are common in minor glands but rare in the major where occasionally they can be clinically mistaken for tumours.

MUCOUS GLAND TUMOURS

EPITHELIAL TUMOURS

Adenomas

PLEOMORPHIC ADENOMA – 'MIXED TUMOUR'

Incidence

The most common tumour of salivary glands. About 70 per cent of parotid gland tumours are of this type and it is 10 times more frequent in the parotid gland than in the submandibular.

Age

Increasing with age from 25 years onwards.

Sex

M:F 3:4.

Macroscopical

A lobulated, firm circumscribed tumour within the salivary gland. The cut surface often glistens and appears semi-translucent.

Microscopical

A very variable appearance of differing arrangements of epithelial cells in ductular or acinar patterns with associated myoepithelial cell proliferation and the presence of luminal mucin and areas of cartilage in the stroma which is probably produced by the myoepithelial cells. There is a thin fibrous capsule through which extensions of new lobules of tumour grow, rendering complete excision by enucleation impossible.

Results

Growth is slow and by expansion and if surgical excision is performed with a margin of salivary gland tissue, cure results. Local recurrence is quite frequent following enucleation and may be subsequently very troublesome and difficult to effect a cure without severe mutilation. Malignant change can infrequently occur (see p. 180).

MONOMORPHIC ADENOMAS

Adenolymphoma

Incidence – about 8 per cent of parotid gland tumours, rare in the submandibular and minor salivary glands.

Age – 35–80 years.

Sex – M:F 5:1.

Macroscopical – variably cystic, smooth surfaced, ovoid and moderately firm, usually situated near the gland surface and not uncommonly multiple.

Microscopical – the cystic spaces are lined by papillary adenomatous tissue with variable amounts of lymphocytic infiltration, including follicles, in the stroma. The epithelium is double-layered with a tall, very regular, characteristic eosinophilic inner layer.

Results – these tumours are benign. Similar lesions are occasionally found within lymph nodes adjacent to the parotid gland and in the upper cervical groups. These also behave innocently.

Oxyphilic adenoma

This benign, encapsulated, uncommon tumour is composed of regular acini of large eosinophilic cells – *oncocytes*. It is nearly always in the parotid where it forms 1 per cent of tumours of this gland.

Other adenomas

Rare benign epithelial tumours include: tubular, clear cell, basal cell, trabecular and sebaceous adenomas.

Mucoepidermoid tumour

INCIDENCE

About 8 per cent of major salivary gland tumours, 90 per cent in the parotids and nearly all the remainder in the submandibular gland.

AGE

Most 20–60 years but occasionally in children.

SEX

M:F equal.

MACROSCOPICAL
Solitary, locally infiltrative, solid or partially cystic.

MICROSCOPICAL
A mixture of mucus-secreting and squamous epithelial cells with cysts containing thick mucin.

RESULTS
Radical removal leads to cure in 85 per cent. In some patients growth and local infiltration is rapid and in others cervical lymph node or visceral metastatic spread may occur.

Acinic cell tumour
This rather rare tumour accounts for about 2 per cent of parotid gland tumours and is even less common in the submandibular. More frequent in males (3 : 1) they may occur at almost any age. The tumour is composed of epithelial cells resembling the salivary serous cells and with basophilic granular cytoplasm. Results of surgical removal are good with 80 per cent 5-year survival, but local recurrence and, in 5–10 per cent of patients, local lymph node or distant metastases, indicate the malignant potential.

Carcinomas

ADENOID CYSTIC CARCINOMA – CYLINDROMA
– ADENOCYSTIC CARCINOMA
An infiltrative malignant tumour of characteristic cribriform pattern composed of two cell types, duct-lining cells and myoepithelial cells. The fibrous stroma is commonly very hyaline and marginal and perineural lymphatic invasion is usually prominent. The tumour is more common in females in the 40–60 age group and forms 1.2 per cent of parotid gland tumours. It is relatively more common in submandibular gland (17 per cent) and forms 15 per cent of tumours of minor salivary glands, e.g. palate, lip, tongue and respiratory tract. Growth is slow and lymphatic and blood-borne metastases are late, with 5-year survival figures of 70 per cent but 20-year survival of 13 per cent. The best results occur in patients in whom the tumour is widely locally excised at the first attempt.

OTHER CARCINOMAS
Adenocarcinoma, squamous cell and undifferentiated carcinomas arise *de novo* or on the basis of a pre-existing pleomorphic adenoma. They are obviously infiltrative and of poor prognosis with 5-year survival of only 25 per cent and 50 per cent of these patients die from distant metastases.

NON-EPITHELIAL TUMOURS

Connective tissue tumours within the glands are uncommon with the exception, in young children, of haemangioma and lymphangioma; lipomas and neurofibromas occasionally occur.

Congenital

Abnormalities of the septum
The oesophagus develops with the trachea as a single structure, being later separated by the intervention of a longitudinal septum. Abnormalities of development of this septum lead to malformations at various levels, most of which have fistulous communications – *tracheo-oesophageal fistulae*, resulting in the inhalation of milk or gastric contents into the lungs.

Congenital narrowing
Narrowing of the lumen may be due to a segmental area of atresia of to a congenital mucosal web.

Congenital shortening
Most cases of so-called congenital shortening are associated with hiatus hernia. True congenital shortening is very rare.

Ectopic gastric mucosa
The oesophagus is normally lined throughout its

length by squamous epithelium; occasionally single or multiple foci of gastric mucosa may occur in the lower end of an otherwise normal oesophagus.

Achalasia of the cardia – 'cardiospasm'

Age
Most cases present in early adulthood.

Aetiology
The physiological sphincter at the cardia fails to relax and the proximal oesophagus loses its normal peristaltic rhythm. There are demonstrable abnormalities of argyrophil neurones with loss of ganglion cells throughout but more marked in the proximal segment.

Effects
The cardia become thickened, producing obstruction to the passage of food so that the oesophagus above becomes distended, lengthened, hypertrophic and slightly tortuous. The mucosal surface may become ulcerated.

Results
Progressive dysphagia which requires treatment by intermittent dilatation or by surgery. The results of the operation are good although recurrence of symptoms is not uncommon. Complications due to aspiration of material from the dilated oesophagus

into the respiratory tract are common, e.g. lipid pneumonia, lung abscess (see p. 663). There is also an increased incidence of oesophageal carcinoma subsequently.

Hiatus hernia

Nature
An abnormality of the oesophageal hiatus in the diaphragm whereby there is partial herniation of the stomach into the thorax.

Aetiology
This is unknown but there may be a congenital weakness of part of the diaphragm, abnormalities of the crura, or neuromuscular inco-ordination of the muscular parts of the diaphragm.

Types
1 *Sliding* (see Fig. 29).
2 *Rolling*.

Appearances
There is enlargement of the hiatus with variable amounts of stomach in the posterior mediastinum.

Effects
The condition is commonly asymptomatic, being found incidentally on radiological examination. Many of those presenting with symptoms referable to the hernia have had the condition present for

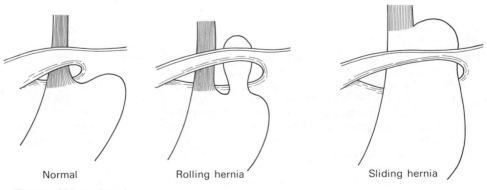

Normal   Rolling hernia   Sliding hernia

Fig. 29. Types of hiatus hernia.

many years, attention being drawn to the area by pain, commonly associated with pregnancy or increasing obesity. The important effects are caused by oesophageal reflux of gastric juice producing oesophagitis, ulceration, fibrosis and stricture of the lower oesophagus. Bleeding is commonly associated with these complications and the condition may present as chronic iron deficiency anaemia.

Diverticula

Pharyngeal pouch – 'pulsion diverticulum'

NATURE
A pulsion diverticulum of the lower pharynx occurring at an area of weakness of the inferior constrictor muscle.

MACROSCOPICAL
A pouch develops which is directed anterolaterally and downwards.

MICROSCOPICAL
A squamous-lined pouch with a fibrous wall containing scanty muscle fibres.

RESULTS
Swallowed food is directed into the pouch which therefore enlarges further and may cause dysphagia. Regurgitation of food contents and aspiration into the lungs may cause pneumonia or lung abscess.

Traction diverticulum

NATURE
Traction on the wall of the oesophagus externally due to adherent tuberculous lymph nodes in the mediastinum.

SITE
Usually in the lower third.

MACROSCOPICAL
The pouch is directed upwards and anteriorly.

MICROSCOPICAL
A small squamous-lined pouch.

RESULTS
Usually asymptomatic as they empty spontaneously.

Vascular

Varices

NATURE
Varicosities of the oesophageal veins, especially at the gastro-oesophageal junction.

AETIOLOGY
Portal hypertension, usually due to cirrhosis of the liver (see p. 562), results in reversal of blood flow from the portal venous system into the systemic circulation and thus distension of the oesophageal veins occurs.

MACROSCOPICAL
The veins of the oesophagus, especially at the lower end and in the upper portion of the stomach, are prominent and grossly varicose.

RESULTS
Ulceration of the covering mucosa is followed by leakage of blood of slight or catastrophic amounts. A haematemesis from this source is the most common presenting feature of portal hypertension.

Plummer–Vinson syndrome – sideropenic dysphagia – Paterson–Kelly syndrome

This syndrome occurs in females and consists of dysphagia, glossitis – smooth glazed tongue, koilonychia and iron deficiency anaemia.

The dysphagia is probably due to abnormal oesophageal peristalsis which may show as a 'web' in the post-cricoid region of the upper oesophagus. This initially can only be demonstrated radiologically, but later has a structural basis of narrowing with increased fibrosis of the wall. There is a constant relationship to chronic iron deficiency, hence sideropenia, although the degree of anaemia may be slight.

In longstanding cases in females there is increased incidence of carcinoma of the tongue and of the post-cricoid region.

Oesophageal ulceration

Traumatic
This may follow the swallowing of sharp foreign bodies, e.g. bones, etc., or follow instrumentation. In some cases perforation may occur with ensuing mediastinitis.

Corrosives
Accidental or suicidal ingestion of corrosive poisons, e.g. strong acids and alkalis, phenol, cresol, etc., is followed by oesophageal ulceration. In non-fatal cases, fibrotic stricture may follow.

Tuberculosis
A tuberculous ulcer due to swallowing infected sputum is extremely rare.

Peptic ulceration
Ulceration occurring in the lower third of the oesophagus in ectopic gastric mucosa has the typical appearance of a peptic ulcer (see p. 188). The ulcer may produce pain, haematemesis, perforation, or a stricture due to fibrous scarring of the healed lesion.

Oesophagitis
Reflux of gastric juice in hiatus hernia and prolonged vomiting may cause digestion of the squamous epithelium and ulceration.

Squamous cell carcinoma

Carcinoma of oesophagus

Incidence
About 2 per cent of all malignant disease, but much higher in Japan, France, Switzerland, parts of Africa and in Chinese.

Age
Rare below 50, the average age is about 65 years.

Sex
Ninety per cent occur in men, except in the post-cricoid region where the sex incidence shows marked female predilection.

Sites
The middle third, lower third and then upper third, in order of frequency.

Predisposing factors
The one definite predisposing factor is the Plummer–Vinson syndrome, but this only applies to the post-cricoid region in females. Other predisposing factors are speculative and include carcinogenic foods, hot drinks, nicotine; leukoplakia, achalasia of

the cardia and mucosal ulceration at the mouth of diverticula are established but rare causes.

Macroscopical
Solid, pale and frequently nodular growths which extend in the submucosa and in the wall of the oesophagus and eventually ulcerate. This results in dysphagia with eventual complete obstruction of the lumen.

Microscopical
The vast majority of the tumours are squamous cell carcinomas of varying grades of differentiation and only a small minority are adenocarcinomas; these latter may arise from ectopic gastric mucosa in the lower third of the oesophagus or by direct extension of gastric cancers.

Spread
The cancers spread directly through the wall to involve adjacent mediastinal structures, e.g. trachea to produce a tracheo-oesophageal fistula. They also show a predilection to spread vertically in the submucosa and form multiple satellite submucosal nodules. By the time the diagnosis is made, the regional lymph nodes are usually invaded, e.g. cervical nodes from the upper third, mediastinal nodes from the middle third and abdominal nodes from the lower third. Blood dissemination also occurs to any organ, but especially the brain and liver.

Prognosis
This is very poor and even in operable cases the 5-year survival figure is only about 5 per cent. Most die within 1 year.

Oesophageal obstruction

Lumen
Impaction of foreign bodies.

Wall
(*a*) Congenital stenosis.
(*b*) Scarring from traumatic or corrosive ulceration.
(*c*) Scarring from peptic oesophagitis.
(*d*) Cardiospasm – achalasia of the cardia.
(*e*) Hiatus hernia.
(*f*) Plummer–Vinson syndrome.

(g) Scleroderma (see p. 726).

(h) Carcinoma.

External

Pressure on the oesophagus due to tumours, aneurysms, goitres, pharyngeal pouch, abscess, etc.

Results

The oesophageal obstruction is usually progressive, involving firstly solid foods and finally even liquids.

Dysphagia

All the previously mentioned causes of oesphageal obstruction may produce dysphagia. In addition, neurological disorders, e.g. poliomyelitis and bulbar palsy, may cause similar difficulties in swallowing.

Oesophageal perforation

Lumen

Foreign bodies, instruments (dilators, bougies), fish bones, etc.

Wall

Carcinoma, especially when eroding into the aorta or trachea, peptic ulceration or 'spontaneous' perforation.

'SPONTANEOUS' PERFORATION – MALLORY–WEISS SYNDROME

Nature

This usually occurs during violent or 'resisted' vomiting in elderly males, especially following a large meal.

Appearances

There is a linear split in the lower end of the oesophagus and gastric contents pour into the chest.

Results

This is usually a fatal condition unless the diagnosis is made at an early stage and the perforation sutured or the haemorrhage arrested.

External

Tumours especially carcinoma of the bronchus, aneurysms and abscesses.

Results

Oesophageal perforation is followed by pleurisy with effusion, empyema, mediastinitis, pericarditis and pneumonia. The mortality rate is very high.

Chapter 36
Alimentary System – Stomach

Congenital pyloric stenosis

Nature
Achalasia of the pylorus due to 'neuromuscular inco-ordination'.

Appearances
There is a firm, thickened pyloric sphincter with distension of the stomach. Histologically, there is hypertrophy of the pyloric muscle fibres, but the mucosa is normal. Abnormalities of myenteric ganglion cells are consistently found.

Results
Projectile vomiting, usually in a first-born, 6-weeks-old, male infant, followed by electrolyte and nutritional disturbances unless a muscle-splitting operation is performed. This abnormality may run in families but some cases do not become clinically apparent until adult life. In this adult type of congenital pyloric stenosis the changes are similar.

'Gastritis'

Nature
A vague and ill-defined term in which the relationship of the clinical manifestations to the pathological changes is commonly obscure.

ACUTE GASTRITIS

Aetiology
This is extemely variable. It may be caused by dietary indiscretions, aspirin, alcoholic excess or be part of a systemic infection, whilst extemely florid examples are seen in suicidal patients swallowing corrosive fluids.

Macroscopical
The stomach is thickened, oedematous, congested and may show ulceration of the tips of the rugae. In severe cases, the ulceration may be more extensive, especially following corrosive poisons.

Microscopical
There is a polymorph infiltration of the submucosa with variable congestion, oedema and mucosal ulceration. A particularly exuberant example occurs in *phlegmonous gastritis* when the inflammatory reaction extends into the muscle coat which shows severe necrosis with profuse organisms but only a relatively scanty inflammatory cell infiltration (see p. 26).

Effects
This pathology may account for some forms of indigestion, but it is probable that in many instances the stomach returns to normal, except in the corrosive cases and in phlegmonous gastritis, both of which are frequently fatal.

CHRONIC GASTRITIS

Superficial gastritis
Only the superficial zone of antral or body mucosa is affected by loss of surface cells but preservation of normal mucosal thickness. There is some loss of acid and pepsin secretory cells and relative increase in mucus-secreting cells with a variable inflammatory cell infiltrate of the lamina propria. The lesion is associated with a considerable fall of acid and pepsinogen output and may proceed to atrophic gastritis.

Atrophic gastritis
This follows the superficial type and shows marked loss of chief and parietal cells in the deeper parts of the body mucosa with, usually, some thinning. Increase in mucus-secreting cells often occurs – *pseudopyloric metaplasia*. Lymphoid aggregates or follicles may develop – *follicular gastritis* and microcyst formation and regenerative polyps may also occur. Secretory functions are markedly impaired and production of B_{12} binding material is deficient. The condition is associated with intestinal metaplasia and increased risk of carcinoma.

Intestinal metaplasia
An important change associated with atrophic gastritis and gastric atrophy in which focal or diffuse areas of the superficial zone show goblet mucus-secreting cells of histological and histochemical appearances of colonic epithelium. This condition is precancerous.

Gastric atrophy
Atrophy of diffuse distribution may follow atrophic gastritis or be idiopathic. The mucosa is grossly thinned with absence of chief and parietal cells and replacement by simple epithelial cells and intestinal metaplastic areas.

Stomach in pernicious anaemia
Patients with this disease (see p. 482) have superficial gastritis, atrophic gastritis or gastric atrophy at various stages and also, in a high proportion, complement-fixing antibodies against microsomes of parietal cells whilst 60 per cent have specific anti-intrinsic factor antibodies.

Peptic ulceration

ACUTE PEPTIC ULCER

Aetiology
Some are associated with severe burns (Curling's ulcer), cerebral haemorrhages, steroid therapy, pituitary tumours (Cushing's ulcer), uraemia, irritative chemicals particularly when ingested in tablet form, e.g. aspirin. The majority of acute ulcers, however, have no known predisposing factors and most examples are seen in young adults.

Sites
Frequently multiple, they may be located in any region of the stomach and occasionally in the duodenum.

Macroscopical
Single or multiple small round areas of surface

mucosal ulceration which are sometimes called 'gastric erosions'.

Microscopical

There is a small area of non-specific surface ulceration which extends down to, but not through, the muscularis mucosae. These is a mild inflammatory cell infiltration but no vascular changes.

Effects

The majority heal rapidly without scarring but a small minority may produce an haematemesis or rarely perforate. Of practical significance is the absence of induration or peritoneal involvement, thus, at operation, they are frequently difficult to find even on opening the stomach. These acute gastric erosions probably play no part in the pathogenesis of chronic peptic ulceration.

CHRONIC PEPTIC ULCER

Incidence

Approximately 20 per cent of the adult population have, or have had, a peptic ulcer.

Sites and age

Duodenal:gastric:7:2·5.

Gastric ulcers more common in men up to 40 years, equally common 40–50, more in females after 50.

Duodenal ulcers much more in males in 30–40 age group, decreasing to sex equality by 55–60 years.

Aetiology

The exact aetiology is still wrapped in mystery and conjecture but certain facts are known and there is a definite but multifactorial genetic predisposition.

SITES

Peptic ulcers only occur in five sites – stomach, duodenum, oesophagus, Meckel's diverticulum and at a gastro-enterostomy stoma – i.e. at sites where the mucosa is bathed by gastric juice.

GASTRIC JUICE

The presence of gastric juice appears essential for the formation of a peptic ulcer, i.e. pepsin + acid *versus* the mucosa.

ACID CONTENT

Peptic ulceration does not occur with complete achlorhydria and should this develop in an ulcer patient or the acid-producing regions of the stomach be surgically removed, the ulcer rapidly heals. Conversely, there is evidence of increased acid secretion in many patients with duodenal ulcers. Likewise, in the stomach, ulcers are mostly pyloric, i.e. ulcers occur adjacent to, but not in, acid-secreting areas. Gastrin production may be intermediary in stimulating hypersecretion, and, in this respect, the acid hypersecretion and intractable peptic ulceration in patients with the *Zollinger–Ellison* syndrome (see p. 636) who have a gastrin-secreting D-cell tumour or hyperplasia of the pancreatic islets, is significant.

DECREASED MUCOSAL RESISTANCE

There is no real evidence that trauma from food or vasospasm produce mucosal damage. Irritant foodstuffs and tobacco are also probably not very significant factors. Lack of mucin or excess of mucolytic enzymes has been postulated, without good evidence, for reduction in the mucosal protective effect of mucin.

NEUROGENIC

Vagal stimulation increases acid secretion and vagotomy decreases production. Stress stimulation of the vagus has been suggested as an important factor.

Location

In the duodenum, they are in the anterior or posterior wall of the first part, rarely in the second part and almost never beyond this site. The second commonest site is astride the lesser curvature of the antral region or the margenstrasse of the stomach. Duodenal and gastric ulcers together account for 97 per cent of all peptic ulcers, the small remainder being stomal ulcers, in the oesophagus (see p. 184), or in a Meckel's diverticulum (see p. 194).

Size

Peptic ulcers are commonly small and the majority are less than 3 cm diameter. Larger ones are, however, not infrequent and do not necessarily imply malignancy.

Macroscopical

They have a relatively constant appearance with a

round or oval outline, a deep, rather punched-out, appearance and slightly sloping sides, the edges being flat and at the same level or only slightly raised from the surrounding mucosal surface. Their depth varies, being shallow in the healing cases, but very deep in the penetrating examples. The floor is usually smooth, but thrombosed or patent blood vessels may be apparent. Externally, there is induration and the peritoneal coat commonly shows fibrous puckering.

Microscopical
The following zones are visible:
1 A superficial ulcer floor of necrotic inflammatory granulation tissue.
2 Beneath this there is a zone of active and non-specific inflammatory granulation tissue.
3 The base is composed of dense fibrous tissue which may contain endarteritic blood vessels, chronic inflammatory cells and extensive fibrous tissue. The latter usually replaces the muscle completely and often extends to the peritoneal surface.
4 The epithelium of the margins may show proliferation in an attempt at healing but remains superficial to the muscularis mucosae.

Results

HEALING
The defect is filled by granulation tissue and epithelium grows in from the margins to cover the surface. The healed area becomes a puckered, stellate, firm, fibrous scar covered by thin epithelium.

PENETRATION
The ulceration may progress and penetrate to adjacent tissues, e.g. pancreas, liver or omentum. The base of the ulcer is then formed by these structures.

PERFORATION
The ulcer base may give way with resulting perforation and peritonitis.

HAEMORRHAGE
Haematemesis or melaena is a common complication due to erosion of the large vessels in the gastric wall or adjacent structures, e.g. splenic artery. Endarteritis obliterans, which occurs in vessels in the ulcer base, is seldom sufficiently complete to prevent considerable leakage of blood and furthermore it prevents efficient retraction of an eroded vessel.

STENOSIS
The fibrous scar tissue may extend widely from the ulcer base to produce obstruction, at the pylorus – pyloric stenosis, at the cardia, or in the body – 'hour-glass' stomach.

MALIGNANCY
Malignancy may supervene to produce an '*ulcer-cancer*', but there is much controversy regarding its frequency. The essential criteria for this diagnosis are:
(*a*) There must be histological evidence of a pre-existing chronic gastric ulcer with fibrosis of the muscle coat.
(*b*) The carcinoma must arise from the epithelium at the margins of the ulcer and the cancer cells invade the underlying wall deep to the muscularis mucosae.

The incidence of this complication is difficult to assess and varies from 0 per cent by those who deny the existence of 'ulcer-cancer' to 10 per cent. It seems probable that the incidence of cancer developing in a proven peptic ulcer and the presence of unequivocal evidence of previous peptic ulcer at the site of a proven carcinoma, are both less than 1 per cent.

Prognosis of peptic ulcers
1 *Heal.* The majority of ulcers heal with medical treatment and only about 15 per cent fail to do so. Vagotomy and pyloroplasty are very successful in causing healing to occur in those in whom conservative measures have failed.
2 *Recurrence.* There is recurrence of ulcer symptoms in about 50 per cent of cases within 3 years and in 75 per cent within 5 years, in those patients treated by a medical regime.
3 *Haemorrhage.* Haemorrhage, producing melaena with a positive occult blood test, is extremely common, but overt haemorrhage with an haematemesis or severe melaena necessitating hospitalization is much less frequent and probably occurs in only about 5 per cent. The mortality of severe bleeding from gastric ulcers is about 20 per cent and from duodenal ulcers about 30 per cent, many of the fatal cases occurring in the older age groups. It will be recalled that severe haematemesis may also be

due to acute gastric erosions, carcinoma of the stomach and oesophageal varices.

4 *Perforation.* This occurs in 1 per cent of male peptic ulcer cases and 0.1 per cent of females in the ratio of eight duodenal ulcers to one gastric ulcer. The prognosis of treated cases varies according to the age of the patient and the interval between perforation and operation, but carries a mortality of at least 5 per cent.

Tumours

BENIGN

Connective tissue
Leiomyomas, fibromas, lipomas and neurofibromas are uncommon but are being diagnosed with increasing frequency. These benign tumours produce a smooth projection into the lumen of the stomach with a central apical ulcer to result in a characteristic radiological appearance.

Epithelial
Papillomas and adenomas rarely occur in the stomach but are important in that they slowly increase in size and eventually become malignant in a significant proportion of cases when more than 2.0 cm diameter. Hamartomatous or regenerative (inflammatory) polyps are not pre-cancerous.

MALIGNANT

Carcinoma

INCIDENCE
This is a common cancer and is responsible for approximately 15 per cent of all cancer deaths, a figure which is exceeded only by lung and large bowel cancers. The tumour is even more common in Japan and Scandinavia; rare in Malays and common amongst the Chinese in Indonesia.

AGE
Rare below 30; the commonest age group is 60–70 years.

SEX
M:F 2:1

PREDISPOSING FACTORS
1 *Peptic ulcer.* Occasionally, careful microscopic examination will reveal evidence of malignant change at the epithelial edge of a chronic peptic ulcer with invasion of the underlying wall (see below).
2 *Ingested foods.* Alcohol, fried foods, nicotine, spices and other miscellaneous foodstuffs, have been postulated as factors but so far without confirmatory evidence.
3 *Benign tumours.* Gastric papillomas and adenomas are progressive tumours which slowly increase in size; a high proportion of them eventually becoming carcinomatous.
4 *Intestinal metaplasia and atrophic gastritis.* Intestinal metaplasia and, to a lesser extent, atrophic gastritis are pre-cancerous. Carcinoma is 3 to 4 times more common in patients with pernicious anaemia, almost certainly due to the presence of intestinal metaplasia (see p. 187).

SITES
Approximately 50 per cent of gastric cancers arise in the pyloric region or the pyloric antrum, but 25 per cent occur on the lesser curvature. The remainder are diffuse, at the cardia, or at any other site, including the greater curvature.

MACROSCOPICAL
1 *Nodular* – about 45 per cent. Raised nodules of growth, discrete or confluent but not polypoid, which may secondarily ulcerate.
2 *Ulcerating* – about 40 per cent. Shallow ulcers, usually single but multiple in 5–10 per cent, with raised rolled edges and infiltrated indurated adjacent stomach wall. The ulcer base is normally raised above the surrounding mucosal surface.
3 *Fungating* – about 6 per cent. Protruberant, bulky, solid, often partly ulcerated, tumours.
4 *Diffusely infiltrative* – Linitis plastica – about 7 per cent. The 'leather-bottle' stomach shows diffuse induration, rigidity of the wall and thickening.
5 *Superficial carcinoma* – *early gastric cancer* (EGC) – about 2 per cent. These grow in the mucosa and submucosa which may show slight thickening or wrinkling with some rigidity and, later, superficial ulceration, or they may be grossly inconspicuous.
6 *Ulcer-cancer* – less than 1 per cent. An apparently benign gastric ulcer which may, on close inspection, show slight marginal firmness or atypicality (see above).

MICROSCOPICAL

All are of glandular origin and show varying grades of differentiation as adenocarcinomas, papillary carcinomas, spheroidal cell carcinomas, signet-ring cancers or any mixtures of these descriptive varieties. Rarely, squamous metaplasia may result in a squamous cell carcinoma.

SPREAD

Gastric cancer is usually diagnosed at a comparatively late stage by which time spread has usually occurred:

1 *Direct*. Spread in the submucosa and through the wall to the peritoneal coat. Penetration of adjacent organs, e.g. pancreas or large bowel to produce a gastro-colic fistula, may occur.

2 *Lymphatic*. Involvement of the regional lymph nodes on the lesser or greater curvatures, the coeliac or other abdominal nodes. Mediastinal or cervical nodes (Virchow's gland) are frequently involved.

3 *Transcoelomic*. Spread following invasion of the serosa will produce multiple tumour nodules in the omentum or peritoneum and on the serosal coats of abdominal viscera. The ovary is frequently involved by a 'signet-ring' type of cancer – Krukenberg tumour (see p. 440). The mode of spread may be transcoelomic but spread via the lymphatics in the retroperitoneal tissues has also been suggested as a possible mechanism.

4 *Blood*. This is common by the time of diagnosis and may be widespread in any organ but especially the liver, lungs and bones.

PROGNOSIS

Only about half of all patients with gastric carcinoma are suitable for surgical resection but of these 20 per cent survive 10 years. Favourable features are small tumours, lack of lymph node metastases and the presence of a mixed fibroblastic and lymphocytic plasma cell marginal reaction. Superficial carcinoma carries a good prognosis (70 to 90 per cent at 5 years) and improved results can be anticipated by improved techniques of earlier diagnosis by fibreoptic instruments and cytological diagnosis in high risk groups.

Other types of tumour

MALIGNANT CONNECTIVE TISSUE

Fibrosarcoma, neurofibrosarcoma and leiomyosarcoma are all rare primary tumours of the stomach which usually form large fungating and highly malignant masses.

LYMPHOMA

Both Hodgkin's and non-Hodgkin's lymphomas occur in the stomach either as manifestations of systematized disease or as primary site of presentation. On gross appearances they may be difficult to differentiate from carcinoma particularly of the diffusely infiltrative type. The prognosis is now known to be similar to lymphomas of similar types presenting in a more classical manner in lymph nodes (see p. 580).

Chapter 37
Alimentary System – Intestines: Congenital: Diverticula: Vascular

Congenital

There are a large number of congenital abnormalities which may affect the bowel. Some of the more common conditions are:

Microcolon
The whole or part of the colon is small and underdeveloped.

Reduplication
The small intestine, particularly the ileum, or the large bowel, may rarely show reduplication of the lumen – 'double-barrelled'.

Abnormal rotations
Variable anatomical abnormalities may result from a failure of normal gut rotation. These range from complete transposition of all the abdominal viscera

to partial abnormalities. All are rare but one of the more common manifestations is the failure of the caecum to descend to the right iliac fossa, remaining in the region of the liver; this may be of considerable surgical importance.

Abnormal mesenteries

These are common. A long duodenal mesentery may produce pathological mobility of this structure. There may be a long mesentery of the pelvic colon and in both cases there is an increased likelihood of volvulus.

Atresias

Segmental areas of narrowing may occur anywhere in the alimentary tract but are especially liable to occur in the duodenum at the level of the ampulla of Vater, at the level of Meckel's diverticulum, or at the anus – *imperforate anus*. This latter condition is due to a defect in the union between the endodermal hind-gut and the ectodermal anal canal. The defect is of variable degrees of completeness and the rectum may also be deformed. In severe cases, there may be associated fistulous communications with the urinary tract or the genital canal in females.

Megacolon

NATURE
Gross distension of the colon and sometimes the rectum; there are two types.

'IDIOPATHIC' AND ACQUIRED MEGACOLON
There is no histological abnormality of the wall of the colon or rectum but there is distension of the whole large intestine by faeces, down to the anal canal. The aetiology is unknown and the disorder usually presents in childhood with persistent constipation and abdominal swelling due to the massive colonic distension. Adults with chronic constipation or mental or neurological disorders may present a similar picture – *acquired megacolon*.

HIRSCHSPRUNG'S DISEASE

Nature
There is a block of normal intestinal peristalsis by an aganglionic segment. The aetiology is partly genetic. When the aganglionic segment is short and no higher than the pelvic colon, the risk to brothers is 1 in 20 and to sisters less than 1 in 20. If the

segment is long (at least ascending colon) the risk to brothers is 1 in 6 and to sisters 1 in 8.

Macroscopical
There is a narrowed segment, usually in the lower rectum and anal canal, beyond which the anus is normal. Proximal to this area there is gross dilatation of the lumen, hypertrophy of the wall, and mucosal ulceration of stercoral origin is commonly seen.

Microscopical
The narrowed segment shows absence of the ganglion cells of Meissner's and Auerbach's plexuses and reduction in number in the first 1–5 cm of the proximal funnel-shaped portion. Abnormally thick non-myelinated nerve bundles are present in the affected segments.

Results
Cure is effected by removal of the aganglionic segment and re-anastomosis of the bowel to restore its continuity.

Diverticula

Meckel's diverticulum and small gut diverticula are described below.

Volvulus neonatorum

Volvulus occurring in the neonatal period due to abnormalities of attachment of the intestinal mesentery (see above).

Diverticula

TRUE DIVERTICULA

Nature
Pouches which contain all layers of the bowel wall. These are congenital in origin and usually occur in the upper small intestine, especially in the duodenum, and as a Meckel's diverticulum.

Duodenal diverticula
These are comparatively rare and seldom produce symptoms as the intestinal contents are fluid at this level. Sometimes an enterolith (a mass of inspissated bowel content) may form in the pouch and can produce intestinal obstruction if it is extruded into the bowel lumen.

Meckel's diverticulum

ORIGIN
Persistence of a remnant of the omphalo-mesenteric (vitelline) duct.

SITE
Attached to the anti-mesenteric border of the terminal ileum, 60–90 cm from the ileo-caecal valve.

INCIDENCE
Occurs in 2–3 per cent of the general population.

MACROSCOPICAL
May be merely a fibrous cord extending from the ileum to the umbilicus but more usually has a pouch up to 5 cm long at the ileal end.

MICROSCOPICAL
The wall is composed of ileal tissue but ectopic pancreatic or gastric mucosa is commonly present.

COMPLICATIONS
1 *Diverticulum*
(a) The neck of the sac may become obstructed.
(b) The sac may undergo torsion.
(c) A peptic ulcer may form in the ectopic gastric mucosa with bleeding or perforation.
(d) The ileum may be narrowed at the level of attachment of the diverticulum.
(e) Intussusception.
2. *Cord.* The cord connecting the sac to the umbilicus may contain, in any part of its length, remnants of intestinal mucosa. Enterocystoma may be produced by cystic dilatation of these epithelial structures, or an adenoma may form at the umbilicus.
3 *Extrinsic.* A volvulus or strangulation of a loop of bowel may be caused by the cord.

FALSE DIVERTICULA

Nature
Pouches consisting of gut mucosa without muscle in the wall. These hernias pass through congenitally weak points of the muscle wall between the taeniae of the colon, usually at the sites of blood vessel entry.

Small gut
The commonest are jejunal diverticula. These are solitary or few in number and are relatively common incidental post-mortem findings, the majority remaining symptomless. Occasionally they are numerous and have been reported as producing a malabsorption state with B_{12} deficiency anaemia on rare occasions (see p. 482).

Large gut
False diverticula of the large gut result in the important condition of diverticular disease.

Diverticular disease of colon

Nature
A disease characterized by a colonic muscular abnormality and by the presence of hernial protrusions of mucosa into and through the wall. The uncomplicated lesion was formerly named *diverticulosis* and, when attended by complications, *diverticulitis*.

Incidence
Rare below 40 years; 1 in 10 of Western populations in 50–70 age group; 1 in 3 of over sixties; slightly more common in females. Less common in Southern Europe and South America and rare at any age in Africa, India and the Orient.

Sites
Confined to sigmoid colon in the majority with a small number of cases where varying lengths of proximal colon are also involved. The rectum is always spared.

Macroscopical
Typical pulsion-type pouches of mucous membrane with muscularis mucosae projecting through the circular layer of muscle to pericolic fat. Usually two rows are seen on each side of the bowel wall between the mesenteric and antemesenteric taenia at the site of entry of blood vessels, i.e. weak points. A constant associated feature is thickening and excessive fasciculation of circular muscle and thickening of longitudinal muscle causing mucosal corrugations, between which rather narrow diverticular mouths are seen. The muscle abnormality can occasionally be seen without diverticula, lending support to the view that the muscle changes are the primary disorder. The pathogenesis is, however,

obscure though there seems to be some correlation with dietary habits in respect of increased frequency in those with low residue diet.

Microscopical

The mucosal pouch is covered by a thin layer of longitudinal muscle. The thickened muscle shows no evidence of hyperplasia or individual fibre hypertrophy and is condensed in the circular layer into a number of interdigitatory processes forming semi-lunar areas.

Complications

1 *Inflammation – diverticulitis.* There follows stasis of faecal contents in the diverticula with mucosal abrasion and bacterial infection of the wall and pericolic fat of variable severity. Local peritonitis occurs early and pericolic abscess is common. Subsequently, generalized peritonitis with free perforation is a dangerous and relatively common complication.
2 *Haemorrhage.* Some degree of blood loss is usual. More commonly this is occult but occasionally massive and fatal.
3 *Fistula formation.* Following inflammatory changes and adhesion to adjacent tissues, fistulous tracts may form, e.g. to abdominal wall, vagina, bladder, small intestine.
4 *Obstruction.* Inflammation with pericolic fibrosis increases the thickening and lack of distensibility of the colonic wall. Luminal narrowing may become severe and cause intestinal obstruction, usually subacute rather than acute.
5 *Portal pylephlebitis.* Inflammatory complications may rarely cause septic thrombophlebitis with portal pyaemia and pylephlebitis.

Vascular

When the intestine is deprived of blood, changes occur which are very variable and which form a spectrum of conditions, pathological and clinical, depending on the severity of the resultant anoxia and on its acuteness. This group of lesions has become very complex and, whilst in many there is clear evidence of an ischaemic origin, in others the pathogenesis is more speculative. Demonstrable arterial or venous obstruction to blood flow clearly explains some of the clinico-pathological states, but reduction of blood flow by hypoperfusion in hypotension and other clinical syndromes is less readily

defined. In the present state of knowledge the conditions have been grouped according to the appearance of the intestinal lesions.

INFARCTION AND GANGRENE

Nature

Death of variable thickness of the intestinal wall, complete in the case of gangrene.

Aetiology

ARTERIAL
(a) *Thrombosis* of the superior or inferior mesenteric artery or large branches, usually superimposed on atheroma and common in the elderly or in diabetics. May occasionally be due to arteritis, e.g. polyarteritis.
(b) *Embolism* of arteries from the left atrial appendage in atrial fibrillation or mitral stenosis or mural thrombus overlying a myocardial infarct or in valvular endocarditis.

VENOUS
Occlusion of major mesenteric veins can occur due to pressure from external lesions, e.g. margins of hernial sacs, enlarged lymph nodes, tumours, abdominal injuries and infections including appendicitis, peritonitis and pelvic and colonic inflammatory diseases. This can occasionally be frankly infected – *portal pylephlebitis.*

STRANGULATION
Mechanical occlusion of venous and/or arterial supply to a segment of intestine and often associated with luminal obstruction.
(a) *Incarceration in a hernial sac*, e.g. inguinal, femoral, incisional, umbilical, or internal hernias.
(b) *Kinking of mesentery,* e.g. around peritoneal adhesions, fibrous bands, congenital abnormalities.
(c) *Volvulus*; twisting of loop of large or small intestine (see p. 220).
The vascular occlusion is initially venous but, if unrelieved, arterial obstruction and thrombosis supervene.

Appearances

Plum-coloured congestion of a variable length of small and/or large intestine depending on the aetiology. Frank changes of haemorrhagic infarction develop with mucosal, followed by full thickness, necrosis and thrombosis in smaller vessels. Gangrene and perforation rapidly develop. When due to strangulation the margin of infarction is usually sharply demarcated.

Results
Surgical removal of the cause of the vascular obstruction may occur in time for reperfusion of the bowel and a return to viability. Once full thickness necrosis and vascular thrombosis in the wall have occurred then only resection of the affected intestine can prevent death from perforation and peritonitis.

ACUTE ISCHAEMIC ENTEROCOLITIS

Nature
An uncommon but important condition in which patchy or widespread areas of ischaemic mucosal necrosis occur in small or large intestine or both and, in some areas, involve also the deeper layers, leading to gangrene and perforation.

Pathogenesis
In only a small proportion of cases can significant disease or obstruction of larger mesenteric vessels be demonstrated. In the majority, large vessels are normal but, in severe cases in particular, fibrin and platelet thrombotic occlusion can be seen in small veins and arteries particularly in the submucosa. Many of the patients have an identified episode of hypotension, e.g. shock, haemorrhage, septicaemia, and others have abnormal circulation due to congestive cardiac failure, diabetes and other serious and often debilitating conditions. It is likely, but unproven, that hypoperfusion and hypoxia are the common denominators.

Incidence
The condition may complicate the respiratory distress syndrome, congenital heart disease and other prostrating diseases of neonates particularly when premature – *Necrotizing or haemorrhagic enterocolitis of infancy*. Most other cases occur in the elderly.

Macroscopical
In less severe cases, rather non-specific patchy foci of mucosal necrosis and ulceration of variable distribution are seen, the intestine otherwise appearing normal. The more severe examples show extensive areas of sloughing mucosa usually of a segmental distribution and seldom uniform. The necrotic mucosa may have the appearance of a membrane. The very severe cases show areas of infarction and gangrene in addition.

Microscopical
In the abnormal areas there is ischaemic necrosis of the tissues and associated congestion and oedema. Sometimes only tips of villi will be involved but more commonly most of the mucosa is replaced by necrotic tissue forming a surface membrane. Inflammatory cells are usually very scanty. The necrosis can extend to the muscular layers. In later stages the necrotic tissue is shed with resulting ulceration.

Results
The less severe cases heal without scarring by mucosal regeneration. If there is full thickness mucosal loss scarring of varying extent may follow. In segmentally penetrating cases or with severe widespread lesions there is a high mortality rate from circulatory failure, 'toxaemia', electrolytic disturbances and blood loss whilst gangrene, perforation and peritonitis may also ensue. Secondary invasion of devitalized ischaemic tissues by organisms which are normal bowel commensals, particularly *Clostridia*, is almost always fatal – this is sometimes called *gangrenous colitis* but the infective element is always secondary.

CHRONIC ISCHAEMIA – ISCHAEMIC STRICTURE

Nature
A localized area of narrowing of the gut lumen due to stricture formation from fibrosis of the wall following ischaemia.

Aetiology
This can follow identified clinical episodes of segmental acute ischaemic enterocolitis which recover but heal by scarring or it can develop *de novo* from an acute subclinical episode of ischaemia, or a slowly developing chronic blood flow reduction.

Sites

Small intestine, where they are commonly multiple, or colon, particularly at the junction of the superior and inferior mesenteric artery territories in the descending part.

Macroscopical

A segment, usually short, but occasionally quite long (more than 10 cm) shows marked luminal narrowing commonly with mucosal ulceration or an atrophic scarred appearance. The deeper layers of the wall are variably fibrous in appearance.

Microscopical

The mucosa shows an atrophic but regenerative appearance or may be ulcerated with a base of granulation tissue containing macrophages laden with haemosiderin. There is consistently dense submucosal fibrosis which may also involve the muscular layers and the serosa. Mesenteric vessels may show evidence of arterial disease, e.g. atheroma or previous thrombosis, but are commonly normal.

Results

Usually presents with intestinal obstruction but occasionally, in the small intestine, with malabsorption. Resection of the stenosed segments is usually curative.

'Thiazide' or 'Potassium' ulcers

Solitary or multiple ulcers and strictures of the small bowel have been sometimes identified as associated with the taking of enteric-coated tablets of potassium chloride with hydrochlorthiazide. The appearances are very similar to ischaemic ulcers and strictures and it is believed that an ischaemic mechanism is operative.

PORTAL HYPERTENSION

Portal venous hypertension due to intrahepatic obstruction, e.g. cirrhosis of the liver, or extrahepatic obstruction, e.g. portal vein thrombosis, causes congestion of veins and dilatation at the sites of anastomoses with systemic veins. In addition to oesophageal varices (see p. 183), varicosities are common in the lower rectum – *haemorrhoids*, and sometimes around the umbilicus – '*caput Medusae*'.

Pneumatosis intestinalis

Macroscopical

The colon, or small intestine, shows multiple nodules in the submucosa which on section are found to be unilocular gas-filled cysts. Some of these cysts may be large enough to produce intestinal obstruction or mimic carcinoma.

Microscopical

These submucosal gas-filled cysts contain nitrogen and are lined by fibrous tissue. It is agreed that the spaces are lymphatics.

Nature

This remains in doubt and the origin of the gas is also debatable; it may be due to gas entering the wall through breaches in mucosal continuity. It has also been suggested that the air may be derived from the lungs, especially in chronic bronchitics. Air may track down into the retroperitoneal tissues and then follows the course of the lymphatics to the bowel wall.

Melanosis coli

Macroscopical

Deep brown pigmentation of the colonic mucosa which may be diffuse and intense.

Microscopical

A brown pigment in macrophages in the colonic mucosa.

Nature

The pigment is melanin or a closely related compound and the aetiology is obscure; furthermore the condition is of no clinical importance. There is a correlation with use of anthracene purgatives.

Chapter 38
Alimentary System – Intestines: Inflammations I

INTESTINAL TUBERCULOSIS

Primary
This site for primary infection following ingestion of infected milk is now very rare. At one time it was a common site for the primary complex of a small ileal lesion with large caseous mesenteric lymph nodes – *tabes mesenterica*. This frequently calcified.

Tuberculous enteritis
Circumferential ulcers of the terminal ileum may occur as a complication of advanced pulmonary tuberculosis and ingestion of heavily infected sputum. Surface tubercles are usually seen but lymph nodes are seldom significantly enlarged.

Hyperplastic ileo-caecal tuberculosis
Most cases formerly diagnosed histologically as tuberculosis with gross thickening of the caecal and terminal ileal walls are probably Crohn's disease (see p. 200). Differential diagnosis may be difficult and in the last resort require identification of *Mycobacterium tuberculosis*.

Yersinia infection

Nature
Infection with *Yersinia pseudotuberculosis* or *Y. enterocolitica*, pleomorphic coccobacilli of the Enterobacteria family and which more commonly affect animals.

Sites
The commonest presentation is as acute mesenteric adenitis, particularly in children and young adults. The small intestine or appendix may also be involved.

Appearances
Lymphoid tissue is hyperplastic followed by histiocytic proliferation, formation of epithelioid

198

granulomas and central necrosis. The necrotic granulomas are of irregular outline and resemble those of lymphogranuloma venereum (p. 406) and cat-scratch disease (see p. 579).

Prognosis
Occasional fatalities are reported from septicaemia but it usually resolves without specific therapy. Symptoms mimic other inflammatory conditions, particularly acute appendicitis and so laparotomy is often performed.

Typhoid fever

Aetiology
Ingestion of *Salmonella typhi* from infected contaminated food or drink. The contamination is often caused by asymptomatic 'carriers'.

Geographical distribution
Although only sporadic cases or minor epidemics occur in this country, this disease is of world-wide distribution and is only kept in check by general preventive and hygienic measures. In some areas of the Middle and Far East, where public and personal hygiene is less advanced, the disease is extremely common and major epidemics are of frequent occurrence due to contamination of communal water and food supplies.

Pathogenesis
Incubation. Ingested organisms are mostly destroyed by acid in the stomach but sufficient survive to reach the intestine where they penetrate the mucosa and enter the lymphoid tissue in which they multiply. In this incubation stage of about 10 days there are no symptoms.

Septicaemia. A frankly septicaemic picture is associated with the clinical onset and is due to generalized infection of the body by the organisms. This lasts for 7–10 days.

Localization. Localization of organisms in the lymphoreticular system with particular preference for Peyer's patches in the ileum, the spleen, mesenteric lymph nodes and bone marrow.

Recovery. Lysis occurs, usually after about 3 weeks.

Macroscopical
The lymphoid tissue of the terminal ileum, particularly the Peyer's patches, is swollen and raised in a plateau manner. Necrosis occurs at about the tenth day of the clinical disease and ulceration is seen between the fourteenth and twenty-first days with separation of a slough of overlying mucosa. When the disease subsides, healing occurs without scarring. The ulcers are in the longitudinal axis of the bowel and the mesenteric nodes are enlarged and fleshy.

Microscopical
The cellular reaction is mononuclear and these cells phagocytose both organisms and red cells. The same mononuclear inflammatory cell infiltrate is seen in the other affected organs, e.g. spleen, lymph nodes, bone, gall bladder and liver.

Effects
1   *Gut.* Separation of the sloughs may cause intestinal haemorrhage (5–10 per cent of cases), whilst the very sinister complication of perforation may occur in about 5 per cent.
2   *Spleen.* The spleen is soft and enlarges rapidly due to congestion and an infiltration by mononuclear cells. The enlarged organ may spontaneously rupture.
3   *Liver.* The liver is enlarged, shows scattered areas of focal necrosis and focal areas of Kupffer cell proliferation and mononuclear cell infiltration.
4   *Bone marrow.* The mononuclear cell infiltration is associated with a leucopenia. The organisms may remain in one or more bones to produce typhoid osteitis as a late manifestation (see p. 717).
5   *Muscle.* A toxic coagulation of skeletal and occasionally cardiac muscle may occur – Zenker's degeneration (see p. 107).
6   *Lymph nodes.* There may be generalized enlargement in addition to the considerable enlargement of the mesenteric nodes.
7   *Lungs.* At the beginning of the infection bronchitis is common; this may later progress to bronchopneumonia.
8   *Gall bladder.* Infection of the biliary tract may occur and a residual cholecystitis may result in a chronic carrier state.
9   *Veins.* Thrombophlebitis is common.
10   *Nerves.* A peripheral neuritis is also common.
11   *Skin.* In the septicaemic stage a rash of rose-red spots on the trunk is usually a noticeable feature.

Diagnosis

ISOLATION OF THE ORGANISM
Blood culture – first and second weeks.

Urine culture – second week.
Faeces culture – second week onwards.

A rising titre of serum agglutinins is usually diagnostic from the second week onwards but single tests may be misleading, especially if the patient has been previously immunized.

OTHER INFECTIONS WITH SALMONELLAE

ENTERIC FEVER GROUP
The most severe enteric fever is caused by *Salmonella typhi*. Other organisms causing identical but less severe lesions are *S. paratyphi* A and B, and *S. cholerae-suis*.

FOOD POISONING GROUP
There are very numerous strains, including *S. typhi-murium, S. enteritidis, S. newport*, etc., which give rise to a non-specific clinical picture of acute gastro-enteritis. The incubation period following ingestion of contaminated food is short, usually 8–25 hours, and is followed by violent diarrhoea and vomiting due to superficial inflammation of the gastro-intestinal tract. In severe instances, invasion of the lymphoreticular system may produce clinical and pathological appearances similar to enteric fever. Diagnosis is by isolation and identification of the organisms from faeces, the latter commonly being a complex procedure based on minor differences in their antigenic structure.

Crohn's disease – regional ileitis – regional colitis

The disease is frequently known as regional ileitis as this is the commonest site, but the jejunum and stomach are sometimes affected and the colon may also be involved – regional colitis. Appearances are similar in all sites.

Incidence
A relatively common disease which appears to be increasing in frequency.

Aetiology
This remains entirely unknown but agents and processes suggested include: sarcoidosis, atypical tuberculosis, viral infection, non-specific bacterial infection, a psychosomatic disorder, reaction to certain particulate ingested materials, e.g. some toothpastes.

Macroscopical
Single or multiple sharply demarcated areas in the terminal ileum stopping abruptly at the ileo-caecal valve are the most common appearances. The lesion produces thickening and rigidity of the bowel wall with narrowing of the lumen. On section, the bowel wall is thickened by firm, pale tissue maximally involving the mucosa and submucosa, commonly with mucosal ulceration – *Cobblestone* pattern. The adjacent mesentery is also firm and thickened and contains enlarged lymph nodes. When there are multiple areas of involvement the intervening 'skip' areas are normal. In two-thirds of cases, the small intestine only is involved, in half the remainder there are lesions in both large and small intestine and in others in large gut only. Some cases may present with fistula-in-ano or perineal ulceration and may only develop bowel lesions several years subsequently.

Microscopical
The early lesions show lymphoedema, increased vascularity and fibrosis. At a later stage, the fibrosis becomes marked and the tissue is less vascular with a non-specific chronic inflammatory cell infiltrate. The fibrous tissue is maximal in the mucosa and submucosa but also involves the peritoneal coat and to a lesser extent the muscle i.e. the inflammation is transmural. Multiple sections may reveal non-caseating foci of epithelioid cells and giant cells reminiscent of sarcoidosis; similar lesions may be found in the lymph nodes. A characteristic of relatively early lesions is the presence of fissures in the mucosa with focal collections of lymphocytes and plasma cells at their apices.

Effects
The lesions produce varying degrees of intestinal obstruction due to narrowing of the affected areas – radiological 'string' sign. Complications which may occur include:
1   *Intestinal obstruction.* Usually subacute.
2   *Fistula formation.* Ileo-ileal; ileo-colic; external (faecal) fistulae; rarely ileo-vesical. This occurs in about 10 per cent.
3   *Malabsorption syndrome.* Usually occurs late and commonly as a sequel to by-pass operations or

fistula formation. In the late stages malnutrition may be clinically dominant.

4 *Perforation.* Rare.

5 *Haemorrhage.* A degree of anaemia from blood loss is common.

6 *Carcinoma.* There is a slight but definite association with development of malignancy in affected portions of the intestine.

7 *Others.* Occasional associated conditions include, ankylosing spondylitis, polyarthritis, iridocyclitis, cirrhosis of liver, amyloidosis.

Results

The course is extremely variable and unpredictable.

1 Lesions may regress and not recur.

2 Lesions may regress but new sites of involvement appear at irregular time intervals.

3 Multiple lesions, especially those requiring surgery, may pursue a progresssive course with malnourishment leading to death.

4 The death rate is twice that expected for a control group of same age and sex.

Chapter 39
Alimentary System – Intestines: Inflammations II

Ulcerative colitis

Nature
An inflammatory disease, confined to the colon, of unknown aetiology but with specific appearances and very common in Western populations.

Age
Peak incidence in third decade but wide range from infancy to the elderly.

Sex
M:F 2:3

Pathogenesis
In spite of extensive research and numerous hypotheses, the pathogenetic mechanism is not known. It seems likely, however, that there is a muscle factor of abnormal motility and a vascular component with secondary damage from invading bacteria. No evidence of an initiating hypersensitivity or other immunological process has been identified.

Sites
The disease nearly always commences in the rectum with subsequent proximal involvement of

variable amounts of colonic mucosa, sometimes with 'total colitis'. The changes are almost invariably most severe in the distal part.

Macroscopical

The earliest stages of mucosal congestion and haemorrhagic foci are followed by ulceration. The ulcers are variable in distribution, shape and size but are commonly linear along the long axis of the bowel. They are usually shallow but often irregular in outline with ragged margins, undermining and mucosal bridges. Pseudo-polyps of granulation tissue and 'polyps' of residual epithelial islands are often synchronously seen with active ulcers, healing ulcers and scars. In the more chronic cases some luminal narrowing associated with rigidity of the wall may occur. Occasionally, a small segment of terminal ileum may show congestion or ulceration – 'backwash ileitis'; otherwise the small intestine is normal.

Microscopical

The early stages show vascular congestion and oedema and an inflammatory cell infiltrate of polymorphs, eosinophils, plasma cells and lymphocytes confined to the mucosa. 'Crypt abscesses' are conspicuous, though not specific for this disease, and the epithelial cells show marked depletion of mucus. Later, ulceration occurs, usually superficial but, in severe cases, full thickness of mucosa. Inflammatory involvement of the muscular coats is uncommon except in the most severe forms. In the more chronic cases, the mucosa shows pseudo-polyps of inflammatory granulation tissue. Paneth cells appear in the epithelium and there is only a slight increase in submucosal fibrous tissue. Regeneration of the epithelium with healing of ulcers can frequently be identified.

Complications

1 *Haemorrhage.* Some degree of anaemia is almost invariably found and occasionally is severe with frank blood loss.

2 *Malnutrition.* Weight loss, hypoproteinaemia and considerable nutritional disturbances are common in acute widespread disease.

3 *Electrolytic disturbance.* Common and often severe.

4 *Perforation.* This is uncommon except in toxic megacolon.

5 *Toxic megacolon.* A segment of acutely affected colon, usually transverse, becomes acutely dilated with marked thinning of all coats, extensive ulceration and marked fragility, often with single or multiple perforations. Emergency colectomy is often necessary otherwise this complication carries a very high mortality.

6 *Stricture formation.* True fibrous stricture does not occur. The presence of a segmental area of narrowing usually indicates malignancy.

7 *Fistula formation.* Very uncommon.

8 *Malignancy.* There is a significant risk, 5–10 times greater than the general population. This risk is particularly high in patients with total colonic disease and when disease has been present for more than 10 years and is chronic and continuous rather than acute and relapsing.

9 *Liver damage.* Liver function is often abnormal and biopsy may show fatty change or pericholangitis or periportal inflammation which may progress to biliary cirrhosis.

10 *Miscellaneous.* Skin lesions, particularly pyoderma gangrenosum, polyarthritis, iridocyclitis and amyloidosis can occur.

Results

The natural history is very variable depending in part on the development of complications. Additionally however, the disease may be mild, localized and transient or severe, acute and extensive with all grades in between. Remissions, either spontaneous or induced by therapy, are commonly followed by relapses of variable severity. The course in any individual patient is somewhat unpredictable.

Dysentery

Nature

A clinical syndrome characterized by diarrhoea, blood and mucus in the stools. The pathological use of the term dysentery is here restricted to infection by the specific organisms described below as producing bacillary and amoebic dysentery.

BACILLARY DYSENTERY

Aetiology

Caused by the Shigella group of Gram-negative,

non-motile bacilli: *Shigella shigae*, *S. flexneri* and *S. sonnei*.

Mode of infection
Ingestion of contaminated food or water, commonly infected by a chronic carrier.

Macroscopical
An acute superficial suppurative inflammation of the colon and terminal ileum. Early, there is intense congestion of the mucosa which is swollen, oedematous and congested. Later, there is necrosis of the mucosal surface with slough formation and separation producing ulceration of the tips of the mucosal folds. These ulcers coalesce to produce ragged but shallow larger ulcers which, however, do not penetrate the muscularis mucosae.

Microscopical
Acute, suppurative, mucosal inflammation with congestion, oedema, fibrin, polymorphs and numerous organisms. The sloughs separate as membranes which are passed in the fluid faeces together with mucus, blood and inflammatory debris.

Results
In most cases the mucosa rapidly regenerates without scarring. In a few cases the organisms may persist to result in chronic carriers. The organisms do not invade the blood stream and the diagnosis depends upon cultural isolation of the specific organisms from the faeces.

AMOEBIC DYSENTERY

Aetiology
Caused by *Entamoeba histolytica* – a protozoon which, in vegetative form, is actively and purposefully motile and actively phagocytic. The encysted form contains four nuclei.

Mode of infection
The disease is spread by the ingestion of cystic forms, usually from food contaminated by a 'carrier'. It has been estimated that up to 10 per cent of the population of some countries have these amoebae in the stools but that they live in symbiosis with the host. Invasion of the mucosa may occur due to minor bacterial infection or some other, but unknown, cause of breakdown of the normal defence mechanisms. There may be a delay of many months or years between infection and the development of colonic disease.

Sites
The pelvic colon and caecum are the most commonly affected areas.

Macroscopical
The vegetative amoebae burrow into the colonic glands and release a proteolytic ferment which digests the submucosal tissues, resulting in undermined flask-shaped ulcers with narrow orifices and ragged undermined edges. The intervening mucosa appears normal.

Microscopical
Numerous amoebae are seen in the edges of the ulcers, in mucus and in the portal venous radicles of the submucosa. There is only a mild inflammatory cell reaction, abundant mucus secretion but no pus formation.

Diagnosis
1 Examination of faeces for amoebae or cysts.
2 Rectal biopsy for organisms.
3 Fluorescent antibody studies on serum.

Results
The infestation may involve a large area of the large intestine and produce severe diarrhoea with blood and mucus. Occasionally, a localized area of granulomatous reaction occurs – 'amoeboma'. As noted microscopically, the amoebae are commonly present in the veins and are carried to the liver to produce amoebic hepatitis or an amoebic 'abscess' (see p. 557).

GIARDIASIS
Infestation of the small intestine by the flagellated *Giardia lamblia*, is common in children and warm climates and particularly so in the immunodeficient. It may be a cause of malabsorption and partial villous atrophy of the mucosa (see p. 208)

Actinomycosis

Aetiology
Actinomyces israeli.

Sites

Twenty-five per cent of cases of actinomycosis occur in the ileo-caecal region. The cases frequently present as acute appendicitis or as pain associated with a mass in the R.I.F.

Macroscopical

A hard, fibrotic mass with 'honeycomb' abscesses containing the characteristic 'sulphur granules'.

Microscopical

The fungus is identifiable in the tissues, surrounded by dense fibrous tissue and polymorphs.

Results

The cases are frequently operated upon as acute appendicitis, the true diagnosis only being apparent from the large fibrotic mass and the histological appearances of excised tissues. Direct spread may occur to involve the caecum, anterior abdominal wall, hip, spine, right paracolic gutter or kidney and skin sinuses may form. Blood spread to the liver, producing honeycomb abscesses in the hepatic substance, may occur. The prognosis has improved with antibiotic therapy but is still poor.

Staphylococcal enterocolitis

Nature

An extremely severe intestinal inflammation, usually in hospitalized patients who are the victims of cross-infection and caused by the profuse multiplication of *Staphylococcus pyogenes* within the lumen of the gut. This condition should not be confused with the food poisoning caused by ingestion of pre-formed staphylococcal enterotoxin in food nor with pseudomembranous colitis (see below).

Pathogenesis

The infection usually follows administration of antibiotics either by mouth or parenterally and is also commonly associated with abdominal operations, particularly gastrectomy. *S. pyogenes* is not usually present in normal persons in any significant numbers in the bowel, due to their destruction by stomach acid and by competition from normal bowel inhabitants. In infected patients, it is therefore suggested that reduction of gastric acid in abdominal operations and absence or reduction of the normal commensal bacterial population induced by broad-spectrum antibiotics, are responsible for the profuse multiplication of staphyloccoci associated with the condition.

Macroscopical

There is an intense mucosal inflammation with sloughing of the entire mucous membrane. The bowel contents are of 'rice-water' appearance containing enormous numbers of staphylococci. A Gram's stain of this material is usually sufficient to provide the diagnosis. Healing at the sites of surgical anastomoses is prejudiced and usually results in their disintegration followed by peritonitis.

Microscopical

Intense vascularity with mucosal necrosis but little inflammatory cell reaction.

Results

There is profound electrolytic disturbance and toxaemia with a mortality of well over 50 per cent.

Antibiotic-associated colitis – pseudomembranous colitis

Nature

An uncommon but very characteristic lesion of large intestine occurring as a complication of oral antibiotic therapy. Originally associated with lincamycin and neomycin, a much wider range of antibiotics including synthetic penicillins has now been implicated.

Pathogenesis

Cultural and serological studies have disclosed the consistent presence of *Clostridium difficile* which is considered to be the aetiological agent once bacterial competition has been eliminated by the constantly related oral antibiotic therapy.

Macroscopical

Oedema with loss of mucosal pattern occurs initially followed by the appearance of a false membrane of mucus, cell debris and necrotic superficial mucosa. This may then be shed leaving an ulcerated surface.

Microscopical

In the early stages mucosal oedema is accompanied by characteristic 'explosions' within the mucosa with abundant mucus production and death of superficial layers to form the membrane. This appearance may be diagnosed at sigmoidoscopic biopsy.

Results

Symptoms of diarrhoea, loss of mucus and fluid and toxaemia may be severe and fatal if untreated. If therapy is instituted, healing occurs, normally without scarring.

Cholera

Nature

A very severe, acute and often fulminating enteritis caused by *Vibrio cholerae* and characterized by a severe necrotizing but superficial ulceration of the gut mucosa.

Incidence

This is predominantly a disease of hot climates and poor hygiene and is thus most common in the Far East where very severe epidemics occur in addition to sporadic cases.

Mode of infection

Ingestion of the organism in food, water or milk, contaminated by active subclinical or convalescent cases. A true chronic carrier state does not occur.

Clinical

The short incubation period of 1–5 days is followed by violent watery diarrhoea – 'rice-water' stools, with toxaemia and severe electrolytic disturbances.

Appearances

There is intense oedema, hyperaemia and polymorph infiltration of the mucosa with desquamation of the surface epithelium, but full thickness mucosal ulceration is rare.

Diagnosis

Isolation of *V. cholerae* from the stools.

Results

There is no invasion by the organisms and the mortality, 5 per cent in sporadic cases but up to 20 per cent in epidemics, is due to the electrolyte disturbances and to a lesser extent the toxaemia. Recovery is attended by complete regeneration of the intestinal mucosa.

URAEMIC COLITIS

Patients in renal failure commonly develop diarrhoea and, in fatal cases, some show necrotic, haemorrhagic ulceration of the intestine, predominantly colonic. It is likely that this is of ischaemic type (see p. 196) and is non-specific otherwise.

STERCORAL ULCERATION

Nature

Ulceration due to the impaction of faeces following chronic intestinal obstruction from any cause.

Appearances

Intestinal obstruction is present with impaction of hard faecal material within the dilated bowel proximal to the obstruction. The mucosal surface shows multiple discoloured shallow ulcers of non-specific appearance, probably resulting from physical pressure necrosis by the faecal masses.

FISTULA-IN-ANO

Nature

A fistulous communication between the anal canal and the perineum. This is a common condition.

Pathogenesis

The fistulae arise following infection of the anal glands. These mucus-secreting glands are situated in the submucosa, in muscle and between the longitudinal and circular muscle layers and communicate with the anal canal by long and narrow ducts. Inflammation of these glands by bowel commensals, or more rarely by *Mycobacterium tuberculosis*, which find their way down the ducts, is followed by suppuration or caseation within the wall. An abscess is formed which may penetrate directly through the remaining outer layers of the bowel wall to form a low fistula, or may track upwards between the muscle layers and then rupture outwards into the ischio-rectal fossa and thence to the perineum to produce a high level fistula. Many of the cases formerly considered to be tuberculous in origin are manifestations of Crohn's disease.

Appearances
The fistulous track is lined by inflammatory granulation tissue which is usually non-specific but occasionally of giant cell granulomatous appearance. By the time of surgical excision little or no epithelial glandular tissue remains.

Results
An abscess pointing in the ischio-rectal fossa or perineal skin bursts and the fistula may temporarily heal on the surface. Persistence of the fistula or recurrent episodes of acute inflammation usually occur until the track is totally excised and the wound allowed to granulate. When due to Crohn's disease it may be some years before the intestinal disease becomes apparent.

Chapter 40
Alimentary System – Intestines: Malabsorption Syndrome: Diseases of the Appendix

Malabsorption syndrome and steatorrhoea

NATURE
A syndrome associated with malabsorption from the intestine of food-stuffs and products of their digestion. Particularly important are minerals, vitamins, salts, protein and fat. Failure of fat absorption results in pale, bulky, offensive stools which gives the syndrome its name of steatorrhoea, but reflects only one aspect of the multiple deficiencies which may be produced by the condition.

DIFFUSE VILLOUS ATROPHY
Investigation of malabsorption syndromes by peroral biopsy of jejunal mucosa has shown two main types of atrophy of the villi.

(a) *Subtotal.* The villi are virtually absent although the thickness of mucosa is not greatly reduced. There is increase in goblet cells, loss of enzyme-secreting cells and increase in stromal plasma cells and lymphocytes. This type is commonly found in cases of gluten enteropathy, i.e. coeliac disease and idiopathic steatorrhoea, and

rarely in tropical sprue, lymphoma involving the intestine and Crohn's disease.

(b) *Partial.* The villi are shortened and uneven in length with persistence of some as continuous ridges. This partial atrophy is commonly found in tropical sprue and lymphoma and rarely in gluten enteropathy, pancreatic diseases, post-gastrectomy and blind loop syndromes. In Crohn's disease and neomycin therapy partial atrophic changes are occasionally found.

CAUSES

Mucosal or lymphatic disease
Any generalized disease which affects the intestinal mucous membrane or lymphatics. Amongst these diseases are tuberculosis, Crohn's disease, giardiasis, amyloidosis and scleroderma affecting the mucosa, or lymphoma and carcinoma involving the lymphatics.

WHIPPLE'S DISEASE
This rare disorder is a cause of steatorrhoea. It

occurs usually in middle-aged males and is characterized by the deposition of glycoproteins and fat in the intestinal wall and mesenteric lymphatics. It is now considered to be an infection by an, as yet, unidentified micro-organism. At post-mortem examination there is thickening of the pale intestinal mucosa with a 'shaggy rug' appearance of the mucosal villi. Microscopically, there is infiltration of the mucosa and submucosa and of the mesenteric lymph nodes by large granular histiocytes which contain abundant P.A.S.-positive material and organisms. Similar appearances are occasionally found in other groups of lymph nodes and in synovial tissues with the polyarthritis which is occasionally seen associated with the disease. The condition usually responds satisfactorily to antibiotic therapy.

Small gut deficiency

A deficiency in length of available small intestine may result in malabsorption and usually occurs following small gut resections or spontaneous and surgical short circuits and fistulae. Post-gastrectomy steatorrhoea and malabsorption probably occurs as a result of intestinal hurry and loss of gastric mucosa.

Gluten enteropathy: tropical sprue

In coeliac disease of children and the idiopathic steatorrhoea of adults subtotal villous atrophy is commonly observed. It is probable that coeliac disease and idiopathic steatorrhoea are the same disorder manifest in different age groups and are due to gluten sensitivity, since there is commonly a marked improvement with a gluten-free diet – gluten enteropathy. In tropical sprue partial atrophy is usual and this disease is probably due to folic acid deficiency caused by an alteration in the intestinal bacterial flora (see p. 484).

Bacterial causes

Many vitamins, including the B complex, B_{12} and K, are synthesized in the gut by bacteria. If the bacterial flora is changed, the availability of these vitamins for absorption is reduced. Causes include intestinal obstruction, bowel stasis due to the presence of 'blind loops' – *blind loop syndrome* and ingested antibiotics, all of which may alter the normal bacterial content of the bowel.

Pancreatic abnormalities

Destruction of the acinar tissue of the pancreas by tumour, or more commonly due to chronic pancreatitis or cystic fibrosis (see p. 632), reduces the output of pancreatic enzymes and may result in impaired digestion of fat, protein and carbohydrates. Steatorrhoea may thus be produced, most of the fat being present in the faeces in unsplit form. Undigested protein is commonly identifiable in the faeces as muscle fibres.

Biliary abnormalities

Reduction in the amount of bile in the intestine, due to biliary obstruction at any level or to biliary fistula, will lead to failure of emulsification of fat, steatorrhoea and failure to absorb calcium and the fat soluble vitamins, A, D and K.

RESULTS

The malabsorption syndrome may produce deficiency of one or many substances and one or more of the following effects may thus ensue:

Malabsorption of	*Effect*
Fat	Steatorrhoea – excessive fat in faeces
Protein	Loss of weight, hypoproteinaemia with oedema, osteoporosis
Calcium and Vitamin D	Rickets, osteomalacia, hypocalcaemia with tetany
Vitamin B_1	Peripheral neuritis – beri beri
Nicotinic acid	Glossitis, pellagra, etc.
Riboflavine	Cheilosis, keratitis, glossitis, etc.
Vitamin B_{12}	Macrocytic megaloblastic anaemia
Vitamin A	Xerophthalmia, night-blindness
Folic Acid	Macrocytic megaloblastic anaemia
Iron	Hypochromic anaemia
Vitamin K	Hypoprothrombinaemia and haemorrhagic diathesis
Salt and water	Dehydration and salt depletion
Potassium	Hypokalaemia

Diseases of the appendix

ACUTE APPENDICITIS

Nature

An acute non-specific inflammation of the *appendix vermiformis*.

Pathogenesis

The organisms responsible for the inflammation of the wall are derived from the normal intestinal bacterial flora constantly within the lumen of this blind tube. The exact mechanism responsible for the development of inflammation remains debatable, but it is probable that obstruction to the lumen is the major factor.

Macroscopical

In a typical acute appendicitis the following changes may be present:

1 *Lumen.* Contains an obstructing faecolith and is distended by purulent material.

2 *Mucosa.* Hyperaemic, swollen and often ulcerated or completely necrotic.

3 *Wall.* Oedema, congestion and swelling of the muscular wall.

4 *Peritoneum.* Congestion of the serosal vessels and an inflammatory exudate, commonly fibrinous or frankly purulent.

Microscopical

The appearances are those of an acute, non-specific, inflammatory reaction affecting all layers of the wall.

Results

1 *Resolution.* The inflammatory reaction may subside and the appendix return to normal.

2 *Incomplete resolution.* The inflammatory reaction may not completely resolve but results in an appendix with increased fibrous tissue, especially of the peritoneal coat.

3 *Chronic appendicitis.* The inflammatory reaction may persist, recur and become chronic, resulting in an enlarged thickened and fibrotic appendix showing the microscopic features of a non-specific, active, chronic inflammation (see p. 29).

4 *Appendix abscess.* The omentum and adjacent tissues may surround the inflamed appendix to wall-off the spreading inflammation, but local suppuration continues resulting in an appendix abscess.

5 *Gangrenous appendicitis.* In virulent infections, especially when associated with appendicular obstruction, a necrotizing inflammation with vascular thrombosis occurs resulting in death of the tissues of the wall.

6 *Perforated appendicitis.* The gangrenous wall of the appendix perforates with spilling of the infected faecal contents and producing a local peritonitis, an appendicular abscess, or a generalized peritonitis.

7 *Portal pyaemia.* The accompanying septic thrombophlebitis may result in septic emboli and portal pyaemia.

8 *Mucocoele.* If the infection is very mild, the obstruction causes retention of the secreted mucus – mucocoele. Should the contents be spilled into the peritoneal cavity, *myxoma peritonei* may result (see p. 221).

9 *Late sequelae.* The acute manifestations may resolve but intestinal adhesions or intraperitoneal fibrous bands may remain, which later may cause intestinal obstruction by producing volvulus or strangulation of the bowel.

CHRONIC APPENDICITIS

True chronic inflammation of the appendix is uncommon but may occur following an acute appendicitis with continued reaction to a residual infection. Uncommonly, a chronic appendicitis may arise *de novo* due to infection by organisms of low virulence, especially when associated with partial obstruction to the lumen. Clinically, this may give rise to vague abdominal symptoms associated with tenderness over the appendix and the clinical condition is relieved by appendicectomy. On histological examination, these appendices may show increased fibrosis of all layers of the wall and an associated non-specific chronic inflammatory cell infiltration.

OTHER APPENDICULAR DISEASES

In appendicectomy specimens, the following conditions are sometimes encountered.

Actinomycosis
See p. 57.

Tuberculosis
See p. 45.

Threadworms
Multiple threadworms are frequently found in the lumen of the appendix in children; it is doubtful if they have any significant clinical effects in this organ (see p. 67).

Schistosomiasis

As part of an intestinal infestation, especially by *Schistosoma mansoni* (see p. 558).

Crohn's disease

Rarely, regional ileitis may affect the appendix only (see p. 200), or the organ may be involved together with the ileum or colon.

Measles

In the prodromal stage of measles, there is swelling of the lymphoid tissue which may produce the clinical manifestations of an obstructive acute appendicitis. On microscopy, the lymphoid tissue of the appendix contains large giant cells with up to 250 nuclei – Warthin–Finkeldey giant cells, which are diagnostic of measles (see p. 42).

Carcinoid tumour

See p. 212.

Lymphoma

Malignant proliferation of the appendicular lymphoid tissue may result in obstructive symptoms mimicking acute appendicitis.

Carcinoma

Rarely, the obstruction is due to an adenocarcinoma arising from the appendicular epithelium.

Endometriosis

Occasionally, endometrial tubules with stromal cells and surrounding hypertrophic smooth muscle are found, usually on the serosal aspect. This is commonly associated with endometriosis of the ovaries.

Isolated arteritis

Occasionally fibrinoid necrosis and inflammatory cell infiltration of the type seen in necrotizing arteritis (see p. 263) is found in small arteries in the appendix. In the vast majority of such cases this appears to be an entirely local phenomenon and not a manifestation of polyarteritis.

Chapter 41
Alimentary System – Intestines: Tumours

Tumours of the small intestine

BENIGN TUMOURS
These are rarely the cause of clinical disease but fibromas, leiomyomas and neurofibromas are occasionally found and may be the initiating cause of intussusception (see p. 219).

CARCINOID TUMOURS

Nature
Endocrine tumours of Kulschitzsky cell origin which, in the small intestine and appendix, are readily identified in the mucosal crypts by silver stains for argyrophil and argentaffin properties and by diazo-positivity in formalin-fixed tissue.

Macroscopical
Nodules or plaques of yellowish, often infiltrative tumour in submucosa and often with little or no ulceration. They have commonly penetrated to the serosal coat by the time of diagnosis.

Microscopical
In typical cases clumps, columns, strands and rosettes of regular small eosinophilic cells of polyhedral shape are seen, occasionally with glandular acini. Diazo- and argentaffin stains show the typical

granules of 5-hydroxytryptamine. Lead haematoxylin stain also demonstrates the granules.

Behaviour

APPENDIX

Usually removed incidentally they virtually never metastasize and hormone effects are not seen.

A variant at this site is the *goblet-cell carcinoid* in which cells are distended by mucin. This is potentially more aggressive.

SMALL INTESTINE

Although histologically identical this behaves more aggressively than the appendicular counterpart and may have metastasized to lymph nodes and/or liver by time of diagnosis. If there is a sufficient mass of tumour, enough 5-H.T. is produced to give rise to the carcinoid syndrome. The metabolite 5-HIAA (5-hydroxyindoleacetic acid) is excreted by the kidney, and urinary measurements can therefore aid diagnosis. The full syndrome consists of flushing with cyanosis, diarrhoea, bronchospasm, ascites, oedema and heart valve lesions (see p. 247) producing pulmonary stenosis.

LARGE INTESTINE

Carcinoid tumours of colon are usually benign and hormonally inactive.

OTHER GASTRO-INTESTINAL TRACT CARCINOIDS AND RELATED TUMOURS

The mucosa of the gastro-intestinal tract and the pancreas contain large numbers of cells of the 'diffuse endocrine system' sometimes called APUD cells (see p. 145). They elaborate a very large number of peptide hormone substances and hyperplasia or tumours of such cells are often endocrinologically active. Some of the tumours are carcinomas, other are adenomas but many have carcinoid-like features even when frankly malignant.

Immunohistochemical techniques, e.g. immunoperoxidase stains of fixed tissue using specific antisera, are required to demonstrate the specific hormone but hormonal activity in general can be shown by the presence of cytoplasmic granules which are lead haematoxylin positive and are shown to be neurosecretory in type by electron microscopy.

The list of recently identified hormones in this cell system grows rapidly. Amongst the most important in the gastro-intestinal tract are:

Stomach
  G cells producing gastrin (Zollinger–Ellison syndrome).
  A cells producing enteroglucagon.
  D cells producing somatostatin.
Small intestine
  S cells producing secretin.
  D cells producing gastrin inhibitory polypeptide (GIP).
  EG cells producing enteroglucagon.
  N cells producing vasoactive intestinal peptide (VIP).
  D cells producing somatostatin.
Pancreas (Islets)
  B cells producing insulin.
  A cells producing glucagon.
  D cells producing somatostatin.

MALIGNANT TUMOURS

Malignant tumours of the small bowel are all rare; the least infrequent is lymphoma, usually of non-Hodgkin's type, which produces a homogeneous, pale tumour arising from the lymphoid tissue. This may present with intestinal obstruction or be accompanied by intussusception. Primary carcinoma is extremely rare and is an adenocarcinoma which commonly encircles the small gut – 'string' carcinoma. As the bowel contents are fluid at this level, obstructive symptoms occur late and the prognosis is poor due to the presence of metastases at the time of diagnosis.

Tumours of the large intestine

POLYPS

NON-NEOPLASTIC

Types

1 *Benign lymphoid*. Smooth, rounded sessile and rare nodules, usually small and most commonly in the rectum. Histological examination shows a large collection of benign lymphoid tissue in the submucosa. These polyps are usually found incidentally and are harmless.

2 *Inflammatory polyposis*. Pseudo-polyps of inflammatory granulation tissue only or of inflamed mucosal tags are associated with ulcerative colitis

and less commonly with dysentery and Crohn's disease (see p. 200).

3 *Metaplastic polyps.* These small, sessile, flat-topped nodules most common in the rectum, are usually numerous and the same colour as the adjacent mucous membrane. They are very frequently seen and microscopically show elongated tubules, often cystic and with reduction in goblet cells. They are not neoplastic and are quite harmless.

4 *Hamartomatous polyps.* In these polyps there is overgrowth of the smooth muscle of the muscularis mucosa which separates acini of proliferated epithelium. The most common syndrome is *Peutz–Jegher* consisting of gastro-intestinal polyposis, mucocutaneous melanin pigmentation and transmission as a Mendelian dominant. It is doubtful if there is any significant risk of malignant change in hamartomatous polyps of this or the solitary 'juvenile' type.

NEOPLASTIC POLYPS

Nature
Polypoid protruberant tumours of hyperplastic benign large intestinal epithelium which may be solitary, or few in number, or very numerous (often thousands) in *familial polyposis.*

Site
They may occur in any part of the large intestine but are more frequently found in the rectum and pelvic colon.

Age
Wide range from 20 years onwards with a peak incidence of 57 years.

Macroscopical
Lobulated or papillary raised surface lesions which may be variably pedunculated or sessile. The range of size is large from 0.2 cm in diameter to several centimetres, particularly in the more sessile tumours.

Microscopical
As with the gross appearances so there is a wide spectrum microscopically from a lobulated tubular pattern of columnar epithelial overgrowth with, in the case of pedunculated lesions, a core of loose connective tissue, through a tubulo-villous structure to a villous sessile tumour. Classification histologically is into (*a*) tubular, (*b*) tubulo-villous and (*c*) villous. Where the structure and cytological features are regular this variation of pattern seems to be of little significance in respect of behaviour. When atypical foci are present, including areas of *in situ* malignant change, this only becomes clinically relevant if there is invasion deep to the muscularis mucosae. Minor degrees of stromal invasion when superficial to this do not confer a malignant natural history if locally excised.

MALIGNANT CHANGE — THE 'POLYP—CANCER' SEQUENCE

The age distribution curves of neoplastic polyps of the colon and large intestinal carcinomas are very similar but separated by 5 years – earlier in life for the polyps. Patients who have had benign neoplastic polyps removed have a much greater incidence of subsequent development, not only of further polyps, but also of carcinoma, than the general population. The exact number of neoplastic polyps which become malignant is not accurately predictable but is probably of the order of 5 per cent. The inference that most carcinomas arise in pre-existing adenomatous or villous neoplastic polyps indicates that management clinically should be based on the need to remove locally diagnosed lesions as premalignant.

In *familial polyposis*, a dominant inherited condition with 80 per cent penetrance, malignant change in affected members of a family is virtually inevitable unless prophylactic colectomy is performed. In those operative specimens where carcinoma has developed and has been clinically manifest, it is not uncommon to find variable stages of malignancy in several different polyps. The age incidence of malignant change is 40 years, some 10 years earlier than non-polyposis colonic cancer.

CARCINOMA OF THE LARGE INTESTINE

Incidence
In England and Wales this very common form of cancer accounts for nearly 20 per cent of malignant deaths (about 15 000 per annum) and is thus exceeded only in frequency by lung cancer. The incidence is geographically highest in affluent

Western Countries and it is uncommon in African countries, South America and Asia.

Age
Mean 60 years. Range – childhood onwards.

Sex
Colon M:F 1:2.
Rectum M:F 3:2.

Sites

	Per cent
Rectum and recto-sigmoid	50
Sigmoid colon	25
Caecum, ascending, transverse and descending colon	25
Multiple synchronous (usually not more than 2)	4

Subsequent new primary carcinoma after partial resection of intestine – 4 per cent. Average time interval – 8 years.

Predisposing factors
1 *The polyp – cancer sequence with neoplastic polyps.* The very significant risk of malignant change in solitary neoplastic polyps and the even greater incidence in familial polyposis is discussed on p. 214.
2 *Ulcerative colitis.* Total colonic involvement by this condition particularly when long standing, i.e. over 10 years, carries a high incidence of malignant change (see p. 202).
3 *Crohn's disease.* It seems likely that involvement of the colon by Crohn's disease carries an increased risk of malignancy (see p. 200).
4 *Dietary factors.* The much increased incidence in affluent societies of the West has been attributed to reduction in residue in the dietary intake at the expense of richer more completely absorbed food substances. This observation remains to be confirmed.

Macroscopical
Wide range of appearances but the tumours are usually relatively small except in the caecum. Most are papillary or polypoid with central ulceration of classical raised everted malignant features at the margins. Stenosis from a purse-string-like annular tumour commonly leads to intestinal obstruction at an early stage particularly in the left side of the large intestine. About 10 per cent show a grossly mucoid or colloid appearance. Diffuse infiltrating types of tumour are very uncommon.

Microscopical
Most are columnar cell adenocarcinomas, some very mucoid with occasional signet-ring cell types. Differentiated tumours predominate

Low grade	20 per cent.
Average grade	60 per cent.
High grade	20 per cent.

Effects
Variable according to site:
1 *Change of bowel habit.*
2 *Blood loss.* Usually obvious fresh bleeding from left-sided tumours but occult sometimes, particularly when caecal in position and presenting commonly as iron deficiency anaemia.
3 *Intestinal obstruction.* Apparent early in transverse and pelvic colon but late in the caecum and ascending colon where contents are more fluid.
4 *Perforation.* Pericolic abscess if localized or adherent to other structures, otherwise generalized faecal peritonitis.
5 *Fistulae.* For example, to bladder, vagina, uterus, small intestine or stomach.

Spread
1 *Direct.* Restricted to the wall – stage A. Penetrating all coats – stage B.
2 *Lymphatic.* Spread to regional lymph nodes – stage C. More distant groups can also be involved. These two factors have a very important bearing on surgical resection and prognosis (see Fig. 30, p. 216).
3 *Blood.* This can commonly be observed histologically in the submucous venous plexus of the adjacent intestinal wall but appears not to carry a sinister prognosis. Invasion of extramural veins, however, reduces 5-year survival from 55 per cent to 30 per cent. Thirty-five per cent of all patients with large intestinal cancer die from blood-borne metastasis, mostly in the liver but sometimes more widely disseminated.
4 *Transcoelomic.* Penetration of the serosal coat by tumour cells may lead to deposits subsequently appearing anywhere in the peritoneal cavity but most commonly in the pouch of Douglas or on the ovaries – *Krukenberg tumour* (see p. 440).
5 *Implantation:*
(a) *Natural.* Secondary deposits may occur due to implantation of naturally exfoliated malignant

cells on to damaged surfaces, e.g. anal fistula or fissure or haemorrhoids.

(b) *Artificial*. In suture lines of bowel anastomosis or in abdominal or perineal wounds.

Prognosis

The influence of Dukes' staging on prognosis is illustrated by Fig. 30. It should be appreciated, however, that blood spread can occur with any of the illustrated stages and that histological grading also is helpful in this site in assessment of prognosis.

Five-year survival:

Low grade
  80 per cent (75 per cent are stages A & B)
Average grade   60 per cent (50 per cent are stages A & B)
High grade   25 per cent (20 per cent only are stages A & B).

The overall 5-year survival of all surgically resected cases of large intestinal carcinoma is 50 per cent.

Deaths from locally recurrent disease   10 per cent
Deaths from blood spread   35 per cent
Deaths from lymphatic spread   5 per cent.

OTHER TUMOURS OF THE LARGE INTESTINE

Connective tissues

Fibromas, neurofibromas, haemangiomas, leiomyomas and their malignant counterparts are all rare in this region.

Lymphomas

Secondary deposits of Hodgkin's and non-Hodgkin's lymphomas are uncommon. Primary presentation of lymphoma in the colon is even rarer.

Carcinoid tumours

See p. 212.

CARCINOMA OF THE ANAL CANAL

Incidence

This is a rare tumour by comparison with adenocarcinoma of the large intestine, approximately 1 : 50.

Age

55–65 years.

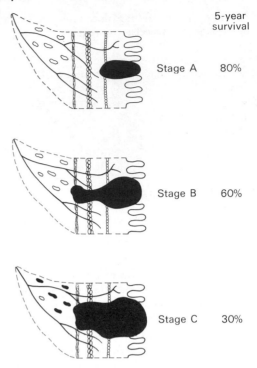

Fig. 30. Carcinoma of the large intestine – staging and prognosis.

Sex

M:F 3:2.

Site

The tumour arises from the squamous epithelium of the anal canal.

Macroscopical

An ulcerating epithelioma of the canal which may extend upwards into the rectum or below to the perianal skin.

Microscopical

Squamous cell carcinomas, frequently with little keratin formation.

Spread

1 *Direct*. Involvement of rectum, perianal tissues and perineum.

2 *Lymphatic*. Metastases to the inguinal nodes

occur in 35 per cent. If the rectum becomes invaded, intra-abdominal nodes may also be involved.

3 *Blood*. This is a late manifestation.

Results

Following surgical resection, 5-year survival is about 50 per cent.

OTHER TUMOURS OF THE ANAL CANAL

Other types of skin tumour can be found in the anal canal or anal marginal skin including: malignant melanoma, basal cell carcinoma, Pagets' disease of the anus, skin appendage tumours and Bowen's disease (intra-epidermal or *in situ* carcinoma). Their behaviour is similar to when they occur at other sites.

Chapter 42
Alimentary System – Intestinal Obstruction: Peritoneum

Intestinal obstruction
Nature

MECHANICAL OBSTRUCTION

Lumen
   Swallowed foreign bodies
   Gall stones
   Enteroliths
   Inspissated barium
   Meconium ileus

Wall
   Tumours
   Ischaemic stricture
   Ulcerative colitis
   Crohn's disease
   Lymphogranuloma venereum
   Diverticular disease of colon
   Congenital
   Intussusception
      Nature
      Macroscopical
      Results

External
   Bands
   External hernias

Internal hernias
Tumours
Volvulus

PARALYTIC ILEUS
Neuromuscular dysfunction
Trauma
Coeliac axis lesions
Vascular
Infection

Peritoneum

Ascites
Nature
Causes

Chylous ascites
Nature
Causes
Macroscopical

Intraperitoneal haemorrhage
Nature
Causes
   Trauma
   Ruptured ectopic pregnancy

Ruptured corpus luteum
   haematoma
Ruptured abdominal
   aneurysm
Haemorrhagic diatheses

PERITONITIS
Nature

Acute
Macroscopical
Causes
   External
   Haematogenous
   Inflamed organs
   Perforated peptic ulcer
   Perforated small or large gut
   Acute pancreatitis
   Biliary perforation
   Strangulated bowel

Chronic

TUMOURS
Primary
Secondary

Intestinal obstruction

Nature
Obstruction to the passage of intestinal contents. This may be due to many causes which are subdivided into mechanical and paralytic.

MECHANICAL OBSTRUCTION

LUMEN

Swallowed foreign bodies

Gall stones
Gall stone ileus (see p. 571).

Enteroliths
From the lumen of a small gut diverticulum (see p. 193).

Inspissated barium
Following radiological investigations.

Meconium ileus
In mucoviscidosis (see p. 632).

WALL

Tumours
Particularly carcinoma of the colon (see p. 215).

Ischaemic stricture
Particularly at the junction of splenic flexure and descending colon (see p. 196).

Ulcerative colitis
Fibrosis of the wall and stricture formation (see p. 202) are uncommon unless malignant change supervenes.

Crohn's disease
Segmental areas of occlusion, especially of the terminal ileum (see p. 200).

Lymphogranuloma venereum
Rectal stricture in females (see p. 406).

Diverticular disease of colon
Association of the thick muscular wall and inflammatory swelling (see p. 194).

Congenital
For example, megacolon, Hirschsprung's disease, atresias, imperforate anus, etc.

Intussusception
Nature. This is the invagination of one portion of the intestine into the lumen of the bowel immediately distal (see Fig. 31).

Macroscopical. The apex passes down the lumen dragging the mesentery and its vessels with it, until strangulation of the vessels occurs and the trapped portion of bowel dies.

Results. This produces a 'sausage-shaped' mass and results in intestinal obstruction. It occurs in infants, when it is of unknown causation, unless there has been a recent dietary change. In adults it is usually associated with a tumour, which forms the apex. The subsequent peristalsis endeavours to extrude the mass, thereby inducing the intussusception.

EXTERNAL

Bands
Fibrous bands and adhesions following previous operations or past intraperitoneal infections. The fibrous band from a Meckel's diverticulum to the umbilicus may also snare loops of bowel and produce intestinal obstruction.

External hernias
The intestine may become obstructed due to incarceration in an external hernial orifice in the inguinal and femoral canals. Incisional hernias through the anterior abdominal wall, at the umbilicus and rarely in the obturator and lumbar regions, may also obstruct the intestines.

Internal hernias
The foramen of Winslow, the duodenal fossa and the diaphragm are all potential orifices through which loops of intestines may pass and become obstructed.

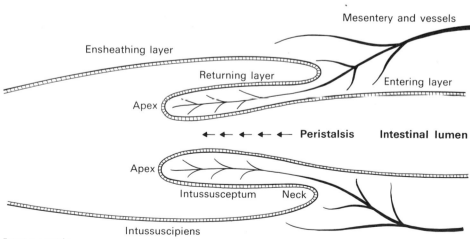

Fig. 31. Intussusception.

The importance of these internal and external orifices is that intestine may pass through the aperture and become irreducible. Strangulation of the herniated bowel may follow as a result of obstruction to the blood supply.

Littré's hernia – contains a Meckel's diverticulum.

Richter's hernia – contains only part of the circumference of the intestinal wall within the sac.

Tumours

Tumours in adjacent organs or in lymph nodes may compress and distort the bowel wall and result in an obstruction.

Volvulus

Torsion of the mesentery of the small bowel or of a long mesentery of the sigmoid colon, may result in vascular obstruction to produce gangrene. A similar process may occur in the small intestine due to a congenitally incomplete attachment of the mesentery, whereby virtually the whole of the small intestine undergoes torsion – *volvulus neonatorum*.

PARALYTIC OBSTRUCTION – PARALYTIC ILEUS

This implies intestinal obstruction without evidence of any mechanical blockage and is due to:

Neuromuscular dysfunction

Absence of normal gut peristalsis commonly occurs in the immediate postoperative period following abdominal operations. There may be an associated dilatation of the stomach.

Trauma

Severe abdominal trauma may be followed by paralytic ileus.

Coeliac axis lesions

A space-occupying lesion causing pressure on the coeliac axis, e.g. haematoma or tumour, may result in paralytic ileus.

Vascular

Superior mesenteric artery or vein obstruction (see p. 195).

Infection

Generalized peritonitis is almost invariably associated with a paralytic ileus.

Diseases of the peritoneum

ASCITES

Nature

An excess of fluid in the peritoneal cavity:
1 *Transudate*. Relative density 1.010. Protein 0.3 g/100 ml or less.
2 *Exudate*. Relative density 1.020 or more. Protein 3 g/100 ml or more.

Causes

1 Cardiac failure
2 Nephrotic syndrome ⎫ Transudate
3 Portal hypertension ⎭
4 Inflammatory – Exudate, i.e. peritonitis.

CHYLOUS ASCITES

Nature

An excess of fluid in the peritoneal cavity containing chyle.

Causes

Any obstructive lesion of the thoracic duct or mesenteric lymphatics. The usual causes are secondary carcinoma or primary malignant lymphoma.

Macroscopical

The peritoneal cavity is filled with milky fluid containing finely emulsified fatty globules.

INTRAPERITONEAL HAEMORRHAGE

Nature

Blood within the peritoneal cavity.

Causes

1 *Trauma*. Especially with rupture of the spleen, liver or kidney.
2 *Ruptured ectopic pregnancy*
3 *Ruptured corpus luteum haematoma*
4 *Ruptured abdominal aneurysm*
5 *Haemorrhagic diatheses*. Including anticoagulant therapy.

Blood-stained fluid may also be found in abdominal tuberculosis, *carcinomatosis peritonei*, strangulated intestines, infarction due to mesenteric vascular occlusion and acute pancreatitis.

PERITONITIS

Nature
An inflammatory reaction in the peritoneal cavity. This may be acute or chronic, sterile or infected, localized or generalized.

ACUTE

Macroscopical
The normally glistening peritoneum is dull, congested and is glued together by exudate and fibrinous adhesions. The exudate may be serous, fibrinous, haemorrhagic, sero-fibrinous or purulent in type and the loops of gut are often distended due to the associated paralytic ileus.

Causes
1 *External*. Resulting from penetrating wounds.
2 *Haematogenous*. A very rare primary form, usually due to pneumococci and occurring almost exclusively in female children.
3 *Inflamed organs*, e.g. appendicitis, salpingitis, cholecystitis, etc.
4 *Perforated peptic ulcer*. Acid gastric contents and food products.
5 *Perforated small or large gut*, e.g. typhoid, Crohn's disease, diverticular disease, carcinoma, etc.
6 *Acute pancreatitis*. The release of proteolytic and lipolytic enzymes induces a marked peritoneal reaction. There are chalky-white areas of fat necrosis and free fat in the peritoneal cavity, producing a diagnostic picture.
7 *Biliary perforation*. Leakage of bile by trauma, surgery, or with cholecystitis, produces a bile-stained peritonitis which is intensely irritating to the peritoneal tissues, although commonly sterile.
8 *Strangulated bowel*. Due to volvulus, hernia, intussusception, etc., resulting in death of the bowel wall and allowing passage of bacteria through the wall into the peritoneal cavity.

CHRONIC

This may occur as a result of a tuberculous peritonitis associated with tuberculous enteritis or salpingitis, or it may be blood-borne. The result is an ascites with an adhesive or plastic type of peritonitis. A special form occurs in Concato's disease – *polyserositis*, probably due to active tuberculosis. In Pick's disease there is a healed tuberculous pericarditis with constriction and the peritoneal fluid is thus a transudate due to the accompanying cardiac failure.

In chronic peritonitis the adhesions tend to be thick and fibrous and increase the risk of subsequent strangulation of the bowel by bands. The serosal surfaces of the liver and spleen are covered with a thick fibrous capsule – 'sugar-icing'.

TUMOURS

Primary
These are excessively rare – *mesotheliomas*. They have a similar structure to the pleural mesothelioma (see p. 680) and nearly all occur in persons occupationally exposed to asbestos.

Secondary
Exceedingly common and deposits of carcinoma on the peritoneum – *carcinomatosis peritonei*, occur with many different types of tumour. They are especially common with carcinoma of the stomach, large gut, ovary and breast and form multiple serosal and omental nodules associated with a peritoneal exudate which is frequently blood-stained – malignant ascites. Examination of removed fluid will frequently reveal the presence of malignant cells.

An allied condition is *myxoma peritonei*, in which the pelvic peritoneal cavity, and sometimes the general peritoneal cavity, becomes filled with gelatinous material. This is usually due to peritoneal seedlings from a ruptured mucinous cystadenoma or cystadenocarcinoma of the ovary, but may rarely follow rupture of an appendicular mucocoele.

Chapter 43
Diseases of the Breast – Benign

CONGENITAL

Congenital abnormalities of the breast are rare and unimportant with the exception of *polymastia* and *polythelia* –accessory breasts and accessory nipples. These may occur anywhere along the 'milk-line' from the chest to the groin and are subject to the same disorders as normally situated breasts.

Disorders of breast growth

Failure of development
Usually due to ovarian agenesis – *Turner's syndrome* (see p. 432) or a relative ovarian deficiency – *premature menopause syndrome*. The breasts remain rudimentary, but a degree of breast development may be induced with oestrogen therapy.

Precocious development
The breasts may develop early as part of the syndrome of precocious puberty, i.e. before the age of 8 or 9 years. Although a small proportion of cases are associated with a granulosa cell or other ovarian tumour (see p. 436), in most cases no causative lesion is found. Surgical intervention is not indicated.

Adolescent hypertrophy
This is the commonest form of true hypertrophy of the female breast. Over a period of 1–2 years the breasts may enlarge so greatly that they become a severe physical and psychological burden. Occasionally the hypertrophy is unilateral. The cause is unknown and the only effective treatment is surgical. Microscopic examination of the breast tissue

shows normal epithelial elements with an increase in adipose and connective tissue.

Massive hypertrophy of pregnancy
Rare cases of massive breast hypertrophy of unknown pathogenesis occurring during pregnancy have been recorded.

INFLAMMATORY LESIONS

ACUTE MASTITIS AND BREAST ABSCESS

Aetiology
This condition is usually, but not always, associated with lactation and a cracked nipple through which staphylococci or streptococci gain entry to the breast tissue.

Macroscopical
There may be a generalized, red, painful and swollen breast due to diffuse involvement of the organ by infection, or a localized abscess may form in a single breast lobule.

Microscopical
Actively lactating breast tissue with acute suppurative inflammation and abscess formation.

Results
Successful treatment results in resolution, but when abscess formation occurs fibrous scarring may result or there may be incomplete resolution followed by true chronic mastitis.

CHRONIC MASTITIS

True chronic inflammation of the breast due to bacterial infection is extremely uncommon. Most cases are due to incomplete resolution of acute mastitis in the lactating breast or to chronic breast abscess. This condition should not be confused with the non-inflammatory conditions often grouped as 'chronic mastitis' and which are of hormonal origin (see below).

TUBERCULOSIS

Tuberculosis is very rare in the breast but may occasionally occur due to secondary involvement via lymphatics from intra-thoracic disease.

SYPHILIS

The nipple is a relatively common site for an extragenital chancre but other forms of syphilis are very rare.

TRAUMATIC FAT NECROSIS

Aetiology
Although less than half the patients give a history of any definite injury, there is good evidence that the lesion results from trauma to an area of adipose tissue sufficient to disrupt the fat cells and allow the escape of fat globules into the surrounding tissue.

Macroscopical
Presents as a hard mass in the breast, sometimes with local fixation and skin tethering. On section, there is a pale, firm, fibrous nodule containing multiple yellow foci some of which contain fluid fatty material.

Microscopical
The disrupted fat cells release their fat content which causes a foreign body giant cell reaction. There is thus an area composed of fat spaces, phagocytic foam cells, foreign body giant cells, inflammatory cells and later dense fibrous tissue.

Results
The hardness of this lesion and the fibrous reaction which may result in fixation to surrounding tissues, produces a close clinical resemblance to carcinoma.

Mammary dysplasia

Nature
Amongst other terms formerly or still used for this condition are *fibrocystic disease*, *cystic hyperplasia*, *chronic mastitis*, and *cystic mastitis*. The condition is the commonest of all breast lesions, and probably affects about 10 per cent of women. It is not, as some of the terms imply, inflammatory, but almost certainly has a hormonal basis. The cyclical changes in the ovary, with alternating oestrogen and progesterone secretion, produce effects not only in the endometrium but also in the breasts. Thus proliferative changes in both epithelial and stromal

elements of the breast lobules occur during the menstrual cycle, with a return to normal at the end of each cycle. Mammary dysplasia is at its peak in the immediate pre-menopausal years and regresses after the menopause. This is the time when hormonal imbalances are most likely to occur, with ovarian function diminishing. As a result, the epithelium and stroma of the breast lobule remain in an abnormal proliferative state, producing nodular, granular, lumpy or cystic breasts.

Macroscopic appearances

The condition may be localized or diffuse, unilateral or bilateral, painful or painless, cystic or solid. It may occur at any time during the childbearing period, but is particularly common premenopausally.

Microscopic components

A spectrum of microscopic appearances may be seen and, apart from cystic change, the microscopic changes cannot be predicted from the gross appearance. Any of the microscopic components may occur in a focal or a generalized distribution, be restricted to one type or show all conceivable combinations in one or both breasts.

CYSTIC CHANGE

Cysts may be visible to the naked eye or apparent only on microscopy – *microcysts*. They may be single or multiple, and contain clear fluid unless haemorrhage or infection causes a change to red, brown or green. The cysts are dilated ducts and are lined by flattened epithelium. Later the epithelium may disappear and the cyst is then lined by the fibrous tissue of the wall. Occasionally, the epithelium may proliferate to give papillary structures, but these have no sinister significance.

FIBROSIS

An increase in interlobular fibrous tissue occurs normally with increasing age. This is exaggerated in mammary dysplasia, and is accompanied by intralobular fibrosis. Both types of fibrosis are frequently associated with cysts.

EPITHELIAL PROLIFERATION

Adenosis

There is increased cellularity due to regular proliferation of the inner epithelial secretory cells and outer myo-epithelial cells of ducts and acini, conforming to a lobular pattern. There may also be proliferation of intralobular connective tissue producing distortion of the acinar pattern and, eventually, sclerosis of the epithelial structures – *sclerosing adenosis*. The end result is one of progressive hyaline fibrosis.

Epitheliosis

The essential feature is an increase in the thickness of the epithelium of lobular ducts and acini due to benign proliferation of the epithelial secretory cells. The cells are several layers in depth and the lumen may be completely obliterated by this solid proliferation. The nuclei are regular with normal polarity, although occasional minor atypicalities may be seen. The lesion must be distinguished from intraduct carcinoma, in which the epithelial proliferation is irregular, with loss of polarity, numerous atypical nuclei and mitotic activity.

Papillomatosis

This is a more florid form of epitheliosis in which ducts, many of which are dilated, are filled by regular epithelial papillary projections from the lining epithelium. The lesion should be distinguished from intraduct papilloma which is a macroscopically visible organoid structure (see p. 225).

Pink cell change

The normal cuboidal epithelial secretory cells are transformed into columnar peg-like cells with abundant eosinophilic cytoplasm. This change is frequently seen in dilated ducts and cysts. It has been termed 'apocrine metaplasia', but ultrastructural studies do not support the pathogenetic implications of this name.

Summary

All these conditions may produce sinister clinical manifestations, commonly with a lump in the breast. Sclerosing adenosis may be mistaken microscopically for invasive carcinoma, and epitheliosis and papillomatosis must not be confused with intraduct carcinoma. Patients with mammary dysplasia have an approximately four-fold increased risk of developing breast carcinoma compared with normal.

MAMMARY DUCT ECTASIA

Aetiology
This condition is a component of mammary dysplasia and appears to be hormonally based being increasingly seen in post-menopausal patients.

Macroscopical
Many ducts are distended by creamy material and the adjacent breast tissue is of increased firmness. The condition may occur in the main breast ducts or be more peripherally situated.

Microscopical
Creamy material distends the ducts and causes a reaction in the surrounding breast tissue with lymphocytes, plasma cells, foam cells, foreign body giant cells and fibroblastic proliferation.

Benign tumours

FIBROADENOMA

Nature
Although these lesions are conventionally classed as benign tumours, there is considerable evidence to support the view that they are not true neoplasms, but rather focal areas of lobular hyperplasia caused mainly by overgrowth of intralobular connective tissue.

Age
Occurs at any age after puberty, but most commonly before 30 years.

Macroscopical
Firm rubbery, lobulated, sharply defined, pale and occasionally multiple nodules in the breast.

Microscopical
The nodules are composed of branching ducts and associated acini with surrounding proliferating connective tissue, often resembling hyperplastic lobules. There are two characteristic patterns, both of which are usually seen in the same nodule, although one may predominate:
1 *Pericanalicular*. The connective tissue is arranged in whorls around groups of acini.
2 *Intracanalicular*. The epithelial element is arranged in elongated clefts which appear to be compressed by the surrounding connective tissue.

The epithelial cell nuclei are regular and normal in appearance.

Results
At operation the nodules are easily enucleated. Further nodules may develop, but individual lesions do not recur. If not removed, they become sclerotic with age. Neoplastic change does not occur.

CYSTOSARCOMA PHYLLODES — PHYLLODES TUMOUR — GIANT FIBROADENOMA

Age
Mostly occur in the middle-aged or elderly.

Macroscopical
They form very large, lobulated, circumscribed tumours which cause massive enlargement of the breast. Ulceration of the skin may occur by pressure necrosis due to their rapid growth. On section they are firm, pale and lobulated, but areas of cystic or myxomatous change and cleft-formation are commonly seen.

Microscopical
They have a similar structure to fibroadenomas of intracanalicular pattern, but the stroma is cellular, sometimes extremely so, with nuclear atypicality and numerous mitoses. The clefts are lined by epithelial cells of regular appearance, and nuclear abnormalities are uncommon.

Results
The majority of these lesions, in spite of their rapidity of growth, behave as benign tumours, and local mastectomy is curative. However, sarcomatous behaviour of the stroma occurs in about 5 per cent and about 10 per cent recur locally after excision by enucleation.

PAPILLOMA — INTRADUCT OR INTRACYSTIC

Nature
A few epithelial papillary breast lesions are part of the more generalized 'papillomatosis' (see p. 274). However, solitary benign papillary tumours occur as a distinct entity and are much more common.

Age

Most occur in the 20–30 age group and papillomas are extremely rare above 50 years of age.

Sites

Most commonly situated in one of the main ducts near the nipple.

Macroscopical

Distension of the duct of origin by a papillary tumour protruding into the lumen. Frequently, there is blood-stained material in the duct which may cause bleeding from the nipple.

Microscopical

A columnar cell papilloma with a narrow pedicle and covered by regular cells arising from duct epithelium.

Results

The duct may become cystic and the papilloma increase in size, thus forming an intracystic papilloma.

The vast majority of these papillomas pursue a benign course but, occasionally, carcinoma may develop in the lesion, usually many years later.

OTHER BENIGN TUMOURS

A rare benign epithelial tumour is the *adenoma of nipple* – a slowly growing adenomatous tumour arising from a main duct and distorting the nipple. Local removal is usually curative. Benign connective tissue tumours are uncommon but include lipoma, angioma and leiomyoma.

Chapter 44
Diseases of the Breast – Malignant

Carcinoma of the breast

Incidence

Carcinoma of the breast is the commonest malignant tumour in women (20 per cent) and approximately 11 000 women die of this disease annually in England and Wales. It is exceeded overall only by carcinoma of the lung, stomach and large intestine. The frequency is increasing and this is not entirely due to increase in the 'at risk' population.

Age

Any age group can be affected but it is rare below 30 and the majority of cases occur between 40 and 70 years.

Sex

F:M 100:1 Carcinoma of the male breast is extremely uncommon.

Aetiology

PREDISPOSING FACTORS

Racial
A lower incidence is reported in Japanese and Chinese women, but this is probably due to environmental rather than racial factors.

Parity
Parous women have a lower incidence of breast cancer than non-parous women. There is a slight

protection when the first child is born early in the reproductive age span. Breast feeding probably affords no protection.

Menstrual factors

There is a slightly increased risk of developing breast cancer in women who have an early menarche and in women with a late menopause. There is no association with endometrial cystic hyperplasia (see p. 413).

Hormonal activity

No consistent oestrogen abnormalities have been associated with breast cancer. Low levels of excretion of androgenic metabolites have been recorded, but the significance is uncertain. No increased risk has yet been demonstrated in women receiving exogenous oestrogen.

Heredity

There is a slight but definite increased risk for females if a family member has had carcinoma of the breast, and the risk is as great for paternal as maternal relatives. In addition there are rare 'breast cancer families', affecting successive generations, e.g. grandmother, mother, daughter.

Mammary dysplasia

Women with histologically proven mammary dysplasia have a four-fold increased risk of subsequent breast cancer (see p. 223).

EXPERIMENTAL

Heredity

As a result of many years of research Maud Slye was able to breed true strains of mice: (1) a 'high' breast cancer strain in which over 95 per cent of female mice developed breast cancer, and (2) 'low' strain in which less than 1 per cent developed breast cancer. Several further 'high' and 'low' mouse strains have since selectively been bred.

Viral factors

In 1936 Bittner showed that, in addition to heredity, a transmissible agent also played an important part in the aetiology of mouse mammary tumours. Mice from a 'low' carcinoma strain suckled by a mother of 'high' strain developed the disease with a high frequency, and vice versa. This Bittner 'milk factor' has now been identified as an RNA virus.

Hormonal activity

Removal of the ovaries in female mice of 'high' carcinoma strain entirely prevents the development of mammary carcinoma. Administration of exogenous oestrogen will only induce mammary carcinoma in males of 'high' carcinoma strain.

SUMMARY

No single aetiological agent has been shown to cause human breast cancer, and the predisposing factors such as parity, heredity and mammary dysplasia only have a slight effect. Experimental work in mice has shown that an RNA virus is the main aetiological agent, but no convincing evidence has yet been produced to implicate a virus in human breast cancer.

Sites

Any part of the breast substance which contains epithelium, including the axillary tail. The upper outer quadrant is, however, the most frequent site of origin.

Macroscopical

Breast carcinomas vary in size from 0.5 cm to several centimetres in diameter. They may be as follows.

INTRADUCT OR COMEDO

Usually multiple ducts contain yellowish secretion, including the proliferating epithelium, which can be expressed from the cut surface on pressure like a 'blackhead' – *comedo*.

SCIRRHOUS·

The most frequent type. The tumours contain a variable amount of connective tissue, making them hard and gritty – they cut like an 'unripe pear'. The margin may be clearly or ill-defined.

MUCOID

Uncommon. These are relatively soft tumours with a jelly like mucoid appearance due to excessive mucin secretion by the tumour cells.

PAPILLARY

Rare. An intracystic papillary tumour with a solid area of carcinoma invading the wall.

Microscopical

IN-SITU CARCINOMA

There are two types of in-situ carcinoma.

Intraduct

A variable number of ducts are filled by a disorderly proliferation of large epithelial cells with evidence of nuclear atypicality and increased mitotic activity. The epithelial basement membrane is intact, and there is no invasion of the adjacent breast tissue.

Lobular carcinoma-in-situ

This type is characterized by the proliferation of small epithelial cells within the acini of a group of lobules, obliterating the acinar lumen. The lobular units are distended, and the specialized intralobular connective tissue is crowded out. Basement membranes remain intact, with no invasion.

It is important to examine many areas of both these types of tumour to exclude the possibility of early stromal invasion.

INVASIVE CARCINOMA

Ductal

The majority of invasive carcinomas arise in the ducts from a pre-existing intraduct carcinoma, and are composed of cords and sheets of large epithelial cells infiltrating in a connective tissue stroma. Three grades of differentiation can be recognized, based on the amount of tubule formation, variation in size of nuclei and mitotic activity: grade 1, well differentiated; grade 2, moderately differentiated; grade 3, poorly differentiated. This system of histological grading has a bearing on prognosis (see p. 230).

Infiltrating lobular

This is the invasive counterpart of lobular carcinoma-in-situ. Typically there are dissociated linear cords of small epithelial tumour cells infiltrating diffusely in connective tissue – 'indian filing'. There is often a concentric 'targetoid' arrangement around preserved normal ducts.

Medullary

These tumours have a sharply demarcated edge and are composed of anastamosing sheets of tumour cells forming syncytial masses, with a conspicuous lymphoplasmacytic infiltrate in the stroma. Despite the poorly differentiated appearance of the tumour cells, these tumours have a relatively favourable prognosis.

Mucoid

This variant of adenocarcinoma produces excessive mucin so that islands of tumour cells appear to float in a sea of mucin.

Papillary

When malignancy supervenes in an intracystic papilloma the surface epithelium of the papillary lesion becomes atypical. The stroma of the stalk and the adjacent breast tissue are invaded.

Metaplastic

Very rarely metaplastic changes occur in breast carcinomas, e.g. squamous cell carcinoma, chondromatous change, osteosarcomatous change.

Routes of spread

DIRECT

Direct spread of the infiltrating tumour cells involves a progressive amount of the breast tissue and eventually results in either skin involvement and ulceration or attachment to muscle and chest wall.

LYMPHATIC

(a) Blockage of the local dermal lymphatics by tumour produces thickening of the skin with a *'peau d'orange'* appearance.

(b) Dermal lymphatic invasion may produce multiple tumour nodules and a dense reactive dermal fibrosis *'cancer en cuirasse'*.

(c) Axillary lymph nodes are involved in 50–60 per cent of patients with 'operable' breast cancer.

(d) The internal mammary lymph nodes may also be involved, particularly from tumours in the medial quadrants.

(e) Later, widespread involvement of mediastinal, abdominal and other groups of lymph nodes may occur.

BLOOD

Blood-borne spread is extremely common and is present in virtually all fatal cases. The lungs, liver and bones are the most frequent sites, but many other organs may be involved.

TRANSCOELOMIC

Once the tumour has spread to a body cavity, e.g. parietal pleura or peritoneum, transcoelomic spread may occur.

TUMOUR IMPLANTATION

'Spilling' of malignant cells from the tumour into the wound at the time of the initial operation may result in the continued growth of these cells in the scar tissue – *scar recurrence*. However, many recurrences in the region of the scar are in fact due to previous lymphatic permeation.

BREAST DUCTS

In some cases the ducts adjacent to an invasive breast carcinoma are filled with malignant cells. This may be due to spread of the tumour along the duct lumen, but more often they represent separate foci of intraduct carcinoma. This method of spread along the lumen of the duct towards the nipple is important in Paget's disease (see below).

Staging

Most attempts at staging the extent of spread in breast cancer, such as the International T.N.M. classification are based on clinical assessment only. They are inaccurate because (*a*) they assume that all enlarged axillary lymph nodes contain metastatic tumour, and (*b*) they do not take into account the possibility of distant occult microscopic metastases. A more accurate form of staging is based on pathological assessment of the breast and associated nodes; together with clinical and radiological examination for distant metastases. A simple staging is:
Stage 1 Tumour confined within the breast and not fixed to skin or fascia. Axillary and internal mammary lymph nodes not involved.
Stage 2. Tumour within the breast, fixed or not, with axillary or internal mammary node involvement.
Stage 3 Tumour in the breast, with distant metastases.

Prognosis

The two main factors which influence the prognosis of a patient with invasive breast cancer are:
1 The grade of histological differentiation of the tumour.
2 The stage of the tumour at the time of presentation.

SURVIVAL

All cases untreated – 22 per cent at 5 years – 5 per cent at 10 years.
All cases treated – 40 per cent at 5 years – 25 per cent at 10 years.
Histological grade 1, treated – 80 per cent at 5 years.
Histological grade 3, treated – 25 per cent at 5 years.

All grades, lymph nodes uninvolved – 75 per cent at 5 years.
All grades, lymph nodes involved – 30 per cent at 5 years.
Patients with intraduct carcinoma (*in situ* carcinoma) only, and no evidence of invasive carcinoma have an excellent prognosis – over 95 per cent at 5 years.
Carcinomas occurring during pregnancy and lactation have a particularly poor prognosis.

Even in the small group of patients who survive for 20 years or more, death may still occur from breast cancer, indicating that the disease may never be entirely cured.

Hormone dependency

The progress of some breast cancers may be influenced by alterations in the hormonal background of the patient. This forms the rationale for anti-oestrogen therapy and oophorectomy and adrenalectomy in pre-menopausal women, and the giving of oestrogens in post-menopausal women. Oestrogen receptor sites have been identified in normal and malignant breast tissue, and it may be possible to use this fact to assess which tumours are likely to respond to treatment.

Paget's disease of the nipple

Nature

A red, scaly, eczematous lesion of the nipple, associated with carcinoma in the breast.

Macroscopical

There is an eczematous lesion of the nipple, but the underlying breast tumour may not be palpable.

Microscopical

1 *Nipple*. Thickening of the squamous epithelium with prolongation of the rete pegs and an underlying inflammatory cell infiltration with increased fibrosis. Within the epidermis of the nipple there are multiple clear cells with a 'halo' appearance around atypical and often hyperchromatic nuclei – *Paget's cells*.
2 *Underlying breast*. This shows a carcinoma which is usually of the intraduct type involving the main ducts and extending along the lumen to the nipple surface. This intraduct cancer may not be palpable on clinical examination.

Pathogenesis

The precise nature and origin of the Paget's cells remain in dispute. The two main conflicting views are as follows.

1 The Paget's cells are mammary cancer cells which have extended along the main ducts from the primary breast tumour and become implanted in the epidermis. This is the most widely held view.

2 The Paget's cells are epidermal cells and the appearances are those of a 'carcinoma *in situ*' (intra-epidermal carcinoma) of the skin and that the breast carcinoma is merely an expression of malignant disease occurring in two adjacent epithelial structures simultaneously. This seems an unlikely explanation, as the cells, both within the ducts and within the thickened skin of the nipple, appear microscopically identical and usually can be shown to contain mucins.

Prognosis

This condition should be considered as carcinoma of the breast and treated as such. The prognosis depends on the nature of the underlying tumour. If this is intraduct then the prognosis is excellent, but if invasion has occurred, then the prognosis is that of invasive carcinoma of the breast.

Diagnosis of breast cancer

Most patients with breast cancer present with a 'lump in the breast'. However, numerous other pathological processes, such as mammary dysplasia, fibroadenoma and fat necrosis, may also give rise to a lump in the breast, and a definite tissue diagnosis must be established before the surgeon proceeds to mastectomy. The conventional way to achieve this is for the surgeon to take an operative biopsy, and whilst the patient is still under anaesthesia for the pathologist to make an immediate diagnosis on a rapid frozen section. Recently, out-patient needle biopsy techniques have been developed, which give a pre-operative diagnosis, and allows the surgeon and patient to have a full discussion of the nature of the lesion before definitive treatment is determined.

Male breast lesions

Lesions of the male breast are rare, but epithelial hyperplasia, gynaecomastia, fibroadenoma, carcinoma and sarcoma all occasionally occur. Enlargement also occurs in oestrogen therapy for carcinoma of prostate.

Other malignant tumours

Other malignant tumours which occur in the breast include sarcomas, such as fibrosarcoma, liposarcoma and angiosarcoma, but these are exceedingly rare.

Chapter 45
Cardiovascular System – Heart: Pericardium: Myocardium

Pericardium

INFLAMMATIONS

ACUTE PERICARDITIS

Nature
Primary pericarditis is very rare. Most cases are due to direct involvement from myocardial or endocardial disease, or by extension from neighbouring tissues, e.g. lungs.

Aetiology
1 *Infective*. Bacterial – e.g. staphylococci, streptococci, pneumococci; septicaemic or pyaemic; tuberculous.
2 *Aseptic*. Rheumatic; uraemic; secondary to myocardial infarction; tumour infiltration; systemic lupus erythematosus.

Appearances
The usual inflammatory phenomena occur, with hyperaemia, loss of lustre and exudates of varying appearance.

Types
1 *Serous*. Occurs particularly with non-bacterial inflammations. The fluid is clear, straw-coloured, protein-rich and has a relative density of 1.020 or more, with small numbers of polymorphs, lymphocytes and shed mesothelial cells. The volume is usually small (50–200 ml) and when formed slowly, produces little effect on cardiac function. With

remission of the underlying disease, the fluid reabsorbs with minimal adhesion formation.

2 *Sero-fibrinous or fibrinous*. This is the most frequent type and occurs with rheumatic fever, myocardial infarction and in uraemia. There is an abundant fibrin-rich exudate with variable amounts of fluid and the 'bread and butter' appearance on separating the parietal and visceral layers. With remission of the underlying cause there is:

(*a*) Resolution with digestion of the fibrin.

(*b*) Organization with variable obliteration of the pericardial sac which may result in an adherent pericardium.

The condition only rarely leads to embarrassment of cardiac action or to other sequelae.

3 *Purulent or suppurative*. The cause is almost always pyogenic bacterial invasion:

(*a*) Direct extension from neighbouring inflammations, e.g. empyema, pneumonia.

(*b*) Blood spread from other sites in septicaemia or pyaemia.

(*c*) Lymphatic spread from neighbouring sites, including subdiaphragmatic inflammation, e.g. subphrenic or hepatic abscesses.

(*d*) Penetrating injuries which become infected.

There may be large volumes of watery turbid fluid or thick creamy pus from which the organisms can be cultured. Variable amounts of fibrin are present on the surfaces and the inflammatory process may extend into the myocardium. Death may occur, but in survivors, complete resolution is unusual; more commonly, organization and an adherent pericardium ensue.

4 *Haemorrhagic*. This is blood mixed with inflammatory exudate and has to be differentiated from haemopericardium. It is usually due to invasion by tumour but sometimes occurs in fulminating bacterial infections. When due to tumour, malignant cells may be identified in aspirated fluid.

TUBERCULOUS PERICARDITIS

Origin

1 Miliary spread, i.e. blood-borne.

2 Extension from pulmonary disease or from mediastinal lymph nodes.

Appearances

Fibrinous exudate with granulation tissue covering the pericardial surfaces, visible tubercles and sometimes areas of caseation. It may occasionally be haemorrhagic with copious amounts of fluid. Microscopically, tuberculous caseating giant cell systems are seen.

Results

Resolution does not occur and the process heals by gross fibrosis often followed by calcification. Not only is the pericardial sac obliterated, but the dense fibrous tissue layer contracts and restricts filling of the heart in diastole – *constrictive pericarditis*.

CONSTRICTIVE PERICARDITIS — PICK'S DISEASE

Aetiology

Most cases are due to healed tuberculous pericarditis but a few may follow suppurative bacterial disease or, rarely, connective tissue diseases.

Macroscopical

There is a thick, firm layer of fibrous tissue obliterating the pericardium and completely ensheathing the heart. The tissue frequently contains plaques of calcification and may be firmly adherent internally to the myocardium and externally to the lung, anterior chest wall or diaphragm. In addition, there is often a particularly dense fibrous area around the orifices of the inferior and superior vena cavae as they enter the right atrium.

Microscopical

Hyaline fibrous tissue with plaques of calcium in which there is rarely any significant inflammatory cell infiltration. Only occasionally is there histological evidence of residual active tuberculosis.

Effects

The fibrous tissue impedes venous return, resulting in an enlarged liver, ascites and distended neck veins. In addition, direct mechanical embarrassment to cardiac action may occur.

Results

Excision of the constricting fibrous and partially calcified tissues leads to relief, but this may be technically exceptionally difficult.

POLYSEROSITIS — CONCATO'S DISEASE

In this rare condition of childhood there are

inflammatory serous effusions of pleural, peritoneal or pericardial sacs. Some are caused by tuberculosis, in others the aetiology is unknown. Organization in the later stages results in hyaline fibrosis with 'sugar-icing' plaques on the surface of liver and spleen and constrictive pericarditis.

HYDROPERICARDIUM

Nature
Accumulation of a transudate with a low r.d. of 1.012, low protein content and usually containing only very scanty mesothelial cells.

Aetiology
1 Cardiac failure.
2 Chronic renal disease.
3 Hypoproteinaemia.

Appearances
The pericardial surfaces remain smooth and glistening and the fluid is clear and faintly straw-coloured.

Effects
There may be very large amounts of fluid which eventually interfere with the heart's action.

Results
Absorbs with removal of the cause, leaving a normal pericardium.

HAEMOPERICARDIUM

Nature
Pure blood in the pericardial sac.

Aetiology
1 Rupture of the heart
(*a*) Traumatic – e.g. stab wound.
(*b*) Spontaneous – e.g. myocardial infarct.
2 Rupture of the intrapericardial portion of the aorta.
(*a*) Dissecting aneurysm.
(*b*) Syphilitic aneurysm.
(*c*) Traumatic.
3 In haemorrhagic diatheses – e.g. purpura, scurvy, hypoprothrombinaemia, anticoagulant therapy.

Effects
In most cases, death occurs rapidly due to cardiac tamponade, as little as 200–300 ml commonly being sufficient.

PNEUMOPERICARDIUM

Nature
Air in the pericardial sac.

Aetiology
1 Trauma.
2 Perforation of the lung or the oesophagus into the pericardium.
3 Pericarditis due to gas-forming organisms.

TUMOURS OF THE PERICARDIUM

Primary
Extremely rare – lipoma, fibroma, mesothelioma.

Secondary
Fairly common.
1 Direct extension from adjacent organs – e.g. lung, oesophagus, etc.
2 Blood-borne or lymphatic metastases – e.g. malignant melanoma, malignant lymphomas, etc.

Myocardium – Vascular

CORONARY INSUFFICIENCY

There are two factors of importance in respect of reduction of blood flow of the coronary arteries:
1 The rate at which the flow is decreased, i.e. gradual or sudden occlusion.
2 The amount of the decrease in the flow.

GRADUAL OCCLUSION — ARTERIOSCLEROTIC HEART DISEASE

Nature
Slowly progressive ischaemia of the heart muscle, usually due to atheroma, commonly associated with hypertension and resulting in replacement fibrosis of the myocardium.

Age
Extremely common over the age of 50 years, particularly in males.

Appearances

1 *Myocardium*. Varying amounts of diffuse or patchy fibrous tissue replacing the myocardium, which, however, may be thicker than normal due to associated hypertension.

2 *Coronary arteries*. Ninety per cent show atheroma with narrowing of the lumen, usually affecting all branches, but variable in severity and distribution.

3 *Valves*. These are commonly involved by slight fibrous thickening or distortion but they are of little clinical significance unless there is severe senile calcific aortic stenosis (see p. 248).

Effects

1 Angina pectoris – slow progression in severity often extending over many years.

2 Arrhythmias due to involvement of the conducting tissue.

3 Congestive heart failure.

4 Superimposed sudden occlusion of the coronary vessels with myocardial infarction.

SUDDEN OCCLUSION – MYOCARDIAL INFARCTION

Incidence

Extremely common though recently with a 10–15 per cent fall in incidence. This condition causes about 60 per cent of sudden unexpected deaths and is directly responsible for 10–15 per cent of all deaths.

Sex

Under 50 years M:F 5:1; increasing incidence in women post menopausally but there is a 'time-lag' of 10–20 years between the sexes.

Age

Predominantly middle-aged between 50–60 years, but 10 per cent occur in the younger age groups, 35–50. The average age of onset appears to be decreasing.

Pathogenesis

Occlusion of a coronary artery, usually a major branch, with inadequacy of the collateral circulation. Although some infarcts appear to be precipitated by sudden and unaccustomed exercise, emotional crises, following large meals or in extremes of climate, many occur during sleep.

Aetiology

Atheroma. Ninety-eight per cent or more are associated with coronary atherosclerosis.

1 Thrombosis superimposed on atheroma. This is probably the commonest cause.

2 Haemorrhage into an atheromatous plaque.

3 Ulceration of a plaque with discharge of its degenerate material.

4 Atheroma uncomplicated by the above factors.
Other causes. These include:

1 Coronary embolism – very rare.

2 Ostial narrowing due to syphilic aortitis (see p. 244).

3 Dissecting aneurysm with involvement of coronary ostia.

4 Polyarteritis nodosa affecting the coronary arteries.

Contributory factors

1 Vascular insufficiency due to deranged coronary filling:

(*a*) Aortic stenosis.

(*b*) Aortic incompetence.

(*c*) Shock with hypotension.

(*d*) Arrhythmias, bradycardia and extreme tachycardia.

2 Vascular insufficiency due to alteration in the general circulation:

(*a*) Severe anaemia.

(*b*) Anoxia.

3 Relative insufficiency due to myocardial hypertrophy:

(*a*) Hypertension.

(*b*) Rheumatic heart disease.

Sites of occlusion

First 1–2 cm of the main left and right arteries – rare.

Next 2–3 cm – common.

Branches 1 Anterior descending, left – most common.

2 Circumflex branch, left – common.

3 Main trunk, right – common.

4 Other branches – rare.

Sites of infarction

Almost always involves the left ventricle; the right ventricle and both atria are very rarely affected. The sites within the left ventricular myocardium correspond to the distribution of the artery occluded:

1 Anterior descending, left – anterior wall and anterior part of the interventricular septum.

2 Circumflex branch, left – left border of the heart and left side of the posterior surface.

3 Main trunk, right – posterior wall of the left venticle and posterior part of the interventricular septum.

Appearances

Small infarcts may be confined to a central area of muscle or be principally subendocardial or subpericardial. When larger, the infarct usually involves adjacent surfaces, particularly the endocardium including the columnae carnae and papillary muscles.

Stages

1 0–12 hours – slight pallor and flabbiness, but may appear normal.

2 12–24 hours – pallor but indistinctly defined and slightly friable.

3 2–4 days – marked yellow-grey pallor and loss of structure with softening. The margin is hyperaemic and fairly sharply outlined with an irregular contour.

4 4–10 days – yellow structureless soft area with foci of haemorrhage or streakiness and an intensely haemorrhagic margin – *myomalacia cordis*.

5 10 days–6 weeks – progressive fibrous replacement from the margins to form an area of greyish-white colour. By 6 weeks most or all of the area is fibrotic, eventually leading to an area of thinning of the wall.

Effects

1 Sudden death, probably due to ventricular fibrillation.

2 Death from shock or heart failure during the first few days.

3 Intractable congestive heart failure, usually with pulmonary oedema.

4 Healing with fibrous replacement of the infarcted area of myocardium.

5 Complications.

(*a*) Pericarditis over the infarcted area – friction rub.

(*b*) Rupture of the heart with haemopericardium.

(*c*) Mural thrombosis of the left ventricle which may cause embolism, e.g. cerebral.

(*d*) Aneurysm – the weakened area may dilate and subsequently rupture.

(*e*) Extension of the infarcted area, commonly by retrograde propagation of the thrombus.

(*f*) Arrhythmias including heart block, due to interruption of the conducting tissue.

Microscopical

Coagulative necrosis with a polymorph infiltration. Later, macrophages remove the dead material and fibroblastic and capillary proliferation at the margins leads to fibrous organization, ultimately producing a hyalinized and avascular scar.

Results

The immediate mortality is about 15 per cent but is increased to nearly 50 per cent when serious arrhythmias occur. There has been a considerable reduction in mortality in the early stages in recent years. Of the survivors, 25 per cent live for 10 years or more. The others die from complications or, more commonly, from a further cardiac infarct.

Chapter 46
Cardiovascular System – Heart: Myocardium: Rheumatic Fever

Degenerations and infiltrations

BROWN ATROPHY
Aetiology
Appearances
Microscopical

CLOUDY SWELLING
Aetiology
Macroscopical
Microscopical

FATTY HEART

Obesity

Fatty change
Nature
Aetiology
Macroscopical
Microscopical

AMYLOIDOSIS
Macroscopical
Microscopical
Effects

GLYCOGEN INFILTRATION

Cardiomyopathy
Nature
Types
  Familial
  HOCM
  COCM
  Nutritional
  Alcohol
  Pregnancy
  Systemic diseases

Inflammations

SUPPURATIVE
Nature
Origin
Macroscopical
Microscopical
Effects

NON-SUPPURATIVE

'Toxic myocarditis'
Nature
Aetiology
Appearances
Effects

Viral Myocarditis
Aetiology
Appearances
Effects

Acute idiopathic myocarditis
Nature
Appearances
Effects

Rheumatic fever
Nature
Incidence
Aetiology
Age
Sex
Clinical

HEART

Pericardium

Myocardium
Macroscopical
Microscopical

Aschoff node
Exudative phase
Proliferative phase
Healed phase
Effects

Endocardium
Mural
Valvular
  Sites
  Appearances
  Effects

JOINTS
Macroscopical
Microscopical

SKIN
Sites
Macroscopical
Microscopical
Fate

BLOOD VESSELS

LUNGS

BRAIN (CHOREA)
Clinical
Appearances

RESULTS

Syphilis of the heart
Incidence
Age
Appearances
  Aortitis
  Myocardium

Hypertensive heart disease

237

Degenerations and infiltrations

BROWN ATROPHY

Aetiology
Unknown, but is frequently associated with wasting diseases and old age.

Appearances
The heart is small and the surface wrinkled with loss of epicardial fat, tortuous coronary vessels and brown-coloured friable muscle.

Microscopical
The muscle fibres are shrunken and contain brownish pigment at the nuclear poles – *lipofuscin* (see p. 118).

CLOUDY SWELLING

Aetiology
Infections and many toxic states, e.g. typhoid, influenza, septicaemia, etc.

Macroscopical
Soft, pale and friable myocardium.

Microscopical
The muscle fibres are swollen with granular fragmentation of the cytoplasmic mitochondria (see p. 103).

FATTY HEART

OBESITY

Increased epicardial deposition of fat associated with generalized adiposity. This may extend into the fibrous septa and between the muscle fibres and cause interference with heart action, but the myocardial fibres are normal (see p. 105).

FATTY CHANGE

Nature
Represents damage to myocardial cells as a result of which there is accumulation of fatty material within the cell cytoplasm.

Aetiology
Any of the many causes of cell damage (see p. 106).

Macroscopical
There is a pale mottling of the muscle, particularly of the subendocardial fibres and especially in the left ventricle – 'thrush breast' or 'tabby cat' appearance.

Microscopical
Fine fatty droplets in the muscle fibres most marked in those situated furthest from the blood vessels and therefore at the sites of maximal anoxia.

AMYLOIDOSIS

Cardiac involvement is mostly seen in primary amyloidosis, when it may be the only organ involved.

Macroscopical
Firm, waxy, thickening of the myocardium.

Microscopical
Hyaline, eosinophilic, amyloid material identifiable by the specific stains in the interstitial tissue and in the walls of blood vessels; degeneration of muscle fibres may be marked (see p. 108).

Effects
Cardiac involvement may be the dominant lesion with weakening of the heart's action and death due to congestive failure.

GLYCOGEN INFILTRATION

The heart is involved in von Gierke's disease, a systemic derangement of glycogen metabolism. Glycogen accumulates in the myocardial fibres with enlargement of the heart and disturbance of function (see p. 112).

Cardiomyopathy

Nature
A heterogeneous group of diseases each of which may present as different syndromes but which have in common abnormality in structure and/or function of the myocardium. By common consent,

however, the term excludes disease of the heart due to hypertension, coronary insufficiency, valvular malfunction or rheumatism.

Cardiomyopathies may be present in families or be sporadic. The cardiac lesion may be the only demonstrable abnormality or many other systems may be affected. The illness may arise associated with a particular disease, after or during the main presenting factor, e.g. in haemochromatosis (see p. 562), occur in an alcoholic or in malnourishment or pregnancy. It may occur in a family with a known illness, e.g. a myopathy, and thus be classifiable. More often, however, the patient presents with the cardiac illness without any clue to the aetiology and this may not be determinable even at post-mortem examination; in the present stage of knowledge regarding treatment, this is of little importance.

TYPES

FAMILIAL CARDIOMYOPATHY

Specific
(a) In hereditary ataxic neurological disease, e.g. Friedreich's ataxia, cardiomegaly with diffuse interstitial myocardial fibrosis may be prominent (see p. 617).
(b) Myopathies – the myocardium may be severely affected, particularly in the pseudohypertrophic and myotonia atrophica types (see p. 589).
(c) Glycogen storage disease – deposition of large amounts of glycogen (see p. 112).
(d) Gargoylism – deposition of mucopolysaccharides.
(e) Pseudoxanthoma elasticum – fibroelastosis may be seen.
(f) Cystic fibrosis – myocardial fibrosis may occur (see p. 632).

Non-specific
Occasional cases of idiopathic familial cardiomyopathy have been described.

HYPERTROPHIC OBSTRUCTIVE CARDIOMYOPATHY — HOCM

Idiopathic and often familial. Outflow tract obstruction of either right or left ventricles or both. Diffuse, often asymmetrical, hypertrophy of muscle and connective tissue but valves are normal.

NON-SPECIFIC NON-FAMILIAL CONGESTIVE CARDIOMYOPATHY – COCM

FIBROELASTOSIS

This presents in infancy as fibrous endocardial thickening, with or without increase in elastic tissue, involving the mural endocardium of the left side of the heart with or without involvement of aortic and mitral valve cusps and rings. The aetiology is debatable but many cases show a high titre of antibodies to the mumps virus which may be causatively involved as a foetal infection.

ENDOMYOCARDIAL FIBROSIS—EMF

Most commonly found in East Africa but more recently described from other countries including West Africa and the West Indies. Marked progressive cardiomegaly, gross endocardial fibrosis without elastosis, organizing mural thrombus and dilatation of chambers. The fibrous tissue encroaches on to the myocardium and involves papillary muscles, chordae and sometimes the mitral and tricuspid valves. Usually more severe on the left side of the heart. Aetiology unknown but high serotonin levels induced by high banana consumption has been implicated.

OTHER NON-FAMILIAL IDIOPATHIC CARDIOMYOPATHIES

Bearing some features in common with the above conditions and reported in individual cases.

NUTRITIONAL

Heart failure with atrophy or dilatation of the heart in severe, non-specific, generalized nutritonal deficiency and in kwashiorkor and beri-beri.

ALCOHOL

Chronic alcoholic poisoning may cause severe cardiac dilatation with myocardial degeneration, oedema and fine fibrosis, arrhythmias and characteristic disturbances of the E.C.G.

PREGNANCY

Puerperal myocarditis, which is a debatable entity, may occur as cardiac malfunction and enlargement of non-specific appearance occurring in the last trimester of pregnancy or the puerperium. Some patients improve after delivery but others progressively deteriorate.

SYSTEMIC DISEASES

Myocardial involvement may be severe in connective tissue diseases (see p. 280), amyloidosis, particularly of primary type (see p. 108), thyroid disease, both myxoedema and thyrotoxicosis (see pp. 312 and 309), and some other generalized disorders.

Inflammations

SUPPURATIVE

Nature
Infection of the myocardium by pyogenic organisms. This is a rare condition.

Origin
Usually via the blood stream in septicaemia and pyaemia; occasionally by direct spread from the pericardium or endocardium, e.g. heart valves.

Macroscopical
Focal areas of inflammation progressing to abscess formation.

Microscopical
Acute inflammation in the interstitial tissue, usually focal, with destruction of the muscle as the disease progresses to frank suppuration.

Effects
If widespread, it may cause arrhythmias or myocardial failure.

NON-SUPPURATIVE

'TOXIC MYOCARDITIS'

Nature
Focal areas of toxic degeneration or necrosis associated with a wide variety of infective and toxic conditions.

Aetiology
1 Particularly common with diphtheria, pneumonia, typhoid and streptococcal infections. No organisms are present in the heart lesions.
2 Chemical – e.g. carbon monoxide, arsenic, sulphonamides, phosphorus, chloroform.

Appearances
These are variable. There may be fatty change, or necrotic foci, with interstitial oedema and a cellular infiltration by lymphocytes, plasma cells, eosinophils, polymorphs or macrophages.

Effects
There is seldom sufficient damage to interfere seriously with cardiac function, but occasionally death may result when the myocarditis is extensive, e.g. diphtheria.

VIRAL MYOCARDITIS

Aetiology
Many viral diseases including poliomyelitis, psittacosis, yellow fever, influenza and infective hepatitis, occasionally cause myocarditis.

Appearances
Diffuse interstitial inflammation with an infiltrate of lymphocytes, plasma cells and macrophages. The viral agent is presumed to be present in the lesions.

Effects
Occasionally, in severe examples, the myocardial involvement may cause death.

ACUTE IDIOPATHIC MYOCARDITIS

Nature
Whilst some cases of myocarditis with heart failure and death may have identifiable toxic or infective cause, in many others the aetiology remains obscure. A presumption of a virus cause is often made but intensive efforts to find supportive evidence fail. Many of these cases were previously recorded as *Fiedler's myocarditis* and most occur in early adult life.

Appearances
There are two types:
1 Diffuse inflammatory cell infiltration in interstitial tissue.
2 A granulomatous focal infiltrate often with numerous giant cells – *giant cell myocarditis*.

Effects
In both types the heart's action is compromised by injury to muscle fibres with degeneration, necrosis and failure.

Rheumatic fever

Rheumatic affection of the heart involves the pericardium, myocardium and endocardium – *pancarditis*.

Nature
A systemic inflammatory process of connective tissues affecting joints, tendons, serosal membranes, skin, respiratory system and blood vessels in a comparatively transient or benign manner, but with common and frequently fatal sequelae in the heart.

Incidence
Rheumatic heart disease forms a significant but decreasing proportion of cases of organic heart disease. The incidence of acute rheumatic fever is impossible to establish, as many cases, severely debilitated in later life by the heart complications, give no clear history of a previous acute attack.

Aetiology
Epidemiological, clinical, and experimental evidence suggests that the disease is closely related to group A haemolytic streptococcal infections. Organisms are not present in the lesions and the evidence points to an indirect hypersensitivity response on the part of the affected tissues to the presence of circulating streptococcal toxins. Other factors which may predispose are:
(a) Climate. Increased frequency in temperate, damp climates.
(b) Social. More common in urban than in rural areas and in those with poor living conditions and inadequate nutrition.

Age
Ninety per cent of the first attacks occur between the ages of 5 and 15 and a first attack of acute rheumatic fever is rare above the age of 20.

Sex
M:F equal.

Clinical
Insidious onset of fever 2–3 weeks after a sore throat or other streptococcal infection. Symptomatic evidence of involvement of several systems follows:
85 per cent – have a migratory polyarthritis, usually of large joints.
65 per cent – have pancarditis.
30 per cent – have chorea.
Subcutaneous nodules and pulmonary symptoms less commonly occur. This initial acute attack subsides after a few weeks and may remain quiescent, but clinical exacerbations may occur at intervals, usually within the first 5 years. With each exacerbation, the risk of carditis increases, so that eventually 75 per cent of all patients show evidence of cardiac involvement.

HEART

PERICARDIUM

Diffuse fibrinous inflammation with adhesion of the two layers and a 'bread and butter' appearance. Little fluid is present. This may resolve by fibrinolysis, but is more commonly organized to produce relatively thin fibrous plaques on the visceral layer but little adhesion formation.

MYOCARDIUM

Macroscopical
There may be little or no gross abnormality visible. Occasionally, scattered pin-head-sized pale grey foci may be seen.

Microscopical
The characteristic Aschoff nodes are seen in the connective tissues of the atrial and ventricular myocardium, particularly in the subendocardial fibrous tissue and around blood vessels in the intermuscular fibrous septa.

ASCHOFF NODE

Exudative phase
There is focal mucoid degeneration of the collagen with surrounding polymorphs, plasma cells and histiocytes. This histological appearance is seen only transiently in the early stages.

Proliferative phase
The characteristic Aschoff node consists of:
(a) Central focus of fibrinoid collagen necrosis.
(b) Surrounding granulomatous reaction with:
　(i) Fibroblasts.
　(ii) Plasma cells and lymphocytes but scanty polymorphs.
　(iii) Multinucleate giant cells – Aschoff cells, composed of two to five centrally arranged nuclei and a basophilic cytoplasm.
　(iv) 'Anitschkow' myocytes. These cells are characteristically oval-shaped with a central chromatin bar from which fine projections are visible, mimicking the legs of a caterpillar – 'caterpillar cells'. Their origin is disputed, being either modified fibroblasts or altered muscle cells.

Healed phase
Progressive hyalinization and fibrosis with disappearance of Aschoff and Anitschkow cells. The last elements to disappear are the plasma cells and lymphocytes at the periphery.

The Aschoff node is diagnostic of rheumatic myocarditis. It is present in a recognizable form in 40–50 per cent of atrial appendages removed from patients at mitral valvotomy for mitral stenosis, in whom there has been no clinical or laboratory evidence of rheumatic activity for many years. This paradox raises problems which are at present unanswerable as to the exact significance of Aschoff nodes in relation to the disease process as a whole.

Effects
The scarring from the healed lesions causes a diffuse fibrosis and injury to adjacent myocardial fibres. Death may occur in the acute stage due to this myocarditis or, in the later stages, the heart's action may be impeded. Generally, however, the endocardial sequelae overshadow those of the myocardium.

ENDOCARDIUM

Mural
Patchy involvement of the atrial endocardium with subendocardial Aschoff nodes leads to scarring and to MacCallum's patch, usually situated just above the posterior cusp of the mitral valve.

Valvular

SITES
The valve lesions are distributed as follows: mitral alone – 40 per cent; mitral and aortic – 40 per cent; aortic alone – 10 per cent; mitral, aortic and tricuspid – 5 per cent; tricuspid alone – rare; pulmonary alone – very rare.

APPEARANCES
Sequence. Similar for all valves:
1　Red, swollen and thickened, particularly at the free margins.
2　Vegetations form due to erosion of the inflamed surfaces at the lines of closure and on the chordae tendinae. Small (1–2 mm), firmly adherent, rubbery, low, warty nodules are seen along the lines of closure and on the surfaces exposed to blood flow. They consist of platelets and fibrin.
3　The valve cusps show mucoid degeneration or fibrinoid necrosis of the ground substance, with occasional Anitschkow myocytes and mononuclear inflammatory cells, but well-formed Aschoff nodes are rare.
4　Organization with vascularization of the valve cusps. The valves are thickened, deformed, opaque and inflexible with thickening at the sites of the vegetations. Fibrous tissue bridges across the commissures, resulting in fusion of the valve cusps. In the mitral valve this commissural fusion produces the slit-like, 'button hole' type of mitral stenosis. In addition the chordae tendinae are thickened and fused.
5　Contracture of fibrous tissue increases the deformity of the valves. At the mitral valve, the fibrous contraction of the chordae tendinae results in anchoring of the valve cusps on the ventricular aspect and produces the 'funnel-shaped' type of mitral stenosis, when viewed from the atrial aspect.
6　Deposition of calcium in the damaged valves further increases the deformity and inelasticity.

EFFECTS
The later stages progress slowly over many years.

The two main effects of the valvular deformities result in:

1 Stenosis of the orifice.
2 Incompetence of valve cusps.

There is a variable mixture of one or both effects in individual cases and in individually affected valves (see p. 248).

JOINTS

The lesions are transient and very rarely give rise to residual disability.

Macroscopical
Swelling, redness and heat with subsidence in a few days. The larger joints are usually involved and arthritis is often multiple and symmetrical. The synovium is thickened, red and granular, later resolving to normal.

Microscopical
Aschoff nodes, or alternatively mucoid or fibrinoid degeneration, are seen in the connective tissues and similar changes are found in the joint capsules, affected tendons, fascia and muscle sheaths, frequently accompanied by a lymphocytic infiltrate.

SKIN

Sites
Subcutaneous tissues, particularly over bony prominences of wrist, elbow, ankle, knee or occiput.

Macroscopical
Circumscribed mobile subcutaneous nodules of firm consistency with erythema but no ulceration of the overlying skin.

Microscopical
Massive central area of fibrinoid necrosis with a palisade of radially arranged histiocytes at the margin and a surrounding inflammatory cell infiltration.

Fate
Gradually replaced by dense fibrous tissue which may subsequently calcify.

BLOOD VESSELS

An acute vasculitis, confined to the intima, may rarely occur and is usually inconspicuous with little or no effect on the involved organ. It may be widespread and affect the coronary, pulmonary, renal, mesenteric and cerebral arteries and the aorta.

LUNGS

A few cases show focal areas of interstitial inflammation with fibrinous exudate into the alveoli and histiocytic and lymphocytic infiltration of the alveolar septa. The affection is mostly mild, transient and of doubtful specificity.

BRAIN – CHOREA – SYDENHAM'S CHOREA

Clinical
Nearly 30 per cent of patients with acute rheumatism show clinical evidence of cerebral irritability or sudden, involuntary, irregular, rapid movements with muscular inco-ordination and weakness – St Vitus' dance. Only very rarely are these manifestations serious and the majority recover completely, usually in a few months.

Appearances
Variable and inconspicuous lesions are found in the rare fatal cases in the corpus striatum and cerebral cortex. Perivascular lymphocyte infiltration, hyperaemia and, rarely, Aschoff nodes may be seen.

RESULTS OF RHEUMATIC FEVER

In cases where valve lesions are not surgically corrected thirty per cent are dead within 20 years: 10 per cent in the first 5 years; 10 per cent in the next 5 years; 10 per cent in the next 10 years. However, surgical replacement of valves is often very successful and has markedly reduced mortality. A further 30 per cent have signs of rheumatic heart disease at the end of 20 years and these patients have a considerably reduced life expectancy.

Syphilis of the heart

Incidence
At one time this was a common cardiac disorder but now accounts for only 1 per cent or less of organic heart disease.

Age
Average 40–55 years, usually 15–20 years after the primary infection.

Appearances

AORTITIS
The irregular fibrous replacement of the media leads to intimal thickening, scarring around the mouths of the coronary arteries and weakness of the aortic wall (see p. 260).
(a) Stretching of the valve ring and separation of the commissures leads to aortic incompetence.
(b) Narrowing of the coronary ostia leads to coronary insufficiency.

MYOCARDIUM
(a) A rare form of cardiac involvement with solitary or multiple myocardial gummas of variable size.
(b) Very rarely, a diffuse form of interstitial myocardial inflammation with endarteritis obliterans and fibrosis occurs in congenital syphilis.

Hypertensive heart disease

The effect of sustained systemic hypertension on the heart is to produce hypertrophy of the left ventricle. As long as the cardiac reserve is not exhausted and the hypertrophic myocardium maintains a normal output, a compensated state exists. Eventually, the reserve may be exhausted when the ventricle will dilate and congestive heart failure supervenes. The disease is commonly associated with coronary atherosclerosis, depriving the thickened cardiac muscle of essential oxygen and myocardial infarction is a common complication.

Death in 50–70 per cent of hypertensive patients is due to heart failure from myocardial or coronary insufficiency. There is commonly a sudden fatal termination with ventricular fibrillation (see p. 267).

Chapter 47
Cardiovascular System – Heart: Endocardium: Tumours

Endocardium

ENDOCARDITIS

Rheumatic

Infective
Nature
Types
  Acute
    Organisms
    Origin
    Age and sex
    Aetiology
    Appearances
  Subacute
    Organisms
    Origin
    Sites
    Appearances
Complications
  Local
  Embolic
  Mycotic aneurysms
Diagnosis
Other infections

Atypical verrucous
Nature
Sites
Macroscopical
Microscopical
Effects

Carcinoid syndrome
Nature
Macroscopical

Floppy valve syndrome
Nature
Macroscopical
Effects

Senile calcific aortic stenosis
Nature
Appearances
Results

Valvular lesions

STENOSIS AND INCOMPETENCE
(REGURGITATION)

Mitral valve
Stenosis
  Causes
  Effects
Incompetence
  Causes
  Effects
Results

Aortic valve
Stenosis
  Causes
  Effects
Incompetence
  Causes
  Effects
Results

Tricuspid valve
Stenosis
  Causes
  Effects
Incompetence
  Causes
  Effects
Results

Pulmonary valve
Stenosis
  Causes
  Effects
Incompetence
  Causes
  Effects
Results

Myocardial hypertrophy
Nature
Types
  Concentric
  Eccentric

LEFT VENTRICLE – 'COR BOVINUM'
Causes
  Obstruction to outflow
  Increased output

RIGHT VENTRICLE – 'COR PULMONALE'
Causes
  Pulmonary hypertension
  Pulmonary stenosis
  Tricuspid incompetence

ATRIA

EFFECTS

Dilatation of the heart
Nature
Causes
  Inability to expel all the blood
  Reflux
  Other conditions

Lesions of conducting tissue
Causes
  Myocarditis
  Coronary artery disease
  Digitalis
  Tumours

Tumours

BENIGN
Connective tissues
Myxoma
  Incidence
  Macroscopical
  Microscopical
  Nature
  Effects
Rhabdomyoma

MALIGNANT
Primary
Secondary
  Direct
  Metastatic

Endocardium

ENDOCARDITIS

When used as an unqualified term, it implies inflammation of the valves. Mural endocarditis is inflammation of the lining of the heart chambers.

RHEUMATIC ENDOCARDITIS

(See p. 242).

INFECTIVE ENDOCARDITIS

Nature

Formerly called bacterial endocarditis, the recognition that rickettsiae, fungi and other organisms may cause endocardial inflammatory damage, has led to abandonment of this term.

All types are uncommon except in the special circumstances of previous injury by rheumatic disease or by congenital abnormalities, or in septicaemia or generally reduced resistance to infections.

There are two main clinical types related to pathogenicity of the infecting agent and the rapidity of progression of the damage, but overlap is common.

Types

ACUTE, MALIGNANT OR ULCERATIVE ENDOCARDITIS

Organisms
Coagulase-positive staphylococci, β-haemolytic streptococci, pneumococci, gonococci, coliforms, meningococci.

Origin
Usually as a complication of septicaemia or primary disease at another site but rarely may follow cardiac surgical procedures.

Age and sex
A wide age range, usually adults, with a 3:1 male preponderance.

Aetiology
Usually occurs on previously normal valves.

Appearances
Large, globular, soft, friable, easily detached vegetations on the valve cusps often extending on to the mural surface or into adjacent myocardium. Ulceration of valve cusps, rupture of chordae or perforation of cusps is commonly seen and local destruction can be extensive and rapid.

The vegetations are composed of fibrin with bacteria and polymorphs.

SUBACUTE ENDOCARDITIS

Organisms
Seventy-five per cent are due to *Streptococcus viridans:* other causes include enterococci (*S. faecalis*), brucellae, haemophilus species and *Coxiella burnetti* (Q fever, see p. 44).

Origin
Many of these organisms are commensals but may gain entry to the blood following surgical procedures, particularly dental extractions. In most normal persons the bacteraemia is cleared but in those with congenital abnormalities or damage to endocardium the bacteria are more likely to cause endocardial inflammation. Increasingly in recent years the condition has been recognized as occurring in the elderly, in particular on previously normal valves.

Sites
The mitral valve either alone – 40 per cent – or combined with involvement of the aortic valve – 40 per cent – are the most frequent sites. Other valves are uncommonly affected, alone or in combination.

Appearances
There may be evidence of pre-existing rheumatic or congenital disease. Vegetations which are friable, polypoid and easily detached but less florid than with the acute type are present, usually at the site of contact of cusps. Microscopically they are composed of fibrin and platelets with scanty inflammatory cells and usually rather few organisms. Ulceration occurs late and perforation and destruction of cusps, chordae or adjacent myocardium is unusual. Progression is slower but functional effects of valvular distortion may be severe.

Complications of endocarditis

LOCAL

Functional impairment due to failure of closure of valves, perforation and distortion.

EMBOLIC

Portions of vegetation may break off and produce embolic effects, either septic in the case of the more acute infections with high grade pathogens, e.g. septic infarction, or non-suppurative in the sub-acute type. In this case the low grade pathogenicity of the organisms results in splinter haemorrhages and Osler's nodes in the skin, 'flea-bitten' kidney of a focal nephritis (see p. 359), bland infarcts in brain, kidney, spleen, etc.

MYCOTIC ANEURYSMS

These are also seen in the subacute type following weakening of the arterial wall by a combination of infection and embolic lodgement. They occur particularly in cerebral, mesenteric, renal and limb arteries.

Diagnosis

1   *Blood culture.* The responsible organisms can usually be recovered from blood cultures though multiple specimens may be necessary. They should preferably be taken whilst pyrexia is rising or during embolic episodes and before antibiotics are administered.

2   *Blood.* There is always a high sedimentation rate, a variably marked leucocytosis and anaemia. The latter can be severe.

Other infective causes of endocarditis

Increasingly, opportunistic infections complicating immunosuppressive or corticosteroid therapy are recognized. Responsible organisms include fungi, e.g. *Candida albicans, Histoplasma capsulatum* and a wide range of normally non-pathogenic bacteria, chlamydia (see p. 43), etc.

ATYPICAL VERRUCOUS ENDOCARDITIS – LIBMAN–SACKS ENDOCARDITIS

Nature

The endocardial manifestations of systemic lupus erythematosus (see p. 281).

Sites

Seen in 50 per cent or more of cases of S.L.E. The mitral and tricuspid valves are commonly affected and the pulmonary valve only occasionally.

Macroscopical

Small warty excrescences, firmly adherent anywhere on the valve cusp. They are usually multiple and on either aspect of the cusp, whilst frequently they extend on to the atrial or ventricular endocardium.

Microscopical

The vegetations are composed of fibrin with necrotic debris, fibrinoid material and entangled fibroblasts with mononuclear cells. The valves show fibrinoid necrosis of the ground substance with vascularization, fibroblastic proliferation and scanty mononuclear and polymorph inflammatory cell infiltration. Haematoxyphil bodies may be found in the fibrinoid material (see p. 281).

Effects

Clinical evidence of cardiac involvement is common, but the valvular changes seldom give rise to any appreciable functional deficiency.

CARCINOID SYNDROME

Nature

Some cases of carcinoid tumour, usually of the small intestine and with metastases in the liver, have a symptom complex associated with secretion of excessive amounts of 5-hydroxytryptamine. In such cases, endocardial lesions of the tricuspid and pulmonary valves are commonly present (see p. 213).

Macroscopical

No vegetations are seen, but the valves, especially the pulmonary cusps, are thickened, fibrotic and distorted, resulting in stenosis or incompetence.

FLOPPY VALVE SYNDROME

Nature

This *'floppy valve'* lesion results from myxoid degeneration of the ground substance of cardiac valves, usually and most severely the mitral cusps. Chordae are also affected and may rupture. The condition is increasingly seen with advancing years but also occurs associated with Marfan's syndrome and in some congenital cardiac lesions.

Macroscopical

The affected valve cusps are thickened, opaque, slightly nodular and stretched with irregular free margin. Stretching or rupture of chordae may cause prolapse into the left atrium – *parachute deformity*.

Effects

Mildly affected valves are very commonly found in the elderly and usually appear to cause little effect. Less often mitral regurgitation, which may be severe and intractable, results.

SENILE CALCIFIC AORTIC STENOSIS

Nature

A condition of the elderly in which degenerative changes, predominantly atheroma, cause deformity and stenosis of the aortic valve.

Appearances

In severe cases, there is marked fibrous thickening of the valve cusps with deformity and rigidity. Large nodular masses of calcium may be found subendothelially within the sinuses of Valsalva behind the aortic cusps. Ulceration over the calcified areas may occur and some adhesion of the cusps at the commissures may increase the rigidity and the degree of stenosis. Calcified material is also found in the valve ring.

Differentiation from the more common rheumatic form of aortic stenosis may be difficult, but the age, the predominance of calcification on the side away from the blood flow and the lesser degree of commissural adhesion, are factors in favour of this arteriosclerotic type.

Results

1 Left ventricular hypertrophy.
2 Coronary insufficiency.
3 Syncopal attacks or sudden death due to acute heart failure.

Valvular lesions

STENOSIS AND INCOMPETENCE (REGURGITATION)

Both may be present together but one is usually dominant. The mitral and aortic valves are the most frequently affected; the tricuspid and pulmonary valves only infrequently.

MITRAL VALVE

In 40 per cent this is the only valve affected; in 40 per cent there are combined mitral and aortic lesions.

Stenosis

CAUSES
1 Rheumatic.
2 Infective endocarditis.

EFFECTS
1 Dilated, slightly hypertrophied left atrium which may be grossly distended – giant left atrium. Thrombus commonly forms in the left atrial appendage.
2 Normal-sized left ventricle, unless mitral incompetence is also present.
3 Right ventricular hypertrophy.
4 Chronic passive congestion of the lungs – *brown induration*.
5 Pulmonary hypertension.
6 Functional tricuspid incompetence.
7 'Nutmeg' liver and congested kidneys, etc.

Incompetence

CAUSES
As for stenosis above together with myxomatous degeneration – floppy valve.

EFFECTS
1 Dilated, hypertrophied left ventricle.
2 Dilated left atrium.
3 Chronic passive venous congestion of the lung.
4 Pulmonary hypertension and right ventricular hypertrophy, but less marked than in mitral stenosis.

Results of mitral disease

Death from:

1 Congestive heart failure.
2 Emboli from left atrial thrombus.

The results of mitral valve surgery by valvotomy or prosthetic replacement are good in selected patients.

AORTIC VALVE

Forty per cent show aortic and mitral involvement: 10 per cent aortic alone.

Stenosis

CAUSES

1 Congenital – uncommon.
2 Rheumatic – common.
3 Calcific aortic stenosis.
4 Infective endocarditis.

EFFECTS

1 Hypertrophy of left ventricle.
2 Coronary artery insufficiency.
3 Cerebral vascular insufficiency – syncopal attacks.
4 Sudden death, probably due to ventricular fibrillation.

Incompetence

CAUSES

1 As for stenosis above.
2 Syphilitic aortitis (see p. 260).

EFFECTS

1 Left ventricular dilatation.
2 Later left ventricular hypertrophy.

Results of aortic disease

Death from acute heart failure with pulmonary oedema. The results of surgery in aortic valve disease by prosthetic replacement are only moderately good.

TRICUSPID VALVE

Stenosis

This is rare.

CAUSES

Rheumatic and the carcinoid syndrome.

EFFECTS

1 Right atrial dilatation.
2 Right heart failure.

Incompetence

Uncommon.

CAUSES

1 Functional. Distortion of the valve ring in mitral stenosis.
2 Structural:
(*a*) Rheumatic – nearly always associated with mitral and aortic involvement.
(*b*) Atypical verrucous endocarditis (S.L.E.).

EFFECTS

1 Right atrial dilatation.
2 Right-sided heart failure.
3 Chronic venous congestion with a pulsatile liver and 'nutmeg' appearance leading to cardiac fibrosis and derangement of function.

Results of tricuspid disease

Death from right-sided heart failure. Prosthetic replacement may be successful.

PULMONARY VALVE

Stenosis

CAUSES

1 Congenital
(*a*) isolated valvular stenosis.
(*b*) Fallot's tetralogy (see p. 254).
2 Rheumatic, very rare.
3 Carcinoid syndrome (see p. 213).

EFFECTS

1 Right ventricular hypertrophy.
2 Pulmonary oligaemia with cyanosis.

Incompetence

CAUSES

1 Functional. Distortion of the valve in mitral stenosis – Graham Steell murmur.
2 Structural – very rare – congenital with superimposed endocarditis.

EFFECTS
1 Right ventricular dilatation and hypertrophy.
2 Pulmonary hypertension.

Results of pulmonary valve disease
Right-sided heart failure. Surgical correction may be possible particularly in the true valvular type.

Myocardial hypertrophy

Nature
Increase in size of individual myocardial fibres as a result of prolonged increased work.

Types

CONCENTRIC
Thickening of the wall, the lumen of the chamber appearing decreased in size.

ECCENTRIC
Thickening of the wall and dilatation of the chamber.

LEFT VENTRICLE – 'COR BOVINUM'

Causes

OBSTRUCTION TO OUTFLOW
(*a*) Structural: aortic stenosis, coarctation of aorta.
(*b*) Functional: systemic hypertension.

INCREASED OUTPUT
(*a*) Aortic incompetence.
(*b*) Mitral incompetence.
(*c*) Hypermetabolic states, e.g. thyrotoxicosis.
(*d*) Vascular anomalies including shunts, e.g. in Paget's disease of bone.

RIGHT VENTRICLE – 'COR PULMONALE'

Causes

PULMONARY HYPERTENSION
(*a*) Mitral stenosis.
(*b*) Left to right shunts – mostly congenital (see p. 256).

(*c*) Pulmonary fibrosis, e.g. pneumoconioses (see p. 668).
(*d*) Emphysema (see p. 654).
(*e*) Multiple pulmonary infarcts or emboli.
(*f*) Idiopathic – primary pulmonary hypertension (see p. 649).

PULMONARY STENOSIS
(*a*) Valvular stenosis.
(*b*) Fallot's tetralogy.

TRICUSPID INCOMPETENCE

ATRIA

Although hypertrophy of the atria occurs in mitral and tricuspid stenosis, this is overshadowed by the gross degree of atrial dilatation in each case.

EFFECTS

1 Very considerable degrees of hypertrophy occur and may be present for long periods. The hypertrophic myocardium is, however, more likely to fail due to relative insufficiency of the coronary blood flow.
2 Sudden death due to the development of arrhythmias, notably ventricular fibrillation, are common in hypertensive patients and particularly so in cases of pulmonary hypertension which is less well tolerated than the systemic type.
3 Relief of the causative factors may result in a diminution of the size of the myocardial fibres and a return to normal chamber size.

Dilatation of the heart

Nature
Increased capacity of the chambers which may be associated with hypertrophy or occur alone.

Causes

INABILITY TO EXPEL ALL THE BLOOD IT RECEIVES
(*a*) Myocarditis – including rheumatic carditis.
(*b*) Myocardial infarction.
(*c*) The atria in mitral or tricuspid stenosis.

REFLUX
(a) Left ventricle in aortic incompetence.
(b) Left atrium in mitral incompetence.
(c) Right atrium in tricuspid incompetence.

OTHER CONDITIONS – CARDIOMYOPATHIES
(See p. 238).

Lesions of the conducting tissue

Interruption of the conducting tissue gives rise to arrhythmias, complete or partial heart block.

Causes

MYOCARDITIS
(a) Acute, e.g. diphtheria, influenza, pyaemic abscesses, rheumatic fever.
(b) Chronic: rheumatic carditis, syphilis.

CORONARY ARTERY DISEASE
(a) Myocardial fibrosis.
(b) Myocardial infarction.

DIGITALIS
Overdosage.

TUMOURS
Usually secondary.

Tumours

BENIGN

Connective tissues
Fibroma, lipoma and angeioma are all very rare.

Myxoma

INCIDENCE
The commonest primary heart tumour but even this is rare.

MACROSCOPICAL
A globular or polypoid mass arising from the endocardial surface of the left atrium, usually from the septum, but occasionally from the valve cusps. It projects into the chamber and is commonly pedunculated, having a soft and gelatinous appearance. Some may attain a large size and even extend through the mitral valve orifice.

MICROSCOPICAL
Myxomatous fibrous tissue containing thin-walled blood vessels.

NATURE
Most are probably myxomatous degeneration in organized thrombus, but some may be hamartomatous malformations which may recur locally after surgical removal.

EFFECTS
May cause interference with the blood flow or act as a 'ball-valve' obstruction, especially in the mitral valve.

Rhabdomyoma
A rare hamartomatous malformation of cardiac muscle fibres, usually associated with tuberose sclerosis (see p. 593).

MALIGNANT

Primary
Rhabdomyosarcomas and fibrosarcomas exist but are extremely rare.

Secondary

DIRECT
Extension of tumours from adjacent structures, e.g. lung, oesophagus, etc.

METASTATIC
Malignant melanoma, carcinomas from any site, lymphomas. However, secondary tumours in the heart are surprisingly uncommon.

Chapter 48
Cardiovascular System – Congenital Heart Disease

Introduction
Many of these disabling congenital abnormalities of the heart and blood vessels are now surgically correctable and thus the subject is no longer of mere academic interest.

Incidence
Two per cent of all organic heart disease. Ten per cent of all heart disease in children.

Aetiology
Definitive development of the heart from a simple tube occurs in the fifth to eighth weeks of intra-uterine life and it is in this period that most of the congenital abnormalities are produced. The precise causation is unknown but factors include the following.

INTRINSIC
Heredity – a defect of the germ plasm; 20 per cent show congenital lesions in other organs.

EXTRINSIC
1 Virus infections – rubella during the first 3

months of pregnancy carries a 25–50 per cent risk of congenital heart disease or cataracts. Other maternal virus infections have come under suspicion, including influenza, but positive proof is still lacking.

2 Vitamin deficiency in pregnancy.

3 Foetal endocarditis and other intra-uterine infections.

4 Heavy metals – especially lead.

5 Syphilis.

With the exception of rubella infection, however, there is little evidence to support any of the other postulated extrinsic factors.

Classification

The lesions vary in severity, from those which are incompatible with life, to those completely asymptomatic and which cause no appreciable interference with a normal life span.

The older classifications into cyanotic and acyanotic disease are not satisfactory and the only tenable classification is one based on the anatomical features present.

Disorders of the whole heart

Ectopia cordis

Failure of development of the anterior chest wall, the heart lying outside the chest or subcutaneously. This is incompatible with life and is fortunately extremely rare.

Dextrocardia

(a) Complete mirror image with transposition of all viscera – *situs inversus*. The incidence is 1 in 5000 births and causes no significant disability.

(b) Partial transposition of the viscera. This is associated with other serious congenital heart abnormalities.

(c) Isolated dextrocardia with normally positioned viscera. This is usually associated with other grave cardiac abnormalities.

Defects of the septum

INTERATRIAL SEPTAL DEFECT – A.S.D.

Patent foramen ovale

Functionally, the foramen ovale normally closes within a few hours following birth, but structurally may not be completely fused for a year. Minor degrees of probe-patency at one margin of the membrane are extremely common, but these are non-functional, and are clinically insignificant.

Ostium secundum type

This is persistence of the foramen ovale and is of variable size and always functional. This type is readily closed by sutures without recourse to a 'patch'.

Ostium primum type

The defect is large and involves the lower portions of the septum. It is commonly associated with abnormal attachments of the septal cusps of the mitral and tricuspid valves or with a deficiency of the membranous portion of the interventricular septum. Surgical correction requires interposition of a 'patch' of foreign material and may be technically extremely difficult owing to the associated valvular anomalies.

Lutembacher's syndrome

Atrial septal defects of the secundum type associated with congenital or acquired mitral stenosis and gross dilatation of the pulmonary artery.

INTERVENTRICULAR SEPTAL DEFECT – V.S.D.

As a solitary lesion

There may be single or multiple defects in the muscular part of the septum, but more commonly there is a solitary defect restricted to the upper membranous portion. When the defect is very large – *trilocular heart*.

Associated with other abnormalities

For example Fallot's tetralogy.

Abnormalities of the great vessels

Truncus arteriosus

The abnormalities vary in degree from common pulmonary and aortic trunks to fistulous communications between the two. A further rare abnormality is the failure of development of the pulmonary arteries involving the main trunk or one or both branches. The lungs are then supplied by enlarged bronchial arteries.

Transposition

COMPLETE

The aorta and pulmonary arteries arise from the right ventricle and the left ventricle respectively and the ventricles are also transposed, i.e. the bicuspid mitral valve is on the right side and the tricuspid valve is on the left. Unless a septal defect is present or the great veins are also transposed, the condition is incompatible with life.

PARTIAL

The great vessels are transposed but the ventricles are normally situated. In both instances surgical correction may be possible and successful.

Abnormalities of valves and outflow tracts

SUPERNUMERARY CUSPS

Extra aortic or pulmonary cusps.

MISSING CUSPS

Bicuspid aortic or pulmonary valves.

AORTIC STENOSIS

(*a*) Valvular.
(*b*) Subvalvular.

PULMONARY STENOSIS

(*a*) Isolated valvular stenosis.
(*b*) Fallot's tetralogy.

FALLOT'S TETRALOGY

Incidence
This is the commonest (70 per cent) of the congenital heart lesions causing cyanosis at rest.

Lesions
1 *Pulmonary stenosis.* This is usually of the subvalvular type with muscular thickening of the narrowed infundibulum; rarely it may be valvular as a diaphragm formed by fusion of the cusps.
2 *Ventricular septal defect.* The defect is in the upper membranous part of the septum.
3 *Dextraposition and overriding of the aorta.* The aorta overrides the V.S.D. and receives blood from both ventricles.
4 *Right ventricular hypertrophy.* The right ventricular hypertrophy, with a concavity along the left border of the heart due to the absence of the pulmonary conus, produces the 'boot-shaped' deformity seen radiologically.

Effects
Most of the blood from the right ventricle passes into the aorta and the pulmonary blood flow is diminished. The aortic blood is thus mixed and unsaturated and cyanosis is therefore marked in all but the very mildest cases.

Operation
The principle of Blalock's operation is to by-pass the pulmonary obstruction and produce an artificial anastomosis through which an adequate amount of blood will pass from the systemic to the pulmonary circulation for oxygenation. The left subclavian artery is usually used and is anastomosed to the left pulmonary artery. In most cases, an improvement ensues with increased oxygenation of the blood and disappearance of the cyanosis. However, the anastomosis becomes inadequate with the progressive growth of the child and cyanosis returns after an interval, usually of some years. Increase of the pulmonary blood flow by enlargement of the infundibulum may then produce further improvement, but the pulmonary circulation is unable to deal adequately with the large amount of blood associated with a left to right shunt through the V.S.D. Pulmonary hypertension therefore results. A one-stage operation with pulmonary valvotomy and closure of the V.S.D. is now favoured; there is a significant operative mortality but in survivors the results are good.

EISENMENGER COMPLEX

This is Fallot's tetralogy without the pulmonary stenosis – *trilogy*. The blood from the left ventricle passes through the V.S.D. into the pulmonary circulation resulting in pulmonary hypertension.

TRICUSPID ATRESIA

Failure of development of one or more cusps of the tricuspid valve, sometimes associated with a complete septum across the valve orifice and a rudimentary right ventricle. In such cases a V.S.D. is usually present, otherwise the lesion is incompatible with life.

Patent ductus arteriosus

Nature
In intra-uterine life, the blood passes from the pulmonary circulation through the ductus arteriosus into the aorta. In the normal infant, contraction of smooth muscle very soon after birth produces functional occlusion of the lumen of the ductus followed by permanent obliteration, usually by about 8 weeks. Failure of occlusion leads to a patent ductus arteriosus.

Results
A patent ductus arteriosus is compatible with life but, as the aortic systemic pressure is higher than the pulmonary pressure, there is a persistent left to right shunt through the ductus which produces the 'machinery' murmur. In cases with a large ductus, there follows hypertrophy of the left ventricle and left atrium, with engorgement of the pulmonary vessels and pulmonary hypertension.

If untreated, the majority of patients (about 70 per cent) will succumb to either cardiac failure or to *Streptococcus viridans* infection at the site of the ductus. Operative ligation of the patent vessel obviates both serious sequelae and carries only a small mortality.

Coarctation of the aorta

Nature
A segmental area of narrowing of the aortic lumen between the left subclavian artery and the site of the ductus arteriosus.

Results
The stenosis of the aorta jeopardizes the blood supply below the area but compensation occurs by:
1 Left ventricular hypertrophy producing a raised systemic pressure.
2 Opening up of collateral vessels thus by-passing the obstruction, e.g. via the subscapular to the intercostal arteries thus reaching the thoracic aorta and producing radiological 'rib notching'; via the internal mammary artery to anastomose with the epigastric vessels.

These two mechanisms occur in the 'adult' form of coarctation when there has been closure of the ductus arteriosus.
3 In the 'foetal' type of coarctation there is a patent ductus arteriosus and this allows a by-pass of the coarctation by permitting a flow of blood from the pulmonary artery to the aorta below the level of the obstruction. However, this pulmonary arterial blood is unsaturated.

Effects
The defect produces:
(a) An increased blood pressure in the arms, head and neck.
(b) Prominence of collateral blood vessels.
(c) Diminished pulses and blood pressure in the legs.

These abnormalities predispose to:
1 Severe hypertension in the head and neck with heart failure or cerebral haemorrhage.
2 *Streptococcus viridans* infection at the site of the coarctation.
3 Aneurysm formation above or just below the coarcted segment.
4 Rupture or dissecting aneurysm of the aorta.

These sequelae can be avoided by the surgical removal of the narrowed aortic segment and re-anastomosis or interposition of a graft of human aorta or of synthetic material.

Veins

Persistent left superior vena cava
Usually opens into the coronary sinus or left atrium.

Abnormal pulmonary veins
Usually all four are present, but one or more may open into the right atrium, particularly if an A.S.D. is also present.

Coronary vessels

Many variations in the relative sizes of the right and left arteries and their branches are frequently found and there may be anomalies also in situation, distribution or origin.

Other congenital abnormalities

Numerous other variations and abnormalities exist which may be of considerable practical importance in relationship to surgical correction. However, the important common lesions are:
1   Septal defects – A.S.D. and V.S.D.
2   Patent ductus arteriosus.
3   Fallot's tetralogy.
4   Coarctation of the aorta.

Dangers of congenital heart disease

Heart failure
Abnormalities of blood flow lead to increased strain on one or both ventricles with hypertrophy, but ultimately failure, of one or both chambers. Septal defects and patent ductus arteriosus cause left to right shunting of blood and pulmonary hypertension with resulting right ventricular hyptertrophy. Ultimately shunt reversal (right to left) occurs, which is of sinister significance.

Pulmonary hypertension
Particularly in septal defects and ductus arteriosus but also in the Eisenmenger complex, severe progressive pulmonary hypertension results in structural arterial changes in the pulmonary circulation and this increases the pulmonary resistance. Sudden heart failure is common in these circumstances (see p. 269).

Endocarditis
Congenital abnormalities, particularly patent ductus and valvular lesions, predispose to the development of bacterial endocarditis (see p. 246).

Predisposition to infections
Resistance to infections is low and may be the presenting feature, e.g. frequent upper respiratory infections in patients with septal defects. The infections increase the strain on the already abnormal circulation.

Functional disabilities
These may be severe, e.g. in Fallot's tetralogy, where exercise tolerance is very poor and squatting may occur after walking a few steps. The disabilities become progressively severe with increasing age.

Cyanosis
Interference with oxygenation leads to mental and physical retardation. The cyanosis may be manifest at all times or only appear on taking exercise.

Results

Untreated
1   Minor abnormalities may cause no interference with the normal life span and are found incidentally at post-mortem examination, even in ripe old age.
2   The more serious disorders cause variable degrees of decreased life expectancy, death occurring in many during infancy, childhood or adult life.

Treated
Many of the more common conditions can be surgically corrected although not without risk, which in some cases is considerable. Complete correction of most forms of septal defect, patent ductus arteriosus and coarctation of the aorta can be carried out and should be performed before serious complications or secondary structural changes are too far advanced.

More recent developments of cardiac surgery include excision of congenital or acquired diseased valves and stenoses and replacement by either cadaveric or artificial prostheses. Further improvements of extra-corporeal circulatory techniques allow of these and other more sophisticated procedures.

Chapter 49
Cardiovascular System – Arteries I: Atheroma: Syphilis

NORMAL ARTERIES

There are three groups of arteries.

Large elastic
The aorta and its major branches.

Medium muscular
Distributing arteries, e.g. renal, femoral and brachial.

Small arteries and arterioles
Mostly within the substance of tissues and organs.

NORMAL STRUCTURE

There are three layers present in all these vessels but in differing proportions.

Intima
An endothelial cell lining with subendothelial avascular connective tissue.

Media
This is of variable thickness and is composed of muscle and elastic tissue. The latter is widely distributed in the large elastic vessels; largely condensed into internal and external elastic laminae in the medium muscular arteries; less well defined in the small vessels.

Adventitia
A poorly defined layer of connective tissue external to the media and containing nerve fibres and the vasa vasorum. These nutrient arteries are derived from branches of the same artery, pass through the adventitia into the wall and can be identified in the outer third of the media. In the inner layers, they are poorly formed and fail to enter the intima. The amount of adventitia is relatively large in the small arteries but contains very few recognizable vasa vasorum.

CAPILLARIES

Begin as a rather sudden transition from arterioles and consist of a layer of endothelium supported by a scanty fibrous tissue framework. The diameter varies from 5 to 20 μm. Blood flow through them is controlled by a sphincter-like action of the innervated muscle of the arterioles, so that, in health, only 2–5 per cent of the capillary bed is open and in action at any one time.

Arterial disease

General
Arterial disease may be due to:
1 Primary vascular disease.
2 Affection of vessels by diseases of adjacent structures.
   The general effects of vascular damage may be:
1 Weakening of the vessel walls with dilatation or rupture.
2 Narrowing of the lumen producing ischaemia in the tissue supplied.
3 Damage to the endothelial lining provoking intravascular thrombosis.

Incidence
Some form of vascular disease affects virtually every individual at some stage during his life and, together with cardiac disease, is responsible for 50–60 per cent of deaths over the age of 50 years and 20–30 per cent of deaths in the 5–50 age group.

ATHEROSCLEROSIS – ATHEROMA

Incidence
Found in some degree in virtually every adult over the age of 40 years and in many younger individuals. The incidence has probably not significantly increased in recent years but the seven-fold increase in deaths resulting from the disease during the period 1909–49 is due to the increased frequency of the complications, particularly thrombosis.

Age
Increases with advancing age.

Sex
Up to 45 years, M:F 2:1. Over 45 years (postmenopausal), M:F equal.

Sites
The arteries principally affected are:
1 Aorta. Particularly the abdominal aorta.

2 Coronary arteries.
3 Cerebral arteries.
   Other large and medium-sized vessels are affected less commonly and the pulmonary arteries only very rarely, unless pulmonary hypertension is also present.
   The lesions are patchy along the length of a vessel and are usually most marked at the origin of branches, i.e. at the points of maximal stress. The lesions are variable in severity from one artery to another in the same individual.

Aetiological factors

DIET AND FAT METABOLISM
It is well established that accelerated atherosclerosis occurs in those with hypercholesterolaemia particularly in diabetes, hypothyroidism and certain types of familial xanthomatosis.
   Experimentally, in certain animals atheromatous-like lesions can be readily produced by feeding with prolonged lipid-rich diets, particularly with saturated fats.
   Less certain is correlation between known human cases of severe atherosclerosis and identifiable abnormalities of blood lipids. In most, cholesterol levels are normal but certain lipoproteins, particularly β and very low density lipoproteins (LDL) and triglycerides, when raised, may show better correlation between severity of atherosclerosis and its complications and blood levels.
   Blood levels of HDL, *when low*, indicate a high risk factor.
   It has yet to be demonstrated, however, that reduction in blood levels of such lipids by dietary or other biochemical factors decreases risks, though lowered intake of animal fats and reduction of obesity are probably desirable and helpful. This effect may, however, be more related to reduction of complicating thrombosis than of control of the atherosclerotic process.

THROMBOGENIC FACTORS
It is suggested that deposits of fibrin and platelets on the endothelial surface of the intima are organized and 'incorporated' into the wall with formation of fibrous tissue, vascularization and some iron pigment from trapped erythrocytes. Fat is believed to be derived from the blood by 'insudation', or possibly as a result of fatty degeneration of incorporated thrombus and haemorrhage.
   Fibrin can be identified by special techniques in

early fatty streaks but it seems more likely that encrustation by thrombus is more important in building up previously established lesions and in producing the later stages.

DISTURBANCES OF BLOOD COAGULATION
Encrustation may be related to enhanced deposition of fibrin and platelets by change in some parameters of blood coagulation or altered fibrinolytic activity. High blood fat content has an *in vitro* effect on decreasing clotting time. Alterations in platelet adhesiveness may also be important in this context.

MECHANICAL FACTORS
Local alterations to the vessel wall resulting in some sort of injury by haemodynamic shearing strains, endocrine, metabolic, immunological, hypoxic or toxic damage, may predispose both to increased permeability of the walls to lipids and/or to encrustation by fibrin and platelets.

Such factors may relate more to distribution of lesions than to severity in individuals.

SEX
Pre-menopausal females are 'protected' compared with men but post-menopausally atheroma tends to develop more rapidly. Oestrogens may be the significant factor, though long-term oestrogen therapy in young women (oral contraceptives) has a significantly higher complication rate of arterial disease and thrombotic complications than controls.

RACE
There are wide variations in incidence of atheroma in different countries, much of which is explicable as dietary differences, though other factors cannot be excluded. The condition is relatively uncommon in Chinese, Japanese and Africans.

HYPERTENSION
High blood pressure, though not apparently a causative factor, appears to accelerate the progress of the disease and may also relate to accentuation of mechanical factors at certain sites.

EMOTIONAL AND PHYSICAL
The impact of stress and level of physical activity are well recognised as conferring a higher risk but seem to relate more to complications of atheroma than to the primary disease process.

FAMILIAL AND HEREDITARY PREDISPOSITION
There is no doubt that this is a powerful factor identifiable in epidemiological studies.

Stages of development

FATTY STREAKING OF INTIMA
Mononuclear cells filled with lipid substances immediately beneath the endothelium. The cells are histiocytes and smooth muscle cells and the lipids are rich in cholesterol.

The streaks are best seen in the aorta and its branches and may be found as parallel 0.1 cm or so wide, yellow, longitudinal streaks, sometimes at a very early age. It is probably that they are capable of absorption or dispersion or alternatively serve as a focal point for increasing fatty accumulations, which may or may not be the starting point of the next stage.

THE ATHEROMATOUS PLAQUE
The uncomplicated plaque appears as a smooth yellow or white button-like lesion of circular outline and variable in size and number. Microscopically fat, partially intracellular but also more centrally extracellular forming a structureless mass, is present in and thickens the intima. With age the lesions not only increase in size but develop a layer of intimal hyaline fibres with increasing pallor and fibrosis. At the base of the plaque pressure effects cause secondary change in internal elastic lamina and later the media.

THE FULLY DEVELOPED LESION
The further development of plaques is very variable. Extension is accompanied by increasing fibrosis and intimal vascularization. Severely affected vessels may also show calcification, ulceration, mural thrombus formation and progressive surface occlusive thrombosis. The lesion remains predominantly intimal in situation, but with increasing effect on deeper layers.

Effects
1 Narrowing of the lumen – ischaemia.
2 Predisposition to thrombosis – occlusion.
3 Weakening of the wall – aneurysm formation.

SYPHILIS

Large arteries

SITES

1 *Aorta*. Virtually always confined to the thoracic portion, particularly the ascending part of the aortic arch.
2 *Medium muscular arteries*. Rarely affected.

PATHOGENESIS
Although the spirochaetes are disseminated during the primary stage of the disease and are present in the aorta from this time, the aortitis is a manifestation of the tertiary stage (see p. 54).

MACROSCOPICAL
Pearly-grey raised plaques on the thickened intimal surface together with puckering of the intima to give stellate or longitudinal scarring, classically of 'tree bark' appearance. The plaques are maximal around the origin of vessels, e.g. coronary ostia, and the lumen is commonly dilated, with or without local aneurysm formation.

MICROSCOPICAL
1 Endarteritis of the vasa vasorum with a perivascular cuffing by lymphocytes and plasma cells in the adventitia.
2 The inflammatory process and the endarteritis extend into the media with progressive ischaemia.

3 Fragmentation of the elastic tissue due to ischaemia.
4 Degeneration of the muscle due to ischaemia.
5 Replacement fibrosis.

RESULTS
1 *Aneurysm formation*. Localized – saccular (see p. 271). More diffuse – fusiform (see p. 271).
2 *Narrowing of coronary ostia*. Coronary insufficiency (see p. 234).
3 *Aortic incompetence*. Due to stretching of the valve ring (see p. 249).

Small arteries

At all stages of congenital or acquired syphilis, small arteries may be involved in affected organs. The resulting endarteritis is responsible for the degenerative changes in the C.N.S. and for the necrosis and fibrosis seen in gummas.

MICROSCOPICAL
The microscopical appearances of the vessels are identical in all sites – endarteritis obliterans and perivascular cuffing with plasma cells and lymphocytes.

RESULTS
Ischaemia due to the vascular narrowing with subsequent degenerative changes and replacement fibrosis.

Chapter 50
Cardiovascular System – Arteries II: Other Diseases

Mucoid medial degeneration – idiopathic cystic medial necrosis

Incidence
Mild localized changes are common and are found in about 30 per cent of autopsies but severe and extensive medial degeneration is uncommon.

Aetiology
This is unknown, but the following factors have been suggested:
1 *Hereditary*. Metabolic or biochemical abnormalities of the ground substance. The disease is sometimes associated with congenital heart disease and Marfan's syndrome (see p. 16).

2 *Toxic*. Due to bacterial toxins. There is no confirmatory evidence for this aetiological factor.
3 *Experimental*. Lathyrism is a condition occurring in rats fed on extracts from sweet peas in which fundamental abnormalities occur in the chemical composition and structure of various connective tissues. One of these changes is medial degeneration and is commonly followed by a dissecting aneurysm. Similar changes also occur experimentally when aminonitriles are administered.
4 *Anoxia*. Epinephrine-induced constriction of the vasa vasorum produces medial degeneration. Similarly, experimentally induced thrombosis of the vasa vasorum also causes the lesion. The suggestion is that interference with oxygenation of the media may cause the degeneration to develop.

261

5 *Hypertension*. Dissecting aneurysms most commonly occur in hypertensive patients, but there is no evidence to suggest that the medial change results directly from hypertension.

Age
Usually 40 years of age and above, but is occasionally manifest in younger age groups.

Sex
M:F 2:1.

Site
Confined to the aorta and to the origins of its major branches.

Macroscopical
Seldom noticeable unless complicated by a dissecting aneurysm.

Microscopical
Focal degeneration of the elastic tissue and muscle of the media with poorly delineated areas of basophilic amorphous material of rather myxomatous appearance. Small cyst-like spaces are filled with this mucopolysaccharide which stains red with P.A.S. The distribution is variable but is usually in the outer half of the media. The intima may show unrelated atheroma but the adventitia is normal.

Results
Dissecting aneurysm, when the disease is extensive (see p. 273).

Mönckeberg's medial calcific sclerosis – Mönckeberg's medial degeneration

Incidence
A common disease. The frequency increases with advancing age and it is rare under the age of 50 years.

Sex
M:F equal.

Sites
Medium-sized muscular arteries, particularly of the limbs; the genital arterial supply is commonly involved, e.g. uterine vessels after the menopause.

Aetiology
This is obscure. There is no relationship with atheroma, although the two diseases may co-exist.

Macroscopical
Tortuous, hard, calcified vessel walls but with no diminution of the lumen – 'pipe stem' arteries.

Microscopical
The media only is affected. There are deposits of calcium in the hyalinized media. Bone may form in these calcified areas which are initially patchily distributed in rings or plaques but later become more continuous.

Effects
There is no narrowing so the disorder does not, by itself, produce ischaemia. It commonly co-exists with atheroma when ischaemia may follow.

Thrombo-angiitis obliterans – Buerger's disease

Nature
The disease is a segmental, thrombosing, chronic inflammation of arteries and other structures in the neurovascular bundle, in the legs of young or middle-aged males. The true incidence is rare.

Age
25–40 years.

Sex
Almost exclusively males.

Sites
Muscular arteries of the legs; very rare in other vessels.

Aetiology
This is obscure, but factors include an increased frequency in Jews, heavy smokers and those in sedentary occupations. An infective agent has been postulated but not isolated and although cold aggravates the condition, it is not primarily causative.

Macroscopical
Segmental in distribution, affecting initially the anterior and posterior tibial vessels and subsequently the popliteal and femoral arteries. Small

arteries are very rarely affected. The involved segment is thickened and indurated, binding all the components of the neurovascular bundle together. The lumen is thrombosed and subsequently replaced by pale, firm, fibrous tissue. The large proximal vessels may show gross narrowing by atheroma.

Microscopical

Early. There is an inflammatory cell infiltration of the intima with endothelial and fibroblastic proliferation.

Late. The process extends to other coats of the wall but does not destroy the architecture. The lumen is thrombosed and is followed by organization and attempts at recanalization. Usually the vein is similarly involved and thrombosed. In the late fibrous stages, dense collagen binds the nerves and vessels together.

Results

There is progressive ischaemia of the limbs:
1   Intermittent claudication.
2   Trophic skin changes.
3   Gangrene.

Amputation is necessary at some stage of the disease in at least 30 per cent of cases.

Arteriolosclerosis

Nature

Thickening of the walls with narrowing of the lumen of small arteries and arterioles in systemic hypertension. The hypertension precedes these structural changes (see p. 267).

Sites

Small arteries and arterioles anywhere in the body, but particularly in the kidneys, pancreas, gall bladder, small intestines, adrenals and the retina.

Macroscopical

The vessels pout from a cut surface and the lumen is narrowed.

Microscopical

HYALINE ARTERIOLOSCLEROSIS – BENIGN HYPERTENSION
Hyaline and fibrous thickening of the walls with loss of muscle and narrowing of the lumen. There is

also increased elastic tissue in the distributing arteries, with reduplication of the internal elastic lamina.

HYPERPLASTIC ARTERIOLOSLEROSIS – ACCELERATED HYPERTENSION
(a) Concentric, laminated, 'onion-skin' appearance, due to cellular proliferation of the endothelium, intimal fibroblasts and medial muscle cells.
(b) Fibrinoid necrosis of the arterioles with an intensely eosinophilic and smudgy appearance. Haemorrhages may occur into the surrounding tissues, e.g. glomeruli.

Non-specific arteritis

Causes

Injury by bacterial toxins, bacteria, trauma, ionizing radiation, chemicals.

Sites

Usually localized to a particular segment of an artery, adjacent to, or involved in a non-specific inflammatory process, e.g. in the base of a gastric ulcer, in ulcerative colitis, in tuberculous granulation tissue, etc.

Appearances

ACUTE
Non-specific inflammatory changes in the vessel wall, commonly accompanied by thrombosis.

CHRONIC
Fibroblastic overgrowth with lymphocytic infiltration and a progressive, but usually incomplete, occlusion of the lumen – *endarteritis obliterans*.

Results

Ischaemic changes resulting from both the acute and chronic types may materially worsen the prognosis of the underlying condition or result in infarction, perforation, haemorrhage and other complications.

Necrotizing arteritis

Nature

A group of conditions characterized by necrosis of

the wall of small vessels with or without a cellular inflammatory reaction. They are all of similar appearance although varying in distribution and many have the aetiological factor of hypersensitivity in common.

Most of the examples are described in the chapter on connective tissue disease (see p. 280), into which group they logically belong.

POLYARTERITIS NODOSA

Multiple system and organ involvement of medium muscular and small arteries (see p. 282).

LOCALIZED VASCULITIS

Affects both veins and arteries and is found in four skin conditions:
1 *Erythema nodosum* (see p. 726).
2 *Erythema induratum* (see p. 726).
3 *Nodular, non-suppurative, febrile panniculitis – Weber-Christian disease* (see p. 727).
4 *Nodular vasculitis* (see p. 726).

Appearances
There is active vasculitis of the dermal or subcutaneous vessels with obliterative intimal proliferation, cellular infiltration of the media or medial destruction. Fibrinoid necrosis is slight or absent but there are commonly secondary changes in the overlying epidermis.

HENOCH–SCHÖNLEIN PURPURA

In addition to the capillary damage leading to the purpuric manifestations in the skin and gastro-intestinal tract, renal involvement with a focal glomerulonephritis and occasionally a necrotizing arteritis, occurs in a substantial proportion of cases (see p. 361).

SYSTEMIC LUPUS ERYTHEMATOSUS

Arterioles and small arteries in many organs, particularly the spleen and kidney, commonly show necrosis and inflammatory reaction (see p. 281).

THROMBOTIC MICROANGIOPATHY – THROMBOTIC THROMBOCYTOPENIC PURPURA

A progressive and fatal disease, mostly occurring in young adults. There is thrombocytopenic purpura, haemolytic anaemia, fever and fluctuating neurological signs. Pre-capillary arterioles in many organs are plugged by structureless material with necrosis and dilatation of the wall to form micro-aneurysms. There is no inflammatory cell infiltration (see p. 531).

Temporal arteritis – Giant cell arteritis

Incidence
An uncommon condition occurring in the older age groups and equally in both sexes.

Clinical
Fever with severe headache and palpable, nodular thickening of the temporal arteries.

Sites
One or both temporal arteries, with occasional involvement of the occipital, carotid or cerebral arteries including the ophthalmic branch. The aorta may rarely be involved in a more generalized form of the disease.

Aetiology
Unknown; infective and hypersensitivity aetiological agents have been suggested, but lack positive proof; however, very high sedimentation rates are usual together with increase in serum globulins. There is an association with cases of polymyalgia rheumatica (see p. 286).

Macroscopical
The temporal artery is thickened, nodular, indurated and tender, forming a readily palpable cord.

Microscopical
Necrosis of the inner media with fragmentation of the elastic lamina and giant cells aggregated around the fragments of the degenerated elastic fibres.

There are inflammatory cells in all layers and fibroblastic proliferation of the intima. The lumen is narrowed and is usually occluded by thrombus.

Results

The disease is controlled by corticosteroid therapy.

1 *Healing*. With fibrous organization; usually the disease remains clinically active for 6 months or more.

2 *Blindness*. Occurs in 30 per cent of untreated cases due to involvement of the ophthalmic artery.

3 *Death*. This is rare but may occur from:

(*a*) Cerebral ischaemia.

(*b*) Rupture of the aorta.

(*c*) Generalization of the disease to involve visceral arteries.

Pulseless disease – aortic arch syndrome – Takayashu's disease

Nature

A rare disease of young women (90 per cent females, mostly in 20–30 age group), in which there is an arteritis of unknown aetiology affecting all coats of the innominate, carotid and subclavian arteries and the aorta. As a result of the intimal thickening and superimposed thrombosis, occlusion with absence of the pulses occurs.

Rheumatoid aortitis

A small number of patients with rheumatoid arthritis, and more particularly with ankylosing spondylitis, show characteristic and specific lesions of the ascending aorta. There is chronic inflammatory cell infiltration of all coats of the wall around the vasa vasorum and degenerative changes in the media reminiscent of syphilitic mesaortitis. Following weakening of the wall, aortic incompetence may result, occasionally associated with aneurysm (see p. 286). Rheumatoid granulomas, similar to the appearances of rheumatoid nodules, may also occur in the walls of the aorta and other arteries.

Chapter 51
Cardiovascular System – Hypertension

Systemic hypertension

Definition
A sustained rise of the systemic blood pressure above 140 mm Hg systolic and 90 mm Hg diastolic.

Types

PRIMARY OR ESSENTIAL
(a) Benign hypertension.
(b) Accelerated or malignant hypertension.
Ninety per cent of hypertensives are of this type with no known cause.

SECONDARY
That is, follows a number of known conditions, many of which are renal.

PRIMARY ESSENTIAL HYPERTENSION

BENIGN HYPERTENSION

Clinical
An extremely common condition in which there is a slowly progressive rise in the blood pressure over a period of many years. Five per cent of such patients enter an accelerated phase after many years of benign progression.

Age
Usually 50 years or above.

Sex
More common in males.

Effects

The hypertension precedes and produces arteriosclerosis (see p. 263) and mild renal damage. In addition other organ changes result.

Organ changes

CARDIOVASCULAR

Heart. Concentric left ventricular hypertrophy (see p. 250).

Large arteries. Although not causative, atheroma is potentiated by hypertension, particularly in the aorta, coronary and cerebral vessels.

Muscular arteries. Medial hypertrophy and intimal thickening.

Small arteries. Arteriolosclerosis (see p. 263).

(*a*) Hyaline thickening of the wall.

(*b*) Increased elastic tissue with reduplication of the elastic lamina.

BRAIN

The combination of hypertension and potentiated atheroma commonly leads to cerebral vascular accidents (see p. 598).

KIDNEY

Results in benign nephrosclerosis. Renal function is unimpaired in the large majority of cases (see p. 367).

Prognosis

From the time of diagnosis the average course in untreated cases is in excess of 10 years, but much longer when therapy effectively controls the pressure. The additional mortality of a blood pressure of 150/100 mm Hg is 125 per cent. Men with blood pressure higher than 178 mm Hg systolic and 108 mm Hg diastolic, have an excess mortality of 600 per cent.

Death may be due to:

1 Congestive heart failure – 45 per cent.
2 Coronary insufficiency or infarction – 35 per cent.
3 Cerebral vascular accident – 15 per cent.
4 Renal failure – 5 per cent.

ACCELERATED – MALIGNANT HYPERTENSION

Nature

Most cases arise *de novo*, but some are due to a malignant termination of benign hypertension.

Clinical

A more rapidly progressive form of hypertension in which very high levels are commonly reached, e.g. 280 mm Hg systolic and 180 mm Hg diastolic. This is accompanied by severe headaches, papilloedema and other hypertensive retinal changes, severe renal functional impairment, albuminuria and haematuria.

Age

Mostly occurs in patients younger than 45 years of age.

Organ changes

CARDIOVASCULAR

Heart. The degree of left ventricular hypertrophy depends upon the duration of the disease. In rapidly progressive cases it may be minimal.

Vessels. Usually uncomplicated by any significant degree of atheroma. The small arteries show malignant arteriolosclerosis (see p. 263) with:

(*a*) Fibrinoid necrosis.

(*b*) Hyperplasia of the 'onion-skin' type.

KIDNEY

Accelerated nephrosclerosis (see p. 367).

BRAIN

Cerebral vascular accidents are relatively uncommon.

Prognosis

This is poor in untreated cases, but well-managed and treated cases have a good survival. Untreated patients die from:

1 Renal failure – 90 per cent.
2 Heart failure.
3 Cerebral vascular episode.

SECONDARY HYPERTENSION

Nature

This is hypertension secondary to a pre-existing disease.

Causes

RENAL DISEASE

(*a*) *Parenchymal.* Chronic pyelonephritis; glomerulonephritis; polycystic kidneys; amyloidosis; infarction; toxaemia of pregnancy.

(b) *Renal vessels.* Vascular obstruction: thrombosis; atheroma; ligatures; pressure from tumours; dissecting aneurysm involving renal vessels; polyarteritis nodosa

(c) *Obstruction.* Hydronephrosis.

Whilst more common in bilateral disease, unilateral renal lesions may also result in hypertension.

BLOOD

Polycythaemia (see p. 458).

ENDOCRINE

(a) Cushing's syndrome due to pituitary or adrenal hypersecretion or steroid therapy (see p. 291).

(b) Phaeochromocytoma – the hypertension is commonly intermittent (see p. 293).

(c) Diabetes with renal involvement – Kimmelstiel-Wilson disease (see p. 358).

(d) Conn's syndrome due to hyperaldosteronism (see p. 294).

CEREBRAL

(a) Increased intracranial pressure due to: trauma; tumours; haemorrhage; inflammations.

(b) Lesions of the hypothalamic region.

(c) Lesions of the brain stem.

DRUGS

Adrenaline and related sympatheticomimetic drugs.

CARDIOVASCULAR

Coarctation of the aorta; arteriovenous fistulae and shunts.

MECHANISMS OF CAUSATION OF HYPERTENSION

Experimental procedures

A large number of differing procedures will cause sustained hypertension in animals.

INFUSION OF PRESSOR SUBSTANCES

(a) *Renin.* Only mild elevation of pressure is possible.

(b) *Angiotensin* – particularly angiotensin II, which has a marked vasoconstrictive effect.

(c) *Adrenaline and noradrenaline* – potent vasocon-

strictive effects which can be sustained for long periods of time.

OVERDOSAGE WITH SALT AND ADRENAL CORTICAL HORMONES

(a) *Salt* – high dietary salt intake causes sustained hypertension in some animals but not in others.

(b) *Deoxycorticosterone acetate (D.O.C.A.)* – administered to rats with high dietary salt produces sustained hypertension.

INTERFERENCE WITH KIDNEYS

Hypertension can be produced by renal irradiation or removal of both kidneys or wrapping kidneys in silk or cellophane.

More relevant however to disease in man is the effect of interference with renal arterial flow.

(a) *Unilateral renal artery constriction.* Man appears to behave like the rat in producing prolonged severe hypertension associated with rise in renin and probably maintained and potentiated by angiotensin II.

(b) *Unilateral renal artery constriction after nephrectomy on other side.* This produces a persistent, usually very high level of hypertension not associated with excess renin or angiotensin II.

Secondary hypertension in man

(a) Renal diseases
  i. Excess renin.
  ii. Sodium and water retention.

(b) Adrenal diseases
  i. Aldosterone excess induces sodium retention.
  ii. Glucocorticoid excess probably operates similarly.
  iii. Adrenaline and nor-adrenaline produce vasoconstriction.

Primary or essential hypertension in man

The mechanism in benign hypertension is not understood but the condition may be initiated by response to emotional stress in genetically susceptible individuals via the sympathetic nervous system, with resulting renal vasoconstriction and sodium retention. If sufficiently prolonged, organic vascular narrowing of renal vessels will effect a permanent rise in the threshold for sodium excretion and further vaso-constriction.

In accelerated hypertension it is thought likely that renin and angiotensin II have a role initiated by damage to renal afferent arterioles caused by a severe and steep rise in arterial pressure. The primary initiating factors may also be related to genetic predisposition and nervous and emotional causes.

Pulmonary hypertension

Nature
Pulmonary arterial pressure in excess of 30 mm Hg.

Normal pulmonary vasculature
Normal pulmonary blood flow – 5–8 litre/min at rest. Normal pressure – 16–17 mm Hg. With exercise, the flow increases up to 16 litres/min but the pressure does not rise significantly.

The requirement of the pulmonary circulation is to transmit the total right ventricular output with the minimum of resistance through the lungs. The vessels are therefore capacious and thin-walled. Elastic arteries extend as far as the end of the cartilaginous bronchi and the muscular arteries are short, ending at the level of the respiratory bronchioles and are thinner than their systemic counterparts. The arterioles soon lose their muscle and consist mostly of intima, external elastic tissue and adventitia. They end in the capillaries which are in close relationship to the alveoli.

MECHANISMS IN THE PRODUCTION OF PULMONARY HYPERTENSION

1 *Passive*. Back pressure from the left atrium.
2 *Increased flow*. In excess of the vascular capacity.
3 *Organic obstruction*. Impeding the blood flow.
4 *Increased arterial tone*. Producing increased peripheral resistance of vascular origin.

Usually, more than one of these factors are involved in each individual case of pulmonary hypertension.

PASSIVE PULMONARY HYPERTENSION

Causes
1 Chronic left ventricular failure.
2 Mitral stenosis or incompetence.

Effects
1 *Chronic left ventricular failure*. The degree of pulmonary hypertension is seldom marked. There is slight atheroma and increased thickening of the muscle in the muscular arteries.
2 *Mitral valve disease*. More severe changes occur:
(*a*) Atheroma is usually marked as superficial fatty streaking.
(*b*) Muscular hypertrophy of elastic and muscular arteries.
(*c*) Arterial thrombosis may occur.
(*d*) Embolism may also be found.

PULMONARY HYPERTENSION DUE TO INCREASED BLOOD FLOW

Causes
1 Atrial septal defect (A.S.D.)
2 Ventricular septal defect (V.S.D.)
3 Other left to right shunts, e.g. ductus arteriosus, Blalock's operation etc. (see p. 254).

Effects
1 *A.S.D.* Left to right shunt with a massive increase in the blood flow and a marked rise of pressure. Initially, the increased pressure is reversible, but later is constant. In the late stages, the resistance increases to a sufficient degree to reverse the shunt from right to left. The changes include:
(*a*) Dilatation of elastic arteries which may become aneurysmal.
(*b*) Atheroma which is often severe.
(*c*) Thrombosis, mainly arterial.
(*d*) Muscular arteries are thickened with increased fibrosis and may be obliterated.
2 *V.S.D.* The pulmonary vessels are exposed to the full force of the left ventricular pressure from birth. As a result the pressure is higher and the damage is greater. Thus, the effects are similar to those occurring with an A.S.D., but are even more severe.

PULMONARY HYPERTENSION DUE TO ORGANIC VASCULAR OBSTRUCTION

Causes
1 Multiple pulmonary emboli.
2 Loss of pulmonary tissue:
(*a*) *Pulmonary fibrosis*. From any cause, but particularly in progressive massive coal miners' pneumoconiosis (see p. 670).
(*b*) *Emphysema*. Partly due to spasm but also to

compression of the alveolar blood vessels by the raised intra-alveolar tension and to loss of tissue with reduction of the capillary bed.

(c) *Lung resection.* More than a third of the lung tissue needs to be removed before hypertension is likely to result.

Effects

The degree varies with the extent of the causative lesions but may be severe.

Atheroma and muscular hypertrophy are present in the vessels.

PRIMARY PULMONARY HYPERTENSION

This is due to increased arterial tone with a raised peripheral resistance of vascular origin and is thus analogous to essential systemic hypertension.

The diagnosis is made only after careful exclusion of all the known causes and thus this primary form of hypertension is rare. There is muscular hypertrophy of the elastic and muscular arteries and fibrous thickening of the small arteries and arterioles.

The aetiology is unknown but the mechanism is presumed to include an initial period of increased vascular tone without organic structural changes such as is seen in the systemic type of hypertension.

Chapter 52
Cardiovascular System – Aneurysms

Definition
Abnormal localized dilatation of an artery.

Types
1 *True*. The wall is formed by one or more layers of the affected vessel.
2 *False*. The wall is formed by connective tissue which is not part of a vessel. They are usually due to traumatic or infective openings in vessels limited by the surrounding tissues.

True aneurysms

Macroscopical
1 *Fusiform*. Spindle-shaped area of dilatation due to a long segment of the vessel wall being affected around the whole circumference.
2 *Saccular*. Part of the circumference only is involved to produce a globular sac, usually with a narrow neck in the early stages.
3 *Dissecting*. Blood tracking along a false lumen within the arterial wall.

General Features

Aneurysms form as a result of weakening of the wall due to a variety of causes. Loss of elasticity and contractability due to a deficiency in the media is the most important factor.

Once the wall starts to stretch, the process is usually progressive under normal or abnormal (hypertensive) pressure forces, with increasing thinning of the wall until eventual rupture may occur. Build-up of laminated thrombus within the lumen of the aneurysmal sac is protective but only rarely is this process sufficient to repair the defect and reconstitute a normal lumen to the artery of origin.

The purely descriptive terms of the macroscopic types above give no idea of the underlying process responsible and thus a classification largely based on aetiology is more satisfactory.

CONGENITAL ANEURYSMS

'BERRY' ANEURYSMS

Incidence

This is the most common cause of subarachnoid haemorrhage and is only rarely found incidentally when death has occurred from unrelated causes.

Age

The average age at presentation is 50 years.

Sex

M:F 1:1.2.

Site

The vessels around the circle of Willis, particularly at the junctions of the communicating arteries. They are much more common in the anterior part of the circle (75 per cent) than posteriorly (25 per cent).

Pathogenesis

A congenital defect of the media in the angles formed by the junctions of vessels. The defect involves both the muscle and elastic tissue, thus, with increasing age and particularly with hypertension, this area of weak artery stretches and forms the aneurysm.

Macroscopical

They may be solitary or multiple or even symmetri-cal and form small (seldom more than 1 cm dia) sessile or pedunculated thin-walled sacs. The aneurysm is frequently obscured by surrounding blood clot when rupture has occurred.

Microscopical

The wall usually consists only of fibrous tissue with an endothelial lining.

Results

BEFORE RUPTURE
(a) Pressure symptoms, which may produce locali-zing signs.
(b) Ischaemia of adjacent brain.

LEAKAGE
Blood staining of C.S.F.

RUPTURE
(a) Subarachnoid haemorrhage.
(b) Rupture into the ventricles
(c) Intracerebral haemorrhage.

Prognosis

With the first bleed, untreated: 60 per cent die; 20 per cent disabled; 20 per cent recover.

Treatment by direct attack or by tying the carotid artery considerably improves this prognosis, e.g. there is about a 25 per cent immediate mortality, but of the survivors, 75 per cent are alive, well and at work 5 years later.

ARTERIOVENOUS MALFORMATIONS

Rare congenital conditions showing localized groups of poorly formed blood vessels, involving both arteries and veins. Many occur in the brain – so-called 'angioma', and at many other sites, e.g. limbs, lungs, etc. When large, they cause problems by the shunting of blood and cardiac strain. The small lesions may be symptomless or may rupture with haemorrhage.

CIRSOID ANEURYSMS

A mass of dilated, elongated, pulsating and inter-communicating arteries and veins – 'bag of worms'. Eighty to ninety per cent are congenital and the remainder traumatic in origin. Most occur in the scalp connected with the frontal or temporal arteries. They increase in size gradually and may cause destruction of the surrounding tissues or rupture with haemorrhage.

ATHEROMATOUS ANEURYSMS

Incidence
Common in the older age groups where they form the most frequent type of aneurysm.

Sites
The abdominal aorta and the common iliac arteries particularly, but any atheromatous artery may also be affected.

Appearances
Usually fusiform dilatation of the wall due to involvement of the media by the advanced atheromatous process (see p. 259). They only occur therefore in the late stages of the disease, mostly in elderly males and are frequently multiple; they are by far the most common cause of abdominal aortic aneurysm. Most of them are situated below the origin of the renal arteries and are thus amenable to resection and replacement by a graft.

Results
There is a gradual increase in size and they may eventually rupture with a fatal outcome. The aneurysm may be surgically excised and continuity of the vessel restored by a graft or prosthesis. The prognosis is then that of the severity of atheroma present in other organs, e.g. coronary and cerebral arteries.

SYPHILITIC ANEURYSMS

Incidence
Formerly common, but now rare.

Sites
The thoracic aorta, particularly the ascending and transverse portions of the arch.

Appearances
Mostly saccular in type. The wall of the adjacent vessel shows the scarring of syphilitic aortitis (see p. 260).

Effects
1 Pressure on surrounding structures, e.g. trachea and oesophagus.
2 Erosion of the sternum by pressure necrosis with the production of a pulsatile subcutaneous swelling.

Results
May reach an enormous size and eventually rupture. They are often associated with aortic incompetence due to dilatation of the valve ring.

DISSECTING ANEURYSMS

Incidence
Fairly common.

Site
Aorta

Aetiology
Due to medial degeneration (see p. 261).

Pathogenesis
Entry of blood into the diseased media whence it separates the wall into an inner layer of intima and part of the media and an outer layer of part of the media and the adventitia. Blood may enter this false lumen via:
1 Intramural haemorrhage from the vasa vasorum.
2 A break in the intima at a site of particular weakness, often in the ascending portion or arch of the aorta and rarely at the site of an atheromatous plaque.

The false lumen may be long but inevitably must rupture:
1 *Internally*. To recommunicate with the true lumen or
2 *Externally*. To produce a catastrophic haemorrhage. This is more common and results in:
(a) Intrapericardial haemorrhage – haemopericardium with cardiac tamponade.
(b) Mediastinal haemorrhage.
(c) Pleural cavity – haemothorax.
(d) Abdominal haemorrhage.

Appearances
A double-barrelled aorta, often extending from its origin to the bifurcation, but it may not involve the whole circumference of the wall. Acute cases show

little blood in the false lumen due to its escape into the para-aortic tissues; in the rarer, more chronic, forms which re-enter the true lumen, variable amounts of blood clot are present in the lumen of the sac. In other rare cases, the entire aortic blood flow may pass through the area of dissection in the wall, the original lumen of the aorta having been blocked due to the pressure of blood in the false lumen.

Effects

1 *Rupture*. With rapid death.
2 *Chronic dissecting aneurysm.* When re-entry occurs. This usually ruptures after a short period of time, e.g. months.
3 *Obliteration of branches.* As the blood extends in the wall it dissects the origins of branches resulting in their occlusion and thus causing renal or mesenteric infarction or gangrene of the lower limbs. The carotid and subclavian vessels are usually spared.

MYCOTIC ANEURYSMS

Nature
Formed by weakness of the wall due to bacterial infection.

Causes
Nearly all are associated with 'subacute' infective endocarditis (see p. 247) and the low-grade inflammation which accompanies impaction of embolic material.

The process is also seen in vessels in the walls of tuberculous cavities, abscesses and rarely adjacent to foci of acute or chronic non-specific inflmmation.

Appearances
Usually small saccular dilatations with destruction of the muscle and elastic tissue by the inflammatory process, the wall then being formed by thin, stretched, fibrous tissue in which there may be scanty residual inflammatory cells.

Sites
Aorta, coronary, cerebral and mesenteric arteries are most commonly affected.

Effects
1 *Rupture*. Uncommon, except as a late manifestation.
2 *Thrombosis.* In the lumen of the aneurysms and

later involving the lumen of the vessel of origin, thus resulting in ischaemic changes in the region supplied.

LOSS OF SUPPORT

Destruction of soft tissues around blood-vessels may occasionally lead to loss of support and aneurysmal dilatation. This is stated to occur in the brain substance following cerebral softening and in the lungs as a sequel to pulmonary destruction, e.g. tuberculosis. However, other factors causing damage to the vessel wall are usually also present, e.g. inflammation.

POLYARTERITIS NODOSA

A common sequel to the necrotizing arteritis is the dilatation of weakened arterial walls (see p. 282).

Appearances
Usually multiple and commonly numerous along the course of vessels as nodules of about twice the normal diameter. They frequently become filled with firm thrombus.

Sites
Small arteries, but the disease may affect medium-sized muscular vessels. The classical sites are the kidneys, heart, intestines and lungs.

Effects
1 *Thrombosis.* Producing infarction.
2 *Rupture.* Producing haemorrhage; however, this is unusual.

False aneurysms – traumatic aneurysms

PULSATING HAEMATOMA

Nature
A false aneurysm resulting from a small perforation in the wall of an artery.

Aetiology
Trauma, usually due to a sharp instrument.

Pathogenesis

The small aperture is sufficiently large to permit the escape of blood into the surrounding tissues where it collects until the pressure within the haematoma approaches that of the blood pressure. At this point, the haematoma no longer enlarges as the blood then re-enters the artery in diastole and refills in systole resulting in a 'to-and-fro' murmur.

Appearances

The walls of the haematoma are formed by the compressed adjacent tissues, e.g. muscle and fascia of the arms and legs. The lumen is filled with laminated clot externally and fluid blood in the centre.

Results

The false aneurysm may be removed and the arterial perforation sutured. If the haematoma persists, pain due to pressure or ischaemia due to progressive pressure on the vessel, may ensue.

ARTERIOVENOUS FISTULAE

Nature

A false aneurysm communicating with both an artery and a vein.

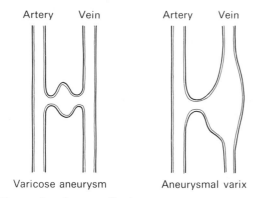

Fig. 32. Arteriovenous fistulae.

Aetiology

Trauma, penetrating the walls of both an artery and a vein.

Pathogenesis

The haematoma communicates with the lumen of both the artery and the vein so that there is a fistulous communication between the two via the haematoma. A continuous murmur is produced due to the arterial blood flowing constantly into the vein.

Appearances

Usually there is a false aneurysm containing blood, situated between the artery and the vein and through which blood flows – '*varicose aneurysm*' (see Fig. 32).

Sometimes there is only a small haematoma when the trauma has resulted in an immediate communication between the artery and the vein. The pressure of the arterial blood then distends the vein – '*aneurysmal varix*' (see Fig. 32).

Results

1 Increased blood flow in the artery above the fistula causes dilatation and hypertrophy of the wall with subsequent degenerative changes.
2 Decreased blood flow in the artery distal to the fistula may result in peripheral ischaemia.
3 Venous enlargement at the site of the fistula due to excessive blood flow and pressure. The vein dilates and the wall hypertrophies until it attains the histological features of an artery – venous arterialization.
4 Gross enlargement of the false aneurysm to produce pressure symptoms.
5 Cardiac hypertrophy due to the shunting effect of the arteriovenous communication which may terminate in heart failure if the fistula is not closed.

Chapter 53
Cardiovascular System – Diseases of Veins and Lymphatics: Tumours of Endothelium

Veins

VARICOSE VEINS

Nature
Abnormally dilated tortuous veins.

Sites
1 Systemic – Usually leg veins.
2 Portal – In portal venous hypertension, e.g. oesophagus, haemorrhoids, umbilicus.

Incidence
Common in legs; 10–20 per cent of the general population develop this disorder at some age.

Age
Increasing incidence with age, most common above 50 years.

Sex
M:F 1:4

Pathogenesis
Factors involved include:
1 *Relating to support of the venous wall.*
(a) *Familial.* A relative weakening of the wall. There is a familial incidence in about 40 per cent of all cases.
(b) *Obesity.* Poor support by the adipose tissue of the leg.
(c) *Age.* Loss of support by degenerative changes in the surrounding tissues and decreased activity of the muscles.
(d) *Posture.* The dependent position is a predisposition and occupations involving prolonged standing or sitting show an increased incidence.
2 *Increased pressure within the lumen.*

276

(*a*) *Pregnancy.*
(*b*) *Intravascular thrombosis.*
(*c*) *Tumour masses pressing on veins*, e.g. uterine fibroids and ovarian tumours.
(*d*) *Garters and other constrictions.*

Appearances

More common in the superficial veins where support is least effective, but they may occur at any site where local obstruction is present. Asymmetrical dilatation and tortuosity of the veins occurs with elongation and varying thickness of the wall. Later, there is hypertrophy of the muscle but this is ineffectual and the valves become incompetent due to the uneven stretching and deformity of the wall.

Complications

1 Oedema.
2 Trophic skin changes – varicose or gravitational ulcers.
3 Thrombosis.
4 Haemorrhage.
5 Infection – thrombophlebitis.
6 Embolism.

VENOUS THROMBOSIS

PHLEBOTHROMBOSIS

Bland thrombosis of non-inflammatory origin but with secondary inflammatory changes in the vessel wall.

THROMBOPHLEBITIS

Thrombosis initiated by inflammation.

In most cases, the differentiation between the two types is impossible and is of little significance, although sometimes the embolic sequelae may be different due to the presence or absence of infection within the thrombus.

Incidence
Common.

Predisposing Factors
Cardiac failure; pregnancy; prolonged bed rest; immunobilization; varicose veins.

Although these factors which give rise to stasis are the most important, direct injury or infection

may be the precipitating cause. The condition may also occur in young and otherwise healthy ambulant individuals in whom the aetiology is obscure.

Sites
Anywhere, but most common and important in:
1 Legs – 95 per cent, particularly the lower leg where the deep veins are often involved.
2 Skull and dural sinuses – this is now rare.
3 Portal venous tributaries.
4 Pelvic veins.

Appearances
Similar in both types; the veins are distended by laminated thrombus. The bland type of thrombus is only locally attached to the wall in the early stages whereas the thrombi seen in pre-existing inflammation are usually more firmly adherent. Later, organization of the thrombus and subsequent recanalization may occur.

Complications

EMBOLISM
(*a*) *Phlebothrombosis.* More common, causing infarction by aseptic thrombus.
(*b*) *Thrombophlebitis.* Less common, resulting in septic infarcts or pyaemic abscesses.
   In many cases of fatal pulmonary embolism, the venous thrombosis of the legs or pelvis has remained clinically 'silent'.

THROMBOPHLEBITIS MIGRANS

An uncommon disease characterized by transient venous inflammation which migrates from one area of the body to another. The aetiology is unknown but a number of cases are associated with malignant disease, particularly carcinomas of the bronchus and pancreas.

Lymphatics

LYMPHANGITIS

The lymphatic channels draining any focus of inflammation are inflamed, dilated and contain inflammatory cells. They may be responsible for the spread of the infection in some cases, e.g. in tuberculosis, and sometimes the inflammation is very marked clinically with tender swelling of the regional lymph nodes (see p. 579).

Appearances
Usually only seen in the subcutaneous channels as red streaks. When chronic, there may be fibrous blockage of the lymphatics resulting in lymphoedema.

LYMPHOEDEMA

Nature
Brawny induration of tissues due to blockage of the lymphatics. When severe, the thickening of the skin and the overgrowth of the dermal connective tissues results in elephantiasis.

Causes
1   Malignant tumours with mechanical blockage by tumour cells.
2   Radical surgery with resection of lymphatics.
3   Post-irradiation fibrosis.
4   Filariasis (see p. 69).
5   Post-inflammatory fibrosis – e.g. lymphogranuloma venereum (see p. 406).
6   Primary lymphatic disorders.
(a) *Milroy's disease.* A inherited lymphoedema in which there is faulty development of the lymphatic channels, usually of the lower limbs. It is present from birth but is frequently not clinically apparent until after puberty.
(b) *Lymphoedema praecox.* A rare condition of females aged 10–25 years, remaining localized to the feet or extending on to the trunk. The aetiology is obscure.

Effects
In addition to the swelling, which may be very gross, the oedematous part is very susceptible to attacks of lymphangitis and to ulceration. Surgical treatment may produce considerable improvement.

Tumours of vascular and lymphatic endothelium

Nature
Tumours or malformations of vascular and lymphatic endothelium. Many have been described previously on p. 155.

HAEMANGIOMA

Capillary
A lesion composed of capillary blood vessels.

Cavernous
A lesion composed of cavernous, endothelial-lined spaces.

Sclerosing
Produced as a result of fibrosis or sclerosis of a capillary haemangioma; a predominantly fibrous nodule containing iron pigment remains.

GLOMUS TUMOUR — GLOMANGIOMA

Nature
Rare tumours arising from the cells of the glomus organ.

The Glomus Organ
This is a convoluted arteriovenous anastomosis with modified muscle cells – glomus cells, in the walls, which have a cuboidal epithelial-like appearance. The glomus organ is richly supplied with nerves and is believed to be responsible for temperature regulation by modifying the calibre of the vessels and thus blood flow through the area. The glomus organs are situated predominantly in the peripheral parts of the limbs, but also are widely distributed throughout many viscera.

Age
Usually present in adult life and only very rarely in children.

Sites
Periphery of the limbs, especially the fingers, but rarely elsewhere.

Macroscopical
Painful red or purple tumours on the fingers usually less than 2 cm dia.

Microscopical
Multiple, small, vascular spaces surrounded by sheets of uniform glomus cells; special stains reveal a profuse nerve supply to the tumour, which possibly accounts for the pain.

Results
Local excision is curative and the pain disappears; the tumours are benign.

HAEMANGIOPERICYTOMA

This is a very rare tumour occurring in relation to a blood vessel which appears to be a variant of the glomus tumour, being derived from the haemangiopericytes. These are contractile cells in close relation to capillary walls. They form well-defined tumours in the limbs, mediastinum, retroperitoneal tissues or elsewhere and are composed of multiple vascular spaces surrounded by the plump polyhedral pericytes. Though formerly regarded as benign, it is now quite clear that these can be malignant tumours though the course is variably prolonged.

ANGIOSARCOMA

A rare but true tumour of endothelial origin composed of highly atypical vasoformative tissue.

The tumour invades locally and commonly metastasizes widely (see p. 155).

LYMPHANGIOMA

These are almost identical to the haemangiomas in type and structure but the lumen contains lymph.

Simple or capillary
Masses of small lymphatic channels.

Cavernous
Cavernous lymph spaces, rare but most common in the spleen.

Cystic
Results in a 'cystic hygroma'.

LYMPHANGIOSARCOMA

This malignant tumour is very rare and almost exclusively arises in areas of lymphoedema, the neoplasm being derived from the endothelium of the dilated lymphatics.

Chapter 54
Connective Tissue Diseases

Introduction

A group of diseases of connective tissues affecting many organs and systems and predominantly, but not exclusively, showing changes in collagen. Because of this feature the diseases were, until recently, known as 'collagen diseases', on the basis that the commonest features shown were mucoid degeneration, fibrinoid necrosis and hyalinization of collagen. However, a wider appreciation of the diseases included in this group and their natural history and systemic lesions has indicated that the term used now is more applicable.

Aetiology

It is by no means certain that this is a homogenous group of diseases and it should not necessarily be inferred that they all have identical aetiologies. There is considerable evidence to support the view that some or all arise as immunological disorders largely on the basis of demonstrable antibodies in patients. Experimental reproduction of the diseases has proved difficult however, and proof of an auto-immune origin is still lacking.

It should be further understood that, although in many cases the connective tissue diseases are divisible into clear-cut clinical entities, there is considerable overlap, with a minority of patients showing features of more than one disease of the group.

Systemic lupus erythematosus – S.L.E.

Incidence

At one time uncommon, the disease is now diagnosed more frequently. This is probably a real increase but possibly only apparent, due to improved diagnostic tests and increased awareness of the condition.

Aetiological factors

1 *Genetic.* Definite predisposition in relatives. There is a high incidence – 33 per cent, of tissue antigen HL-A8 and also increase in antigen W15.
2 *Auto-antibodies.* Several types of anti-nuclear antibody are found in most cases (ANA). These are nearly all anti-DNA but are neither organ nor species-specific.
3 *Virus infection.* There is a remarkable resemblance to the probable virus infection of the auto-immune disease of NZB mice.
4 *Drug-induced.* Substances implicated include, hydralazine, anti-convulsants, some antibiotics and reserpine.

Sex
Predominantly females.

Age
Twenty to forty years.

Organ changes

1 *Serous membranes.* Acute, subacute or chronic pericarditis, pleurisy and peritonitis occur in 70 per cent. It may be generalized or focal with, in the acute stages, a slight fibrinous exudate overlying areas of mucoid or fibrinoid degeneration in the submesothelial connective tissue. The end result is healing with slight scarring and adhesions.
2 *Heart.* Non-bacterial verrucous endocarditis – Libman–Sacks endocarditis, with vegetations on the mitral and tricuspid valves in 50 per cent or more of the cases (see p. 247). Lesions may also occur in the myocardial interstitial tissue in up to 30 per cent.
3 *Kidney.* Involved in most cases with variable appearances which are described on p. 358.
4 *Blood vessels.* In most cases, blood vessels in various organs, but particularly in the kidney and the spleen, show acute necrotizing arteritis and arteriolitis with fibrinoid necrosis and marked surrounding inflammatory cell reaction. At a later stage, thrombosis occurs and is followed by healing and organization of the thrombus. Ischaemic changes may result.
5 *Skin.* Eighty per cent have a skin rash which is classically of 'butterfly' distribution on the face around the bridge of the nose and is of erythematous maculo-papular type. Sometimes the rash is more generalized (see p. 726). About 5 per cent of patients with chronic discoid lupus erythematosus may eventually progress to the systemic disease.
6 *Joints, muscles and tendons.* Commonly involved with an atypical rheumatoid clinical picture and seldom with any great degree of deformity.
7 *Blood.* Eighty per cent of cases show the characteristic 'L.E. phenomenon' (see p. 510). Suitably prepared specimens of bone marrow or peripheral blood show the presence of 'L.E. cells' which are polymorphs with engulfed, large, basophilic, haematoxylin-staining masses. These are identical with '*haematoxyphil bodies*', characteristically seen in cells of many tissues affected by the disease process. 'False' positives occur in a few cases of chronic discoid lupus erythematosus, rheumatoid arthritis, scleroderma, dermatomyositis, hepatitis and some examples of drug sensitivity, e.g. to penicillin. A false positive Wasserman reaction occurs in a few cases.

Microscopical

The affected organs and tissues show changes which comprise mucoid degeneration, fibrinoid degeneration and necrosis, acute vasculitis and collagenous fibrosis and hyalinization. Inflammatory cell reaction is usually slight but the presence of haematoxyphil bodies is diagnostic.

Clinical

An insidious onset with a protracted course and exacerbations and remissions. Irregular fever is often present together with muscle and joint pain and swelling and a skin rash. Effusions into serous cavities, cardiac murmurs, albuminuria and haematuria, weight loss and prostration denote severe organ involvement.

Diagnosis

1 Blood
(a) L.E. cell test – positive.
(b) Anti-nuclear antibodies (ANA). Nearly all cases show a diffuse homogeneous or peripheral ring pattern of indirect immunofluorescence. DNA-binding levels are more specific and can be used, with complement levels in the blood, to monitor progress. Cases with renal involvement usually have particularly high anti-DNA titres.
(c) Proteins – γ-globulin raised.
(d) A normochromic anaemia and neutropenia.
(e) Very high sedimentation rate.
2 *Biopsy. Kidney or skin rash*. Immunofluorescent coarse granular deposits of IgG or sometimes IgA or IgM can be consistently demonstrated at the dermal–epidermal junction in skin lesions and also in light-exposed areas of normal skin.

Prognosis

Remittent but progressive deterioration with death in severe untreated cases in 2–5 years from:
1 Cardiac involvement and congestive heart failure.
2 Renal involvement and renal failure.
3 Intercurrent infection.
   The progress of the disease may be arrested by administration of corticosteroids and the ultimate prognosis is markedly improved.

Polyarteritis nodosa

Nature

A subacute or chronic, remittent, disseminated, vascular disease, characterized by focal necrotizing inflammation of the walls of arteries.

Incidence

Uncommon and apparently decreasing.

Age

Twenty to sixty years.

Sex

M:F 3:1.

Aetiological factors

1 There is no real evidence of an auto-immune origin and antibodies are usually not found. Clinical and experimental evidence points to a hypersensitivity reaction to external antigens either microbiological or chemical. These may be initiating factors which are possibly subsequently perpetuated by an immune reaction. Agents implicated include the sulphonamides, penicillin and streptococci.
2 Some cases follow longstanding rheumatoid arthritis.
3 Hepatitis B antigen – HB$_s$Ag is found in as many as 50 per cent of cases.

Macroscopical

The distribution of the lesions is very variable but any artery of medium or small size or any arteriole in any organ or system may be affected: Kidneys 80 per cent; heart 70 per cent; liver 65 per cent; gastro-intestinal tract 50 per cent.

   Less commonly, the pancreas, lung, voluntary muscle, C.N.S. and peripheral nerves may be involved. There is a random distribution in sharply localized segments of the vessels and the lesions may also be asymmetrical. The gross appearances may be inapparent or minimal, but in marked cases the affected vessels have nodular swellings along their course with aneurysmal dilatations.

   Petechial haemorrhages or haematomas from rupture, intravascular thromboses and infarcts or areas of ischaemic atrophy are also commonly seen (see p. 235).

Microscopical

STAGES
1 Mucoid degeneration and fibrinoid necrosis, starting in the media and extending usually to the other layers. This necrosis may affect only part of

the circumference of the vessel and there is oedema of the wall.

2 Intense polymorph infiltration of all coats in which eosinophils are commonly prominent.

The elastic tissue of the vessel is destroyed and there is marked narrowing of the lumen, often with thrombosis.

3 Fibroblastic proliferation with subsidence of the inflammatory cell infiltrate leaving lymphocytes and plasma cells but only scanty polymorphs. Organization of the damaged wall and any contained thrombus follows.

4 Fibrous healing with disappearance of all the inflammatory cells, muscle and elastic tissue, so that the wall becomes weakened and predisposes to aneurysm formation.

All vessels are not synchronously involved and therefore all these different stages may be seen in an affected organ at the same time.

Clinical
The picture is varied. Most characteristically, general symptoms with an acute, subacute or insidious onset of low-grade fever, weakness, malaise, associated with a leucocytosis and with evidence of concomitant involvement of several systems, particularly the kidney, gastro-intestinal tract and C.N.S. Hypertension is usually present.

Diagnosis
1 *Blood.* Leucocytosis, often with an eosinophilia and a high E.S.R.
2 *Biopsy.* This is the only certain way of making a diagnosis but, due to the random distribution of the lesions, a negative biopsy does not exclude the diagnosis. The best sites for biopsy are muscle, particularly from areas of tenderness or swelling, and from the kidney.
3 *Antibody tests.* Are inevitably negative.

Prognosis
The original concept of the disease was widespread and inevitably progressive to a fatal termination in about 5 years has required modification. Some cases appear localized and self-limiting and treatment with corticosteroids and/or immunosuppressive drugs, e.g. azathioprine, commonly produces dramatic clinical remission and may considerably alter the eventual prognosis. Where there is evidence of generalized disease, death is due to renal or cardiac failure or to haemorrhage from rupture of an aneurysm. Evidence of renal involvement is the most serious prognostic feature.

OTHER TYPES OF NECROTIZING ARTERITIS

1 Wegener's granulomatosis (see p. 640).
2 Allergic granulomatosis
3 Other forms of arteritis
(*a*) Giant cell arteritis (see p. 264).
(*b*) Takayasu's disease (see p. 265).
4 Arteritis in other diseases
(*a*) Rheumatic fever (see p. 243).
(*b*) Rheumatoid arthritis (see p. 708).
(*c*) S.L.E. (see p. 281).
(*d*) Serum sickness (see p. 285).
(*e*) Accelerated hypertension (see p. 263).

Scleroderma – progressive systemic sclerosis

Nature
An insidious chronic disorder characterized by progressive fibrosis of skin and subcutaneous tissues and frequently with subsequent involvement of internal organs – hence progressive systemic sclerosis.

Incidence
Uncommon.

Age
Thirty to fifty years.

Sex
M:F 1:2.

Aetiology
Unknown but some support for an immune basis:
1 Anti-erythrocyte antibodies are sometimes found.
2 Some cases show complement-fixing antibodies.
3 Speckled type of antinuclear antibody in low titre in 80 per cent. Rheumatoid factor positive in 30 per cent.
4 There is some evidence that fibrin deposition and diminished fibrinolysis may be implicated.

Organ changes

1 *Skin.* Most cases show widespread involvement of skin and subsequently the viscera, but occasionally the disease remains localized to areas of skin and there is no visceral involvement – *scleroderma circumscripta*.

Stages
(a) Thickened, oedematous, 'doughy' areas.
(b) Thickening, with induration and adhesion of the epidermis to subcutaneous structures.
(c) Atrophy of the skin, dense adhesions and loss of subcutaneous fat and elasticity.

Later
(d) The fingers become clawed and tapered with limitation of movements of these and other joints, e.g. jaw opening is often considerably restricted. Flexion contractures may develop.
(e) Alterations in pigmentation with loss in some areas and excess in others.
(f) Ulceration, particularly of the fingers. The disease may be associated with a Raynaud's phenomenon, i.e. arterial spasm.

2 *Other organs.* Muscles, heart, oesophagus, intestine, kidneys, lungs and blood vessels may show areas of fibrosis with stricture formation in the hollow viscera and a 'honeycomb' appearance in the lung (see p. 673).

Microscopical

1 *Skin*
(a) Mucoid degeneration–fibrinoid necrosis is seldom prominent but there is a scanty inflammatory cell infiltrate.
(b) Increased collagenization, with progressive atrophy of fat and of special structures, e.g. the sebaceous glands and hair follicles.
(c) Complete collagenization with loss of adnexae and encroachment on neighbouring structures. Epidermal atrophy follows (see p. 726).
2 *Other organs.* Patchy fibrosing changes of a similar type occur.
3 *Blood vessels.* A very characteristic intimal mucoid fibrous thickening is seen in arteries, particularly in the kidneys. The lumen is very greatly reduced and there is marked increase of elastic tissue in the media. Secondary ischaemic changes follow at affected sites.

Clinical

An insidious onset involving the skin of the face, neck, extremities and trunk; this may remain localized or more commonly extends to involve large areas of the skin surface. There is impairment of chewing and swallowing, marked loss of strength and limitation of muscular activity. Joint movements become restricted and signs of generalized involvement follow, usually many years later.

Diagnosis

Biopsy of skin.

Prognosis

Although disabilities and deformities occur, it is uncommonly a primary cause of death. In only 5–10 per cent is death due to the disease, from cardiac or pulmonary involvement or rarely from intestinal or renal manifestations.

Dermatomyositis

Nature

An acute, subacute or chronic disease affecting skin and skeletal muscles, usually symmetrically.

Incidence

Rare.

Age

Thirty to fifty years.

Sex

M : F equal.

Aetiological factors

About 25 per cent are associated with the presence of an underlying visceral tumour which may be occult. Anti-nuclear antibodies are only present, in low titre, in about 30 per cent of cases. Clear evidence of an immunologically mediated basis is lacking.

Appearances

1 *Muscle.* Pale and of firm consistency but later flabby and atrophic. There is swelling of the muscle cells with coagulative necrosis and degeneration accompanied by oedema and mucoid and fibrinoid degeneration of the interstitial connective tissue. Considerable diffuse lymphocytic and plasma cell infiltration occurs throughout the muscle (see p. 590).
2 *Skin.* The most prominent feature is perivascu-

lar lymphocyte and plasma cell infiltration in the dermis and subcutaneous tissues with a slight mucoid or fibrinoid degeneration of the dermis.

3 *Other organs.* Uncommonly involved. Changes in the heart may occur similar to those in voluntary muscle but this is rare. The serosal membranes may be inflamed and subsequently become fibrous and adherent.

Clinical
There is often a rather acute onset with fever, malaise, marked weakness and pain, swelling and tenderness of muscles. The most common muscles involved are those of the proximal regions of the extremities, especially the upper arm, shoulder, girdle, neck and upper thighs. The involvement is usually symmetrical. Loss of activity occurs so that contractures may develop.

Raynaud's phenomenon is associated in about 30 per cent.

Diagnosis
Muscle biopsy may be helpful but is not always diagnostic. Muscle enzymes – serum creatine phosphokinase and aldolase, are usually markedly raised.

Prognosis
This is unfavourable. When the onset is acute, there is a rapidly progressive course with death in a few months. In the more chronic types, there are periods of remission which may be permanent. However, 50 per cent of all cases are dead within 2 years of diagnosis.

Serum sickness

Nature
An acute, self-limiting disorder, subsiding promptly with or without treatment.

Aetiology
An hypersensitivity reaction to foreign protein, e.g. antisera (see p. 100).

Clinical
The intensity varies with the degree of sensitization. When extreme, it may be fatal within a few hours or be delayed 8–12 days after the administration of the foreign substance.

Age
Any age.

Appearances
Only a few fatal cases have been fully studied. There is mucoid and fibrinoid degeneration of collagen, particularly in the heart, blood vessels and kidneys, but any organ may show these changes.

Prognosis
Only a very small number die. The majority of the survivors show complete clinical recovery.

Rheumatoid arthritis

Nature
A chronic inflammatory systemic disease of connective tissues, predominantly affecting joints, but frequently involving many other sites.

Incidence
A common disease of worldwide distribution but most frequently occurring in temperate climates.

Age
Twenty to forty-five years.

Sex
M:F 1:3.

Aetiology
Unknown, but considerable evidence points to an immunological disorder, probably auto-immune but possibly requiring additional initiating factors.
1 *Microbiological agents.* Many differing bacteria and viruses have been implicated from time to time but supportive evidence is unconvincing.
2 *Endocrine factors.* There is a marked predisposition for females in whom the disease may remit clinically most dramatically if they become pregnant.
3 *Genetic.* Relatives show a considerably increased risk of developing the disease and serum rheumatoid factors are found in relatives in a significantly higher proportion than in controls.
4 *Immunological*
(*a*) Known hypersensitivity reactions, e.g. serum sickness, show clinical and histological features of similarity.
(*b*) Experimental injection of foreign fibrin produces very similar lesions in animals and in a

few instances the same appearances have been produced by the animals' own fibrin.

(*c*) Antibodies against IgG are present in the serum in 95 per cent of patients although these produce no effects if given to normal individuals and high titres may persist long after the disease has become clinically dormant. Moreover, rheumatoid factors have no effect on synovial cells in tissue culture. However, the factors are present in cells in synovium of affected joints and in plasma cells.

(*d*) Both type B and type T lymphocytes are present in rheumatoid lesions.

Organ changes

1 *Joints*. The polyarticular lesions are described on p. 708, and the spine lesions of the allied ankylosing spondylitis on p. 716.

2 *Skin*. Rheumatoid nodules. Areas of fibrinoid necrosis of dermal collagen surrounded by a palisade of fibroblasts and histiocytes.

3 *Muscle*. Foci of inflammation and degeneration of the interstitial tissue with degenerative changes in adjacent muscle fibres and a focal mononuclear cell infiltration – *polymyositis* (see p. 589).

4 *Heart*. Many cases show focal Aschoff nodes similar in appearances to those of rheumatic fever (see p. 242). More common, however, is a more diffuse inflammatory reaction and interstitial fibrosis associated with areas of fibrinoid necrosis.

5 *Lymphoid tissue*. There may be enlargment of lymphoid tissue with focal areas of collagen necrosis and reactive hyperplasia. This may produce lymphadenopathy or splenomegaly – *Felty's syndrome* or *Still's disease* in children.

6 *Blood vessels*. The aorta, particularly the ascending part, may show medial degeneration and inflammatory cell infiltration which is most marked around the vasa vasorum – *rheumatoid aortitis* (see p. 265).

7 *Lung*. Foci of collagen degeneration with subsequent fibrosis – Caplan's syndrome or rheumatoid lung (see p. 673).

Complications

Although the joint disease is clinically dominant, some cases may develop:

1 *Amyloidosis*. Not uncommon in longstanding and severely affected cases.

2 *Polyarteritis nodosa*. This may develop after many years, particularly in younger individuals (see p. 282).

3 *Systemic lupus erythematosus*. Some cases of typical rheumatoid arthritis subsequently develop all the classical features and findings of S.L.E. (see p. 281).

4 *Aortic incompetence or aneurysm*. Due to the aortic lesion.

Prognosis

In the absence of the complicating factors described above, which occur in only a small proportion of cases, the disease eventually 'burns out' after some years leaving disability and deformity. There is usually no significant interference with the normal life span of these patients

Diagnosis

1 *Blood*

(*a*) Mild or moderate normochromic or hypochromic anaemia with a high E.S.R.

(*b*) R.A. factors: Rheumatoid factor is present in 90 per cent of cases and is an IgM active against IgG.

   (i) Rose–Waaler test – differential agglutination of sheep red cells sensitized by coating with rabbit anti-sheep antibody. Positive at a titre of 16 or over in 95 per cent of cases.

   (ii) Latex tests – a more sensitive and easily performed but less specific test using latex particles coated with human γ-globulin. False positives occur in cases of syphilis, sarcoidosis, viral hepatitis and 3 per cent of normal population. In these the Rose–Waaler is negative. Occasional false negatives in 'non-joint' type of disease.

   (iii) Anti-nuclear antibody – ANA. This is positive in 15 per cent of cases of RA with nodules.

2 *Biopsy*. Usually of a skin nodule or of the synovium which may show characteristic changes.

Rheumatic fever

This has been considered on p. 241.

Polymyalgia rheumatica

A disorder of middle-aged and elderly with diffuse and generally symmetrical muscle pain and stiffness in the absence of weakness and wasting. The

E.S.R. is raised, but muscle enzymes and biopsy are normal. Some cases have associated giant cell arteritis (see p. 264). The condition usually responds dramatically to low-dosage corticosteroid therapy.

Mixed connective tissue disease

There is clearly considerable overlap between a number of the diseases of connective tissues. In some cases there is evidence of progression from one clear-cut type to another.

Other instances can be identified where, from the beginning the disorder was of 'mixed' features.

Under this heading groups of patients have been described with arthralgia, swelling of hands, Raynaud's phenomenon, lymphadenopathy, myositis and abnormal oesophageal motility. Consistently present are high-titre speckled ANA antibodies with an RNA component.

Though many of the features are of systemic sclerosis there is a good response to corticosteroid therapy.

This concept is not as yet universally acceptable.

Other connective tissue diseases

HENOCH – SCHÖNLEIN PURPURA

In this hypersensitivity disorder, capillaries, particularly of the skin, gastro-intestinal tract and kidneys, show necrosis and inflammatory changes (see p. 361).

HYPERSENSITIVITY ANGIITIS

A rare disorder clinically related to sera, drugs, etc., and which may affect many organs, particularly the kidneys and heart. Affected organs show necrotizing inflammation of arteries and veins. The involvement of veins is an important factor of differentiation from polyarteritis nodosa.

WEGENER'S GRANULOMATOSIS

This rare, giant cell granulomatous disorder with necrotic vessels predominantly affects nose and lung often with a complicating severe renal glomerular lesion (see p. 640).

THROMBOTIC MICROANGIOPATHY – THROMBOTIC THROMBOCYTOPENIC PURPURA

A condition in which capillaries are plugged by structureless material with necrosis of their walls in the absence of any inflammatory reaction. Platelets are consumed in the thrombotic process leading to haemorrhage.

Rather than a connective tissue disease, the condition is better identified as *disseminated intravascular coagulation – D.I.C.* It is probably pathogenetically related to the Shwartzman reaction in experimental animals and is considered in more detail on p. 531.

Chapter 55
Diseases of the Endocrine Glands – Adrenals

Each adrenal is composed of two structurally, functionally and embryologically distinct parts: cortex and medulla. The combined normal weight of the adrenals is 12–14 g.

CORTEX

Of mesodermal origin from the urogenital ridge. It is composed of three zones (Fig. 33).

1 *Outer – glomerulosa.* Small nests of cells.
2 *Intermediate – fasciculata.* Parallel cords of cells.
3 *Inner – reticularis.* Interlacing cords.
The cells are similar in appearance, having a polygonal shape with a foamy cytoplasm containing large amounts of lipid which imparts the yellow colour to the cortex.

MEDULLA

The brown central portion of the gland derived from neuroectoderm, which is composed of small clusters of large chromaffin cells, nerve fibres, sympathetic ganglion cells and supporting tissue.

HORMONES

Cortex

GLUCOCORTICOIDS
Mostly produced in the zona fasciculata. The most important glucocorticoid is hydrocortisone which:
1 Stimulates gluconeogenesis from protein.
2 Inhibits peripheral utilization of glucose.
3 Antagonizes some actions of insulin.
In addition to these effects on carbohydrate metabolism, the glucocorticoids have some mineralocorticoid action and also cause:
4 Involution of lymphoid tissue and a fall in blood lymphocytes.
5 Reduction of the blood eosinophil count.
6 Suppression of some aspects of the inflammatory response, and of fibroblastic activity.
  They also interfere with antigen–antibody reactions:
7 By suppressing protein synthesis in tissues other than the liver.
8 By suppressing ACTH secretion by the pituitary.

MINERALOCORTICOIDS
Mainly formed in the zona glomerulosa. The most potent mineralocorticoid is aldosterone which:

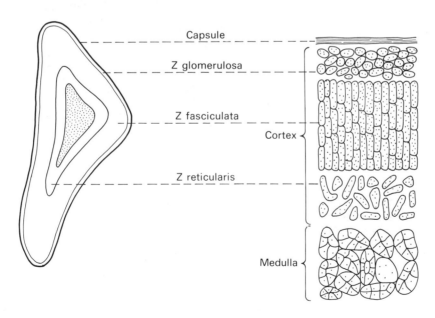

Fig. 33. Adrenal gland structure.

1   Increases sodium reabsorption by the renal tubules.
2   Increases renal potassium excretion.
3   Decreases sodium loss at other sites, e.g. sweat, bowel.

SEX HORMONES

Produced in the zona reticularis. They are mostly androgens with smaller amounts of oestrogen. Adrenal sex hormones are probably responsible for most of the early changes of puberty.

Medulla

Produces adrenaline and noradrenaline in the proportion of approximately 4 : 1. It may also produce neurotransmitter peptides such as enkephalins.

ADRENALINE

By stimulating both α and β adrenergic receptors, it increases cardiac output but has a less marked effect than noradrenaline on peripheral arteriolar resistance. It increases glycogenesis, increases the metabolic rate and causes bronchodilatation.

NORADRENALINE

Stimulates predominantly α adrenergic receptors causing vasoconstriction and increased blood pressure.

Cortical hypofunction

PRIMARY

Nature

As a result of necrosis, replacement or atrophy of adrenal cortical tissue, inadequate amounts of adrenal cortical hormones are produced, thus limiting the ability to resist stressful stimuli.

Causes

1   Addison's disease:
(a) Atrophy – idiopathic or autoimmune – 80 per cent.
(b) Tuberculosis – 20 per cent.
2   Metastatic carcinoma.
3   Previous adrenalectomy.
4   Treatment with adrenolytic drugs, e.g. ortho-para-DDD (opDDD, mitotane).
5   Haemochromatosis, and other infiltrations.
6   Infections – particularly in children with meningococcal septicaemia (Waterhouse–Friderichsen syndrome), influenza, diphtheria.

7   Haemorrhage – traumatic, haemorrhagic diatheses including anti-coagulant therapy.
8   Burns.
9   Abrupt withdrawal from longstanding corticosteroid therapy.

Adrenal

Appearance depends on the cause, with glands either atrophied or replaced by other tissue. Haemorrhages commence in the medulla with little or no inflammatory reaction.

CHRONIC CORTICAL HYPOFUNCTION – ADDISON'S DISEASE

Nature

The destruction of the adrenal cortices in Addison's disease may proceed over months or years. The symptoms and signs are equally insidious and only become marked when crisis is imminent.

Effects

1   Pigmentation. Due to increased secretion of ACTH and related peptides by the pituitary, in response to decreased negative feedback by corticosteroids.
2   Hyponatraemia with hyperkalaemia.
3   Decreased plasma volume with raised blood urea and postural hypotension.
4   Eosinophilia.
5   Hypoglycaemia.

Incidence

Rare.

Age

Any age, but usually early adult life.

Adrenal

Atrophied with variable lymphocytic infiltration. In tuberculous cases replaced by caseous and partly calcified material.

Other organs

Skin pigmentation affecting particularly exposed and pressure areas, scars, finger nails, palmar creases and buccal mucosa. Slight lymphadenopathy with enlargement of the thymus. Wasting and atrophic changes are found in many other organs.

Results

Replacement therapy with glucocorticoids (hydrocortisone or cortisone acetate) and mineralocorticoids (fludrocortisone) must be maintained indefinitely.

ACUTE CORTICAL HYPOFUNCTION – ADDISONIAN CRISIS

May occur spontaneously or in patients with preexisting Addison's disease. The predominant clinical feature is of hypotensive shock although any of the features of chronic cortical hypofunction (see above), and also low grade fever may be present.

Treatment

Urgent administration of intravenous saline and commencement of corticosteroid substitution therapy is life-saving.

SECONDARY

Nature

Adrenal atrophy may be caused by chronically inadequate secretion of ACTH. This may result from hypothalamic or pituitary tumours, or may be iatrogenic – following destructive treatment to the pituitary, or treatment with drugs such as corticosteroids which suppress ACTH secretion.

Effects

Are those of primary adrenal atrophy, although pigmentation does not occur and the tendency to hyponatraemia and hyperkalaemia may be less.

Results

Substitution therapy with glucocorticoids alone is required since the zona glomerulosa is independent of ACTH stimulation.

Medullary hypofunction

Removal or destruction of the adrenal medulla produces no functional disturbance.

Cortical hyperfunction

Over production of hormones may result from excessive stimulation by the trophic hormones, ACTH and renin, or it may result from autonomously functioning adrenal tumours.

GLUCOCORTICOID EXCESS – CUSHING'S SYNDROME

Causes

1 Adrenal adenoma or carcinoma – commonest cause of Cushing's syndrome in children.
2 Adrenal hyperplasia secondary to excessive secretion of ACTH by the pituitary gland (Cushing's disease).
3 Adrenal hyperplasia secondary to excessive secretion of ACTH by a non-pituitary source (ectopic ACTH syndrome).
4 ACTH or corticosteroid therapy.
5 Alcohol-induced pseudo-Cushing's syndrome.

Effects

The effects of sustained elevation of glucocorticoid secretion are:
1 Central obesity and moon face.
2 Muscle wasting and weakness.
3 Osteoporosis – may cause collapse of vertebrae, rib fractures (see p. 692).
4 Atrophy of skin and dermis – paper thin skin with bruising tendency, purple striae.
5 Impaired glucose tolerance.
6 Relative polycythaemia – lowered plasma volume results in high haemoglobin concentration.
7 Hypertension.
8 Ankle swelling.
9 Hirsutism.
10 Menstrual disorders.
11 Hypokalaemia – especially in the ectopic ACTH syndrome.
12 Pigmentation – may occur, but only if plasma ACTH levels are elevated.

Adrenal

In the overactive gland there is increase in the *Zona fasciculata* and to a lesser extent the *Z. reticularis*. (For adrenal tumours see p. 294.)

Pituitary

In Cushing's syndrome irrespective of aetiology, areas of the pituitary are replaced by pink, hyaline material (Crookes' hyaline change). In pituitary dependent Cushing's disease there may be a small adenoma (microadenoma) – large tumours are uncommon. Immunofluorescent or peroxidase techniques may show increased pituitary content of ACTH, β-lipotrophin, endorphins and related peptides, sometimes with increased prolactin.

Ectopic ACTH syndrome
Benign or malignant non-pituitary tumours may secrete sufficient ACTH to cause Cushing's syndrome. Those most commonly involved are:
1   Oat cell carcinoma of the lung.
2   Carcinoid tumour of foregut origin – situated in thymus, thyroid, lung, upper intestine, pancreas (see p. 212).
3   Adrenal medullary tumours.
4   Ovarian and other tumours – rarely.

Results
The prognosis in untreated Cushing's syndrome is poor. The object of treatment is:
1   To lower elevated plasma cortisol – by bilateral adrenalectomy or with enzyme blocking drugs such as metyrapone.
2   Treatment of the cause.

MINERALOCORTICOID EXCESS

Causes
1   Primary hyperaldosteronism – Conn's syndrome, due to single or multiple adenomas of the *Zona glomerulosa*, with or without surrounding glomerulosa hyperplasia.
2   Secondary hyperaldosteronism:
(a) Renin-secreting tumours – rare.
(b) Conditions associated with secondary hyper-reninaemia: congestive cardiac failure, cirrhosis with ascites, renal disease.

Effects
1   Hypertension – in primary type only, which is usually severe.
2   Hypokalaemia – usually marked in Conn's syndrome. Associated with alkalosis and muscle weakness.
3   Sodium at the upper limit of normal, or slightly raised.
4   Raised plasma aldosterone with, in Conn's syndrome, suppressed plasma renin.

Results
Tumours are rarely, if ever, malignant and hyperaldosteronism is cured by their removal. Hyperten-

sion may persist if arteriolar changes and renal damage have already occurred. The aldosterone antagonist, spironolactone, may be used.

SEX HORMONE EXCESS

Virilization may occur as a result of excessive androgen production in women with Cushing's syndrome. Purely virilizing and feminizing (in men) tumours are exceedingly rare. Most cases of virilization and of feminization occur as part of mixed syndromes (see below).

Effects of excessive androgens
1   *Males*. Boys will pass through a phase of rapid growth with well developed muscles, increasing body hair and with enlargement and maturation of the penis and scrotum (precocious pseudopuberty). As a result of early epiphyseal fusion, growth ceases early and final adult height is stunted. Testes remain pre-pubertal. In adult men the effects of increased androgens would probably not be detected.
2   *Females*. Girls pass through a phase of rapid growth with muscular 'tom-boy' development. Final adult height will be stunted. Body hair will be male in pattern with frontal balding, facial hair, chest, shoulder and abdominal hair, hair on the thighs and increased hair growth on forearms, lower legs and digits. Breast development may be normal, although menstruation is absent or infrequent. There may be clitoromegaly and acne. The voice may deepen.

Effects of excessive oestrogens
1   *Males*. Gynaecomastia may occur in adults or children. Although this may rarely be the result of an adrenal tumour, most cases of gynaecomastia are of uncertain aetiology (see p. 231).
2   *Females*. The effect of increased oestrogens are usually those of menstrual irregularity, with menorrhagia and breakthrough menstrual bleeding.

MIXED SYNDROMES

CONGENITAL ADRENAL HYPERPLASIA

A rare inborn autosomal recessive enzyme deficiency resulting in deficiency of glucocorticoids, with or without deficiency of mineralocorticoids – 'salt-losing' type. The tendency to low plasma cortisol leads to raised ACTH. This in turn causes adrenal hypertrophy and excessive production of androgens.

Effects
See effects of androgens, above.
1 Rapid growth in children but premature epiphyseal fusion.
2 Precocious pseudopuberty in boys.
3 Masculinization of girls with delayed or absent menstruation.
4 Pseudohermaphroditism of genetically female infants (see p. 409).

Adrenal
Both adrenals are hyperplastic.

Results
Replacement with glucocorticoids, and mineralocorticoids if necessary, results in normal development although external genitalia may require corrective surgery in girls.

POLYCYSTIC OVARY SYNDROME – STEIN–LEVENTHAL SYNDROME

Variants of this complex adrenal-ovarian disorder are common in women. Increased secretion of androgens occurs from the adrenal or ovary or both, with increased peripheral conversion of androgens to oestrogens.

Effects
1 Menstrual irregularity.
2 Infertility.
3 Mild virilization.
4 Acne.
5 Occasional galactorrhoea.

Adrenal
The adrenal is histologically normal.

Ovary
In any condition associated with increased serum levels of androgens, multiple small follicular cysts develop beneath a thickened white ovarian capsule.

Medullary hyperfunction

PHAEOCHROMOCYTOMA

Incidence
Rare.

Age
Any age, but commonly young adults.

Macroscopical
Usually well encapsulated, unilateral, red-brown or haemorrhagic tumours arising in the centre of the adrenal gland. They are bilateral in 10 per cent and may very rarely arise outside the adrenal, in the carotid body, the organ of Zuckerkandl, etc., in which sites they are also hormonally active. Tumours may reach 5–6 cm in diameter. They become dark brown in colour when fixed in bichromate solutions.

Microscopical
Nests of cells resembling the normal adrenal medullary chromaffin cells.

Effects
Those of hypersecretion of catecholamines:
1 Hypertension – this is usually intermittent but is sometimes sustained (see p. 268).
2 Hypermetabolism.
3 Hyperglycaemia.

Results
Most of the tumours are histologically and clinically benign and the hypertension is usually relieved following their removal. Five per cent are malignant, metastasizing to the other adrenal and to lymph nodes, lungs, liver and bone. Occasionally phaeochromocytomas occur as part of multiple endocrine adenomatoses, especially associated with medullary (calcitonin-secreting) carcinoma of the thyroid (see p. 315). In von Recklinghausen's disease, phaeochromocytoma or medullary carcinoma of the thyroid may be associated with multiple cutaneous neurofibromata (see p. 620).

Tests of adrenal function

The details given below are meant only as a simple guide. In each case the need for a test, and its subsequent interpretation, are dependent on the clinical circumstances.

CORTICAL HYPOFUNCTION – ADDISON'S DISEASE

1 Hyponatraemia, hyperkalaemia and raised blood urea.
2 Occasional eosinophilia.
3 Plasma cortisol may be normal but is diagnostic if less than 220 nmol/l at 9 a.m., or in the stressed patient.
4 Plasma ACTH and β-lipotrophin are grossly elevated.
5 Synacthen test – absent or diminished rise in plasma cortisol following administration of a synthetic analogue of ACTH – *Synacthen*.

CORTICAL HYPERFUNCTION – CUSHING'S SYNDROME

Diagnosis
1 Loss of circadian rhythm in ACTH and/or cortisol.
2 Elevated 24-hr urinary excretion of cortisol and metabolites.
3 Overnight, or low-dose dexamethasone suppression tests.
4 Hypoglycaemia stress test – Insulin tolerance test-no rise in ACTH and/or cortisol.

Differential diagnosis
1 Plasma ACTH – suppressed in adrenal tumour.
2 High dose dexamethasone test – partial suppression in pituitary dependent disease, but not in adrenal tumour or ectopic ACTH syndrome.
3 Metyrapone test – exaggerated rise in cortisol precursors in pituitary dependent disease.
4 Hypokalaemia – if marked, usually indicates the ectopic ACTH syndrome.
5 Procedures, such as X-rays and isotope scans, to demonstrate directly the presence or absence of adrenal, pituitary or other tumours.

CONN'S SYNDROME

1 Hypokalaemia, with high normal or slightly elevated sodium.
2 Alkalosis.

3 Raised aldosterone levels, with suppressed renin.
4 Adrenal isotope scan.
5 Selective adrenal vein sampling for aldosterone.

CONGENITAL ADRENAL HYPERPLASIA

In the commonest form (21-hydroxylase deficiency) any of the following may be used to diagnose the condition and to monitor response to therapy:
1 Raised ACTH or β-lipotrophin.
2 Raised urinary 17 oxo- or oxogenic-steroids.
3 Raised urinary pregnanetriol.
4 Raised 17 hydroxyprogesterone in blood.
   Most agree, however, that the best way to monitor therapy in children is clinically, by documentation of growth rate.

MEDULLARY HYPERFUNCTION – PHAEOCHROMOCYTOMA

1 Estimation of excretion of catecholamines or their metabolites.
2 Effect on blood pressure of sympathetic blocking agents, such as phentolamine.
3 Demonstration of adrenal tumour, e.g. radiographically.
4 Selective adrenal vein sampling for catecholamines.

Tumours

CORTICAL ADENOMA

Incidence
Extremely common as an incidental finding in up to 30 per cent of all post-mortem examinations.

Macroscopical
Small, encapsulated, yellow nodules which are unilateral or bilateral, single or multiple.

Microscopical
The adenomas resemble the normal cortex although the zonal arrangements may be disorderly.

Effects

1 Inactive – the vast majority have no clinical effects.
2 Functional – these tumours are usually larger:
(a) Cushing's syndrome.
(b) Conn's syndrome.
(c) Virilization or feminization.

There are histological differences apparent between the adenomas found in the various syndromes but functional activity is not always predictable on histological appearances alone.

CORTICAL CARCINOMA

Incidence
Rare.

Age
All ages, but in children functional cortical carcinoma is the commonest cause of Cushing's syndrome.

Macroscopical
Globular, large, soft, lobulated, yellow tumours with a soft, haemorrhagic and necrotic cut surface. Adjacent organs, particularly the kidney, are commonly invaded. The tumour is bilateral in 10 per cent.

Microscopical
Very variable, from tumours showing a close resemblance to normal cortical cells to anaplastic types containing bizarre giant cells. The best guide to the malignancy of a functioning adrenal tumour is its size, not its microscopical appearance: those less than 40 g are benign, whereas those greater than 100 g are malignant in their behaviour.

Effects
1 Endocrine
(a) Inactive – the tumours have no functional activity.
(b) Functional – Cushing's syndrome, often with particularly marked tendency to virilization in females.
There are no differentiating histological features between these two groups.
2 Local. There is normally a large mass with invasion of neighbouring organs.

Spread
1 *Direct*. Kidney, posterior abdominal wall, diaphragm, liver, spleen, etc.
2 *Lymphatic*. Invaded regional lymph nodes are commonly seen by the time of diagnosis.
3 *Blood*. Spread to the other adrenal is common, as are metastases to the lungs, bone and brain.

Prognosis
Extremely poor; most are dead within 2 years and a 5-year survival is very uncommon.

MEDULLA

PHAEOCHROMOCYTOMA
See p. 293.

NEUROBLASTOMA

Nature
A tumour of neuroectodermal origin derived from neuroblasts, cells normally found in the intermediate stages of development of the sympathetic nervous system.

Age
Children are almost exclusively affected. The tumour is rare above the age of 5 years, but adult cases do very occasionally occur.

Incidence
Rare, although neuroblastoma is one of the commoner malignant tumours in children.

Sites
1 Adrenal medulla.
2 Mediastinum – posteriorly. Usually in the posterior mediastinum in relation to the sympathetic chain (see p. 586).
3 Coeliac plexus and other sites of autonomic nerve tissue within the abdomen.

Macroscopical
Bulky, fleshy, greyish-white masses which may be bilateral when arising in the adrenals. They attain a large size and obliterate the cortical tissue. On section they are soft, and often show areas of haemorrhage, necrosis and calcification.

Microscopical
The cells are small with hyperchromatic nuclei and

very little cytoplasm. They may be arranged in sheets or, more typically, in rosettes. Ganglion cells may sometimes be present – *ganglioneuroblastoma*. This tumour is thus intermediate between the differentiated ganglioneuroma and the undifferentiated neuroblastoma (see p. 621).

Spread

1   *Direct*. Early invasion of the adjacent organs and tissues.
2   *Lymphatic*. Regional lymph nodes are commonly invaded.
3   *Blood*. Occurs early and widely but with a particular predilection for bone, liver and the other adrenal.

Results

A highly malignant tumour which is usually inoperable. It is very radiosensitive but long-term results are poor.

GANGLIONEUROMA

Ten per cent of these tumours arise in the adrenal medulla (see p. 621).

Secondary tumours

The adrenal gland is a common site for carcinomatous metastases, especially from the bronchus and from the breast, but less commonly from other tumours. Only rarely do they cause hormonal insufficiency due to complete cortical destruction.

Chapter 56
Diseases of the Endocrine Glands – Pituitary

DEVELOPMENT

1   From the stomodeum – Rathke's pouch – to form the adenohypophysis – anterior pituitary.
2   From the brain – a downgrowth from the floor of the third ventricle to form the neurohypophysis – posterior pituitary.

Structure

This is illustrated in Fig. 34. Unlike the majority of mammals humans do not usually have a pars intermedia sandwiched between the anterior and posterior lobes. There is evidence, however, that a pars intermedia is present in the foetal pituitary, as well as in the pituitary of pregnant women.

ANTERIOR LOBE – ADENO-HYPOPHYSIS – PARS ANTERIOR

Anatomically divided (*a*) pars distalis (PD) and (*b*) pars tuberalis (PT) – surrounding the infundibular stem. The blood vessels of the pituitary stalk represent an extensive portal system carrying releasing and inhibitory factors down from the hypothalamus, as well as pituitary hormones up from the pituitary.

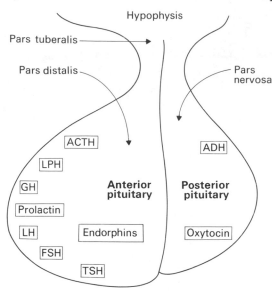

Fig. 34. Anatomical structure of pituitary gland.

Cell types

Formerly characterized on the basis of staining reaction (acidophil, 40 per cent; basophil, 10 per cent; chromophobe, 50 per cent). Now cells are more usually characterized on the basis of immuno-histochemistry and the specific hormones which they elaborate.

POSTERIOR LOBE – PARS NERVOSA – NEUROHYPOPHYSIS

The posterior lobe is connected to the hypothalamus by the supra-optico-hypophyseal and tubero-hypophyseal tracts. These fibres end in perivascular arborizations in all parts of the neurohypophysis.

Hormones

ANTERIOR LOBE

Hormones are synthesized in the pituitary and their release is controlled by hypothalamic releasing or inhibiting factors carried in the hypothalamo–hypophyseal portal tract.

1 *Corticotrophin.   Adrenocorticotrophic   hormone – ACTH.* Probably released by hypothalamic corticotrophin releasing factor – *CRF.*

2 *β-lipotrophin – β-LPH.* Made in the same cells as ACTH, cleaved from the same precursor molecule and controlled by the same factor(s).

3 *The opioid peptides, the endorphins.* Are structurally related to β-LPH and are probably released from the anterior pituitary in man.

4 *Growth hormone – GH.* Release apparently under inhibitory control by somatostatin from the hypothalamus.

5 *Prolactin.* Phylogenetically and structurally very similar to GH. Also under dominant inhibitory control, by prolactin inhibitory factor (almost certainly dopamine).

6 *Thyrotrophin – TSH.* Released by the hypothalamic tripeptide, thyrotrophin releasing hormone – *TRH.*

7 *Follicle stimulating hormone – FSH and luteinizing hormone – LH.* Are both released by the same hypothalamic factor – *LHRH.* Like TSH, they are glycoproteins, whereas the other pituitary hormones are all peptides.

Functions

Undoubtedly our present understanding of pituitary hormones is simplistic. It is not known what role GH plays in the adult, or what role prolactin plays except in the initiation of normal lactation.

1 ACTH releases cortisol and other corticosteroids.

2 β-LPH – function unknown.

3 Endorphins have actions similar to morphine but their physiological role in plasma is not known.

4 GH. Necessary for normal growth.

5 Prolactin. Necessary for the initiation of normal lactation. Like ACTH, β-LPH, endorphins and GH, prolactin is released in response to stress.

6 TSH stimulates the thyroid gland to release thyroid hormones, thyroxine and triodothyronine. These in turn exert feedback inhibition on TSH release (see p. 305).

7 FSH.

(*a*) Female – stimulates ovarian follicular development in the follicular phase of the menstrual cycle.

(*b*) Male – together with testosterone is essential for spermatogenesis.

8 LH

(*a*) Female – released in a burst at mid-cycle to induce ovulation.

(*b*) Male – stimulates the interstitial (Leydig) cells to produce androgens.

POSTERIOR LOBE

Hormones synthesized in the supraoptic and paraventricular nuclei of the hypothalamus and conducted to the posterior lobe by nerve axons, whence they are released into the blood stream.
1   *Oxytocin.*
2   *Antidiuretic hormone – ADH*, vasopressin.

Functions
1   *Oxytocin*
(*a*) Contraction of the pregnant uterus at parturition.
(*b*) Ejection of milk during suckling by action on the mammary myoepithelial cells.
2   *ADH.* Has a stimulatory effect on water reabsorption by the distal tubule of the kidney, resulting in the excretion of urine with increased concentration.

Hypofunction

ANTERIOR LOBE

Causes
1   Hypothalamic tumour, usually craniopharyngioma, more rarely pinealoma, teratoma or secondary from another site.
2   Pituitary tumour. Expanding to impair production or release from normal pituitary cells.
3   Idiopathic deficiency of one or more pituitary hormones, or of their releasing factors. Isolated GH deficiency is a cause of small stature in childhood. Isolated LHRH deficiency (also called isolated gonadotrophin deficiency) is a cause of hypogonadism presenting either at puberty or in adult life.
4   Spontaneous infarction. Occurs either in pre-existing pituitary tumour, or else following torrential post-partum haemorrhage – Sheehan's syndrome.
5   Iatrogenic. Previous surgery or radiotherapy to the hypothalamus or pituitary.
6   Miscellaneous. Rare causes include:
(*a*) Tuberculosis, sarcoidosis, syphilis.
(*b*) Trauma – with or without skull fracture.

(*c*) Giant cell granuloma of the anterior lobe – a very rare giant cell lesion of unknown aetiology.
(*d*) Metastatic tumour.

Effects
1   Secondary hypoadrenalism – ACTH deficiency.
2   Secondary hypothyroidism – TSH deficiency.
3   Impotence or amenorrhoea – LH and FSH deficiency.
4   Small stature – GH deficiency in childhood.
5   Failure of lactation. If post-partum haemorrhage complicates delivery, the first indication of pituitary infarction – Sheehan's syndrome, is failure of lactation. Paradoxically, in non-pregnant females, as well as in males, the first sign of pituitary tumour may be inappropriate milk production – *galactorrhoea*, due to elevation of serum prolactin.

Apart from failure of lactation, prolactin deficiency is without known effect in man, as is GH deficiency in the adult. Hypogonadism secondary to gonadotrophin deficiency is associated with the development of fine, wrinkled skin, and loss of stature secondary to osteoporotic collapse in the spine. Hypogonadism occurring before epiphyseal fusion in the long bones leads to the development of a eunuchoid habitus (span exceeds height) provided GH reserve is intact.

Tests to exclude hypofunction of anterior pituitary
This list is not comprehensive and as with all tests, the results need to be taken in clinical context.
1   ACTH reserve. Adequate if:
(*a*) Random plasma cortisol > 550 nmol/l.
(*b*) Stress-induced cortisol rise > 550 nmol/l.
2. GH reserve. Adequate if:
(*a*) Random plasma level > 20 mU/l.
(*b*) Stress or otherwise elevated GH peak > 20 mU/l.
3. TSH reserve adequate if serum thyroxine is in the normal range.
4. LH reserve adequate if:
(*a*) Males have a normal testosterone.
(*b*) Females are ovulating.
5. FSH reserve adequate if:
(*a*) Males have normal spermatogenesis.
(*b*) Females are ovulating.
Other tests of gonadotrophin reserve, e.g. LHRH test, clomiphene test, will indicate whether it is possible to elevate serum gonadotrophin levels, but

will not necessarily indicate whether the reserve is adequate.

MIXED SYNDROMES

A number of congenital syndromes are associated with various aspects of hypofunction of the anterior pituitary. This pituitary hypofunction is usually secondary to defective hypothalmic function.

1   *Kallman's syndrome*
Isolated LHRH deficiency with defective or absent sense of smell.

2   *Laurence–Moon–Biedl syndrome*
Isolated LHRH deficiency with mental subnormality, retinitis pigmentosa and syndactyly.

3   *Prader–Willi syndrome*
Isolated LHRH deficiency with hyperphagic obesity, mental subnormality and intrauterine or neonatal hypotonia.

POSTERIOR LOBE

DIABETES INSIPIDUS (CRANIAL)

Causes

1   *Surgical trauma.* Usually involving stalk section.

2   *Head injury.* With or without skull fracture. As with surgical trauma, diabetes insipidus occurring in these circumstances is often transient.

3   *Hypothalamic tumour.* Either primary or secondary.

4   *Infiltrative disease of the hypothalamus.* Sarcoidosis, Hand–Schüller–Christian disease (see p. 691).

5   *Idiopathic.* In approximately 30 per cent no cause is found.

6   *DIDMOAD syndrome.* The acronym, Didmoad, applies to the components of this hereditary syndrome (which has complex and uncertain penetrance): cranial diabetes insipidus, diabetes mellitus, optic atrophy and dementia. Formes frustes occur.

Effects

Inability to concentrate urine leads to passing of copious dilute urine with a tendency to dehydration. The night time (11 p.m.–7 a.m) urine volume nearly always exceeds 1.5 litres. If there is associated disease of the anterior pituitary, diabetes insipidus may be masked since adequate levels of cortisol are required to excrete a water load. Polyuria may then occur when replacement therapy is commenced with corticosteroids. Diabetes insipidus may occur also as a result of renal tubular disease – the tubules being unresponsive to normal levels of ADH (nephrogenic diabetes insipidus). There are no known effects of oxytocin deficiency.

Test of posterior pituitary function
Water deprivation test. The object of the test is to demonstrate progressive haemoconcentration (with unaltered urine concentration) when access to water is restricted. It serves to differentiate diabetes insipidus from psychogenic polydipsia, but is potentially dangerous in patients with diabetes insipidus and should be undertaken only under controlled circumstances.

Hyperfunction

ANTERIOR LOBE

Hyperfunction of the anterior pituitary occurs if functioning adenomas are present. Hypersecretion of the glycoprotein hormones, TSH, LH and FSH is exceedingly uncommon.

GROWTH HORMONE

Effects

1   *Before epiphyseal union.* If a GH-secreting tumour occurs in a child there is excessive growth in a regular and initially well-proportioned manner: *gigantism*. Most giants show some features also of acromegaly, with disproportionate enlargement, e.g. of the hands and jaw.

2   *After epiphyseal union.* Excessive GH in an adult results in *acromegaly*:

(*a*) Large hands and feet.
(*b*) Overgrowth of jaw, and prominence of supra-orbital ridges and malar bones.
(*c*) Increased soft tissue in skin and subcutaneous tissue; increased sweating.
(*d*) Kyphosis.
(*e*) Splanchnomegaly.
(*f*) Hypertension and cardiomyopathy.
(*g*) Diabetes mellitus.
(*h*) Hyperprolactinaemia with associated menstrual irregularity or impotence.
(*i*) Thyroid disorders.

PROLACTIN

Causes

1 Large pituitary adenoma (macroadenoma).
2 Small pituitary adenoma (microadenoma).
3 Drugs.
(a) Oestrogens.
(b) Phenothiazines.
(c) Methyldopa.
(d) Some antidepressants.

Effects

Abnormally increased prolactin secretion is associated with menstrual irregularity or infertility in women, and ejaculatory failure or impotence in men. Galactorrhoea may occur in either sex.

ACTH/β-LPH

Causes

1 Physiological. Decreased plasma cortisol, e.g. Addison's disease, congenital adrenal hyperplasia.
2 Pathological. Cushing's disease.

Effects

When the adrenals are intact, the effect of increased ACTH secretion is to cause Cushing's syndrome (see p. 291). When the rise in ACTH is a physiological response to falling cortisol, as in Addison's disease, the only effect of increased ACTH/β-LPH secretion is increased skin pigmentation.

POSTERIOR LOBE

INAPPROPRIATE ADH SECRETION

The syndrome of inappropriate ADH (SIADH) occurs as a complication of other diseases. Primary hypersecretion of ADH, or of oxytocin, is not recognized.

Causes

1 Head injury.
2 Any intracranial pathology.
3 Any thoracic disease, especially carcinoma of the bronchus, pneumonia, pulmonary embolus.
4 Transiently following major trauma, or general anaesthesia.

5 Idiopathic. In some cases the cause is not known.

Pathogenesis.

Increased ADH secretion may occur from direct hypothalamic derangement, or alternatively from involvement of intrathoracic baroreceptors in disease processes. It is possible that some carcinomas of the lung secrete ectopic ADH.

Incidence

Common

Effects

Water retention with haemodilution. In severe cases cerebral oedema supervenes with impaired consciousness.

Tumours

MACROADENOMA OF THE ANTERIOR LOBE

Incidence

About 15 per cent of all primary intracranial tumours. Adenomas of the posterior lobe do not occur.

Types

1 GH-secreting. Acromegaly, gigantism.
2 Prolactin-secreting. Prolactinoma.
3 ACTH/β-LPH-secreting. Cushing's disease.
4 Mixed. Especially GH with prolactin and Cushing's disease with hyperprolactinaemia.
5 Non-functioning. True non-functioning macroadenomas are uncommon.

Effects

1 Endocrine effects.
2 Local pressure symptoms.
(a) On the remainder of the pituitary, resulting in hypofunction.
(b) On the optic chiasm causing visual field defects, usually bitemporal hemianopia.
(c) On the brain. Large tumours result in distortion of the midbrain with internal hydrocephalus.
(d) On the pituitary fossa. Causing progressive enlargement of the fossa, with erosion of the bones of the sphenoid and of the dorsum sellae.

MICROADENOMA OF THE ANTERIOR LOBE

Incidence
Common. Occurs in approximately 30 per cent of the population.

Effects
The vast majority are functionless, being incidental findings on skull X-ray or at post-mortem. A minority appear to be the source of increased prolactin secretion, presenting clinically with the same symptoms as large prolactinomas.

CRANIOPHARYNGIOMA

Origin
From vestigial remnants of Rathke's pouch.

Macroscopical
Solid, or more commonly part cystic and part solid, tumours anywhere along the craniopharyngeal canal. The cysts are multilocular containing granular brown debris and brown fluid with cholesterol crystals. Calcification in the wall is common.

Microscopical
Nests or cords of squamous epithelium in a loose fibrous stroma. Some have an outer layer of columnar-shaped cells which resemble the adamantinomas of the jaw (see p. 175) whilst others may be reminiscent of a basal cell tumour.

Effects
Pressure effects on adjacent structures, e.g. hypothalamus, optic nerves and the pituitary.

Behaviour
Slowly growing and only very rarely invasive.

Complete removal is technically extremely difficult but decompression and radiotherapy is usually curative.

CARCINOMA

Origin
Most examples arise *de novo* but a few have their origin in a pre-existing adenoma.

Microscopical
Usually of chromophobe type. Very rarely they are of mixed cell type and may have hormonal effects. The cells show nuclear irregularity and mitotic activity with evidence of local invasion of the capsule and adjacent soft tissues and bone.

Effects
1 Local invasion with destruction of surrounding tissues.
2 Only rarely hormonally active.

CHORDOMA

Thirty-five per cent of these tumours occur in the base of the skull and may extend to the pituitary fossa or adjacent tissues with consequential pituitary destruction (see p. 719).

SECONDARY TUMOURS

The pituitary is an uncommon site for metastases although deposits from carcinomas of the lung and breast occasionally occur. The posterior lobe is mostly affected and the anterior lobe only rarely. A secondary deposit is an occasional cause of hypopituitarism.

Chapter 57
Diseases of the Endocrine Glands – Thyroid: Inflammations: Goitre

Normal thyroid
Development
Microscopical
Hormones
Effects
Metabolism of hormones

Congenital
Lingual
Aberrant
Thyroglossal duct
Aplasia

Inflammations

INFECTIVE

Acute bacterial
Incidence
Aetiology
Appearances
Results

Acute viral
Synonyms
Incidence
Age
Sex
Clinical
Aetiology
Macroscopical
Microscopical
Results

NON-INFECTIVE

Hashimoto's disease
Nature
Incidence
Age and sex
Macroscopical
Microscopical
Biochemical
Immunology
Other conditions with thyroid
   antibodies
Association with other diseases
Familial
Results

Riedel's thyroiditis
Nature
Aetiology
Incidence
Age
Sex
Macroscopical
Microscopical
Results

Goitre
Definition
Types

SIMPLE GOITRE
Nature

Endemic
Aetiology

Sporadic
Aetiology
Macroscopical
Microscopical
Results

PHYSIOLOGICAL GOITRE
Nature

COLLOID GOITRE
Incidence
Aetiology
Sex

Diffuse
Macroscopical
Microscopical

Nodular
Macroscopical
Microscopical
Results
Complications

TOXIC GOITRE

Graves' disease
Incidence
Age and Sex
Clinical
Aetiology
Macroscopical
Microscopical
Results

Toxic nodular
Incidence
Age
Macroscopical
Microscopical
Clinical

Others

Normal thyroid

The normal adult gland weighs 20–40 g and consists of two lateral lobes connected by the isthmus, which occasionally has a pyramidal lobe attached to its superior border.

Development
A median outgrowth from the floor of the pharynx – *foramen caecum*, which descends into the neck – *thyroglossal duct*, and proliferates to form the adult gland.

Microscopical
Consists of acini lined by cuboidal epithelium containing colloid. There is a loose interacinar connective tissue containing the blood vessels and there may be a sparse lymphocytic infiltration.

Within the follicular basement membrane are the parafollicular or *C cells*, large rather triangular in shape and 'light' in appearance due to lack of eosinophilia. These are of neural crest, ultimobranchial origin and are part of the diffuse endocrine system of polypeptide-hormone-secreting APUD cells (see p. 145).

Hormones
1 Thyroxine – T4
2 Triiodothyronine – T3
3 Reverse triiodothyronine – rT3 – inactive as a thyroid hormone. Within the thyroid gland these compounds are bound to thyroglobulin. In the plasma, thyroxine (99.97%) and triiodothyronine (99.5%) are bound to thyroid-binding globulin, thyroid-binding pre-albumin, and other proteins. Extensive peripheral conversion of T4 to T3 and rT3 occurs, predominantly in the liver.
4 Calcitonin – produced by the parafollicular, C-cells, of the thyroid. Originally thought to oppose the action of parathyroid hormone by lowering serum calcium and increasing calcium deposition in bone. Physiological role is unknown, although often produced by ectopic hormone-secreting tumours (see p. 676).

Effects of thyroxine and triiodothyronine
They are qualitatively similar and probably both T4 and T3 are active *in vivo*. They play a regulatory role in cell metabolism: thyroid hormone deficiency leads to decreased cell metabolism; in hyperthyroidism cell metabolism is increased.

Metabolism of thyroid hormones
This is illustrated in Fig. 35. Stages which appear to be enhanced by thyroid-stimulating hormone – TSH, are indicated by double arrows.

Congenital

LINGUAL THYROID
Failure of descent, with development of all or part of the gland in the region of the foramen caecum.

ABERRANT THYROID
(a) Mid-line. Anywhere along the line of the thyroglossal duct.
(b) Lateral. True ectopic thyroid tissue may rarely be found medial to the sternomastoid muscle. Thyroid tissue lateral to the sternomastoid, even when of very regular appearance, always represents lymph node metastases from a carcinoma of the thyroid. The primary is often very small and occult which led to the use of the erroneous term 'lateral aberrant thyroid' (see p. 314).

PERSISTENCE OF A THYROGLOSSAL DUCT
This may persist in whole or in part as:
(a) Thyroglossal duct.
(b) Thyroglossal cyst.
(c) Thyroglossal fistula. Usually following inflammation in a thyroglossal cyst.
Any of these lesions may be above, in, or below the hyoid bone and be lined by columnar or squamous epithelium.

APLASIA
This is a rare cause of cretinism (see p. 312).

Inflammations

INFECTIVE

ACUTE BACTERIAL THYROIDITIS

Incidence
Very rare.

Aetiology
Bacterial infection by haematogenous, lymphatic or

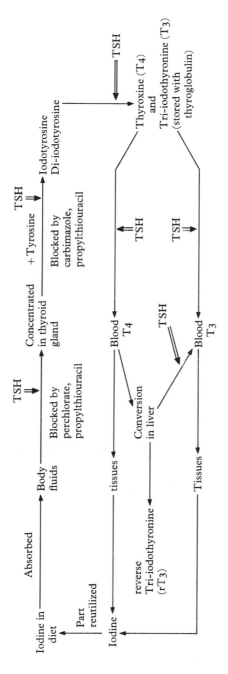

Fig. 35. Metabolism of thyroid hormones.

local spread. The organisms are usually staphylococci or streptococci.

Appearances
Swollen and congested with interstitial inflammation.

Results
1 Resolution, with or without antibiotics – usual.
2 Suppuration with abscess formation – rare.

ACUTE VIRAL THYROIDITIS

Synonyms
Subacute thyroiditis, non-suppurative thyroiditis, de Quervain's disease, granulomatous or giant cell thyroiditis.

Incidence
Rare.

Age
30–50 years, but may occur in the elderly.

Sex
More common in females.

Clinical
An acute, or subacute, onset with fever, malaise, pain in the throat. The thyroid may be enlarged, but is always tender, often markedly. The pain makes swallowing and coughing difficult.

Aetiology
Coxsackie virus infection is the most common, although other viruses have also been implicated.

Macroscopical
The thyroid is enlarged to about twice the normal size. It is smooth, firm and tender; slight adhesion of the gland surface to the adjacent muscles may occur but these adhesions are readily broken down. The cut surface shows focal pale areas poor in colloid.

Microscopical
Focal granulomatous inflammation with numerous foreign body giant cells, often engulfing colloid material – *colloidophagy*, degeneration of the follicles and epithelium and an inflammatory cell infiltration by plasma cells, lymphocytes and histiocytes.

Later, fibrous scarring and thyroid acinar regeneration may occur.

Results
The acute glandular destruction may result in transient elevation of thyroid hormones, with or without thyrotoxicosis. The illness is usually self-limiting and settles in 1–3 weeks. Less often there are relapses, of lessening severity, over a period of several months. Rarely, the patient may become myxoedematous. Severe thyroiditis may be fatal in the elderly and debilitated.

NON-INFECTIVE

HASHIMOTO'S DISEASE
– AUTOIMMUNE THYROIDITIS
– LYMPHADENOID GOITRE
– STRUMA LYMPHOMATOSA

Nature
A disorder characterized by variable degrees of diffuse thyroid enlargement with circulating antithyroid antibodies and showing features of an autoimmune destructive process in the gland.

Incidence
Although detectable thyroid antibodies are found in up to 2 per cent of the population only a relatively small proportion have a clinical goitre.

Age and sex
Maximal between 35 and 55 years, but at any age though rare in children. F:M 12:1.

Macroscopical
The gland is usually diffusely enlarged and commonly 2–5 times normal size, firm and lobulated. The borders are distinct but displacement or slight tracheal compression may occur. Adjacent cervical lymph nodes are often slightly reactively enlarged and rubbery. The cut surface shows marked pale greyish lobulation with diminution of colloid components.

Microscopical
A diffuse process confined within the thyroid capsule, showing:
1 Lymphoid infiltration with lymph follicle formation.
2 A diffuse plasma cell infiltration.

3 Epithelial metaplasia with large, eosinophilic, thyroid epithelial cells – Askanazy cells.

4 Diminished colloid in the disrupted acini.

5 Increased fibrous tissue producing a lobulated pattern.

6 Elements of regeneration and increased activity induced by TSH in non-affected acini.

Biochemical changes

1 Elevated TSH level.

2 Exaggerated TSH response to the intravenous injection of thyrotrophin releasing hormone – TRH (TRH test).

3 Low T_4 level – usual.

4 Low T_3 level – becomes manifest only in later stages.

Immunology

Serum autoantibodies of three types are identified:

1 Precipitin test – detects antithyroglobulin antibodies.

2 Tanned red cell – T.R.C. – also detects antithyroglobulin antibodies and is more sensitive.

3 Complete fixation test – C.F.T. – microsomal antibody.

In Hashimoto's disease T.R.C. levels of 1 in 25 000 or more and a C.F.T. of even 1 in 64 are common and respective titres of 1 in 1 000 000 and 1 in 1000 are not uncommon.

The T.R.C. titre is particularly high in the more fibrotic examples.

Other conditions with thyroid antibodies

1 *Hyperthyroidism* – present in high proportions (65 per cent) usually in low titre but if C.F.T is 1 in 16 or more this indicates a high risk of myxoedema developing after thyroidectomy or radioiodine treatment.

2 *Primary atrophic thyroiditis* – low-titre antibodies are present in 80 per cent of cases of 'primary' myxoedema with thyroid atrophy. However, even though similar pathogenetic factors may operate, it is misleading to define primary atrophic thyroiditis (see p. 312) as 'Hashimoto's disease without goitre'.

3 *Focal lymphocytic thyroiditis* – patchy histological changes of a similar type to that seen in Hashimoto's thyroiditis are seen in 5–10 per cent of autopsy thyroids. Similar focal changes can occur in nodular colloid goitre. There is a spectrum of severity from scattered to diffuse (in 2 per cent of autopsies) and in the more severe forms clinically occult myxoedema is common retrospectively.

Association with other diseases

Other 'auto-immune diseases' are commonly associated with thyroiditis including: S.L.E. (see p. 281), rheumatoid arthritis (see p. 285), Sjögren's syndrome (see p. 178), pernicious anaemia (see p. 482), acquired haemolytic anaemia (see p. 504), adrenal cortical atrophy (Addison's disease) (see p. 294), diabetes mellitus (see p. 634). Antibodies involved in this auto-immune spectrum include, in particular, organ-specific examples e.g. pernicious anaemia (parietal cell antibodies) and Addison's disease (C.F.T. adrenal cortical antibodies) and, additionally, a wide range of antinuclear factors, rheumatoid factors, anti-red-cell antibodies, etc.

Familial

There is a definite genetic predisposition to autoimmune disease development and relatives of Hashimoto's disease patients have a high incidence of circulating thyroid antibodies.

Results

Myxoedema usually results if the condition is not treated, but this may be delayed for many years by compensatory hyperplasia and regeneration of the thyroid epithelium, induced by TSH, which balances to some extent the progressive destruction of thyroid tissue. Thyroxine replacement therapy will reverse the clinical manifestations of myxoedema and will cause regression of any thyroid enlargement which results from TSH stimulation. Thyroid enlargement resulting from the underlying thyroiditis is unaffected by thyroxine treatment.

RIEDEL'S THYROIDITIS – INVASIVE FIBROUS THYROIDITIS – LIGNEOUS THYROIDITIS

Nature

A thyroiditis of distinctive hardness and with involvement of adjacent tissues. There is an association with retroperitoneal and/or mediastinal fibrosis in about 30 per cent of cases.

Aetiology

Unknown, but possibly autoimmune though antibodies are lacking.

Incidence
Very rare.

Age
Variable, but usually in middle age.

Sex
M:F 1:4.

Macroscopical
Irregular enlargement of the thyroid gland with a densely hard and nodular surface inseparable from the surrounding tissues. On section the gland is grey, gritty and fibrous.

Microscopical
Obliteration of the thyroid architecture with replacement by mature collagen containing foci of lymphocytes, plasma cells and scanty polymorphs.

Results
1 Tracheal compression – relieved by wedge resection of the isthmus.
2 Myxoedema – 25 per cent.
3 Part of the gland only involved – rarely.
4 Frequently mistaken clinically for thyroid carcinoma.
5 Thyroid antibody studies inevitably give negative results.

Goitre

Definition
Any enlargement of part or whole of the thyroid gland.

Types
1 Simple goitre.
(*a*) Endemic.
(*b*) Sporadic.
(*c*) Physiological.
2 Colloid goitre.
(*a*) Diffuse.
(*b*) Nodular.
3 Toxic goitre.
(*a*) Graves' disease.
(*b*) Toxic nodular goitre.
(*c*) Other.
4 Infective thyroiditis, including granulomatous.
5 Autoimmune thyroiditis.
6 Riedel's thyroiditis.

7 Adenoma.
8 Carcinoma.

SIMPLE GOITRE

Nature
Diffuse enlargement of the thyroid gland due to an absolute or relative deficiency of iodine, or to goitrogenic agents.

ENDEMIC TYPE

Aetiology
Iodine deficiency in food and water, particularly in geographical areas remote from the sea. In most countries iodine is now added to foods, e.g. bread, salt, but iodine deficiency is still common in the Himalayas and High Andes. The addition of iodine to the diet of schoolchildren in Ohio reduced the prevalence of goitre from 20 per cent to 0.2 per cent.

SPORADIC TYPE

Goitre occurring in individuals where there are adequate supplies of iodine in the food and water.

Aetiology
1 Goitrogens.
(*a*) Ingestion of certain of the cabbage species (Brassicas) is said to be goitrogenic in some, possibly because of their thiourea content.
(*b*) Drugs and chemicals, e.g. perchlorate, resorcinol, paraminosalicylic acid, as well as drugs used in the treatment of thyrotoxicosis.

Macroscopical
A vascular, diffusely and moderately enlarged gland.

Microscopical
Hyperplasia, as evidenced by an increased number of acini, tall columnar epithelium and some colloid deficiency. Later, patchy involutionary changes may occur.

Results
If iodine is supplied, or the goitrogen removed, the gland returns to normal.

PHYSIOLOGICAL GOITRE

Nature
In girls, the thyroid gland may enlarge at the time of puberty, or during pregnancy. The reason is not clear.

COLLOID GOITRE

Incidence
A common disease in districts with endemic iodine deficiency: not uncommon elsewhere.

Aetiology
In endemic districts it represents an end-result of iodine deficiency, and follows involution of the hyperplastic gland. In non-endemic districts the cause is not known although a serum thyroid growth factor has been postulated.

Sex
M:F 1:6.

DIFFUSE COLLOID GOITRE

Macroscopical
Diffuse enlargement with an exaggerated vesicular pattern and a pale brown, glistening colloid appearance on the cut surface.

Microscopical
Less vascular than normal; the epithelium is low cuboidal and there is an increased amount of colloid within the distended vesicles.

NODULAR COLLOID GOITRE

May follow the diffuse type, or may arise *de novo*.

Macroscopical
Nodular enlargement of part, but more usually the whole, of the gland with encapsulated appearance of the nodules. The cut surface is predominantly of a pale brown, colloid appearance with areas of haemorrhage, cyst formation, fibrosis and calcification. Some of these goitres reach an enormous size and they may show retrosternal extension.

Microscopical
The vesicles are distended with colloid and the epithelium is flattened and inactive but a few areas may show residual hyperplastic activity. There may be some areas of focal infiltration by lymphocytes and plasma cells (see p. 307).

Results
The majority of patients are symptom-free and although the gland may enlarge slowly with time, the goitre may be left provided complications do not occur. Plasma levels of T4 and T3 are normal.

Complications
1 *Pressure*. Especially on the trachea or oesophagus, particularly where there is retrosternal extension.
2 *Haemorrhage*. Into the nodules producing a rapid increase in size. This may accentuate the pressure symptoms to a dangerous degree and result in asphyxia.
3 *Toxic change*. One or more nodules may develop secondary toxic changes.
4 *Malignancy*. If this occurs, it is exceedingly rare (see p. 314).

TOXIC GOITRE

GRAVES' DISEASE – EXOPHTHALMIC GOITRE

Incidence
Common.

Age and Sex
Usually 20–40 years. M:F 1:8.

Clinical
Enlargement of the thyroid is usually diffuse or may be slightly nodular. Increased blood flow may be seen, or heard (bruit) pulsing through the enlarged gland. There are associated signs of:
1 Thyroid gland overactivity – weight loss, agitation, tremor, lid lag and stare, atrial fibrillation, etc.
2 The autoimmune process involving other tissues – exopthalmos with or without ophthalmoplegia and, rarely, pretibial myxodema.

Aetiology
An autoimmune process characterized by the pre-

sence of circulating thyroid antibodies. Unlike the antibodies of Hashimoto's disease, these act on the TSH receptor to result in stimulation of the gland. Measurement of these antibodies (variously named thyroid stimulating immunoglobulin – TSI, human thyroid stimulator – HTS, long-acting thyroid stimulator protector – LATSP) is difficult. Thyroid stimulating immunoglobulins may cross the placenta and cause intra-uterine thyrotoxicosis in the infant of a woman who has had Graves' disease.

Macroscopical
Diffuse, vascular, fleshy and moderate enlargement of the gland, with lack of colloid seen on the cut surface.

Microscopical
The epithelium is hyperplastic, tall and columnar, often with papillary processes projecting into the thyroid acini. The vesicles are deficient in colloid and show a 'scalloping' of the colloid margins. There is marked vascularity and a variable lymphocytic infiltration frequently with lymph follicle formation. In addition, the changes of focal thyroiditis are present in scattered areas in 20–30 per cent of cases.

Results
Treatment of Graves' disease is aimed at correcting circulating levels of thyroid hormones.
1 *Surgical removal* – partial or subtotal thyroidectomy.
2 *Antithyroid drugs*
(a) Iodine, Lugol's iodine. The mechanism by which iodine acts is uncertain. Since its effect is only transient (1–2 weeks), it is employed mainly to decrease vascularity of the thyroid gland, prior to thyroidectomy.
(b) Carbimazole, propylthiouracil, etc. These act on both iodine trapping and incorporation into iodotyrosine (see p. 305).
3 *Radioactive iodine*. The isotope is administered orally and is selectively taken up in the thyroid gland, causing local involution. The effects of radioiodine continue for many years, and may cause insidious hypothyroidism years after the patient has been lost to follow-up.

TOXIC NODULAR GOITRE

Occasionally, toxic change occurs in a multinodular colloid goitre. Alternatively, a single autonomous nodule – 'hot nodule', may develop. The aetiology is uncertain although presumed to be autoimmune.

Incidence
Uncommon.

Age
Mostly in the older age group, e.g. middle age and upwards.

Macroscopical
Fleshy areas in one or more nodules of a nodular colloid goitre, or a single, clearly defined nodule.

Microscopical
The changes in multinodular goitre are identical to those found in primary thyrotoxicosis, but arise in a gland also showing changes of a nodular colloid goitre. Areas surrounding a single 'hot nodule' are suppressed.

Clinical
Exophthalmos and pretibial myxoedema do not usually occur. Although antithyroid drugs or radioiodine may be effective, most respond best to partial thyroidectomy.

OTHERS

1 *Trophoblastic tumours*. Tumours of placental origin may secrete large amounts of human chorionic gonadotrophin (HCG) which resembles TSH in being a glycoprotein. Either HCG itself, or closely related glycoproteins may have TSH-like activity and cause thyrotoxicosis.
2 *Pituitary*. Thyrotoxicosis from excessive production of pituitary TSH occurs, but is excessively rare.

Hypothyroidism

CONGENITAL

Nature
Hypothyroidism which is manifest at birth.

(a) *Endemic.* Occurs in the offspring of mothers who have iodine deficiency and who are themselves goitrous.

(b) *Sporadic.* Thyroid agenesis: failure of the thyroid anlage or arrested development during its descent from the floor of the foetal mouth. There is no goitre. Occurs in 1 : 4000 live births.

(c) *Genetic. Dyshormonogenetic goitre* – a rare auto-somal recessive condition characterized by the inability to synthesize thyroid hormones. As blood T3 and T4 levels are low, TSH secretion rises and the gland enlarges. When treated with thyroid hormones, the gland regresses. Dys-hormonogenesis may be associated with con-genital neural deafness – *Pendred's syndrome*.

Appearances

1 Failure of normal mental and bodily develop-ment, particularly of the bones.
2 Dry skin.
3 Coarse facial features with puffed lips.
4 Large tongue.
5 Abdominal distension, often with an umbilical hernia.

Results

Unless treated with thyroid replacement therapy, prognosis is poor. Even when diagnosed early and treated adequately, mental deficiency may still be marked – *cretinism*, as a result of thyroid hormone deficiency *in utero*.

MYXOEDEMA

Nature

Primary hypothyroidism (i.e. not secondary to TSH deficiency) developing after birth.

Age

Mostly occurs in older age groups, but can affect children when it may present with slowed growth or delay in puberty.

Sex

More common in females.

Incidence

Common. If subclinical cases (i.e. diagnosed on basis of biochemistry alone) are included, may affect up to 2 per cent of the population.

Causes

1 *Iodine deficiency*. Very rare. Iodine has to be virtually absent from the diet before myxoedema develops.
2 *Hashimoto's thyroiditis* (see p. 306) and chronic atrophic thyroiditis (see p. 307).
3 *Riedel's thyroiditis* (see p. 307).

4 *Graves' disease*. Approximately 5 per cent of patients with thyrotoxicosis develop hypothyr-oidism in later years, unrelated to any treatment they may have received. Presumably these patients have a spectrum of antithyroid antibodies: some of which stimulate the TSH receptor and some of which are destructive (see p. 310).
5 *Treatment of Graves' disease*. Possibly the com-monest cause of myxoedema. The condition may be transient (caused by antithyroid drugs) or per-manent (following surgery or radioactive iodine). Permanent myxoedema may occur many years after thyrotoxicosis was treated.

Effects

1 *General metabolism*. Metabolism is slowed and patients feel cold and lethargic, constipated and mentally dull. Skin is puffy and facial features are coarsened. Hair is lost and the voice is gruff as a result of oedema of the vocal cords.
2 *Myxoedema*. The condition derives its name from the presence of mucinous, protein-rich extra-cellular material in many tissues. Increased albu-min leakage occurs from the vessels.
3 *Cardiovascular*. Bradycardia is common, as is pericardial effusion.
4 *C.N.S.* Mental slowing, progressing to stupor or coma. Psychosis may occur in some, and may be precipitated by the start of replacement therapy.

Results

Myxoedema usually responds well to thyroxine replacement therapy. However, patients who pre-sent in coma have a high mortality.

Tests of thyroid function

In thyroid disease, as in all of endocrinology, the results of function tests must be interpreted in the light of clinical findings.

THYROXINE (T4)

Total serum thyroxine levels vary from approxi-mately 55–130 nmol/l, but the result is largely dependent on circulating levels of thyroid binding globulin (TBG). TBG levels may be low because of congenital deficiency, liver or renal impairment, and may be elevated by pregnancy and the oral contraceptive pill.

Low serum thyroxine is the best indicator of established hypothyroidism.

TRI-IODOTHYRONINE (T3)

Measured T3 levels are also dependent on TBG concentration, although less so. T3 is depressed in acute ill-health, especially in the elderly, in liver disease as well as in a variety of other conditions (those in which preferential formation of the biologically inactive, reverse T3, is formed). In myxoedema T3 is usually maintained in the normal range until late in the illness. For these reasons low T3 is not a good guide to hypothyroidism.

High serum T3 is the best indicator of thyrotoxicosis.

T3 UPTAKE (T3 RESIN UPTAKE: THYROID HORMONE UPTAKE TEST)

T3 uptake tests measure the number of unsaturated thyroid hormone binding sites, and are thus used to indicate TBG concentration. TBG may be measured directly.

FREE T4 (AND FREE T3) INDEX

Mathematical correction of measured total T4 (and T3) dependent on result of T3 uptake test. The free indices do not, however, correct adequately for large alterations in TBG concentration.

FREE T4 (AND FREE T3)

Techniques are becoming available to measure only that concentration of thyroid hormone which is unbound (and hence the metabolically active fraction). It seems likely that these techniques will replace the calculated free indices in due course.

TSH

Elevated TSH levels occur in primary hypothyroidism. Because the TSH assay is relatively insensitive, it is not possible to discriminate the suppression of basal TSH which occurs in thyrotoxicosis from normal.

TRH TEST

The intravenous injection of hypothalamic thyrotrophin releasing hormone (TRH) releases TSH, with a peak at 20 min. Although an exaggerated response may be sought to confirm the diagnosis of myxoedema, the test is usually reserved to confirm thyrotoxicosis: there is no response to TRH in this condition.

Tumours

BENIGN
THYROID ADENOMA

Nature
Solitary or multiple circumscribed nodules in an otherwise normal or, not uncommonly, a multinodular colloid goitre of different histological structure from that of the surrounding distorted, compressed thyroid tissue. They are found in more than 10 per cent of thyroid glands at autopsy.

Types
1 *Follicular adenoma.* These show a varied pattern of large and small, colloid-containing, small-celled microfollicles and columns of somewhat larger cells of alveolar arrangement, mixed or composed wholly of one of these forms. The solid microfollicular nodule is sometimes inappropriately termed *foetal adenoma.*
2 *Hürthle cell adenoma.* Oxyphilic cell metaplasia (resembling the Askanazy cells of Hashimoto's disease) may affect most or all of an adenoma.
3 *Atypical adenoma.* These uncommon cellular examples with foci of cells with bizarre giant nuclei have infrequent mitoses and do not invade veins. Their natural history is benign.
4 *Papillary 'adenoma'.* Although occasional papillary-like foci are seen in follicular adenomas, true papillary lesions are usually regarded as malignant tumours albeit very well differentiated. This term is therefore best avoided.
5 *Toxic adenoma–'hot nodule'.* Some adenomas cause hyperthyroidism unassociated with the presence of thyroid stimulating antibodies in serum (see p. 310).

Behaviour
Histological differentiation of follicular adenoma from well-differentiated follicular carcinoma (see p. 315) can be extremely difficult. Vascular invasion is

the most commonly accepted criterion for a diagnosis of malignancy. Capsular penetration is also significant.

It is generally accepted that malignant change from adenoma to follicular carcinoma is rare and that most examples of follicular carcinoma arise *de novo*.

MALIGNANT

CARCINOMA OF THYROID

Incidence
Geographically variable: in England and Wales 0.3 per cent of deaths from malignant disease with 3 times as many females as males; about twice this frequency in the goitrous areas of Switzerland and higher still amongst the endemic goitrous zones in Columbia. However, though goitre is common, carcinoma is rare.

Predisposing factors
1 *Nodular goitre*. Carries a small increased risk of follicular carcinoma.
2 *Adenomas*. Probably only very rarely undergo malignant change (see p. 313).
3 *Radiation*. It is clear that external radiation to the thyroid area causes increased risk of carcinoma, largely papillary but sometimes follicular.
4 *Dyshormonogenetic goitre*. Adenomas are a consistent feature due to the high TSH levels and atypical hyperplastic features are often seen, though metastatic spread of such lesions is rarely recorded.

PAPILLARY CARCINOMA

Age
Any age including childhood.

Macroscopical
The primary tumour in the thyroid may be single or multiple and can be quite small and occult. Cystic lesions of the gland should always be carefully examined and if they contain even small amounts of papillary tissue in the lining should be regarded as carcinomas. The papillary structure is usually grossly apparent and the lesions are frequently well circumscribed. Cervical lymph nodes are often enlarged by tumour at original presentation and in many cases this is the first symptom. The term *'lateral aberrant thyroid'* was, at one time, used for a very well-differentiated papillary thyroid carcinomatous deposit which had completely destroyed the lymphoid tissue of the node to which it had metastasized and where the thyroid primary was not clinically apparent. Aberrant thyroid tissue does not, however, occur in this anatomical site, posterior and deep to the sternomastoid muscle.

Microscopical
Papillary fronded tumours, usually exceptionally well differentiated and showing little cytological manifestation of malignancy. Calcified laminated 'psammoma bodies' are seen in about 50 per cent. Most papillary carcinomas have cells with a characteristic large, pale, misshapen nucleus.

Spread
1 *Direct*. This is seldom clinically significant.
2 *Lymphatic*. Cervical lymph node metastases occur in about 50 per cent of cases.
3 *Blood*. This is rare in papillary tumours.

Prognosis
Eighty per cent are alive and well at 10 years. The prognosis is less good in older age groups. Most tumours grow slowly and therapy can be conservative with local removal of lymph node metastases.

FOLLICULAR CARCINOMA

Age
Rare under 30 years.

Macroscopical
Most are slowly growing and encapsulated varying from a few cm to massive tumours. Usually solid, fleshy and opaque, sometimes with foci of necrosis but uncommonly haemorrhagic.

Microscopical
1 *Slightly invasive*. Resembles follicular adenoma but has evidence of sparse vascular invasion, usually after prolonged scrutiny, at the capsular margin and sometimes foci of necrosis.
2 *Overtly invasive*. This type is less common and occurs in older age groups. Direct extension outside the capsule is usually obvious histologically and sometimes grossly. Solid pleomorphic foci,

numerous mitotic figures, foci of necrosis and marked venous invasion are usual features.

Spread

1 *Direct.* Important in the overtly invasive type.
2 *Lymphatic.* Relatively common.
3 *Blood.* Metastatic deposits in bone or lungs are not infrequent but may themselves be very slowly growing.

Behaviour

Thyroidectomy is the treatment of choice. The long-term prognosis is excellent in the slightly invasive tumours but 5-year survival is only 50 per cent in the overtly invasive and 25 per cent at 10 years.

RADIOACTIVE IODINE THERAPY IN DIFFERENTIATED CARCINOMA

Therapy by radioiodine may be very effective in both papillary and follicular differentiated thyroid carcinomas. Uptake by the tumour, both primary and metastatic, is considerably assisted if the normal thyroid tissue is first ablated by total thyroidectomy.

ANAPLASTIC CARCINOMA

This highly malignant tumour accounts for 10–15 per cent of thyroid carcinomas. It is most frequent in the elderly and usually presents with a short history and a clinically obviously malignant local appearance. Lymphatic and blood spread is common and death is usually inevitable 6–12 months after diagnosis.

Histologically, though follicular elements may be seen, the dominant features are of either a spindle-cell tumour with or without giant cell areas or a small cell pattern which may be difficult to differentiate from lymphoma (see p. 000).

MEDULLARY CARCINOMA

Nature

A malignant tumour of C cells (see p. 304) and thus hormonally active in production of calcitonin and other substances.

Age and Incidence

About 5 per cent of thyroid carcinomas—mostly in persons over 40 years but also in the young where it is commonly familial, multiple and associated with other endocrine tumours (see p. 317).

Macroscopical

Grey, discrete but not encapsulated and sometimes multiple. Mostly 2–3 cm and with cervical lymph node metastases in about 50 per cent of cases.

Microscopical

Nests and masses of closely packed eosinophilic, granular, polygonal cells with, characteristically, *amyloid* material in the stroma.

Spread

1 *Direct.* Marked tendency to extend into superior mediastinum.
2 *Lymphatic.* Common.
3 *Blood.* Common in fatal cases in bones, lungs and liver.

Prognosis

50 per cent alive and well at 10 years after surgical treatment.

Associated factors

About 5 per cent of medullary carcinomas are familial with autosomal dominant inheritance. These families show high incidence of adrenal phaeochromocytomas, often bilateral, and may also have neurofibromas of skin, ganglioneuromas of intestinal plexuses, parathyroid adenoma and diarrhoea in addition to rather characteristic facies and body habitus.

Some tumours secrete not only calcitonin but also 5-hydroxytryptamine or corticotrophin.

LYMPHOMAS

Primary non-Hodgkin's lymphoma of the thyroid is probably more common than originally believed as many examples were previously included in the anaplastic carcinoma group. The patients are mainly elderly with a short history of fleshy enlargement of one or both of the lobes of the gland. Histologically, these are mostly plasmacytoid and diffuse (see p. 580). It is likely that some cases arise in pre-existing Hashimoto's disease.

In most cases the prognosis is bad with death in a

few months but a few live for some, or many, years after X-ray or cytotoxic therapy.

OTHER TUMOURS

Sarcomas occasionally occur and the thyroid gland may be involved by blood spread in disseminated carcinoma arising from many sites, e.g. breast, lung or malignant melanoma.

PARATHYROID GLANDS

NORMAL

There are usually two pairs of glands, each pale yellow-brown in colour and up to 0.5 cm dia. Together they weigh about 0.1 g. The upper pair are fairly constant in position in relation to the posterior aspect of the superior poles of the thyroid gland. The lower pair are more inconsistent in position, often being found in the carotid sheath or in the mediastinum.

Microscopical
Nests or cords of epithelial cells in a vascular fibro-fatty stroma. With advancing age increasing amounts of fat appear in the glands.

Cell types
1 *Chief cells.* Most numerous, with the 'water clear' cell as a vacuolated variant.
2 *Oxyphil cells.* These increase in number with age.

Functions
Parathyroid hormone (PTH) secreted by the parathyroid glands acts on bone to increase calcium resorption, and on the kidney in three ways:
1 Increase in calcium reabsorption.
2 Increase in phosphate excretion.
3 Increase in 1-hydroxylation, i.e. activation of Vitamin D.
The combined effects of these actions is to raise serum calcium and to lower serum phosphate.

CONGENITAL ABNORMALITIES

Abnormalities in number (2–5), or position, e.g.

mediastinum, are relatively common and are of importance to the exploring surgeon.

Primary hyperparathyroidism

Causes
1 *Tumour.* 90 per cent. Malignancy is rare.
2 *Hyperplasia.* 10 per cent.

Incidence
Common, affecting approximately 0.1 per cent of the population. In many cases the biochemical abnormality induced is very mild.

Macroscopical
1 *Adenoma.* Usually solitary but multiple in 5 per cent of cases; 75 per cent occur in the lower glands. They are orange-brown, well encapsulated nodules of very variable size but are seldom more than 1 cm dia. They have a homogeneous cut surface.
2 *Hyperplasia.* All the glands are enlarged with an average total weight of 19 g.
3 *Carcinoma.* These tumours usually resemble adenomas but are poorly encapsulated or sometimes frankly invasive.

Microscopical
The histological appearances vary markedly. In more than 50 per cent the chief cell is dominant and in most of the remainder there is a mixture of cell types. Only rarely are 'pure' water-clear cell or oxyphil cell lesions found. Hyperplastic glands may be either diffuse or variably nodular in appearance.

Diagnosis of autonomous functional adenoma(s) from hyperplasia is important and may be difficult unless the appearances of all the parathyroids are known. In individual glands a helpful feature may be the presence of a rim of 'normal', though compressed, parathyroid tissue around the capsule of an adenoma. The presence of fat in enlarged glands suggests hyperplasia rather than adenoma.

Effects
Elevated secretion of PTH results in elevation of serum calcium. The elevated calcium may result in rather non-specific symptoms of polyuria, depression, constipation or it may result in calcification in blood vessels, renal substance (nephrocalcinosis) or urinary tract (stone formation) (see p. 372). Most frequently hypercalcaemia is detected as the result of routine calcium measurement. PTH results in

excessive bone resorption by the osteoclasts and this may be detected as subperiosteal erosions in the phalanges. Rarely, the osteoclasts form large aggregations and the resultant swelling (brown tumour, von Recklinghausen's disease of bone) may be the presenting complaint (see p. 703).

Diagnosis

In the majority of cases the diagnosis is biochemical, and not clinical and depends on the demonstration of raised serum calcium with inappropriately elevated PTH, together with any or all of: decreased fasting serum phosphate, decreased tubular reabsorption of phosphate, increased tubular reabsorption of calcium, increased urinary hydroxyproline excretion and increased serum alkaline phosphatase.

Results

Surgical extirpation usually results in cure, although on occasion the disease recurs or it may not be possible to localize all hyperfunctioning glands. Carcinomas are usually slow-growing and tend to spread locally.

Associated conditions

Chief cell hyperplasia is a characteristic finding in patients with the syndrome of *multiple endocrine neoplasia type 1 – pluriglandular 'adenomatosis'*, in which hyperplasia with variable nodularity of the parathyroids is associated with adenomas of the anterior lobe of pituitary, pancreatic islets and adrenal cortex, sometimes with foregut carcinoid tumours (see p. 145).

A further association occurs in *multiple endocrine neoplasia type 2* in which nodular parathyroid hyperplasia is familialy present along with medullary carcinoma of the thyroid and adrenal phaeochromocytomas (see p. 293).

Secondary hyperparathyroidism

Nature

Compensatory hyperplasia of the parathyroid glands occurs in conditions which lower blood calcium or raise the blood inorganic phosphorus level.

Causes

1 Chronic renal failure and some renal tubular disorders (see p. 366).

2 Steatorrhoea and other malabsorption syndromes (see p. 208).
3 Pregnancy and lactation.

Macroscopical

All the glands are enlarged but to a much less degree than in the hyperplastic type of primary hyperparathyroidism.

Microscopical

There is increase in the 'water clear' cells and chief cells, associated with loss of stromal fat cells.

Diagnosis

The diagnosis, which is usually presumptive and only of importance in renal failure, depends upon the demonstration of elevated PTH, alkaline phosphatase and radiological changes – 'rugger-jersey spine' (see p. 695). Serum calcium is low to normal, while phosphate is elevated as a result of the underlying renal disease.

Tertiary hyperparathyroidism

Chronic overstimulation of the parathyroid glands in renal failure may result in one or more becoming autonomous, with resultant hypercalcaemia.

Hypoparathyroidism

Causes

(a) *Surgery.* Temporary or permanent hypoparathyroidism may result from neck surgery, including treatment of hyperparathyroidism.
(b) *Autoimmune hypoparathyroidism.* The presence of circulating antiparathyroid antibodies leads to atrophy of the glands, with decreased PTH secretion and tendency to hypocalcaemia. The disease may pursue an insidious course for many years and non-specific symptoms of dizziness, gastro-intestinal upset, etc., may not point to the diagnosis.

Effects

Hypoparathyroidism may result in:
1 Tetany.
2 Tendency to abdominal discomfort and diarrhoea.
3 Epilepsy.
4 Chronic monilial infection of the skin and nails.

5   Cataract.

Apart from 1 and 2, these are rare in surgically induced hypoparathyroidism, perhaps because the disease is more abrupt in onset and hence more frequently recognized early.

Diagnosis
Depends on the demonstration of hypocalcaemia (which cannot be explained by coincidental hypoalbuminaemia) together with tendency to high serum phosphate and inappropriately low PTH. Parathyroid antibodies may be demonstrated. In the differential diagnosis it is important to exclude hypomagnesaemia.

Results
Treatment with cholecalciferol, with or without oral calcium supplements, leads to resolution of all but cataract and, possibly, any tendency to epilepsy.

Chapter 59
Diseases of the Ear

External ear

INFLAMMATIONS – OTITIS EXTERNA

Inflammations are common in the skin of the ear and the meatus and, if severe, may lead to destruction of the underlying external cartilage, a feature which may occur following furunculosis. Probably the most common causes of inflammation affecting the ear are seborrhoeic dermatitis (see p. 725) and an external otitis secondary to chronic suppurative otitis media.

Other inflammations may be caused by bacterial infections, especially streptococci and staphylococci, or due to fungi, e.g. aspergilli (otomycosis) or viruses, e.g. herpes zoster.

TRAUMA

CAULIFLOWER EAR

Aetiology
Trauma producing a haematoma beneath the skin or perichondrium.

Macroscopical
Irregular and nodular thickening of the ear with deformity.

Microscopical
Blood clot which becomes organized into fibrous tissue and occasionally to cartilage.

CHONDRODERMATITIS NODULARIS CHRONICA HELICIS

Aetiology
The aetiology is not definitely known but multiple minor injuries may be responsible.

Macroscopical
One or more painful and hard nodules on the upper margins of the ear. The surface is hyperkeratotic and may be ulcerated.

Microscopical
1 Hyperkeratosis.
2 Irregular acanthosis.
3 Central ulceration.

4 Chronic inflammatory cell infiltration of the dermis and of the surface of the cartilage – perichondritis.

Results
When the condition is long standing, the overlying skin may show atypical proliferation and mimic a squamous cell carcinoma.

OTHER LESIONS

GOUTY TOPHI

The ear is a classical site of gouty tophi (see p. 111).

TUMOURS

(*a*) *Osteoma.* Of the bony portion of the external auditory canal.
(*b*) *Adenoma.* A benign tumour derived from ceruminous glands.
(*c*) *Basal cell carcinoma.* See p. 731.
(*d*) *Squamous cell carcinoma.* See p. 730.

AURAL POLYP

Nature
The commonest type is a granulomatous polyp originating within the middle ear, but presenting in the auditory canal through a perforation in the tympanic membrane.

Macroscopical
A red, vascular polyp of variable size.

Microscopical
Formed by a core of vascular granulation tissue with a covering of columnar epithelium derived from the middle ear or, more commonly, by metaplastic squamous epithelium. Surface ulceration is frequently seen and the core may contain mucous glands, foreign body giant cells reacting to wax or keratin, and an intense inflammatory cell infiltration.

Tympanic membrane

The tympanic membrane divides the external auditory canal from the middle ear.

MYRINGITIS

This membrane may be infected from the middle ear (see below) or from an external otitis. A special type producing haemorrhagic bullae – bullous myringitis – is probably due to a virus infection and is most commonly seen during influenzal epidemics.

Middle ear

ACUTE OTITIS MEDIA

Nature
An acute non-specific infection of the middle ear.

Aetiology
The infection is usually caused by β-haemolytic streptococci, staphylococci or pneumococci.

Pathogenesis
Any infection involving the upper respiratory tract, especially in children, associated with swelling of lymphoid tissue, e.g. adenoids, predisposes to blockage of the Eustachian tube and thus to otitis media. The condition, therefore, usually occurs as a complication of tonsillitis, pharyngitis, scarlet fever, influenza, measles and the common cold.

Route of infection
Almost always via the Eustachian tube.

Clinical
Earache and pyrexia, associated with hyperaemia and bulging of the drum.

Macroscopical
The middle ear is filled with pus or mucopus.

Microscopical
An intense acute polymorph reaction in the Eustachian tube and in the middle ear, with oedema and desquamation of the surface epithelium.

RESULTS

Resolution
The condition may resolve, especially if the purulent exudate is drained by myringotomy, by re-establishing the patency of the Eustachian tube, or by antibiotics.

Perforation
Of the tympanic membrane.

Organization
Organization of the exudate may result in fibrous adhesions of the ossicles producing permanent impairment of hearing.

Chronic otitis media
Continuation of the infection with persistence of the inflammatory process results in a chronic 'wet' ear with aural discharge. The lining of the middle ear undergoes squamous metaplasia with the production of an aural polyp (see p. 320) or sometimes a cholesteatoma.

Cholesteatoma

NATURE
This is not a true tumour but is an overgrowth of squamous epithelium in the confined space of the cavity of the middle ear. It is virtually always associated with chronic otitis media.

SITES
Either in the middle ear or in the mastoid air cells.

MACROSCOPICAL
A pale, firm, often foul-smelling, nodule with a laminated outer surface and frequently with a pale, soft and cystic centre.

MICROSCOPICAL
Composed of metaplastic squamous epithelium with profuse laminated keratin formation and frequently containing cholesterol crystals.

RESULTS
The cholesteatoma may grow externally through the drum and present as a polyp. More frequently it extends medially from the mastoid or middle ear and progressively erodes the temporal bone to reach vital structures, e.g. the lateral sinus or cranial cavity. Infection is thereby introduced into these areas, e.g. thrombophlebitis of the sinus, meningitis, cerebral abscess.

Local spread
Mastoiditis; petrositis; labyrinthitis.

Thrombophlebitis

Infected thrombosis may occur in the small veins in the petrous bone and the infection thus be extended into the petrosal venous sinuses. These sinuses drain into the sigmoid sinus and thence into the jugular bulb and vein; thus, infection may reach the systemic circulation.

Cerebral involvement

The infection may spread through the temporal bone from the ear to produce a localized epidural abscess, meningitis or cerebral abscess.

MASTOIDITIS

Due to extension of inflammation from the middle ear, with which it is in direct communication.

The mucosa of the mastoid air cells is infiltrated by polymorphs with pus formation. The condition may resolve under treatment or extend. Extension through the bone internally may lead to epidural abscess or meningitis; external spread may lead to an abscess – *Bezold's abscess*, in the upper portion of the neck, or to cellulitis of the overlying soft tissues.

PETROSITIS

Inflammation of the air cells in the petrous portion of the temporal bone by infection extending from the middle ear. This may result in severe headache and oedema of the canal in which the sixth nerve lies and result in its paralysis – *Gradenigo's syndrome*.

Inner ear

INFLAMMATION – LABYRINTHITIS

Aetiology

Usually secondary to an acute or chronic otitis media or associated with a cholesteatoma. The condition may occasionally complicate suppurative meningitis.

Routes of infection

Usually through the oval window, following damage to the foot-piece of the stapes or through the round window, but it may also occur by direct extension through the bone.

Results

Impairment of both hearing and labyrinthine functions. In the acute cases, secondary to an acute otitis media, a meningitis may supervene.

OTOSCLEROSIS

Nature

A rare disease in which there is progressive bilateral deafness, starting at about puberty. The condition is more frequent in females and there is usually a family history.

Clinical

A progressive conduction deafness starting in one ear but subsequently involving the other. Speech is quiet as, due to bone conduction, the patient's perception of his own voice is not impaired.

Appearances

Irregular formation of vascular, spongy new bone around the oval window and the promontory, sometimes extending on to the cochlear side of the oval window. This new bone shows both osteoclastic and osteoblastic activity with the formation of 'cement lines' of irregular bone similar to that seen in Paget's disease (see p. 690). This results in loss of mobility and finally in fixation of the footplate of the stapes.

Results

The stapes ankylosis interferes with transmission of sound waves to the inner ear and the operations for its relief are designed to mobilize the stapes. The results are good.

MÉNIÈRE'S DISEASE

Nature

A disease characterized by sudden attacks of giddiness, vomiting and tinnitus, accompanied by some degree of deafness. The attacks tend to become progressively more frequent and severe.

Appearances

The basic change is an increased pressure of unknown aetiology in the endolymph in the inner ear resulting in dilatation of the endolymphatic system. The hair cells of the organ of Corti show a progressive degeneration following the pressure increase.

Tumours

In addition to squamous cell carcinomas of the external ear and rarely in the middle ear arising from squamous metaplasia, there is also a distinct tumour entity, the non-chromaffin paraganglioma – glomus jugulare tumour.

CHEMODECTOMAS

Nature
Tumours arising from non-chromaffin paraganglia which are chemoreceptors, i.e. sensitive to changes in the chemical composition of the blood. These tumours may arise from the carotid body, aortic bodies and from the glomus jugulare. They should not be confused with the chromaffin tumours of adrenaline-producing cells, e.g. phaeochromocytoma of the adrenal medulla (see p. 293) or in other sites.

GLOMUS JUGULARE TUMOUR

Origin
From the glomus jugulare, a small chemoreceptor organ, situated in the wall of the jugular bulb.

Clinical
The tumour frequently presents as a vascular polypoid tumour in the auditory meatus. It is associated with some deafness and usually occurs in middle-aged females.

Appearances
It is composed of clumps of large polyhedral cells in a fibrous stroma containing many vascular spaces. The tumour cells show no chromaffin reaction.

Results
The tumour slowly spreads from its site of origin in the jugular bulb to invade the petrous portion of the temporal bone and thus invade and destroy the ear to present as a polyp in the external auditory meatus. Biopsy will reveal the true nature of the tumour but its vascularity is such that biopsy, trauma, or any subsequent operative procedure, may be attended by torrential and even fatal haemorrhage. Thus, irradiation is usually employed in an endeavour to restrict further invasion.

CAROTID BODY TUMOUR

Incidence
A rare tumour, but this is the commonest type of chemodectoma.

Origin
From the carotid body at the bifurcation of the common carotid artery.

Age
Usually between 30 and 60 years of age.

Sex
M:F equal.

Macroscopical
Presents as a firm, solid, 'potato tumour' enveloping the carotid vessels at the bifurcation.

Microscopical
Consists of masses of polyhedral, large and often fat-containing cells in a fibrous stroma in which there are large vascular spaces. The cells are regular in formation and show no mitoses.

Results
They are slowly growing and increasingly compress the carotid arteries, but only very rarely are they malignant. Surgical removal may become necessary to relieve the arterial obstruction.

OTHER CHEMODECTOMAS

The other examples elsewhere in the body are very rare; they have similar appearances to the carotid body tumour and behave in a benign manner.

Chapter 60
Diseases of the Eye – Eyelids: Conjunctiva: Cornea

Eyelids

INFLAMMATIONS

Stye

Chalazion
Nature
Macroscopical
Microscopical

Molluscum contagiosum

CYSTS
Sudosiferous
Sebaceous
Dermoid
Meibomian

TUMOURS
Benign
Xanthelasma
  Nature
  Macroscopical
  Microscopical
Neurofibroma
Squamous cell papilloma
Lipoma
Benign calcifying epithelioma of
  Malherbe
Haemangioma
Lymphangioma
Naevus

Malignant
Pre-cancerous melanosis
Bowen's disease
Squamous cell carcinoma
Basal cell carcinoma
Malignant melanoma
Adenocarcinoma
Sarcoma
Lymphoma

Conjunctiva

INFLAMMATIONS

Simple bacterial conjunctivitis
Acute
Chronic

Follicular conjunctivitis
Trachoma
Nature
Macroscopical
Microscopical

Spring catarrh
Nature
Macroscopical
Microscopical

Tuberculosis
Origin
Macroscopical
Microscopical

Phlyctenular conjunctivitis
Nature
Macroscopical
Microscopical

Sarcoidosis
Incidence
Macroscopical
Microscopical

DEGENERATIONS

Ageing

Pinguecula
Nature
Macroscopical
Microscopical

Concretions
Macroscopical
Microscopical

CYSTS
Traumatic
Retention
Lymphatic

TUMOURS
Benign
Papilloma
Epithelial plaque
Naevus
  Cystic naevus of conjunctiva
Haemangioma
Dermo-lipoma

Malignant
Bowen's disease
Squamous cell carcinoma
Basal cell carcinoma
Pre-cancerous melanosis
  Macroscopical
  Microscopical
Malignant melanoma
Benign lymphoma
Malignant lymphoma

Cornea

INFLAMMATIONS – KERATITIS

Ulcers
Marginal
  Simple catarrhal
  Mooren's ulcer
Central
  Hypopyon ulcer
Sequelae of corneal ulcers
  Opacities
  Facet
  Ectatic cicatrix
  Descemetococle
  Perforation
  Anterior staphyloma

Interstitial keratitis
Nature
Origin
Appearances
Results

CORNEAL DYSTROPHIES
Granular
Macular
Lattice

DEGENERATIONS
Arcus senilis
Pannus degenerativus
Pterygium
Keratoconus

TUMOURS
Epithelial plaques
Squamous cell carcinoma
Fibroma
Dermoid

324

Eyelids

INFLAMMATIONS

STYE – HORDEOLUM

Staphylococcal infection of an eyelash follicle and its associated gland of Zeis. There is cellulitis of the lid followed by localization and pointing, usually at the lid margin.

CHALAZION

Nature
A chronic granuloma developing within an obstructed Meibomian gland.

Macroscopical
A firm and painless lump usually in the upper lid.

Microscopical
Composed of granulation tissue rich in epithelioid

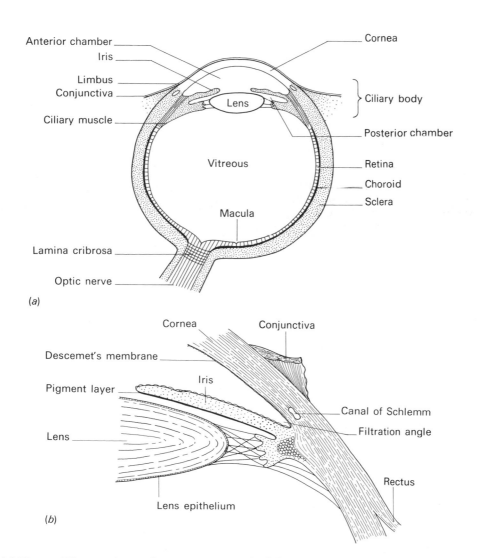

Fig. 36. (a) The eye. Diagram of the main structures.   **(b)** Ciliary body and adjacent structures.

and giant cells. The whole reactive area is surrounded by fibrous tissue, but multiple clear small cystic spaces are present in the main mass containing lipid material. Confusion with tuberculosis may arise but caseation and organisms are not present.

MOLLUSCUM CONTAGIOSUM

This warty swelling with an umbilicated centre is caused by a virus infection of the prickle cells. This skin lesion is described on p. 730.

CYSTS

Sudosiferous
The clear cyst which arises due to duct obstruction of the modified sweat gland of Moll.

Sebaceous
These cysts arise within the sebaceous Zeis's gland.

Dermoid
Inclusion dermoids associated with the suture lines in the orbital bones, may extend into the lids. They are most commonly present at the outer angle of the orbit – *external angular dermoid*.

Meibomian
Blockage of the duct of a Meibomian gland may result in a cyst lined by flattened epithelium.

TUMOURS

BENIGN

Xanthelasma

NATURE
This lesion may be a manifestation of an hypercholesterolaemic condition, e.g. diabetes, or occur as an isolated lesion, particularly in middle-aged women.

MACROSCOPICAL
An elevated yellowish plaque usually situated near the inner canthus – *Xanthelasma palpebrum*.

MICROSCOPICAL
Large foam cells containing cholesterol and phospholipids with a variable fibrous component.

Neurofibroma
In von Recklinghausen's disease, the eyelid is frequently involved by extension of neurofibromas from the fronto-temporal region and orbit.

Squamous cell papilloma
These are simple sessile or pedunculated papillary tumours of the squamous epithelium and are commonly seen on the lids.

Lipoma
Adipose tissue is not normally present in the lid, thus lipomas only occur in this situation as extensions from the orbital fat.

Benign calcifying epithelioma of Malherbe
This uncommon lesion shows calcifying squamous epithelium in the dermis. The condition is entirely benign, occurs at any skin site, especially in children.

Haemangioma
All types occur in the lid, identical to similar lesions in other cutaneous sites. The cavernous variety may be associated with haemangiomas and cysts elsewhere – von Hippel–Lindau disease (see p. 341).

Lymphangioma
Rarely found in the lids.

Naevus
These are common lesions of the lids and occur as compound, junctional and intradermal types (see p. 733).

MALIGNANT

Pre-cancerous melanosis – intra-epithelial melanoma (Ashton)
See p. 329.

Bowen's disease
See p. 730.

Squamous cell carcinoma
This tumour behaves in a similar manner to squamous cell carcinoma elsewhere in the skin. There is an irregular ulcerated area which is capable of causing extensive lid destruction with invasion of surrounding structures.

Basal cell carcinoma – rodent ulcer

This is the most common malignant tumour of eyelids; indeed this is one of the commonest sites for such a tumour to develop. There is at first a small nodule, later an ulcerated centre and a rolled edge. Direct invasion of adjacent structures may result in a very considerable area of destruction involving the globe, orbit and adjacent bone (see p. 731).

Malignant melanoma

This arises in a pre-existing naevus or in an area of pre-cancerous melanosis (see p. 329).

Adenocarcinoma

This is an uncommon tumour which can arise in the sebaceous glands of Zeis, Meibomian glands, sweat glands of Moll or the accessory lacrimal gland of Krause.

Sarcoma

Very rare, but types reported include spindle cell, round cell, angiosarcoma, myxosarcoma, leiomyosarcoma and rhabdomyosarcoma.

Lymphoma

Hodgkin's and non-Hodgkin's deposits and leukaemic tissue are very occasionally seen in the lids.

Conjunctiva

INFLAMMATIONS

SIMPLE BACTERIAL CONJUNCTIVITIS

Acute

Conjunctivitis is extremely common and may be due to a large number of different organisms of variable pathogenicity. The condition usually resolves completely with local treatment.

Chronic

Usually arises as a continuation of acute conjunctivitis with only slight discharge, although the lids feel heavy and gritty. Microscopically, there is a mild chronic inflammatory cell infiltrate and epithelial proliferation.

FOLLICULAR CONJUNCTIVITIS

A response to many irritants including viral and toxic agents. Pinhead-sized elevations, often in rows, occur on the conjunctiva of the lower lid. They are composed of aggregations of mononuclear cells in the subepithelial layer; in those cases due to chalamydial infection, inclusion bodies may be demonstrable.

TRACHOMA

Nature

This important chlamydial infection is the most common cause of blindness in the world, being particularly frequent in Africa and the East. The organism is closely related to that of virus inclusion conjunctivitis.

The sexual partners of trachoma sufferers are frequently found to harbour the infective agent in the urethra or cervix and babies born to mothers with cervicitis and/or trachoma, have been found to have the agent in their conjunctivae.

Macroscopical

In the early stages, there is an acute conjunctivitis but eventually extensive conjunctival and corneal scarring ensures. The diagnosis can be made with certainty in the early stages by the demonstration of inclusion bodies in desquamated epithelial cells.

Microscopical

In the acute stage there is a heavy mononuclear cell infiltration, both diffuse and aggregated into follicles. This is accompanied by epithelial proliferation with invaginations and downgrowths which may become sequestrated to form pseudocysts. Later, the follicles are composed of pale-staining macrophages surrounded by lymphocytes and plasma cells. These follicles eventually rupture through the epithelium, or are absorbed and replaced by scar tissue with resulting lid deformity. Moreover, the inflammatory process extends into the cornea as a pannus starting at the limbus. Bowman's membrane is destroyed and blood vessels migrate into the substantia propria with inevitable scarring and opacity leading to blindness.

SPRING CATARRH – VERNAL CONJUNCTIVITIS

Nature

Occurs in springtime due to a reaction to exogenous allergens, e.g. pollens and moulds.

Macroscopical

The lid conjunctiva shows an hyperaemic 'cobble-stone' appearance, associated with a considerable mucoid discharge rich in eosinophils.

Microscopical

There is proliferation of the goblet cells and the subepithelial tissues. The 'cobbles' and pseudo-cysts are formed from the epithelial invaginations in a similar way to those of trachoma. An infiltration of mononuclear cells and eosinophils is later replaced by fibrous tissue. Follicles are not formed.

TUBERCULOSIS

Origin

Primary lesions are rare and secondary infections uncommon but may occur by extension of disease from the lacrimal gland, lacrimal sac and lids.

Macroscopical

There are three types:
1   Ulcerative – small miliary ulcers.
2   Nodular.
3   Hypertrophic.

Microscopical

The histological appearances are similar to the giant cell systems seen elsewhere in this disease.

PHYLCTENULAR CONJUNCTIVITIS

Nature

Although this condition can occur as an allergic reaction to any protein substance, most cases are caused by tuberculoprotein hypersensitivity.

Macroscopical

Pinkish-yellow spots in the conjunctival epithelium, limbus and cornea with, except in the cornea, surrounding vascular engorgement.

Microscopical

There is an exudate within the subepithelial tissues containing leucocytes and mononuclear cells. No tuberculous giant cell systems are found.

SARCOIDOSIS

Incidence

Ocular involvement occurs in about 25 per cent of cases of this systemic granulomatous disease (see p. 51).

Macroscopical

Although the uveal tract is most commonly involved, the conjunctiva may show pinhead-sized sarcoid lesions in the fold between the bulbar and palpebral conjunctiva – lower fornix.

Microscopical

The absence of caseation and of organisms differentiates the giant cell systems from tuberculosis.

DEGENERATIONS

AGEING

With increasing age, the conjunctiva loses its clear whiteness and becomes slightly roughened and less transparent. The epithelium shows a tendency to keratinization and the subepithelial tissues become hyalinized and thinned.

PINGUECULA

Nature

Exposure to wind and dust enhances degenerative changes, especially at the interpalpebral margin of the cornea.

Macroscopical

A raised, opaque, triangular, yellow spot close to the limbus, usually on the nasal side.

Microscopical

There is patchy atrophy and thickening of the epithelium with proliferation of the subepithelial elastic tissue, subsequent hyalinization and fragmentation.

CONCRETIONS

Macroscopical

White or yellow spots within the tarsal conjunctiva of elderly or debilitated persons.

Microscopical

There are obstructed serous glands containing inspissated epithelial cells and mucus which form concentrically laminated bodies. They may calcify and thus damage the corneal epithelium.

CYSTS

Traumatic
Implanted epithelium, particularly goblet cells, may form a mucinous cyst surrounded by a fibrous capsule.

Retention
These vary greatly in size and may arise from mucous glands, from the epithelial downgrowths of trachoma and spring catarrh, or within Krause's gland.

Lymphatic
Thin-walled dilated lymphatics may rarely be seen on the bulbar conjunctiva.

TUMOURS

BENIGN

Papilloma
These sessile or pedunculated epithelial papillomas frequently arise around the caruncle and are rich in goblet cells.

Epithelial plaque
A whitish area at the limbus consisting of simple and regular proliferation of the epithelial layer, with or without keratinization.

Naevus
In addition to the usual types of naevi seen elsewhere, there is a particular form found only in the conjunctiva:

CYSTIC NAEVUS OF CONJUNCTIVA
A smooth, variably pigmented, mobile nodule composed of downgrowths of epithelium which form cystic structures and are surrounded by naevus cells.

Haemangioma
Capillary or cavernous types occasionally occur.

Dermo-lipoma
A yellow, triangular, congenital tumour which presents between the superior and external rectus muscles. The fatty element is continuous with the orbital fat and, in addition, there are hair follicles, sebaceous and sweat glands. The mass is covered by thickened conjunctival epithelium.

MALIGNANT

Bowen's disease
This condition is similar to Bowen's disease of the skin (see p. 730) and is a pre-invasive condition whilst it remains localized as a reddish-grey plaque at the limbus or lid margin. Eventually, after several years, if untreated, it becomes frankly invasive and subsequently behaves as a squamous cell carcinoma. The irregular and atypical epithelial overgrowth is confined by an intact basement membrane until invasive characteristics appear.

Squamous cell carcinoma
This may arise *de novo*, or from a papilloma, an epithelial plaque or in an area of Bowen's disease. It is seen as a warty non-pigmented tumour in the elderly and is most frequently found at the limbus from whence it may spread across the cornea and invade adjacent tissues.

Basal cell carcinoma
Primary basal cell tumours of the conjunctiva do not occur due to the absence of basal type cells. However, extension from a lid rodent ulcer may cause a secondary tumour.

Pre-cancerous melanosis – intra-epithelial melanoma (Ashton)

MACROSCOPICAL
This may occur in both the skin of the lid and conjunctiva and first appears in middle age. The lesions are flat, irregular and variably pigmented, commonly of a widespread and bespattered 'gunshot' distribution.

MICROSCOPICAL
There is intra-epithelial proliferation of pigmented basal epithelial cells over a wide area resulting in a multilayered structure. Bud-like clusters of cells may extend into the dermis but the lesion remains pre-cancerous for a variable period of time and is analogous to a junctional naevus except for its widespread distribution (see p. 733). Eventually,

anaplasia and frank invasion occurs, the lesion then behaving as a malignant melanoma.

Malignant melanoma
Arises most frequently from pre-cancerous melanosis but may also develop in a previously simple naevus present from birth. Malignancy is high and blood-borne metastases are common.

Benign lymphoma
This is a benign lesion which may be difficult to differentiate from deposits of malignant lymphoma. There is benign overgrowth of conjunctival lymphoid tissue and similar lesions occur in the lids, lacrimal gland and orbit. They are usually bilateral and consist of aggregations of mature lymphocytes.

Malignant lymphoma
Leukaemic deposits, non-Hodgkin's and Hodgkin's lymphoma, are occasionally found in the conjunctiva as a manifestation of generalization of these diseases.

Cornea

INFLAMMATIONS—KERATITIS

ULCERS

Marginal

SIMPLE CATARRHAL
Commonly associated with acute conjunctivitis due to staphylococci or the Koch-Weeks bacillus. A small ulcer develops in the marginal corneal epithelium and is accompanied by an inflammatory cell infiltration. Healing rapidly occurs when the infection is eliminated and corneal perforation is rare.

MOOREN'S ULCER
This occurs in the elderly and is usually bilateral. A shallow ulcer with an overhanging edge forms at the corneal margin and there is a chronic inflammatory cell infiltration with some necrosis of the superficial substantia propria. The ulcer may extend across the entire corneal surface but perforation is uncommon.

Central
Central ulcers usually commence as primary pyo-genic infections of the cornea. An example is the hypopyon ulcer.

HYPOPYON ULCER
Macroscopical. A corneal ulcer associated with cloudy exudate within the anterior chamber.
Microscopical. Acute and chronic inflammatory cells are present in the region of the ulcer and also infiltrate the iris, ciliary body and anterior chamber forming a sterile but cloudy exudate – hypopyon. There is necrosis of the substantia propria, the filtration angles are occluded by exudate and the iris margin frequently adheres to the lens. Thus, anterior and posterior synechiae are formed.
Results. The ulcer either penetrates all layers with resulting perforation or heals with the formation of dense scar tissue.

Sequelae of corneal ulceration

OPACITIES
Due to scarring.

FACET
A shallow surface depression resulting from loss of tissue.

ECTATIC CICATRIX
An outward bulging of scar tissue.

DESCEMETOCOELE
Ulceration may leave only Descement's membrane – the innermost layer, which, as a result of intra-ocular pressure, may bulge outwards.

PERFORATION
Rupture of the cornea, which may be followed by prolapse of the lens and iris through the perforation.

ANTERIOR STAPHYLOMA
If a corneal perforation becomes sealed by the iris and the anterior surface is later epithelialized, intra-ocular pressure may cause bulging of the 'plug' producing the staphylomatous deformity.

INTERSTITIAL KERATITIS

Nature
Inflammation of the deeper layers of the cornea.

Origin

Although sometimes the result of extension from superficial inflammatory lesions, this is more usually syphilitic in origin and is associated with an iridocyclitis.

Appearances

The fibres of the substantia propria become swollen and later necrotic. Vessels and lymphocytes infiltrate from the limbus and there is degeneration of Descement's membrane. Eventually, the vessels within the stroma lose their blood but remain as 'ghosts'. The superficial layers are not involved.

Results

Dense opacity of the cornea follows.

CORNEAL DYSTROPHIES

Hereditary bilateral degenerations of the cornea, usually appearing at the time of puberty. There are three main types.

Granular

Hyaline nodules in all layers with clear intervening zones.

Macular

Central hyaline nodules with opacity of the intervening stroma.

Lattice

Superficial, doubly-contoured, bifurcating lines of granular and hyaline material crossing one another.

DEGENERATIONS

Arcus senilis

This presents in middle age, is caused by fatty infiltration and appears as a pale ring at the periphery. The outer border is sharply defined but the inner margin indefinite.

Pannus degenerativus

This occurs in eyes which are either senile or in which there has been longstanding inflammation. There is vascularization and round cell infiltration in the superficial layers at the margin with overlying epithelial thickening. The central cornea remains unaffected.

Pterygium

A wing-shaped ingrowth of conjunctival epithelium appearing on the nasal or lateral sides of the cornea and progressing towards its centre. There is replacement of degenerate material by vascularized connective tissue.

Keratoconus – conical cornea

Probably has both a congenital and a degenerative aetiology and appears at puberty as apical bulging, rendering the patient grossly myopic. There is thinning of the central cornea.

TUMOURS

The majority of corneal tumours have their origin in the conjunctiva or limbus but primary lesions which have occasionally been described include the following.

Epithelial plaques

Benign overgrowth of squamous cells.

Squamous cell carcinoma

Usually arising within an epithelial plaque.

Fibroma

Following corneal trauma.

Dermoid

A fibro-fatty mass with projecting hairs.

Chapter 61
Diseases of the Eye – Lens:
Uveal Tract: Retina

Lens
Structure

CATARACT
Nature

Lens changes
Nuclear cataract
Cortical cataract

Clinical types
Congenital
Senile
   Absorption without reaction
   Phagolytic glaucoma
   Lens-induced uveitis
Other types
   Traumatic
   Complicated
   Diabetic
   Physical causes
   After (secondary)

PSEUDO-EXFOLIATION OF LENS
   CAPSULE

Uveal tract

INFLAMMATIONS – UVEITIS

Non-specific
Acute
   Origin
   Macroscopical
   Microscopical
Chronic
   Iris
   Ciliary body
   Choroid

Granulomatous
Tuberculosis
   Iris and ciliary body
   Choroid
Acquired syphilis
   Syphilitic iridocyclitis
   Syphilitic choroiditis
Congenital syphilis
   First year of life
   Puberty
   Early adulthood
Sarcoidosis
   Iris and ciliary body
   Choroid
Toxoplasmosis
Toxocara canis
LENS-INDUCED UVEITIS
Nature
Appearances

SYMPATHETIC OPHTHALMITIS
Nature
Pathogenesis
Macroscopical
Microscopical

Retina
VASCULAR DISEASES
Involutionary sclerosis

Arteriolosclerotic retinopathy
Nature
Appearances

Atheroma

Accelerated hypertension

Cytoid bodies

Central retinal vein thrombosis

Diabetic retinopathy
Macroscopical
Microscopical

Eales' disease

Coats's disease

Retrolental fibroplasia
Macroscopical
Microscopical

Senile macular degeneration

Disciform degeneration

DEGENERATIONS

Retinitis pigmentosa
Nature
Macroscopical
Microscopical

Cysts
Nature
Microscopical

CONGENITAL

Coloboma of choroid and retina
Nature
Macroscopical
Microscopical

Persistence of hyaloid artery
Macroscopical
Microscopical

GLAUCOMA
Nature

Primary
Nature
Pathology

Congenital

Secondary
Nature
Aetiology
Results

Lens

Structure

The lens is a unique avascular structure formed entirely by epithelium. It is enclosed by a hyaline capsule, beneath this is the epithelium which produces the keratinized lens fibres. These, as they mature, become packed into the centre to form the 'nucleus' of the lens which inevitably becomes both larger and denser with advancing age.

CATARACT

Nature

Any opacity of the lens.

LENS CHANGES

There are two main senile types.

Nuclear cataract

This is an extension and intensification of the physiological sclerosis which occurs with ageing. The fibres of the nucleus are progressively compressed at the centre into laminated layers which coalesce to form an homogeneous opaque mass.

Cortical cataract

In this type, the changes occur in the cortical fibres that surround the central nucleus. These fibres become oedematous with the deposition of albuminous material which coalesces to form Morgagnian globules: it is this coagulated albuminous material which forms the opacity. Finally the entire lens cortex becomes a pultaceous mass of globules and granular debris enclosed within the capsule.

CLINICAL TYPES

Congenital cataract

This is usually of the nuclear type and the condition may be familial as an autosomal dominant. In other cases, it is associated with multiple intraocular congenital abnormalities, but some cases presenting at birth are due to maternal rubella infection during pregnancy (see p. 43).

Senile cataract

This is the common form of lenticular opacity which becomes increasingly frequent with advancing age. The lens may show either the nuclear or cortical form of cataract. If the latter form occurs, the altered and liquefied lens material may remain within the lens capsule but frequently this ruptures and releases material into the globe resulting in the following:

ABSORPTION WITHOUT REACTION

PHAGOLYTIC GLAUCOMA
Phagocytes appear, ingest the lens material and, in their swollen state, block the filtration angles.

LENS-INDUCED UVEITIS
See p. 335.

Other types of cataract

TRAUMATIC
Following penetration of the lens, the capsule retracts away from the area of injury. The defect is frequently filled by optically dense reparative fibres.

COMPLICATED CATARACT
A cataract following other intra-ocular diseases, e.g. iridocyclitis, retinitis pigmentosa, choroidoretinitis, detached retina, etc.

DIABETIC CATARACT
In severe cases of diabetes in young individuals, a bilateral and rapidly progressive form of cataract frequently occurs. Elderly diabetics are also prone to cataract but it is then indistinguishable from the senile type.

CATARACT DUE TO PHYSICAL CAUSES
Lens opacities may follow exposure to ionizing radiations, lighting or electric shocks; glassworker's cataract occurs due to damage by heat whilst intra-ocular metallic objects, especially iron and copper, may also induce a lens opacity.

AFTER OR SECONDARY CATARACT
This is the development of an opacity in the intracapsular lens residue after nuclear extraction. This is largely due to epithelial proliferation which grows through the capsule incision on to its outer surface and is followed by adhesions to other intra-ocular structures.

PSEUDO-EXFOLIATION OF THE LENS CAPSULE

A collection of fluffy white material of unknown composition which forms within the anterior chamber, on the surface of the iris, ciliary body, zonules and lens capsule. The material shows eosinophilic staining, and is of a feathery shrub-like appearance. It may peel off the lens surface and be carried to the filtration angles resulting in glaucoma.

Uveal tract

The uveal tract consists of the iris, the ciliary body and the choroid.

INFLAMMATIONS – UVEITIS

NON-SPECIFIC

Acute uveitis

ORIGIN
Arising from perforating wounds, corneal ulcers or septicaemic conditions.

MACROSCOPICAL
Purulent infection of the uveal tract – *purulent endophthalmitis*. Localization and abscess formation usually occur with subsequent fibrosis, intra-ocular disorganization, contraction of the entire globe, calcification and ossification – *phthisis bulbi*.

An even more widespread infection of the eye involving the retina and vitreous in addition – *panophthalmitis* – may result in abscess formation within the vitreous with danger of global rupture.

MICROSCOPICAL
The predominant picture is a widespread polymorph infiltration of the affected tissues. When localization takes place fibrosis occurs, its extent varying with the size of the inflammatory mass. If confined to the anterior segment, dense scar tissue may form on the anterior surface of the iris covering the pupil – *occlusio pupillae*, and the filtration angles may become occluded – *peripheral anterior synechiae*. In the posterior segment, localization leads to abscess formation within the vitreous where the

organisms are free from inhibiting structures. Regression is followed by fibrosis in the form of a transverse membrane – *cyclitic membrane*, which, by contraction, may detach the retina, if this has not already occurred due to a subretinal purulent exudate.

Chronic uveitis

The distinction between acute and chronic uveitis is not always clearly defined, but in the usual non-specific infections by organisms of low pathogenicity, the appearances in the uveal tract are as follows.

IRIS
There is a focal chronic inflammatory infiltration, heavy in the region of the sphincter muscles. Adhesions in the filtration angles – peripheral anterior synechiae, commonly develop and eversion of the pupillary margin – *ectropion uveae*, may occur due to fibrosis. Posterior synechiae, adhesions between the iris and lens, usually form and thus the entire pupillary margin becomes adherent to the lens – *seclusio pupillae*. Rising intra-ocular tension is then inevitable and causes the anchored iris to balloon forwards – *'iris bombé'*, narrowing even further the anterior chamber. The pigmented epithelium shows patchy degeneration and proliferation, whilst chronic inflammatory cells wander from the iris into the anterior chamber and aggregate in small clumps on the corneal endothelium – *'keratitis punctata'*.

CILIARY BODY
There is fibrosis and a chronic inflammatory cell infiltration, usually focal and maximal posteriorly.

CHOROID
Dense focal aggregations of lymphocytes and scattered plasma cells which may extend into the retina destroying the pigmented epithelium and outer layers – *choroidoretinitis*. Healing causes dense sclerotic patches within the choroid and overlying retina and the formation of small round hyaline nodules – *colloid bodies*, which may distort the retinal surface.

GRANULOMATOUS

Tuberculosis
This is almost always secondary

IRIS AND CILIARY BODY

An exudate is unusual but pale 'mutton fat' precipitates of endothelial cells may be deposited on the posterior surface of the cornea. Caseation is rare in miliary tubercles but may be present in large, solitary, nodular masses that sometimes occur and which may involve the cornea.

CHOROID

This layer may be involved as part of a generalized miliary tuberculosis but more commonly appears as chronic tuberculous choroiditis. The appearances vary from large masses of granulation tissue, rendering the vitreous and aqueous opaque, to lesions no more than 1 mm in diameter. Both eyes commonly show typical caseating tuberculous granulation tissue, often involving the retina. Healing is prolonged with frequent relapses.

Acquired syphilis

SYPHILITIC IRIDOCYCLITIS

This occurs in the later secondary stages of the disease and is the most frequent ocular manifestation of syphilis. Fleshy pink nodules are situated near the pupillary margin, usually with occlusion of the filtration angles and glaucoma results.

SYPHILITIC CHOROIDITIS

The clinical picture closely resembles that of tuberculous choroiditis but histologically there are gummatous areas and perivascular collections of lymphocytes and plasma cells. The retina and the overlying adjacent sclera are frequently involved.

Congenital syphilis

There are several presentations.

FIRST YEAR OF LIFE

A simple uveitis which may progress to choroidoretinitis.

PUBERTY

Interstitial keratitis and anterior uveitis.

EARLY ADULTHOOD

Choroidoretinitis with fine pigmented scarring – 'pepper and salt fundus'.

Sarcoidosis

IRIS AND CILIARY BODY

Opaque pinkish-yellow nodules of sarcoid tissue, often involving large areas.

CHOROID

Focal or generalized infiltration by sarcoid tissue.

Toxoplasmosis

In both congenital and adult types, the disease is mostly confined to the choroid but with infrequent retinal and scleral involvement. Focal granulomatous lesions may be mistaken for those of tuberculosis. Diagnosis is made by the finding of the protozoon – *Toxoplasma gondii*, either in pseudocysts or extracllularly (see p. 63).

Toxocara canis

The migrating larvae of the dog nematode, *Toxocara canis*, are capable of lodging in the uveal tract of children forming a granulomatous lesion. On ophthalmoscopy this can closely resemble a neoplasm.

LENS-INDUCED UVEITIS – PHAGOANAPHYLACTIC ENDOPHTHALMITIS

Nature

Following the release of lens protein in the opposite eye at an earlier date, release of protein in the second eye may precipitate an anaphylactic anterior uveitis (see below).

Appearances

The eye is acutely inflamed. The iris, ciliary body, anterior choroid and cortex of the ruptured lens are infiltrated by eosinophils, polymorphs, plasma cells, lymphocytes, giant cells, macrophages and endothelial cells. Glaucoma is a common sequel.

SYMPATHETIC OPHTHALMITIS

Nature

This is a bilateral cellular reaction of the entire uveal tract following a penetrating injury to one eye – the 'exciting' eye, 4–8 weeks previously. The response in the non-injured, 'sympathizing' eye, can be avoided if the injured 'exciting' eye is urgently enucleated. If sympathetic ophthalmitis is allowed to proceed, blindness in both eyes is inevitable.

Pathogenesis

It is believed that this is an allergic reaction in both

eyes to uveal pigment released on injury of the 'exciting' eye.

Macroscopical

Clinically, both eyes resemble any of the other granulomatous conditions previously described. Evidence of previous injury to the 'exciting' eye is present but it is the only feature distinguishing the two eyes.

Microscopical

The cellular reaction is contained almost entirely within the uveal tract and consists of:

1 A massive infiltration of lymphocytes.
2 Collections of endothelial cells with scattered giant cells.
3 Eosinophils.
4 Dalen–Fuch's nodules – aggregations of the above cells between the retina and the choroid.
5 Perivascular collections in the sclera and tumour-like cellular aggregations on its outer surface.

The retina remains intact except for slight thinning over the Dalen–Fuch's nodules.

Retina

VASCULAR DISEASES

General features

The central artery of the optic nerve, although structurally similar to other arteries of similar size, loses its elastic tissue after the first and second divisions and the muscle separates into isolated fibres leaving a wall composed of endothelium and adventitia only. Thus vascular disease in the retina varies somewhat from arterial lesions elsewhere. Moreover the vessels are readily visible through an ophthalmoscope so that changes seen in this way may provide important information regarding the state of the vascular system in general.

INVOLUTIONARY SCLEROSIS

An ageing process not associated with hypertension but in which arterioles are narrowed, pale and variable in calibre. Histologically, there is fibrosis and patchy endothelial proliferation.

ARTERIOLOSCLEROTIC RETINOPATHY – DIFFUSE HYPERPLASTIC SCLEROSIS

Nature

Retinal changes associated with hypertension (see p. 267).

Appearances

Early. Narrowing due to endothelial proliferation and deposition of hyaline material. This produces the characteristic 'copper and silver wire' ophthalmoscopic appearance.

Later. Segmental dilatation due to hypertension results in tortuosity and compression at the arteriovenous crossings.

Late. Eventually thin, white, parallel lines of fatty material surround the vessels – 'pipe-stem sheathing'. Retinal haemorrhages occur but are small and are usually rapidly absorbed.

ATHEROMA

Although the retinal artery is not a common site of atheroma, when present it may cause vascular occlusion and serious atrophy of the inner retinal layers. The outer layers are supplied by choroidal vessels and are thus unaffected.

ACCELERATED HYPERTENSION

Papilloedema, exudates and small haemorrhages are present. The vessels show irregular narrowing and areas of fibrinoid necrosis with surrounding extravasated blood.

CYTOID BODIES

These are fluffy white patches in the retina which are found in cases of accelerated hypertension, systemic lupus erythematosus and dermatomyositis. They were originally believed to be varicose nerve fibres, and this has now been confirmed. The cytoid body is actually a nodular swelling on the injured axon – Cajal node, and consists of an eosinophilic pseudo-nucleus lying within a 'cytoplasm' of swollen axon material.

CENTRAL RETINAL VEIN THROMBOSIS – THROMBOTIC GLAUCOMA

Thrombosis of retinal veins at points of arterio-venous crossing. This occurs in hypertensives and frequently at the site of global entry of the optic nerve – *lamina cribrosa*. Retinal degeneration follows and, for an unknown reason, new vessels grow on the surface of the iris and into the filtration angles, thus leading to glaucoma. In the area of the retina drained by the thrombosed vein, haemorrhages occur in great numbers and the veins are engorged. At a later stage, the retinal haemorrhages are absorbed leaving cystic spaces and the thrombus may partially recanalize. Cupping of the optic nerve head follows the glaucomatous rise of intra-ocular pressure.

DIABETIC RETINOPATHY

Macroscopical
Both retinae are affected, the first abnormality being the appearance of 'dot' haemorrhages, now known to be capillary micro-aneurysms. Later, the aneurysms rupture producing 'blot' haemorrhages, accompanied by small yellow-white exudates which may become confluent. Haemorrhages spread into the vitreous provoking development of new blood vessels and fibrous tissue – *'retinitis proliferans'*. This condition frequently leads to retinal detachment and degeneration.

Microscopical
The micro-aneurysms are minute spherical distensions of capillary vessels and are mostly present on the venous side of the network. They lie mainly in the inner layers of the retina but with advanced cases occur in great numbers on both venous and arterial sides. The 'blot' haemorrhages arise from the aneurysms and also from degenerate vessels. Even without haemorrhage, new capillaries may grow into the vitreous – *rete mirabile*, and are frequently the site of fresh haemorrhages. Ultimately *phthisis bulbi* develops.

EALES'S DISEASE

Recurrent vitreous and retinal haemorrhages occurring in young adults; the aetiology is un-known. Absorption of the haemorrhage is followed by vascularization, fibrosis of the vitreous and eventual retinal detachment.

COATS'S DISEASE

A disease of unknown aetiology also occurring in young adults in which haemorrhagic exudation into the subretinal space occurs causing retinal detachment.

Cholesterol crystals with surrounding foreign body giant cells are found within the subretinal exudate. There is a lining of phagocytes lying against the outer surface of the detached retina and the inner surface of the choroid.

RETROLENTAL FIBROPLASIA

Macroscopical
Detachment and fibrosis of the retina, usually bilateral and occurring in premature babies after removal from an incubator in which the oxygen concentration has been greater than 40 per cent.

Microscopical
There is angioblastic activity in the inner retinal layer with haemorrhages and formation of new vessels in the vitreous. This leads to retinal detachment and conversion into the retrolental fibrous membrane.

SENILE MACULAR DEGENERATION (HAAB)

The blood supply of the macula is dependent upon choroidal vessels. Sclerosis of these vessels will result in retinal damage and loss of central vision – *central scotoma*.

DISCIFORM DEGENERATION OF THE MACULA (JUNNIS AND KUHNT)

A degenerative process of the macula of unknown aetiology and characterized by irregular white-yellow swellings. These consist of organized exudates between the choroid and retina, the outer layers of which are atrophic and replaced by glial tissue.

DEGENERATIONS

RETINITIS PIGMENTOSA

Nature
Premature degeneration of the retinal neuroepithelium which commences in early adult life and is manifest by progressive night blindness and loss of visual fields, with total blindness by 50–60 years of age.

Macroscopical
Pigmentary migration and clumping at the fundus, usually more advanced on one side. The arteries are attenuated and the discs pale and waxy.

Microscopical
The rods and cones are almost entirely missing, the outer nuclear and plexiform layers atrophic and the pigmented epithelium disorganized. Cells of this layer migrate haphazardly into the retina and also form proliferating masses. Phagocytes, engorged with pigment granules, are carried towards the retinal perivascular spaces. In many cases the optic disc shows atrophy.

CYSTS

Nature
Cystic change in the peripheral part of the retina occurring in middle age. Rupture of one of these cysts may result in retinal detachment.

Microscopical
Small spaces develop within the outer and inner nuclear layers which fuse forming interlacing channels. At a later stage, all surrounding retinal tissue is destroyed, the channels lying between the internal limiting membrane and a compressed layer of rods and cones.

CONGENITAL

COLOBOMA OF THE CHOROID AND RETINA

Nature
A congenital fissure of the eye.

Macroscopical
May be associated with a similar lesion of the optic nerve, ciliary body and iris. The defect, if complete, extends from the optic disc downwards and inwards to the pupillary margin of the iris. It is due to an anomalous closure of the foetal cleft with ectodermal hyperplasia at the margins.

Microscopical
The sclera and choroid are thin, Bruch's membrane is absent and the fault is covered by atypical retinal tissue.

PERSISTENCE OF THE HYALOID ARTERY – PERSISTENT HYPERPLASTIC VITREOUS

Macroscopical
The remains of the hyaloid artery may be found as a cord stretching from the optic disc to the posterior surface of the lens. Often other congenital abnormalities are also found – microphthalmia, ectopic lens or ectopic pupil.

Microscopical
Posteriorly, the artery may be patent and contain blood. Anteriorly, the fibrotic remnants are adherent to a retrolental membrane which incorporates the posterior lens capsule and stretches across the globe from one retinal surface to the other, frequently detaching it from the choroid.

GLAUCOMA

Nature
Increased intra-ocular tension. The condition may be acute, subacute or chronic and of the following types:

PRIMARY

Nature
Glaucoma presenting without other detectable intra-ocular disease.

Pathology
This is due to failure of the normal drainage mechanisms of the aqueous humour although the exact cause or the site of this failure remains uncertain.

CONGENITAL

This type is due to a congenital anatomical defect in which either Schlemm's canal is absent or in eyes which have an abnormally shallow anterior chamber so that the root of the iris is very close to the corneo-scleral trabeculae of the filtration angle – *closed angle glaucoma*. Any swelling of the ciliary body, e.g. by congestion or oedema, will then block the channels leading to the canal of Schlemm and thus produce glaucoma.

SECONDARY

Nature

Glaucoma occurring secondarily to previous intra-ocular disease which obstructs the drainage of intra-ocular fluid.

Aetiology

1 *Iridocyclitis*. The presence of inflammatory cells, exudate or adhesions – *anterior synechiae*, obstructs the tissues at the filtration angles. A ring adhesion of the pupillary border of the iris with the lens – *iris bombé*, also prevents drainage.

2 *Trauma*. Perforation of the cornea may lead to a diminution of size of the anterior chamber or result in anterior synechiae, with narrowing of the filtration angle. In addition, blood clot may block the drainage channels. Penetration or dislocation of the lens may displace the iris anteriorly, block the pupil or obstruct the drainage channels with disintegrating lens matter.

3 *Intra-ocular tumours*. Space-occupying lesions may push the lens and iris forwards to block the filtration angles. Tumours also predispose to glaucoma by thrombosis of the retinal vein or by producing inflammatory synechiae.

4 *Retinal vein thrombosis*. Thrombosis of the central vein results in the formation of new vessels on the anterior surface of the iris with formation of synechiae – *thrombotic glaucoma*.

Results

Any of these types, if unrelieved, may result in an absolute glaucoma in which the following changes are usually present.

1 Obliteration of the filtration angles by anterior synechiae.

2 Oedema of the cornea.

3 Atrophy of the iris, ciliary body and retina, due to the raised tension and ischaemia.

4 Cupping of the disc with optic atrophy.

5 Cataract.

Chapter 62
Diseases of the Eye – Intra-ocular Tumours: Lacrimal Organs: Orbit: Optic Nerve

Intra-ocular tumours

BENIGN

Benign epithelioma of iris

Benign epithelioma of ciliary body

Naevus

Haemangiomas
Iris and ciliary body
Choroid
Retina

Leiomyoma
Sites
Macroscopical
Microscopical

MALIGNANT

Medulloepithelioma
Diktyoma
   Origin
   Macroscopical
   Microscopical
Malignant epithelioma
   Origin
   Macroscopical
   Microscopical

Retinoblastoma
Origin
Incidence
Aetiology
Macroscopical
Microscopical
Results

Malignant melanoma
Site
Incidence
Macroscopical
Microscopical
   Spindle cell
   Epithelioid cell
Spread
Results

Secondary tumours

Lacrimal organs

LACRIMAL GLAND

Acute dacryoadenitis

Chronic dacryoadenitis

Sjögren's syndrome
Nature
Microscopical

Tumours
Pleomorphic adenoma
Adenocarcinoma
Lymphomas

LACRIMAL PASSAGES

Chronic dacryocystitis
Nature
Microscopical

Tumours of lacrimal sac
Papilloma
Carcinoma
Others

Orbit

CONGENITAL

Cysts
Dermoid
Meningocoele
Encephalocoele

VASCULAR LESIONS

Aneurysms
Saccular
Cirsoid

TUMOURS

Haemangioma
Cavernous
Capillary
Sclerosing

Lymphangioma

Teratoma

Benign connective tissue

Malignant
Sarcoma
Lymphoma
Rhabdomyosarcoma
Meningioma
Secondary tumours

PSEUDOTUMOUR OF ORBIT
Nature
Macroscopical
Microscopical
Results

Optic nerve

INFLAMMATIONS

Perineuritis

Optic neuritis

OPTIC ATROPHY
Causes

PAPILLOEDEMA
Nature
Causes
Appearances
Results

PRIMARY TUMOURS

Glioma
Site
Macroscopical
Microscopical
Results

Meningioma
Macroscopical
Microscopical

Neurofibroma

SECONDARY TUMOURS

Intra-ocular tumours

BENIGN

BENIGN EPITHELIOMA OF THE IRIS

A rare condition which is merely hyperplasia of pigmented epithelium and appears as a pigmented mass, often at the pupillary margin, consisting of overgrown and invaginated pigment epithelium.

BENIGN EPITHELIOMA OF THE CILIARY BODY – ADENOMA

A more frequent but otherwise similar lesion to that of the iris described above. Symptomless and usually found as a round lesion about 1 mm in diameter in an eye removed for some other condition.

NAEVUS

Benign melanomas are seen as elevated, variably pigmented masses on the anterior surface of the iris, in the ciliary body and on the choroid in relation to the ciliary nerves.

HAEMANGIOMAS

Iris and ciliary body
These are rare tumours and are of the capillary type.

Choroid
Usually found posteriorly as flat tumorous masses. They are of cavernous type and ill-defined, tapering off into the surrounding choroid. Calcification and ossification commonly occur.

Retina
Vascular masses in the retina are often associated with angiomas in the brain and there may be associated cysts of the kidney, pancreas, liver and epididymis – von Hippel–Lindau's disease. The tumour is spherical and consists of capillary plexuses in the retina with solid areas of angioblastic cells. Scattered amongst the vessels are swollen endothelial cells containing phagocytosed fat.

Haemorrhages are numerous and may extend into the retina, vitreous or subretinal space.

LEIOMYOMA

Sites
These are rare tumours, usually of the iris where they arise from the sphincter and dilator muscles. Occasionally they occur in the ciliary body.

Macroscopical
Usually present as a vascular mass in the lower half of the iris from which blood may escape into the anterior chamber.

Microscopical
Composed of spindle cells, some of which show 'myoglial fibrils' which are diagnostic and differentiate this benign condition from a non-pigmented malignant melanoma, to which it may otherwise show a close resemblance.

MALIGNANT

MEDULLOEPITHELIOMA OF CILIARY EPITHELIUM

Diktyoma

ORIGIN
Arises in young persons from the non-pigmented epithelium of the ciliary body and is a counterpart of the retinal retinoblastoma.

MACROSCOPICAL
A white non-metastasizing but locally malignant tumour which may fill the entire globe.

MICROSCOPICAL
Non-pigmented epithelial cells are arranged in tubules or rosettes. Mitotic activity is marked and the lesion resembles the early embryonic retina.

Malignant epithelioma

ORIGIN
Occurs in adults, often in chronically inflamed eyes and arises from both layers of the ciliary epithelium.

MACROSCOPICAL
Pigmentation may be heavy. The lesion does not

usually grow to a large size in contrast to the diktyoma and metastases have not been reported.

MICROSCOPICAL

Proliferating epithelium in the form of strands and tubules, resembling a diktyoma but better differentiated.

RETINOBLASTOMA

Origin

A congenital tumour arising from primitive cells in the retina.

Incidence

Presents in early childhood, 75 per cent before 3 years of age; 20–30 per cent of cases are bilateral, the other eye always being the site of an independent focus, i.e. a separate primary tumour.

Aetiology

Most cases develop sporadically, but the influence of heredity is well proven; 50–70 per cent of the children of retinoblastoma survivors will develop the same condition.

Macroscopical

A pink-white lobulated mass extending in several directions:

(*a*) Endophytum – into the vitreous.
(*b*) Exophytum – into the subretinal space.
(*c*) Planum – within the retina.
(*d*) Diffuse infiltrating – within the retina, ciliary body and iris.

All eventually cause glaucoma and fill the entire globe. Extra-ocular spread takes place along the optic nerve into the brain and blood-borne metastases are frequent with a predilection for bone.

Microscopical

Masses of round or carrot-shaped cells with hyperchromatic nuclei and little cytoplasm, arranged in dense sheets, around blood vessels as pseudo-rosettes and as true rosettes of 16 to 30 cells around a central lumen. Mitoses are numerous and necrosis or calcification is frequent; rarely this leads to retrogression of the tumour. Seedling deposits on other intra-ocular structures are common. Pigmentation does not occur.

Results

Five-year survival – 80 per cent. In treated cases death usually occurs in the first year after enucleation, recurrence being exceedingly rare after a 4-year survival period.

MALIGNANT MELANOMA

Site

Eighty-four per cent in the choroid; 10 per cent in the ciliary body; 6 per cent in the iris.

Incidence

This is by far the most frequent intra-ocular tumour.

Macroscopical

Choroid. An elliptical mass, initially confined by the sclera and Bruch's membrane. Eventually, the tumour mushrooms into the subretinal space lifting the retina and causing its destruction. In time, the entire globe may be filled and finally the tumour may burst out of the globe into the orbit. Extra-ocular spread may occur sooner via the channels of the perforating retinal vessels and rarely along the optic nerve. The degree of pigmentation is variable and this feature may be almost absent. Haemorrhages and areas of necrosis are common. Glaucoma may occur due to blockage of the filtration angles by the growing mass or by cellular debris from the neoplasm.

Ciliary body and iris. Glaucoma commonly appears early and the lens may be dislocated and become cataractous. Rarely the lesions spread around the entire iris – '*ring melanoma*'.

Microscopical

Two types are recognized although combinations are usual.

SPINDLE CELL

Elongated cells with oval nuclei which are arranged in groups and bundles. Mitotic figures are scanty.

EPITHELIOID CELL

Large, polygonal and pleomorphic cells with pale nuclei. Mitoses are numerous and giant cells are often present. Tumours predominantly of this type are the most malignant.

The pigment content varies in different areas of the tumour but can be so heavy that bleached sections are necessary for cellular recognition.

Granules of melanin, although produced within the cells, may be phagocytosed to other parts of the globe. Heavy pigmentation is considered to carry a poor prognosis.

Variable amounts of reticulin are formed, the amount being of prognostic significance, i.e. the more reticulin present the more favourable the prognosis.

Spread

1 *Local.* Extension outside the globe to the orbit.
2 *Blood.* As with malignant melanomas elsewhere, blood spread is frequent with metastases to any site, but particularly the liver. This may occur at variable lengths of time after removal of the primary tumour – 'the big liver and glass eye' syndrome.

Results

In most cases, the prognosis is more favourable than with malignant melanomas elsewhere. Overall 5-year survival is about 50 per cent, but deaths from metastases may still occur as long as 20 years later.

SECONDARY TUMOURS

Many forms of carcinoma have been found within the eye. The usual site is the posterior segment of the choroid.

Rarely, deposits of malignant lymphomas are found in the uveal tract.

Lacrimal organs

LACRIMAL GLAND

ACUTE DACRYOADENITIS

May follow virus infections, e.g. mumps and influenza, but 50 per cent are due to *Staphylococcus pyogenes*.

CHRONIC DACRYOADENITIS

Most cases are part of Mikulicz's syndrome, a bilateral, chronic, symmetrical enlargement of the lacrimal and salivary glands due to a variety of conditions (see p. 178).

SJÖGREN'S SYNDROME

Nature

In this condition, there is failure of secretion of the lacrimal and salivary glands resulting in dry conjunctivae, atrophic rhinitis and pharyngitis. The condition chiefly affects post-menopausal women. The cause is unknown but evidence is accumulating in favour of an auto-immune reaction (see p. 98).

Microscopical

The changes are identical to those in the salivary glands (see p. 178).

TUMOURS

Pleomorphic adenoma

The appearances of this tumour in the lacrimal gland are similar to those occurring in the parotid and other salivary glands (p. 179).

Adenocarcinoma

Malignant change occurring in a pleomorphic adenoma.

Lymphomas

All types have been reported in the lacrimal glands which, when bilateral, may cause Mikulicz's syndrome.

LACRIMAL PASSAGES

CHRONIC DACRYOCYSTITIS

Nature

A non-specific chronic inflammation of the tear sac due to stasis in the nasolacrimal duct.

Microscopical

In addition to the non-specific inflammatory cell infiltration, the epithelium shows some areas of hyperplasia with increase of the goblet cells and desquamation.

TUMOURS OF THE LACRIMAL SAC

Papilloma

A benign but potentially malignant papillary overgrowth of columnar epithelium.

Carcinoma
Most are squamous cell carcinomas arising in metaplastic epithelium.

Others
Sarcomas, secondary carcinoma and deposits of malignant lymphomas occur but they are all extremely rare.

Orbit

CONGENITAL

CYSTS

Dermoid cysts
These inclusion dermoid cysts are relatively common and may occur at any site along the cranial suture lines. Peri-orbital dermoids are most frequent at the outer and upper angle – the fronto-malar or the fronto-temporal suture. Intra-orbital dermoids are outside the muscle cone but secondary inflammation may cause adhesion to muscle, optic nerve or other orbital contents.

Meningocoeles and encephalocoeles
Protrusion of meninges – meningocoele, or brain – encephalocoele, into the orbit through a bony defect. They are soft elastic swellings which are sometimes pulsatile but are compressible (see p. 594).

VASCULAR LESIONS

ANEURYSMS

Saccular
Arising from the ophthalmic artery – rare.

Cirsoid or arteriovenous
May be traumatic or congenital (see p. 272).

TUMOURS

HAEMANGIOMA

Cavernous
The most frequent type which is usually encapsulated.

Capillary
Not usually encapsulated.

Sclerosing
Arise by sclerosis of the capillary type.

LYMPHANGIOMA

Rare and of the cavernous type.

TERATOMA

These tumours usually contain representatives of all three germinal layers and thus may contain skin, teeth, bone, muscle, internal organs or almost a complete foetus. They are occasionally found in the orbit where malignant change frequently supervenes.

BENIGN CONNECTIVE TISSUE TUMOURS

These are all rare and are identical to similar tumours occurring at other sites. They include fibroma, lipoma, myxoma, chondroma, osteoma and neurofibroma.

MALIGNANT TUMOURS

Sarcoma
Most arise from the periosteum or fascia and are fibrosarcomas.

Lymphoma
Deposits of leukaemia, Hodgkin's disease and other malignant lymphomas are sometimes found in the orbit.

Rhabdomyosarcoma
A rare striated muscle tumour of young individuals (see p. 150).

Meningioma
See p. 621.

Secondary tumours
Malignant melanoma. Direct extension from the globe (see p. 342).

Carcinoma. Rare, but may occur from many primary sites.

Neuroblastoma. A relatively common site for metastases from an adrenal neuroblastoma – Hutchison's syndrome (see p. 295).

PSEUDOTUMOUR OF THE ORBIT

Nature
A non-specific chronic granuloma of the orbit of unknown aetiology. Some are thought to follow infection of the adjacent sinuses, lacrimal glands or teeth.

Macroscopical
A unilateral lesion, clinically closely simulating a tumour.

Microscopical
The appearances are very variable:
1 Lymph follicles enclosed by fibrous tissue.
2 Focal and perivascular collections of lymphocytes involving the muscles.
3 Diffuse acute or chronic inflammatory cell infiltration of the orbital tissues, frequently with an excess of fibrous tissue and giant cells. Fat necrosis may be found in this type.
4 Dense fibroblastic proliferation with minimal inflammatory cell infiltration.

Results
The great majority regress spontaneously, but occasionally the lesion may persist for a considerable period of time.

Optic nerve

INFLAMMATIONS

PERINEURITIS

Nature
Inflammation of the nerve sheath.

Causes
Usually secondary to inflammation of the meninges or orbit by pyogenic organisms, tuberculosis or syphilis.

OPTIC NEURITIS

Nature
Inflammation of the nerve tissue.

Causes
1 *Pyogenic infections*. Secondary to perineuritis, purulent endophthalmitis, orbital infection or metastatic abscess.
2 *Tuberculosis*. By spread from the choroid or meninges.
3 *Syphilis*. May occur early or in the tabetic stage.
4 *Multiple sclerosis*. Usually retrobulbar in situation.

Results
Destruction of nerve fibres with optic atrophy is common. With multiple sclerosis, which is the commonest cause, pallor of the temporal parts of the disc usually remains, although vision commonly returns to normal.

OPTIC ATROPHY

CAUSES

The more common causes of optic atrophy include the following.

Optic neuritis
Any of its causes as above.

Trauma

Pressure
From glaucoma, aneurysm, etc.

Vascular
Central retinal artery thrombosis.

Papilloedema
Of longstanding.

Poisons
Especially methyl alcohol and tobacco.

PAPILLOEDEMA

Nature
Oedema of the optic disc (papilla).

Causes
1 *Raised intracranial tension.* Due to space-occupying lesions in the skull, e.g. tumour, abscess, haemorrhages, meningitis.
2 *Optic neuritis.*
3 *Accelerated hypertension.*
4 *Venous drainage obstruction.* By thrombosis, e.g. cavernous sinus thrombosis, or by pressure, e.g. from a tumour.

Appearances
Stages:
1 Congestion of retinal veins.
2 Blurring of disc margins.
3 Filling of the physiological cup.
4 Protrusion of the optic disc.
5 Haemorrhages in and around the disc.
6 Optic atrophy with pallor of the disc subsequently.

Results
In addition to deterioration in visual acuity, optic atrophy results when the papilloedema is of long standing.

PRIMARY TUMOURS

The optic nerve should be regarded as part of the brain tissue and most of its tumours are therefore similar to those of cerebral tissue.

GLIOMA

Site
The majority arise in the first decade of life and are usually unilateral. Any part of the optic nerve between the globe and the chiasma may be involved, although most develop within the orbit. Growth anteriorly towards the disc causes unilateral blindness, whereas posterior spread to involve the chiasma results in bilateral blindness.

Macroscopical
There is fusiform enlargement with no clear distinction between the nerve tissue and the tumour.

Microscopical
The appearances are those of infiltrating astrocytomas or oligodendrogliomas (see p. 624). The dura is not penetrated but the pia is ruptured in the early stages so that local extension is usual. Even microscopically, recognition of tumour invasion is not immediately appreciated. However, the nerve septa are separated more widely than usual and contain tumour cells instead of nerve bundles.

Results
Metastases do not occur but cerebral extension may prove fatal. However, resection of the involved nerve at an early stage may be curative.

MENINGIOMA

This tumour arises in later life from the arachnoid of the optic nerve and may grow outwards along the sheath or rarely into the nerve and globe. The majority arise in the region of the optic foramen and either spread forwards into the orbit or backwards as a 'dumb-bell' tumour into the cranium. Metastases do not occur but intracranial spread may be fatal.

Macroscopical
Within the orbit the tumour grows freely until it assumes the shape of the muscle cone; the nerve at its centre is compressed into a thin thread.

Microscopical
The histological appearances are similar to those of meningiomas in other sites (see p. 627).

NEUROFIBROMA

These tumours rarely occur on the optic nerve in neurofibromatosis (see p. 620).

SECONDARY TUMOURS

Direct spread
(*a*) *Retinoblastoma.* The most frequent (see p. 342).
(*b*) *Malignant melanoma.* Rarely spreads into the optic nerve (see p. 733).

Metastases
Very rare but metastases have been reported from the breast, lung, kidney and stomach.

Chapter 63
Genito-Urinary System – Kidney: Congenital: Infections

DEVELOPMENT

The kidneys are of mesodermal origin but arise in two parts:

1 From the ureteric bud of the Wolffian duct – this forms the ureter, pelvis, calyces and collecting tubules.

2 From the urogenital ridge:

(*a*) Pronephros ⎫
(*b*) Mesonephros ⎬ both transient structures.
(*c*) Metanephros – develops at the pelvic brim and forms the nephrons.

After the two parts have united, the organs migrate along the posterior abdominal wall to the loins, obtaining their blood supply successively from the iliac arteries, lower abdominal aorta and finally the upper abdominal aorta.

NORMAL STRUCTURE

Each kidney weighs about 150 g.

NEPHRON

There are about 2 million of these basic units, each formed by a glomerulus and a tubule (see Fig. 37).

Glomerulus

Consists of a mass of capillaries fed by an afferent arteriole, which rejoin to form the efferent arteriole. The capillaries perforate the capsule at the hilum and are lined by endothelial cells lying on a basement membrane. Externally situated are the epithelial cells of the visceral layer which have numerous slender foot processes investing the surface of the capillary tuft. The glomerular epithelium is continuous at the hilum with the parietal layer of epithelial cells which forms the lining of Bowman's capsule. The space between this capsule and the tuft is the capsular space. Between the capillary loops in the stalk of the lobules are *mesangial cells* and the *mesangial substance* (matrix) which they produce. The glomeruli all lie within the renal cortex.

Tubules

1 *Proximal convoluted tubule.* This forms the bulk

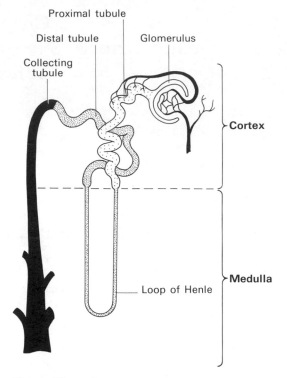

Fig. 37. The nephron.

of the nephron and is composed of cuboidal cells with a brush border; it lies in the cortex.

2 *Descending loop of Henle.* Flattened cuboidal cells; in the medulla.

3 *Ascending loop of Henle.* Low cuboidal cells with a rather dense cytoplasm; also in the medulla.

4 *Distal convoluted tubule.* Cuboidal cells with no brush border; it is found in the cortex.

5 *Collecting tubule.* Low cuboidal epithelium; confined to the medulla.

CORTEX

There is an outer fibrous capsule which strips easily to reveal a smooth surface. It measures about 1.2 cm in depth and is sharply demarcated from the medulla. The pattern is formed by vasa recta, straight lines perpendicular to the capsular surface. In addition to the glomeruli, the cortex contains the convoluted tubules, interlobular arteries and small amounts of loose connective tissue.

MEDULLA

The pyramids end in blunt tips – papillae, which protrude into the calyces. Separating the pyramids are the broad bands of renal substance containing the loops of Henle – columns of Bertini. The medulla also contains collecting tubules, interstitial tissue and the main blood vessels with their arcuate branches at the cortico-medullary junction.

CALYCES AND PELVIS

Lined by transitional epithelium.

SOME ASPECTS OF RENAL FUNCTION

Blood flow

The renal blood flow accounts for 25 per cent of the cardiac output. It passes to the glomeruli where the difference between the hydrostatic and osmotic pressures produces the glomerular filtrate. Blood in the efferent arterioles passes into a capillary bed which then supplies the remaining parts of the nephrons in the cortex at a somewhat lower pressure (see Figs 38 and 39).

Glomerular filtrate

About 170 litres/day. The filtrate passes from the capsular space to the tubules where it is altered by:

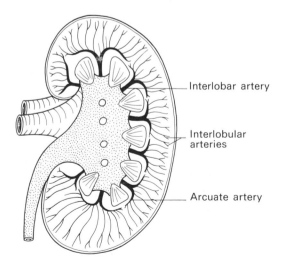

Fig. 38. Kidney – arterial distribution.

Interlobar artery

Interlobular arteries

Arcuate artery

(a) Selective reabsorption – 99 per cent of its bulk.
(b) Tubular secretion – e.g. ammonia.

The altered filtrate then passes to the collecting tubules in which it is carried to the calyces and pelvis as urine – approximately 1700 ml/day.

Renal functions

The chief functions of the kidney are:
(a) Elimination of water.
(b) Excretion of certain substances normally present in plasma when their concentration rises above a certain level – renal threshold.
(c) Selective reabsorption of substances necessary for the body, e.g. sugar, electrolytes, etc.
(d) Excretion of waste products, e.g. urea.
(e) Plays an important role in the regulation of acid-base balance.

Factors necessary for normal renal function

(a) Adequate blood flow and pressure to allow the formation of a normal glomerular filtrate and to maintain tubular function.
(b) Normal glomerular structure to allow the filtrate to form in normal quantities and of normal composition.
(c) Normal tubules to alter the composition of the filtrate according to the requirements of the body.
(d) Unhindered passage of the urine thus formed into the calyces and thence outside the body via a normal lower urinary tract.

Disordered function

This may therefore follow disease processes affecting:
(a) Renal blood flow and blood vessels.
(b) Glomeruli.
(c) Tubules.
(d) Obstruction to the urinary flow at any level.

TESTS OF RENAL FUNCTION

(a) Blood urea (or non-protein nitrogen). Rises above the normal upper limits of 6 mmol/l may be from pre-renal causes, e.g. dehydration, haemorrhage, congestive heart failure, in addition to renal and post-renal obstructive lesions.
(b) Blood creatinine. If this is raised along with the urea, the failure is likely to be of renal origin.
(c) Electrolyte and acid-base blood levels. The

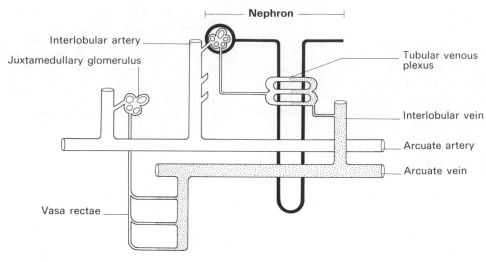

Fig. 39. Diagram of blood supply to the nephron.

interrelationships are discussed in Chapter 15 pages 77 to 86.

(*d*) Clearance rates. Rates of blood clearance of urea, creatinine or inulin are only rarely used in clinical practice.

(*e*) Urine. The volume and R.D. of urine are important, as is the appearance of the centrifuged deposit.

(*f*) Plasma osmolality.

EXAMINATION OF THE KIDNEY

A systematic method of examination of both the macroscopic and microscopic appearances is necessary, not only in respect of local lesions but, more particularly, for diffuse parenchymal disease.

Macroscopical appearances

1 *Size, weight, shape, colour.*
2 *Capsule.* Ease of stripping and appearance of the capsular surface.
3 *Cortex.* Width, demarcation from the medulla, pattern, colour.
4 *Medulla.* Size, pattern, colour.
5 *Pelvis and calyces.* Mucosal appearance, contents, size.
6 *Blood vessels.* Prominence, thickening, occlusion.

Microscopical appearances

1 *Glomeruli.* Tuft and capsule.

2 *Tubules.* Including contents.
3 *Interstitial tissue.*
4 *Blood vessels.*
5 *Calyces and pelvis.*

Congenital

AGENESIS
Failure of development of the kidney.
1 Bilateral – incompatible with life.
2 Unilateral – compensatory hypertrophy of the other kidney occurs.

The ureteric remnants may be present or they too may be aplastic.

RENAL HYPOPLASIA AND DYSPLASIA

Most congenitally small kidneys show evidence of anomalous metanephric differentiation and are termed dysplastic. The renal tissue is disorganized and shows foetal type of structures usually including primitive ducts and cartilage often together with cysts. Other congenital abnormalities of the urinary tract are often present.

FUSION – 'HORSESHOE KIDNEY'

This is quite common – 1 in 500 autopsies, affecting the lower pole in 90 per cent of cases and the upper pole in 10 per cent. The function of the fused organ is unaffected.

ABNORMAL SITES

Development in ectopic foci or, more commonly failure of migration, results in normal kidneys within the pelvis or at the pelvic brim. Kinking of the ureters may occur, predisposing to pyelonephritis.

URETERIC ANOMALIES

1 Double ureter with double pelvis.
2 Stricture.
3 Megaureter – commonly associated with megacolon.

VASCULAR

Anomalous arteries from the iliacs or lower aorta may occur and an additional vessel to the lower pole may cross the pelvi-ureteric junction and be associated with hydronephrosis (see p. 371).

CYSTS

Congenital cysts are of two types, simple cysts and polycystic disease. Additionally, multiple simple retention cysts occur associated with renal scarring, e.g. chronic pyelonephritis, nephrosclerosis.

SIMPLE CYSTS

These are common and occur as solitary, or occasionally multiple, cystic spaces in otherwise normal kidneys. They are usually 1–5 cm in diameter, although they may be 10 cm or more, are filled with clear fluid and lined by a smooth glistening membrane of flattened cuboidal epithelium surrounded by a thin fibrous capsule. They are non-uriniferous and have no communication with the pelvis, usually being cortical in situation. They may cause renal enlargement and distortion and thus require clinical differentiation from tumours.

POLYCYSTIC DISEASE

Nature
An hereditary disease occurring uncommonly and equally between the sexes, in which both kidneys are progressively replaced by numerous cysts lined by flattened cuboidal epithelium. The cysts do not communicate with the calyces or with each other and are non-uriniferous.

Types

ADULT POLYCYSTIC DISEASE
Inherited as autosomal dominant but 50 per cent of cases are new mutants. Present in fourth decade or later usually with very large lobulated loin masses containing cysts up to 5 cm or so in diameter. Associated features are:
(*a*) Berry cerebral aneurysms in 10 per cent.
(*b*) Cysts of liver, pancreas and lung.

INFANTILE POLYCYSTIC DISEASE
Less common than the adult type, this is often autosomal recessive inherited. Usually presents in stillborn or neonates with enlarged kidneys which preserve their reniform outline but on section show radiating, finely cystic pattern in medulla and cortex. The cysts are composed of dilated collecting ducts.

A consistently associated feature is *congenital hepatic fibrosis*.

Effects

ADULT TYPE
1 Hypertension – in 50 per cent.
2 Abdominal swelling – often massive.
3 Renal failure – life may be preserved by dialysis or transplantation.
4 Infection of cysts.
5 Haemorrhage into cysts.

INFANTILE TYPE
1 Most cases die as neonates or are stillborn.
2 A small minority present later in childhood with renal failure or hypertension, or occasionally from the effects of the hepatic fibrosis, e.g. portal hypertension.

Pathogenesis
In both types many theories have been expounded but supportive evidence is lacking for all.

MEDULLARY CYSTIC DISEASE

Medullary sponge kidney
This is a predominantly radiological diagnosis of dilated medullary collecting ducts sometimes with calcification and calculus formation.

Juvenile nephronophthisis – medullary cystic disease
An hereditary nephropathy causing polyuria and renal failure in children. Salt loss, growth retardation and renal osteodystrophy are prominent and a disproportionately severe normochromic anaemia is usual. There is extensive glomerulosclerosis and a variable degree of cystic change at the cortico-medullary junctional area.

Infections

PYOGENIC

BLOOD-BORNE

Pyaemia
In pyaemia, lodgement of infected emboli leads to the formation of multiple abscesses throughout the renal substance. Small, rounded, numerous, yellow areas with a surrounding zone of hyperaemia are visible, maximally in the cortex. The usual organisms are staphylococci.

Carbuncle of the kidney
Blood-borne spread of organisms, usually staphylococci, to the kidney may result in a solitary large abscess in the cortex, sometimes multiloculated. Extensive destruction of renal tissue may occur.

Perinephric abscess
Abscess formation in the perinephric tissue may result from:
(a) Spread from intrarenal inflammation, e.g. carbuncle of the kidney, pyelonephritis.
(b) Primary focus in the perinephric fat without renal involvement.

PYELONEPHRITIS

Definition
Inflammation of the renal pelvis and renal parenchyma. Pyelitis, inflammation of the pelvis alone, is so exceedingly uncommon that the name should be abandoned, as some degree of parenchymal involvement is inevitable.

ACUTE PYELONEPHRITIS

Incidence
Common.

Age
There are three peaks of incidence – childhood, pregnancy and the elderly.

Sex
Females rather more commonly than males.

Organisms
Fifty per cent are due to *Escherichia coli*, others to *Aerobacter aerogenes*, *Proteus vulgaris*, *Streptococcus faecalis*, *Staphylococcus pyogenes*, or *Pseudomonas aeruginosa*, in descending order of frequency.

Pathogenesis
Urinary stasis or urinary tract obstruction is an important and almost invariably predisposing factor, hence the peaks of incidence at the following ages.
Childhood. Major or minor degrees of congenital urinary tract abnormalities and ureteric reflux of urine during micturition.
Pregnancy. Pressure of the gravid uterus on the ureters at the pelvic brim.
Elderly. Women – prolapse of the uterus and cystitis. Men – prostatic enlargement.
Two pathways by which the organisms may reach the kidneys are propounded:
1 Haematogenous.
2 Ascending via the ureters or peri-ureteric lymphatics.
The former is much the more likely usual mechanism.

Macroscopical
The condition may be unilateral or bilateral and the involved organs are enlarged with a tense capsule; small abscesses may be seen beneath the stripped capsule. On section, there are numerous small abscesses in the cortex with linear streaks of yellowish colour in the medulla – 'surgical kidney'. The pelvis is usually hyperaemic and granular with

purulent urinary contents. Earlier cases show less abscess formation and focal areas of hyperaemia.

Microscopical
Acute inflammation with infiltration by polymorphs in the renal tubules and in the interstitial tissue, later causing necrosis and abscess formation. The inflammatory process is focal and a bacterial inflammation is present also in the calyceal and pelvic mucosae.

Results
1 *Resolution.* Before there is frank suppuration; however, some scarring usually occurs.
2 *Healing.* With scarring.
3 *Chronic.* Chronic pyelonephritis.
4 *Suppuration.* If associated with total urinary obstruction will produce a pyonephrosis.
5 *Death.* In uraemia.

HEALED PYELONEPHRITIS

Nature
The end stage of scarring due to a previous acute pyelonephritis or in childhood without demonstrable obstruction, as a result of vesico-ureteric reflux – *reflux nephropathy.*

Macroscopical
The kidneys are small, unequal, and irregularly scarred and contracted. The capsule is thickened and adherent revealing a variably scarred surface with minute and focal or more generalized depressed areas according to the severity of the previous acute inflammation. These scars are irregularly distributed, flat, broad or 'U-shaped' depressions, usually 0.5–2 cm in diameter, which extend into the cortex but do not involve the medulla.

Microscopical
Focal areas of parenchymal replacement by fibrous tissue with occasional lymphocytes. In adjacent areas there are dilated atrophic tubules filled with albuminous material of 'colloid' appearance.

Effects
Although renal function may be unimpaired and the patient remains normotensive in this condition, there is loss of some renal parenchyma which may become significant should further episodes of pyelo-nephritis occur. Reflux nephropathy of childhood often presents as renal failure.

CHRONIC PYELONEPHRITIS

Incidence
Formerly identified as the most common form of fatal primary renal disease, this is now seriously questioned by many authors who suggest that similar renal abnormalities may be caused by non-bacterial agents and processes.

Origin
In only a relatively small proportion of cases is there good evidence of either:
1 Long continued low grade infection, or
2 Recurrent attacks of acute pyelonephritis with scarring.
   Although usually bilateral, unilateral local abnormalities may give rise to involvement of only one kidney.

Macroscopical
The kidneys are small, sometimes very small – 50 g or less. The capsule is firmly adherent and thickened with numerous irregular, wedge-shaped, flat scars on the surface. Occasionally, when the changes are very diffuse, a fine granularity may be seen. On section, the cortex is thinned, particularly at the sites of scarring and the pattern and cortico-medullary differentiation are indistinct. The organs are pale and the medulla is contracted. The pelvic mucosa is usually thickened, pale, fibrotic and granular whilst dilatation of the pelvis and calyces may be present due to a concomitant obstructive lesion. The blood vessels are prominent.

Microscopical
Fibrous replacement in the scarred areas with hyalinized glomeruli and increased interstitial fibrous tissue in which there are dilated atrophic tubules containing albuminous material which mimics colloid – 'thyroid kidney', accompanied by a variable lymphocytic infiltration. There is usually also evidence of inflammatory activity with a focal infiltrate of polymorphs and lymphocytes. The calyces show increased submucosal fibrosis with a lymphocytic infiltration and sometimes cyst-like invaginations of the epithelium – *pyelitis cystica.* The blood vessels are often markedly thickened due

to widespread endarteritic or hypertensive changes. A variant is *xantho-granulomatous* pyelonephritis.

Results

Clinically, some cases give a clear history of past episodes of urinary tract infection or have identifiable predisposing structural abnormalities; in many, however, the disease may remain latent for many years and then present as:

1 Hypertension.
2 Renal failure with uraemia.

Death results from either or both of these sequelae.

In unilateral pyelonephritis associated with hypertension, nephrectomy of the affected kidney may occasionally lead to reversal of the hypertension. More commonly, however, irreversible structural changes have already occurred (see p. 268) and, after a temporary remission following operation, the hypertension returns and progresses.

PAPILLARY NECROSIS AND ANALGESIC ABUSE NEPHROPATHY

Nature

Necrosis of medullary pyramids may occur as a variant of acute suppurative pyelonephritis, particularly in the elderly or in diabetics. The condition is also increasingly recognized in those taking grossly excessive amounts of analgesic substances, particularly those containing phenacetin, over a long period of time. In this situation of analgesic abuse, cortico-medullary interstitial fibrosis is usually also marked.

Macroscopical

The distal portion of the pyramids are brownish or grey or necrotic, separated from the upper medullary tissues by a sharp hyperaemic demarcated zone. Some or all of the papillae may have been shed leaving an ulcer at the apices of the calyces. Scarring of cortex may be considerable in analgesic nephropathy.

Microscopical

The dominant feature is ischaemic necrosis with marginal inflammatory reaction only prominent at the demarcation zone.

Results

Renal failure is inevitable whatever the cause but the time scale is very variable.

Transitional cell carcinomas of the pelvis and calyces, and less commonly of ureter and bladder are increasingly recognized as late complications (see p. 379).

GRANULOMATOUS

TUBERCULOSIS

Miliary

Diffuse involvement of both kidneys as part of generalized haematogenous spread. The organs are usually normal in size and on section show numerous greyish-white pin-head-sized tubercles.

Focal

PATHOGENESIS

Haematogenous; it is probable that all cases are due to blood-borne infection from a distant site. Twenty-five per cent show evidence of active pulmonary tuberculosis, other possible sources being the intestines, tonsils and bone. The concept of ascending infection via the peri-ureteric lymphatics from the bladder and epididymis is now generally discredited.

SITES

Although clinically unilateral, before antibiotic treatment changed the course of the disease 50 per cent of the cases would eventually show active bilateral disease. It seems probable that most cases are bilaterally infected but most commonly the lesion heals in one kidney and progresses in the other. The lesion frequently starts in the cortex and spreads locally to involve the apices of the pyramids and the walls of the calyces.

MACROSCOPICAL

Early. An irregular, pale, yellow, necrotic, caseating lesion is seen near the cortico-medullary junction.

Later. The apices are irregularly ulcerated with the formation of a cavity lined by caseous material and communicating with the pelvis.

Late. The pelvis becomes filled with caseous material and lined by tuberculous granulation tissue. The cavities extend to destroy large areas of renal substance.

Involvement of the pelvi-ureteric junction by tuberculous granulation tissue leads to obstruction and tuberculous pyonephrosis, whilst extension of the tuberculous process down the ureter is common.

MICROSCOPICAL
Caseating tuberculous giant cell systems.

FATE

Untreated
1 Healing with fibrosis and calcification; this only occurs at very early stages.
2 Tuberculous pyonephrosis due to ureteric occlusion.
3 Auto-nephrectomy – the pyonephrosis becomes spontaneously sterile with fibrosis and calcification producing a completely enclosed caseous mass which may partially absorb – '*putty kidney*'.
4 Spread of infection to the lower urinary tract, particularly the bladder, epididymis and seminal vesicles.

Treated (antibiotics)
1 Early lesions heal by fibrosis.
2 If involvement of a calyceal or pelvi-ureteric junction has already occurred before treatment is instituted, healing by fibrosis may still lead to stricture formation, obstruction and subsequent loss of function.

DIAGNOSIS
Urine. Deposit – red cells, pus cells, debris; acid–alcohol fast organisms are commonly seen on Z.N. staining.
  Culture – sterile on ordinary media.
  T.B. cultures on early morning specimens – positive.

RESULTS
Prognosis is good unless diagnosis is delayed and bilateral obstructive complications develop.

ACTINOMYCOSIS

The kidneys are very rarely involved in the disseminated type of actinomycosis (see p. 57).

INTERSTITIAL NEPHRITIS

Nature
True examples of primary interstitial inflammation of the kidney are very uncommon but do occur in:
 (i) Adverse drug reactions, e.g. phenindione and hypersensitivity to some antibiotics (methicillin, etc.)
 (ii) Brucellosis, leptospirosis – Weil's disease (see p. 555) and some cases of glandular fever.
 (iii) Non-infective causes, e.g. irradiation, analgesic abuse nephropathy, hypercalcaemia, etc.
 (iv) Reflux nephropathy.

Additionally the term has been confusingly used in the past as descriptive of the non-specific appearance of chronic inflammatory cell infiltration and interstitial fibrosis occurring in many forms of chronic renal disease, primarily glomerular and leading to tubular atrophy.

Confusion also exists in respect of chronic pyelonephritis (see p. 353) in which the assumed infective element has in the past been overidentified. Interstitial inflammation is, however, invariable in reflux nephropathy (see p. 371) and variably severe in obstructive uropathy.

Chronic interstitial fibrosis of non-infective type is a feature of analgesic abuse nephropathy (see p. 354) and some cases of hypercalcaemia, gout and cystinosis.

Interstitial changes are also marked in irradiation damage to kidneys.

Appearances
Glomeruli are normal or show only mild ischaemic changes. In true interstitial inflammation, interstitial tissue shows patchy infiltration by polymorphonuclear leucocytes with variable admixture of plasma cells and lymphocytes in the more chronic cases. Also related to chronicity is an increasing fibrosis and tubular atrophy.

Chapter 64
Genito-Urinary System – Kidney: Glomerular Lesions

INTRODUCTION

Since Richard Bright's original, and in some ways still classical, description of acute nephritis in 1827, there has been a bewildering succession of classifications of glomerular diseases, particularly of glomerulonephritis. At the time of publication, some of these accurately reflected the current state of knowledge and served a temporary useful purpose. The literature, however, became a confusion of nomenclature with no attempts at standardization. The advances in knowledge of renal pathology which have stemmed from needle biopsy and immunological techniques has led to an awareness that a simplistic approach has considerable advantages, at least until more information is available regarding aetiological factors. The classification given on page 359 has the marked advantage that it enables

356

decisions about patient management to be taken without the necessity of exact pigeon-holing and that it can absorb additional knowledge without needing fundamental alteration.

STEPS IN DIAGNOSIS

Diagnosis based on this classification is made in several steps:
1   Identification of clinical presentation and type of urinary abnormality.
2   Identification of pattern of glomerular response to injury, i.e. histological classification – including electron microscopy where relevant.
3   Immunological abnormalities – deposition of immunoglobulins, complement, fibrin and serological changes.
4   Addition of:
(*a*) Aetiological mechanism, if known.
(*b*) Associated disease process, if present.
(*c*) Specific clinical syndromes.
5   Time scale, i.e. acute or chronic (if known).

Clinical presentation and urinary abnormalities

1   Nephritic – haematuria, proteinuria, often with urinary casts.
2   Nephrotic – proteinuria (usually > 3.5 g/24 hrs) with hypoproteinaemia and oedema.
3   Asymptomatic proteinuria (> 0.3 g/24 hrs) without haematuria.
(*a*) Continuous.
(*b*) Orthostatic.
(*c*) Transient.
4   Haematuria – without significant proteinuria.
(*a*) Continuous.
(*b*) Intermittent.
5   Renal failure.
6   Hypertension.

Histology of patterns of glomerular reaction

Methods
Techniques used in the study of renal histology include:
1   Standard paraffin-wax-embedded needle biopsy material for thin (3 μm) sections. Useful stains, in addition to haematoxylin and eosin are; P.A.S. – for mesangium and basement membrane in particular; silver impregnation, particularly methenamine silver – P.A.S., for basement membrane detail; connective tissue stain, e.g. Mallory trichrome, for collagen, hyaline material, fibrin.
2   Very thin (1 μm) resin-embedded, glutaraldehyde-fixed biopsy material stained with toluidine blue – for deposits.
3   Electron microscopy – for ultrastructural abnormalities and identification of position of immune deposits.
4   Immunoperoxidase techniques – for composition and distribution of immune substances.

Definitions
Diffuse – lesions involving all glomeruli.
Focal – lesions of some glomeruli but not others.
Global – involvement of the whole of the glomerular tuft.
Segmental – segment of glomerular tuft only involved.

MINIMAL GLOMERULAR LESION – LIPOID NEPHROSIS

Appearances
As the name suggests, the essential feature is that glomeruli are normal on light microscopy. On electron microscopy glomerular epithelial cells are swollen by protein droplets and their foot processes are fused – these changes are believed secondary to the escape of protein.

Incidence
This lesion accounts for less than 20 per cent of cases of the nephrotic syndrome in adults but about 50 per cent in children.

Immunology
Appearances on immunofluorescent techniques are non-specific and usually negative for immunoglobulins and complement.

Clinical
Most patients with the disease present with the nephrotic syndrome in which the proteinuria is highly selective. Response to corticosteroid therapy is usually good with occasional relapses requiring a further course of therapy. Lack of remission sug-

gests that the diagnosis was incorrect, particularly in relationship to focal glomerulosclerosis (see p. 362) or early membranous nephropathy (see p. 362). The long-term prognosis is very good.

Aetiology

Virus infection has, along with other factors, been postulated but there is no substantial evidence in favour. There is likewise no evidence of an immune complex origin for the minimal lesion.

OBVIOUS GLOMERULAR LESIONS

SPECIFIC

In this group the glomerular abnormalities are commonly (or usually) sufficiently characteristic to be able to make a definitive diagnosis of a clinical entity.

1 *Diabetic nephropathy.* The characteristic glomerular abnormalities are of diffuse or nodular deposition of eosinophilic, P.A.S.-positive material in basement membranes and endothelial cells. These tend to be maximal towards the central parts of the lobules. Occasionally, quite marked diabetic changes are seen in the absence of overt glycosuria or other manifestations of diabetes. Also specific when present, are the *fibrinoid caps* seen at the periphery of the affected glomerulus and *capsular drops*.

Vascular lesions are also usually present as hyaline arteriolosclerosis or microaneurysms of afferent arterioles. Accelerated atherosclerosis, pyelonephritis and papillary necrosis often complicate the renal diabetic picture (see p. 353).

2 *Amyloid.* The nephrotic syndrome or renal failure are common presenting features of amyloidosis and renal involvement is frequently dominant. Eosinophilic amyloid material of homogeneous appearance is seen variably diffusely or in a more nodular distribution in the intercapillary areas, in blood vessels and in tubular basement membranes. Specific staining by Congo red, Sirius red or thioflavine-T-fluorescence is diagnostic (see p. 109).

3 *Disseminated intravascular coagulopathy (D.I.C.).* Renal involvement in this systemic disorder is usual and oliguria or anuria common, often being responsible for death.

Glomeruli show intracapillary fibrin and platelet plugs with similar changes in arterioles. A variable number of glomeruli may be involved (see p. 531).

4. *Malarial nephropathy.* In endemic areas, particularly for *Plasmodium malariae* infection, the nephrotic syndrome is common. When associated with parasitic infection many cases show a proliferative glomerulonephritis with segmental thickening of capillary walls leading to progressive sclerosis of the tufts. Electron-dense subendothelial deposits are seen and immunofluorescence shows granular deposits of IgM on the epithelial side of the basement membrane. Malarial antigen can be demonstrated in these deposits.

5 *Systemic lupus erythematosus – lupus nephritis.* Renal involvement in S.L.E. is commonly the most important manifestation in respect of therapy and prognosis. Estimates of the frequency of renal involvement vary from 55 per cent to 80 per cent with a mortality from renal failure of 15 per cent or more. The only specific and pathognomonic abnormality is the presence of *haematoxyphil bodies* (see p. 281). Three patterns of involvement are described:

(a) *Minimal glomerular involvement – lupus glomerulitis.* Small focal, proliferative, peripheral foci or endothelial and/or mesangial cells sometimes with minor eosinophilic thickening or fibrinoid change of adjacent capillary walls.

(b) *Lupus glomerulonephritis.* Some glomeruli show focal areas of hypercellularity, necrosis and fibrinoid change. Nuclear pyknosis and karyorrhexis are usually seen. Peripheral capillary loops often show marked thickening by large deposits – *wire loops* and arteriolar fibrinoid may also be present. In more severe forms these lesions are widespread and capsular adhesions are common.

(c) *Membranous lupus nephritis.* Diffuse uniform basement membrane thickening which may be indistinguishable from idiopathic, membranous nephropathy (see p. 362) including the presence of 'spikes'. The other histological abnormalities previously described are usually absent. Electron microscopy shows deposits on the epithelial side of the basement membrane. A mesangiocapillary pattern is also occasionally seen.

Immunofluorescence in lupus nephritis. Whichever type of histological pattern is present in lupus nephritis, immune substances are consistently found in the glomeruli although there is a wide range of appearances. Granular, or occasionally linear, deposits of IgG are almost always present, usually with IgM, IgA, fractions of complement and fibrin.

Levels of complement and anti-DNA antibodies in serum are useful parameters for monitoring activity of the disease.

Prognosis of renal lesion in lupus. Treatment by corticosteroids and/or azathioprine has led to much improvement in prognosis but requires careful monitoring to avoid deaths from complications of therapy rather than disease processes. Overall mortality rates of 2 per cent are achievable.

6 *Infective endocarditis and shunt nephritis.* A range of proliferative glomerular abnormalities can be seen in endocarditis particularly when of *Streptococcus viridans* origin. Similar lesions are found as infective complications of ventriculo-caval and dialysis shunts – usually from coagulase negative staphylococci. Most common is a focal segmental proliferative lesion with fibrin and immune deposits present but no organisms – previously called focal embolic nephritis but *not* embolic. Crescents

are quite common and diffuse global abnormalities may occasionally occur.

NON-SPECIFIC

Nature
Most or all of these glomerulonephritic lesions are the result of immunological disturbances and two types of mechanisms are involved:
1 *Anti-GBM disease.* Specific antiglomerular basement antibodies become fixed to the membrane. Immunological staining techniques show the deposition to be *linear*.
2 *Soluble immune complex disease.* Antigen-antibody complexes in the circulation are incidentally cleared by the kidney and become trapped in glomeruli where they can be demonstrated as *granular* deposits. Their size and position and immunoglobulin composition are very variable in the different subgroups of glomerulonephritis.

Relatively little is known about the nature of the antigen in most cases in this group.

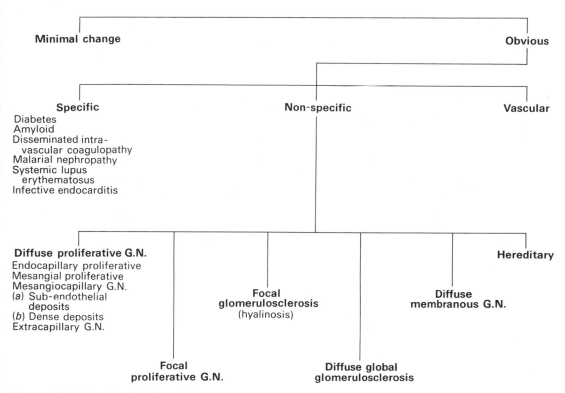

Fig. 40. Histological classification of glomerular lesions.

PROLIFERATIVE GLOMERULONEPHRITIS

DIFFUSE

Nature
Hypercellularity of virtually all glomeruli and all parts of the glomerular tuft.

There are a number of subdivisions depending on:
1 The presence or absence of polymorphs.
2 Increase in mesangial cells and/or matrix.
3 Presence of adhesions to the capsule.
4 Presence or absence of crescents from epithelial cell proliferation and, when present, the percentage of glomeruli thus involved.

ENDOCAPILLARY PROLIFERATIVE GLOMERULONEPHRITIS

Microscopical
In this pattern there is a predominance of endothelial cell proliferation which may be very uniform in appearance in *post-streptococcal glomerulonephritis* and rather more irregular in distribution in bacterial endocarditis, systemic lupus erythematosus and in some other cases where the aetiology is unknown.

In the acute stage there is often an increase in polymorphs – *exudative change*, together with endothelial cell proliferation predominantly axial and loss of capillary lumen with resulting 'bloodless' appearance. Capsular adhesions and some epithelial proliferation may also occur.

Electron microscopy demonstrates subendothelial immune complex deposits in infected children but in adults these deposits of IgG and complement are usually subepithelial – *'lumpy-bumpy'* appearance.

Clinical
Presentation may be as an acute nephritic illness as described originally by Richard Bright with oliguria and hypertension. This is followed in the majority of cases by resolution, which may be complete in 92 per cent of children and 85 per cent of adults, or incomplete with persistent urinary abnormalities and a progressive proliferation and subsequent hyalinization in glomeruli leading to renal failure in a time span varying from a few to more than 30 years. A very small number of patients may die in the acute phase and the clinical pattern may be nephrotic at almost any stage during the progressive illness. In many adult patients the onset is often clinically more insidious.

MESANGIAL PROLIFERATIVE GLOMERULONEPHRITIS

Microscopical
Diffuse expansion of the mesangial regions of the glomerular tufts by mesangial cell proliferation and variable increase in mesangial matrix. The capillary loops appear normal at the periphery.

Clinical
Sometimes associated with systemic diseases, e.g. S.L.E. and Henoch–Schönlein syndrome, this pattern also occurs in the resolving stage of diffuse endocapillary post-streptococcal glomerulonephritis.

May be associated with nephrotic syndrome or the recurrent haematuria syndrome. In the latter case large deposits of mesangial IgA are usually seen, sometimes with C_3 and IgG also (see p. 362).

In most cases of diffuse mesangial proliferative G.N., the course is benign with spontaneous resolution.

Immunology
Many cases are entirely negative but some show mesangial C_3 and IgG in addition to the clear-cut cases of *IgA disease* described above.

MESANGIOCAPILLARY GLOMERULONEPHRITIS – MEMBRANO-PROLIFERATIVE GLOMERULONEPHRITIS

Microscopical
There are two types:
1 *Sub-endothelial deposits.* The characteristic appearances in this condition is of *'double-contour'* basement membranes due to interposition of PAS-positive mesangial matrix. The change is usually diffuse though not necessarily uniform in distribution and is best demonstrated by the PASM (PAS methenamine silver) method. In addition to this feature there is increased cellularity of the tufts due to endothelial cell proliferation. There are considerable variations in appearance and this mesangio-capillary pattern is seen in more than one

disease entity, e.g. also in some cases of S.L.E., bacterial endocarditis; more usually aetiological factors are not identifiable. Sometimes when the mesangial increase is more nodular the term *lobular glomerulonephritis* was previously used.

Immunology. Marked hypocomplementaemia is noted at some stage in nearly all patients. The glomeruli consistently show deposits of complement (C_3) and granular IgG and some have considerable IgA.

2 *Dense deposits.* A further group of patients have very dense intramembranous deposits – these have a worse prognosis. Adhesions and/or epithelial crescents are also frequently seen in this group. Low serum complement levels are associated with C_3 glomerular deposition but other immunoglobulins are usually absent. Some cases are associated with a partial lipodystrophy.

Clinical

Most patients present with insidious renal failure or hypertension. The nephrotic syndrome is a less common feature and appears to confer a worse prognosis. Present methods of treatment appear to influence the course very little. The natural history is not identified with certainty but the prognosis is, on the whole, poor and certainly worse than diffuse membranous glomerulonephritis (see p. 362). There is a rather high recurrence rate in transplants.

EXTRACAPILLARY PROLIFERATIVE GLOMERULONEPHRITIS – CRESCENTIC G.N. – RAPIDLY PROGRESSIVE G.N.

Microscopical

The dominant feature is of proliferation of epithelial cells into the capsular space together with varying degrees of endothelial and/or mesangial proliferation which is usually overshadowed. The capsular space is commonly completely obliterated by these extensive crescents involving 80 per cent or more of glomeruli. Fibrin is often present.

Immunology

Granular deposits of IgG and complement are present in most cases but about one quarter show no significant immunoglobulins and in a minority there is linear deposition of IgG, complement and other immunoglobulins.

Pathogenesis

In many cases aetiological factors cannot be identified but some are due to bacterial endocarditis, polyarteritis nodosa, Henoch–Schönlein syndrome, Wegener's granulomatosis (see p. 640) and, particularly with linear deposits, in *Goodpasture's syndrome* (see p. 363). In this last condition, the deposits are anti-glomerular basement membrane – anti-GBM, a common antigen shared with lung basement membrane hence the haemorrhagic pulmonary lesions. Many cases are however focal rather than diffuse (see below).

Clinical

The onset is acute with severe oliguria, rapidly progressive uraemia and a very high and speedy mortality. Immediate prognosis is related to the percentage of glomeruli with crescents, being particularly grave in those with more than 80 per cent. If transplanted, such patients have a high risk of recurrent disease in the graft.

FOCAL AND SEGMENTAL PROLIFERATIVE GLOMERULONEPHRITIS

Definition

Whilst some cases of diffuse proliferative glomerulonephritis undoubtedly start as focal or segmental lesions, a group of conditions exists where only some glomeruli (focal) or parts of the tufts (segmental) are involved by a proliferative process.

Microscopical

Affected segments show increased cellularity in which endothelial, epithelial and mesangial cells may all take part. One or more lobules may be affected and adhesions and crescents may occur. Fibrinoid areas may be seen and there may be increase in polymorphonuclear leucocytes.

Pathogenetic factors

Focal proliferative lesions may be associated with a wide range of disorders including post-streptococcal glomerulonephritis, bacterial endocarditis, Henoch–Schönlein syndrome, systemic lupus erythematosus, polyarteritis nodosa and other vasculitic conditions. Some are 'idiopathic'. Many cases of Goodpasture's syndrome show focal glomerular disease rather than diffuse, although the linear IgG deposition is diffuse (see above). The focal glomerulosclerosis of children (hyalinosis) needs separation from this proliferative group.

Clinical
The picture is very variable reflecting the range of factors above. Microscopic haematuria is common, particularly so with IgA disease.

Immunology
The syndrome of recurrent haematuria commonly shows deposition of considerable quantities of IgA in the mesangium – *IgA disease*. Whilst this is often associated with focal proliferation, minimal or no proliferation may be seen in patients with marked IgA deposition or they may show diffuse mesangial proliferation (see p. 360). In other cases of focal proliferative G.N., immunoglobulin deposition is usually present and focal but not specific in pattern, usually comprising complement and IgG.

FOCAL GLOMERULOSCLEROSIS – FOCAL AND SEGMENTAL HYALINOSIS

Nature
This is an important cause of the nephrotic syndrome, most commonly occurring in childhood. The pathogenesis is possibly related to fibrin deposition but aetiological factors are not identified.

Microscopical
Segmental adhesions of glomerular tufts to capsule are associated with hyaline eosinophilic subendothelial nodules in the earlier stages. Later, one or more segments show sclerosis and this extends to an increasing number of glomeruli and parts of the tuft. Even in the presence of a grossly nephrotic clinical picture there may be only occasional foci of glomerular involvement and, as a result, some cases are initially misdiagnosed as 'minimal change'.

Immunology
Characteristically, IgM and C_3 are present in glomeruli, often segmentally, and only in the sclerotic areas.

Clinical
The presentation is typically in childhood with the nephrotic syndrome. Progression of the lesion may be rapid and there is steroid-resistance. The overall prognosis is poor and the disease commonly recurs in those initially successfully transplanted.

DIFFUSE GLOBAL GLOMERULOSCLEROSIS

Nature
Diffuse glomerular scarring associated with widespread tubular atrophy and compensatory increase in interstitial tissue.

This occurs with the later stages of any type of glomerulonephritis with masking of differentiating features so that more specific histological identification is not possible.

The term is synonymous with *end-stage nephritis*.

MEMBRANOUS GLOMERULONEPHRITIS – MEMBRANOUS NEPHROPATHY

Microscopical
All glomeruli are uniformly involved and show basement membrane thickening by PAS-positive material which commonly shows 'spikes' of silver-positive material on the epithelial aspect of capillary loops and on electron microscopy shows deposition of proteinaceous material on the outer side of the membrane – *epimembranous*. Progression of the lesion leads to capillary luminal obliteration, hyalinization and renal failure.

Immunology
Capillary loop beaded deposits of granular IgG and C_3, sometimes also with IgM and IgA, are the most typical.

Pathogenetic factors
Most cases are 'idiopathic' but, in adults, about 25 per cent are associated with malignant disease, particularly in the lung, in which case the deposits are of tumour-associated products. The lesion may also occur in systemic lupus erythematosus, with some drugs – gold and penicillamine, and as a result of HB_sAg.

Clinical
The majority of cases present with the nephrotic syndrome and progress to renal failure, often in a 5-year period. About one-third of the cases of the

'idiopathic' type respond to therapy and some patients have a prolonged, rather static course.

HEREDITARY NEPHRITIS

Nature
Glomerular lesions with a familial incidence are relatively common and include most patterns of disease in which more than one member of a family is affected. The pathogenesis of many such cases is obscure and will probably remain so until more is known about glomerular disease antigens. Some are likely to prove to be the result of an infective agent to which sibs are exposed.

Additionally, there are clear-cut inherited conditions.
1 Alport's syndrome.
2 Congenital nephrotic syndrome.

ALPORT'S SYNDROME

Clinical
The fully developed syndrome consists of deafness and progression to renal failure with variably associated features including giant platelets, ocular lesions, neuropathy and bony abnormalities. The renal lesion usually presents as microscopic haematuria and proteinuria appearing in childhood, progressing through a phase of nephrotic syndrome to end-stage failure.

Microscopical
In the early stages, light microscopical appearances are near normal with slight mesangial increase. Electron microscopy is necessary to make the definitive diagnosis by identifying splitting and lamellation of the lamina densa of the basement membrane. Glomerulosclerosis follows.

Inheritance
This is very complex but is basically autosomal dominant with incomplete penetrance in females.

CONGENITAL NEPHROTIC SYNDROME

Classically, this relates to nephrotic syndrome occurring at or shortly after birth often associated with bulky placenta, congenital heart disease and raised α-fetoprotein level in maternal amniotic fluid.

The *Finnish type* shows slight glomerular mesangial proliferation and progressive glomerulosclerosis.

In *non-Finnish type* there is focal and segmental glomerulosclerosis.

Both types progress inexorably to renal failure.

Aetiological mechanisms, clinical syndromes and associated disease processes

In only a relatively small proportion of the patients with glomerular lesions can the exact aetiological mechanism be identified but, in a rather higher percentage, a defined clinical syndrome may be apparent or the renal involvement is part of a more systematized disease. This is true of the group of 'specific' abnormalities identified earlier in this chapter.

Other clinical syndromes include:
1 Henoch–Schönlein – purpura and proliferative glomerulonephritis largely focal (see p. 361).
2 Infective endocarditis – in *Streptococcus viridans* endocarditis in particular (see p. 246).
3 Goodpasture's syndrome – lung haemorrhages and a rapidly progressive type of glomerulonephritis associated with linear deposition of anti-GBM immunoglobulins on the basement membrane (see p. 361).
4 Wegener's granulomatosis – necrotic vasculitic granulomatous lesions affecting upper and lower respiratory tract particularly (see p. 640) and with an associated severe focal proliferative glomerulonephritis with abundant fibrin, crescent formation and no other immune deposition.
5 Post-streptococcal – raised anti-streptolysin and other antibody titres are found in a proportion of cases of focal and diffuse proliferative glomerulonephritis. There may be typical clinical manifestations of infection by particular strains (e.g. Type 12) of β-haemolytic streptococci.

Chapter 65
Genito-Urinary System – Kidney: Tubular and Vascular Disorders

Disorders of tubules

ALTERATIONS IN BASIC TUBULAR MORPHOLOGY

ATROPHY

Tubular loss usually follows glomerular diseases in which there is progressive hyalinization of the tufts. Thus it may follow the various types of glomeru-lonephritis, the specific glomerular lesions identi-fied in Chapter 64 and ischaemic conditions includ-ing hypertension and renal artery atherosclerosis. Shrinkage of tubular lumina is accompanied by reduction in height of the epithelium and loss of specialized features. There is a concomitant in-crease in interstitial tissue by fibrosis and a lympho-cytic infiltrate which is quite non-specific in origin.

Atrophy is also a feature of *obstructive uropathy* (see p. 371).

HYPERTROPHY

A compensatory mechanism involving surviving nephrons where there is progressive chronic renal damage, particularly in hypertension and glomerulonephritis. The enlarged tubules contrast with adjacent patchy areas of atrophy and fibrosis and are responsible for subcapsular granularity.

TUBULAR DILATATION

Distended thin-walled tubules with epithelium of collecting duct type are frequently seen in obstructive uropathy and in many other chronic renal diseases at a relatively late stage.

TUBULAR NECROSIS

Acute necrosis of renal tubules usually occurs in the absence of glomerular abnormalities.

There are two types:
1 Nephrotoxic.
2 Ischaemic.

AETIOLOGICAL FACTORS

1 *Nephrotoxic.* Circulating toxins of chemical or bacterial origin producing a direct effect on tubular epithelial cells, particularly in the proximal convoluted segment. Substances include heavy metal salts particularly mercury and uranium, ethylene glycol and carbon tetrachloride.
2 *Ischaemic.* Usually associated with hypotension or hypoperfusion of glomeruli from other causes. Particularly important predisposing factors are burns, blood loss particularly uterine, traumatic injuries particularly crush injuries – *crush syndrome*, incompatible blood transfusion and the hepatorenal syndrome, seen in cases of severe jaundice or other forms of liver disease often following an episode of operative interference.

Pathogenetic factors

Direct toxic effect of poisons are easy to understand but the exact mechanism in the ischaemic group of cases is more obscure. Reduction of blood flow and of pressure in the tubular vascular plexus appears to be dominant with resulting anoxia and damage particularly to the more sensitive specialized convoluted epithelium.

Macroscopical

Swelling and pallor of the cortex with loss of cortical pattern.

Microscopical

There is considerable variability in morphology of involved tubular segments partly dependent on the cause. A wide range of degenerative changes from swelling, granularity and vacuolation of cytoplasm, to complete necrosis of lining cells and filling of lumina with debris.

Interstitial oedema often with some lymphocytic cellular infiltrate may be prominent but glomeruli are usually structurally intact.

Additional features in specific situations include presence of myoglobin casts in crush syndrome, haematin casts in incompatible blood transfusion kidney and bile staining in hepato-renal syndrome when jaundice is severe.

Secondary calcium deposition is common at an early stage as is the presence of oxalate crystals.

Clinical

Correlation of morphological changes and clinical severity is unrewarding. Severe acute renal failure can be present with little histological evidence of necrosis or cell damage although biopsy evidence of necrotic tubules is also invariably associated with acute renal failure.

Results

1 Acute renal failure with death if untreated.
2 A period of oliguria or anuria is followed by clinical and pathological recovery often heralded by a diuretic phase.
3 Correction of the cause and treatment of the renal failure by attention to fluid and electrolyte balance with or without supportive dialysis usually leads to complete recovery of structure and function.

ALTERATIONS IN TUBULAR CELLS HYDROPIC OR VACUOLAR CHANGE – OSMOTIC NEPHROSIS

Nature

Cytoplasmic swelling with granularity or vacuole formation occurring in tubular epithelial cells, usually in the proximal convoluted tubule. It is believed that this results from disturbance of the normal osmotic relationships within the cells.

Aetiology
Most commonly seen after treatment with sucrose, dextrose and mannitol.

Similar changes are found in some cases of severe or prolonged potassium deficiency.

SUBSTANCES PRESENT IN TUBULAR CELLS OR LUMINA

HYALINE (PROTEIN) DROPLETS

Protein aggregates forming droplets of hyaline eosinophilic, PAS-positive material in tubular cell cytoplasm. These may be found in a wide range of renal diseases in which there is proteinuria.

CALCIUM – NEPHROCALCINOSIS

Deposition of calcium salts can occur in damaged tissues as dystrophic calcification or due to abnormal serum calcium levels – *metastatic calcification* (see p. 115). The most marked examples of nephrocalcinosis are seen in hypercalcaemia due to hyperparathyroidism, malignant disease, sarcoidosis, milk-alkali syndrome and hypervitaminosis D.

MYELOMATOSIS

Renal failure associated with characteristic 'hard' tubular casts and cellular reaction is common in myelomatosis which may also be complicated by secondary renal amyloidosis. The casts are densely eosinophilic usually with multinucleated cells at their periphery which appear to be derived from tubular epithelium (see p. 470).

GOUT

In both primary and secondary gout (see p. 710) renal involvement is common but seldom clinically important. Deposits of urate crystals and surrounding inflammatory reaction including foreign body giant cells may be quite marked. These are usually in the medulla and, whilst starting in the tubules, later appear to be interstitial.

Vascular disorders

HYPERTENSIVE NEPHROSCLEROSIS— ARTERIOLOSCLEROSIS

BENIGN NEPHROSCLEROSIS

Nature
The renal disease associated with benign hypertension (see p. 266).

Incidence
This is the most common form of nephropathy and is found in approximately 75 per cent of autopsies over the age of 60 years.

Aetiology
Most commonly seen in the essential type but it may also be found in cases of hypertension secondary to renal disease and this, therefore, may then complicate the appearances of the kidneys. The hypertension antedates and produces the renal changes in uncomplicated cases.

Kidneys
Diffuse, symmetrical, ischaemic atrophy and scarring in uncomplicated cases of longstanding hypertension.

MACROSCOPICAL
Size. Small and pale.
Capsule. Moderately adherent.
Cortex. Fine, even granularity of the surface, the cortex being pale grey and narrow, with some loss of pattern.
Medulla. Demarcation from the cortex is usually preserved but there is a decrease in size with some pallor.
Blood vessels. The arcuate arteries are particularly affected and are prominent on the cut surface with thickening of their walls.
Calyces and pelvis. Normal.

MICROSCOPICAL
Glomeruli. Progressive fibrosis which is maximal in the periglomerular and capsular interstitial tissues – extracapsular glomerulofibrosis, cf. the intracapsular fibrosis of glomerulonephritis.
Tubules. Atrophic.

Interstitial tissue. Increased fibrosis with a very scanty lymphocytic infiltration.

Blood vessels. Thick-walled arterioles and small arteries which have a markedly decreased lumen. The thickening is due to hyaline material which at first is subendothelial but later replaces the muscle of the media.

These arteriolosclerotic changes are present in other organs and may also be superimposed on other forms of renal disease which cause hypertension, e.g. chronic pyelonephritis and glomerulonephritis.

Results

Not more than 5 per cent of patients with well-developed benign nephrosclerosis die from renal failure. Death in the great majority of cases of benign hypertension occurs from congestive heart failure, coronary insufficiency and cerebral vascular accidents (see p. 598).

ACCELERATED NEPHROSCLEROSIS

Nature

Renal disease produced by accelerated malignant hypertension (see p. 267).

Origin

1 In previously normotensive individuals.
2 Superimposed on pre-existing renal disease or benign hypertension.

Age

In the pure form, the disease usually presents under 40 years of age, but as a complication of benign hypertension is most frequently seen between 60–70 years of age.

Kidney in the pure type

MACROSCOPICAL

Size. Normal or slightly enlarged and congested.
Capsule. Strips easily.
Cortex. Normal pattern and size with small pin-point haemorrhages on the surface.
Medulla. Demarcation from the cortex is preserved and the medullary pattern is normal.
Blood vessels. Normal or slight vascular prominence.
Pelvis and calyces. Normal.

MICROSCOPICAL

Glomeruli. Sometimes focal necrosis may be seen in the capillaries, but more often they appear normal.
Tubules. Minor degenerative changes in the proximal convoluted tubules.

BLOOD VESSELS

1 Fibroblastic proliferation and muscular hypertrophic thickening of the arterioles and small arteries. There is the appearance of concentric fibrous lamination – 'onion-skin'; the lumen is narrowed.
2 Fibrinoid necrosis of the afferent arterioles often with rupture producing haemorrhages or thrombosis; this is the pathognomonic lesion.

Kidney in the secondary type

The appearances are those of a pre-existing renal disease, e.g. chronic pyelonephritis, or of benign hypertension with superimposed fibrinoid necrosis of the blood vessels.

Results

Untreated accelerated hypertension causes death from renal failure in 90 per cent, usually with marked rapidity. If the hypertension is treated adequately before there is evidence of impairment of renal function by a raised blood urea, prognosis is good and subsequent renal failure unusual.

SENILE ARTERIOSCLEROTIC KIDNEY – ATHEROSCLEROTIC NEPHROSCLEROSIS

Aetiology

Atheromatous narrowing of the main renal arteries and branches leading to ischaemic atrophy of the renal substance. Although the renal arteries are not a very common site for atheroma, the mouths of the vessels are frequently involved by aortic atheromatous plaques.

Appearances

1 *Main arteries involved.* Diffuse symmetrical contraction producing a pale, granular, small kidney similar to that of benign nephrosclerosis except that the blood vessels within the renal substance do not show hypertensive changes.
2 *Branch arteries involved.* Asymmetrical, patchy, focal, depressed scars of the cortical surface. These

are pale, granular, wedge-shaped areas of fibrosis extending into the medulla and showing ischaemic atrophy with fibrous replacement of the glomeruli and tubules.

Results

1 Usually there is no interference with renal function.
2 When there is unilateral renal artery obstruction, hypertension may ensue which may occasionally be relieved by removal of the ischaemic organ.
3 Occasionally, severe bilateral main artery involvement may lead to renal failure.

INFARCTION

Incidence
A common site of infarction.

Causes
1 *Arterial*. Ninety-eight per cent.
(a) *Embolic*, e.g. mural thrombus from a cardiac infarct, left atrial thrombus in mitral stenosis.
(b) *Thrombotic*. Due to advanced atheroma, occlusion of renal artery orifices by aortic thrombus, polyarteritis nodosa.
2 *Venous*. Two per cent – renal thrombophlebitis with sudden occlusion is usually associated with perinephric abscess or other intra-abdominal infections.
   Gradual venous occlusion does not cause infarction but may cause the nephrotic syndrome (see below).

Macroscopical
Infarcts in the kidneys are anaemic in type and within 24 hours there is a wedge-shaped, sharply demarcated, pale, yellow-white area with an hyperaemic border, usually confined to the cortex. Later, a V-shaped scar develops.

Microscopical
Coagulative necrosis with a polymorph infiltration at the margins.

RENAL VEIN THROMBOSIS

Nature
This uncommon condition is an occasional cause of

the nephrotic syndrome, usually in adults over 50 years of age. Rapid occlusion of renal veins, e.g. by extension of inferior vena caval thrombus, is likely to produce renal infarction, but the mechanism of a presumed more insidious venous thrombosis is obscure. Some cases are associated with renal amyloidosis, accelerated hypertension, acute pyelonephritis or glomerulonephritis. Extrinsic pressure from metastatic tumour in adjacent lymph nodes is also a frequent cause. Many cases, however, have to be classified as 'idiopathic'.

Appearances
The diagnosis can often be suspected on renal biopsy material when:
1 Tubular damage, atrophy and interstitial oedema and fibrosis are disproportionately greater than glomerular abnormalities.
2 Mild to moderate diffuse basement membrane thickening of glomeruli is present but lacks 'spikes' and other features of membranous glomerulonephritis (see p. 362).

Results
If infarction occurs then renal failure is inevitable. When the presentation is by the nephrotic syndrome, this may be progressive with developing renal failure, or spontaneously improve or improve following anticoagulant therapy.

ACUTE CORTICAL NECROSIS

Nature
Acute massive bilateral symmetrical necrosis of the cortical tissues.

Aetiology
This very rare condition occurs most frequently during pregnancy, but may also follow severe infections, burns and shock.

Mechanisms
1 There is a close association with disseminated intravascular coagulopathy (DIC) and the haemolytic – uraemic syndrome of children (see p. 369).
2 Appearances are very similar to the experimentally produced Shwartzmann reaction.

Macroscopical
Size. Enlarged.
Cortex. The surface shows areas of congestion

and haemorrhage alternating with pale yellow areas of massive necrosis. Double contour (tramline) calcification commonly develops in the subcapsular tissue and at the sharp zone of demarcation between necrotic and normal cortex.

Medulla. Usually completely normal.

Blood vessels. Thrombosed vessels may be seen within the necrotic zones.

Results

When cortical necrosis is bilateral, there is complete anuria and a rapidly fatal outcome. Very rarely the condition may be unilateral and this is compatible with survival, the involved kidney eventually becoming fibrotic and functionless.

HAEMOLYTIC URAEMIC SYNDROME

Nature

The combination of haemolytic anaemia, thrombocytopenia and renal failure mostly in children, usually under 4 years of age. There is often a preceding infective episode.

Clinical

Acute onset of jaundice, thrombocytopenia and haemolytic anaemia with *schistocytes* – fragmented erythrocytes, in the peripheral blood (see p. 531) and acute renal failure, sometimes with hypertension.

Kidney

There is widespread fibrin and platelet deposition in vessels and glomerular tufts with endocapillary proliferation of global or segmental distribution. Apart from fibrin deposition, immunohistological studies are negative.

Arterioles and branch arteries may show intimal fibrous thickening with luminal narrowing, changes which are also notable in *post-partum renal failure*, a rare complication of parturition and probably initiated through fibrin deposition.

In severe cases of the haemolytic uraemic syndrome cortical necrosis occurs (see p. 368).

Pathogenesis

Many of the features are similar to those of disseminated intravascular coagulation (D.I.C.) (see p. 368). The intermediary mechanism may be the Shwartzmann reaction.

Results

The prognosis depends largely on the severity of the acute attack. Recovery is usually possible unless extensive bilateral cortical necrosis has occurred.

POLYARTERITIS NODOSA

Incidence

Renal involvement is common and is often the determining prognostic factor in this multisystem connective tissue disease (see p. 282). The main renal lesion is in the blood vessels, but occasionally a dominant glomerular fibrinoid necrosis sometimes with adhesions and proliferative features, occurs.

TOXAEMIA OF PREGNANCY – ECLAMPSIA

The lesions in the kidneys in this disease are described on p. 428. They consist of diffuse glomerular swelling primarily involving the endothelial cells, deposition of protein material related to fibrin adjacent to the basement membrane and swelling of mesangial cell cytoplasm reducing intercapillary spaces.

The condition usually resolves following evacuation of the uterus but if essential hypertension preceded the pregnancy, its progression may be accelerated.

Chapter 66
Genito-Urinary System – Kidney: Granular Contracted Kidneys: Hydronephrosis: Calculi: Proteinuria: Uraemia

Granular contracted kidneys

Many serious renal diseases lead to renal failure and are associated with small granular contracted kidneys. Characteristic and diagnostic features may be present but often the changes, grossly and histologically, are non-specific.

CHRONIC GLOMERULONEPHRITIS

Diffuse fine granularity with a uniform loss of pattern and prominent blood vessels. The pelvis and calyces are normal.

CHRONIC PYELONEPHRITIS

Irregular granularity with large, flat areas of cortical scarring, the intervening zones often appearing normal. The pelvis and calyces are thickened, pale and granular (see p. 353).

ANALGESIC ABUSE NEPHROPATHY

Cortical scarring pallor and interstitial fibrosis are marked but non-specific. Necrotic papillae, when present, are obvious but identifying the absence of shed papillae is more difficult (see p. 354).

VASCULAR DISEASES

1 *Benign nephrosclerosis.* Fine, even granularity of the cortex with slight loss of the cortical pattern but preservation of cortico-medullary differentiation. The vessels pout from the cut surface and the calyces and pelvis are normal (see p. 266).

2 *Atherosclerotic nephrosclerosis.* Asymmetrical, focal, wedge-shaped cortical scars extending deeply into the medulla with severe atheroma of the large vessels. When the main arteries are involved, however, the kidneys are symmetrically contracted with a fine granularity (see p. 258).

3 *Polyarteritis nodosa.* Petechial haemorrhages and infarcts of varying age are usually seen in addition to a fine cortical granularity. The blood vessels are commonly aneurysmally dilated and may be thrombosed.

DIABETES

Usually a mixed picture due to the common concurrence of pyelonephritis and nephrosclerosis with the rather more streaky and mottled appearance of the Kimmelstiel–Wilson lesion (see p. 635).

Hydronephrosis – Hydrocalycosis

Nature
Dilation of the renal pelvis and calyces.

Mechanism
Due to slowly progressive obstruction at any level of the urinary tract. Ureteric ligation may cause renal atrophy without significant hydronephrosis. However, intermittent, partial, or progressive obstruction leads to distension of the renal pelvis with a rise of pressure, atrophy of the renal parenchyma and subsequent loss of function.

Age and incidence
Common in differing age groups according to the cause.

Causes
These are many and include:
1 *Lumen.* Calculi, blood clot.
2 *Wall.*
 Congenital. Valves, strictures, abnormalities of peristalsis at the pelvi-ureteric junction.

Acquired. Post-traumatic and post-inflammatory stricture, prostatic enlargement, tumours of the renal pelvis, ureter, bladder and urethra.

3 *External.* Gravid uterus; pressure from ovarian or uterine masses; retroperitoneal fibrosis; invasion by tumour from adjacent organs or by enlarged lymph nodes.

An aberrant renal artery crossing the pelvi-ureteric junction probably perpetuates hydronephrosis arising from other causes.

Macroscopical
Hydronephrosis may be unilateral or bilateral. The most severe examples are seen in unilateral lesions due to obstruction proximal to the bladder, especially the pelvi-ureteric type. There is gross enlargement of the kidney with saccular distension of the pelvis, much of which becomes extrarenal in position. The calyces are flattened and the renal parenchyma is thinned and atrophied, in severe cases leaving only a thin rim of recognizable renal tissue. The external surface may be lobulated.

Microscopical
Marked atrophy of the tubules, the glomeruli at first being spared but subsequently becoming hyalinized.

Results
Bilateral. Prolonged bilateral hydronephrosis leads to hypertension and/or renal failure.

Unilateral. The opposite kidney may become hypertrophied and maintain normal function but hypertension may result from the unilateral renal ischaemia (see p. 268).

In both forms, infection is a common complication causing *pyonephrosis*, i.e. pus in the distended pelvis and calyces. Pyelonephritic changes, spreading from the pelvis, speed the progression of the renal atrophy.

Calculi

Nature
Urinary calculi may form in the kidney and bladder but are also seen in passage down the ureter and urethra. These stones are composed of urinary salts in amorphous form bound by a colloid matrix and consist of a nucleus, usually organic, around which are deposited concentric layers of one or more of the salts.

Constituents

PRINCIPALLY
1   Uric acid.
2   Calcium oxalate.
3   Triple phosphates.

OTHERS
4   Amino acids, e.g. xanthine, cystine.
5   Calcium carbonate.
    They may occur in pure form, but are more frequently mixtures.

Types of stone

1   *Primary stone*. No antecedent inflammation. They are usually composed of uric acid, urates or calcium oxalate and the urine is acid.
2   *Secondary stone*. Associated with inflammation. They are mostly triple phosphates or occasionally ammonium urate; the urine is alkaline.

Appearances

1   *Uric acid stones*. May occur alone or more usually combined with urates and oxalates. They are of moderate hardness, light or dark brown in colour with wavy concentric markings.
2   *Oxalate stones*. These are often in pure form and are extremely hard with a dark colour due to blood staining resulting from the production of local injury. They are laminated and show a spiny or prickly exterior – 'mulberry calculus'.
3   *Phosphatic stones*. Occur in a pure form or as a surface covering of primary stones. They are white, smooth and friable.

Pathogenesis

Renal stone formation is of frequent occurrence and the pathogenesis in most cases remains unknown. However, the following factors may be contributory:
1   *Hypercalciuria*. This occurs in hyperparathyroidism due to parathyroid adenoma or secondary hyperplasia (see p. 316).
2   *Urinary infection*. Some urea-splitting organisms cause alkalinity of the urine.
3   *Urinary stasis*. Favours the development of infection and the retention of organic substances.
4   *Vitamin A deficiency*. Suggested as a factor by experimental observations.
5   *Randall's plaques*. Small areas of calcification in the collecting tubules in the apex of the pyramids. These are found, however, in many normal indivi-

duals with no history of stones and are not always present in patients with stones.
6   *Microliths*. Small foci of calcification are commonly seen in the medullary interstitial tissue and within macrophages in lymphatics. They have, however, no constant relationship to the presence or absence of calculi.
7   *pH of urine*. Alkalinity of the urine renders calcium phosphate and triple phosphates less soluble.
    Suggested mechanisms of stone formation include:
1   Deficiency of substances in the urine which normally prevent precipitation and deposition. Possible substances include citrate, magnesium, colloid substances, organic acids, amino acids and urea. There is some evidence that citrate may have a beneficial effect by preventing precipitation.
2   Presence of substances enhancing the precipitation of calcium salts. Mucoprotein, which is usually increased in the urine in hyperparathyroidism, may have such an effect.
3   Disturbance of the mechanism which normally removes calcium precipitated in the kidneys as microliths, which have a similar basic structure to calculi.
    It is suggested that when the mechanism of removal becomes overloaded there is excess calcium deposition leading to stone formation. However, it is possible that this only happens when protective substances, perhaps colloids, become depleted.
    The only clear-cut condition inducing stone formation is hyperparathyroidism. Following removal of the adenoma, further calculi are not formed and those already present do not increase in size. This, however, only accounts for a small but important number of patients – 5 per cent, with urinary calculi.

Sites

RENAL PELVIS
Solitary or multiple, unilateral or bilateral and usually composed of oxalates or urates. Small stones are the commonest but large branched 'stag-horn' calculi may occur and completely fill the pelvis and calyces.

BLADDER
1   Originate in the kidney with subsequent en-

largement in the bladder due to phosphatic encrustation.

2 Formed primarily in the bladder usually of phosphates.

Effects

OBSTRUCTION
1 At the pelvi-ureteric junction.
2 Ureter.
3 Bladder neck.

ULCERATION
Of calyces and pelvic mucosa.

CHRONIC INFECTION
Predisposed to by the stones and by the stasis they cause, thus, pyelonephritis or pyonephrosis are induced if obstruction is present.

Proteinuria

Nature

The term albuminuria, used by many persons to denote the presence of protein in the urine, is technically incorrect but dies hard. Although albumin is the most important constituent of urinary protein loss, normal and abnormal globulins may be present and, indeed, normal persons pass up to 50 mg of total protein daily comprising twenty or more different types, ten closely related to serum proteins.

It is, moreover, true that normal glomerular filtrate contains protein but at a concentration of less than 50 mg/100 ml and that nearly all is reabsorbed by the tubule.

Origin

1 Escape of normal plasma proteins through a defective glomerular membrane.
2 Failure of normal tubular reabsorption.
3 Abnormally increased concentration in the plasma of normal plasma proteins.
4 Abnormal plasma proteins passed in the urine due to small size or failure of tubular reabsorption due to qualitative abnormality.
5 Abnormal secretions of proteins by the cells of the kidney, ureter, lower urinary tract and accessory glands.

In massive proteinuria leading to the nephrotic syndrome (see p. 357) factor 1 is largely responsible because of the glomerular abnormality. Factors 1 and 2 are effective in 'nephrosis' and factor 3 may operate in patients given protein infusion and in certain diseases causing high plasma proteins. Factor 4 is operative in conditions such as haemolytic states with haemoglobinuria and in myeloma and factor 5 comes into play with local abnormalities such as calculi and infections in the urinary tract.

Tests

Prepared test strips are unduly sensitive and often pick up normal amounts of urinary protein as 'trace' which is, therefore, of very dubious significance. Routine chemical tests, e.g. salicylsulphonic acid, are less sensitive and are thus preferable. Urine positive to such a test can be accepted as abnormal and its protein concentration quantitatively determined chemically together with more detailed assessment by electrophoresis.

Causes
The main causes are:

POSTURAL (ORTHOSTATIC) AND EXERCISE PROTEINURIA
The physiological mechanisms are poorly understood but the protein content qualitatively is a reflection of plasma protein levels. If protein is detected in an ambulant or erect person then it should not be detectable after a period of rest or after a time in the supine position for a diagnosis of orthostatic or exercise proteinuria to be acceptable.

The urinary deposit should likewise be normal.

RENAL DISEASES
1 Nephrotic syndrome (see p. 357).
2 Renal vascular disease (see p. 366) and congestive cardiac failure.
3 Glomerulonephritis of all types and stages (see p. 359).
4 As a constituent of escaped blood in any renal cause of haematuria (see p. 379) – red cells identified in urinary deposit.
5 In renal infections (see p. 352) – pus cells and organisms usually identified in urinary deposit together with cultural isolation.

POST-RENAL DISEASES
Disorders of the ureters, bladder and lower urinary tract may cause proteinuria associated with infections, bleeding from these structures, calculi, etc.

Uraemia

Nature
A clinical state associated with a raised blood urea.

Causes
'PRE-RENAL'
1 Acute circulatory failure, e.g. shock.
2 Dehydration and severe electrolyte imbalance; due to excessive loss, e.g. vomiting, diarrhoea and sweating, or to inadequate fluid intake.
3 Bleeding into the gastro-intestinal tract with absorption of breakdown products.
4 Massive tissue necrosis, e.g. gangrene of the leg, large infarcts, etc.

RENAL
The most common causes are:
1 Chronic pyelonephritis and analgesic nephropathy.
2 Vascular disease – accelerated nephrosclerosis, polyarteritis nodosa.
3 Glomerulonephritis – acute and chronic.
4 Diabetes mellitus.
Less common renal causes include:
5 Acute tubular necrosis.
6 Polycystic kidneys.
7 Renal tuberculosis.
8 Myeloma kidney.

'POST-RENAL'
Any severe longstanding obstruction in the urinary tract may produce a bilateral back pressure effect on the kidneys. This is most commonly due to:

1 Hydronephrosis.
2 Calculi.
3 Carcinoma of the bladder.
4 Prostatic enlargement.
5 Carcinoma of the cervix.

Metabolic changes
The most important changes are:
1 *Blood urea and non-protein nitrogen.* Raised.
2 *Metabolic acidosis.* There is a low bicarbonate due to failure of ammonia production and to electrolyte disturbances aggravated by vomiting, diarrhoea, etc.
3 *Electrolytes.* The changes are variable:
(*a*) When the decrease in glomerular filtration rate is dominant, there is sodium and potassium retention with raised blood levels.

(*b*) When failure of tubular re-absorption is dominant, there is sodium and potassium depletion with lowered blood levels. The urinary volume remains large causing excess water loss. This is particularly well seen in analgesic nephropathy.
Chloride levels are very variable.
Phosphate and calcium. Phosphates are retained with increased blood levels. As a result, the ionized serum calcium level falls and secondary hyperparathyroidism may ensue (see p. 317).

Organ changes
These are very variable but some or all of the following may be seen at post-mortem examination:
Heart. Fibrinous pericarditis.
Gastro-intestinal tract. Mucosal or serosal petechial haemorrhages due to damaged capillaries are common. Stomatitis, oesophagitis, gastritis and entero-colitis are frequent, the last named often being associated with a patchy haemorrhagic and necrotizing appearance – 'uraemic colitis' (see p. 206).
Lungs. Pulmonary oedema, often associated with a fibrinous alveolar lining – 'uraemic pneumonitis'.
Skin. Sallow colour with a purpuric rash and frequently an 'uraemic frost'.
Blood. Anaemia, which is commonly severe and of the normochromic normocytic type due to marrow depression in the presence of a raised blood urea, however iron deficiency and macrocytic types may be found. The purpuric manifestations are non-thrombocytopenic and are due to 'toxic' capillary damage (see p. 511).

Renal transplantation

Background to the theoretical considerations of organ allograft transplantation has been considered in Chapter 16.

COMPLICATIONS

It is generally accepted that one of the most successful organs to be transplanted is the kidney and extensive follow-up studies on large number of patients have identified specific problem areas.
1 Technical.
2 Effects of immunosuppression.

3 Graft rejection.
4 Transmission of renal disease to graft.

TECHNICAL

1 Ureteric anastomosis – leakage or pyelonephritis.
2 Venous – venous thrombosis.
3 Arterial – kinking of supply, thrombosis or renal artery stenosis at the anastomosis.

IMMUNOSUPPRESSION

Immunosuppressive drugs may be required in high dosage to control or prevent rejection of the graft. Most commonly used currently are corticosteroids, azathioprine and cyclophosphamide.
   Complications due to this therapy include:
1 Metabolic.
2 Suppression of resistance to infection, particularly normally non-pathogenic *opportunistic* organisms. e.g. aspergillus species, cytomegalovirus, *Pneumocystis carinii.*
Septicaemic episodes by a wide range of micro-organisms are common.
3 Induction of neoplasia – particularly lymphomas but many epithelial tumour associations are now also described.

GRAFT REJECTION

1 *Hyperacute.* This occurs within a few minutes of re-establishing blood flow to the graft. Flow quickly falls and within a few hours urine production ceases. Progressive cortical necrosis appears. Factors responsible include:
(a) Blood group incompatibility.
(b) Presensitization of recipient – from blood transfusions, pregnancy, etc.
   This type of rejection is mediated humorally.
2 *Acute.* Episodes of acute rejection are common in most recipients of grafts in the first few weeks even when immunosuppressed. There is, however, marked variability in severity and the ability to control the episode by treatment.
   There are two types of appearance:
(a) *Cellular (parenchymal) rejection.* Marked oedema and dense focal or more generalized infiltration of the cortex by pyroninophilic lymphoid cells. Tubular degeneration and/or necrosis are usual and there may be endothelial cell swelling in capillaries. IgG and complement are not seen in capillaries or glomeruli. This type is cell mediated.
(b) *Vascular rejection.* Lymphocytic infiltration is slight but platelet aggregates are found in capillaries and small venules later with fibrin and polymorphs. Fibrinoid necrosis is seen in the walls of small arteries and veins with superimposed thrombus deposition. Rupture of the internal elastic lamina of arteries may be seen. The thrombi will show progressive organization if the recipient survives. IgG, IgM, C_{lq}, C_3, fibrinogen can usually be demonstrated in vessel walls and glomerular capillaries. This type is predominantly humoral.
3 *Chronic.* Rejection may occur months or years later presenting as insidious loss of graft function.
(a) *Arterial narrowing.* Thickening of intima by collagen, myofibrils and fatty material often with rupture of internal elastic lamina. IgM and complement are usually present and the lesions are the result of fibrin and platelet deposits. Ischaemic glomerular changes result.
(b) *Glomerular changes.* Basement membrane thickening segmental or diffuse and usually focal. Capsular adhesions sometimes with crescent formation may occur. Immunofluorescence usually shows granular IgM deposition with some C_{lq} and C_3 on capillary basement membranes: occasionally this is linear. The differential diagnosis of 'transplant glomerulopathy' from recurrent disease in the graft may be very difficult.

TRANSMISSION OF RENAL DISEASE TO GRAFT

Changes similar to those seen in the host renal disease may appear after a variable period of time in the graft. In not all of such cases however is it possible to be dogmatic that disease transmission has occurred. A risk of transmission is however identifiable, particularly in focal glomerulosclerosis (see p. 362), crescentic glomerulonephritis and in mesangiocapillary lesions (see p. 360).

Chapter 67
Genito-Urinary System – Kidney: Tumours: Haematuria

Tumours of renal parenchyma

BENIGN

Adenoma
Incidence
Sites
Age
Sex
Predisposing
Size
Macroscopical
Microscopical
Behaviour

Hamartoma

Haemangioma

Other connective tissues

MALIGNANT

Adenocarcinoma
Incidence
Age

Sex
Origin
Site
Macroscopical
Microscopical
   Clear cell
   Granular cell
   Undifferentiated
   Oncocytoma
Grade
Spread
Results

Wilms' tumour
Incidence
Sex
Age
Nature
Macroscopical
Microscopical
Spread
Results

Sarcoma

Secondary tumours

Tumours of renal pelvis and ureter
Incidence
Age
Sex
Site
Predisposing factors
Macroscopical
Microscopical
   Transitional cell tumours
   Squamous cell carcinoma
Spread
Effects
Results

Haematuria
Causes
   'Pre-renal'
   Renal
   'Post-renal'

Tumours of the renal parenchyma

BENIGN

ADENOMA

Incidence
Common, being found in as many as 7 per cent of post-mortems as incidental lesions.

Sites
Cortical, often bilateral and multiple.

Age
Increasing frequency with age.

Sex
M:F equal.

Predisposing factors
Adenomas are most commonly seen in nephrosclerotic and chronic pyelonephritic kidneys.

Size
The majority are very small, i.e. a few millimetres in diameter. When more than 2.5 cm in diameter, their subsequent behaviour is likely to be that of adenocarcinomas.

Macroscopical
Circumscribed cortical lesions, usually yellow in colour and with fibrous bands; small cysts are common.

Microscopical

Solid or papillary regular overgrowths of tubular epithelial cells with a tubular or acinar pattern. There is usually a fibrous capsule, but when the lesions are larger, the cells may merge with the adjacent normal renal tubules.

Behaviour

Usually asymptomatic and are incidental findings. However, it seems certain that adenocarcinomas arise in adenomas and this progression from a benign to a malignant lesion may be very difficult to determine microscopically. Metastases do not occur until such tumours are more than 2.5 cm in diameter; above this size any such tumour should be regarded with suspicion as it is probably a carcinoma.

HAMARTOMA

Although uncommon renal tumours, this is one of the commoner sites in the body for hamartomas. They are probably anomalies of development rather than true neoplasms and are seen in the medullary areas usually as small circumscribed white or yellow nodules containing variable mixtures of smooth muscle, fat, blood vessels and fibrous tissue. Many are the angiomyolipomas of tuberose sclerosis (see p. 593).

HAEMANGIOMA

Capillary and cavernous haemangiomas are rare but may occur in the kidney, usually as small lesions of the pyramids. They may cause haematuria and are thus important in the differential diagnosis of this symptom.

OTHER CONNECTIVE TISSUE TUMOURS

Lipoma
Fibroma
Leiomyoma } Very rare, small, subcapsular, benign, connective tissue tumours; small foci of ectopic adrenal tissue may produce a similar macroscopical appearance.

MALIGNANT

ADENOCARCINOMA – GRAWITZ TUMOUR – HYPERNEPHROMA

Incidence

One per cent of all malignant tumours. Eighty per cent of renal tumours.

Age

Seldom below 40 with an average of 55–60 years of age.

Sex

M:F 2:1.

Origin

The tumours are generally agreed to be of renal tubular origin and many probably arise from pre-existing cortical adenomas. Grawitz's theory of origin from adrenal rests, hence the term hypernephroma, is no longer acceptable.

Site

Originate in the cortex.

Macroscopical

Large, rounded vascular masses, often appearing encapsulated and with a variegated pattern of golden-yellow areas, fibrous trabeculae, cyst formation, areas of necrosis, haemorrhage and sometimes calcification. They seldom cause symptoms until they are large, by which time they have usually destroyed much of the kidney substance, ulcerated the renal pelvis and produced haematuria or invaded through the renal capsule. Macroscopic invasion of the renal vein is seen in approximately 20 per cent with masses of tumour tissue occasionally extending from the renal vein into the lumen of the inferior vena cava.

Microscopical

1 *Clear cell carcinoma.* Large cells with abundant pale foamy cytoplasm containing large amounts of lipid material and glycogen. Variable degrees of an alveolar arrangement, papillary structure, or tubule formation, are seen.
2 *Granular cell carcinoma.* The cytoplasm is more eosinophilic and granular thus resembling convoluted tubular epithelium. A papillary arangement may be evident.
3 *Undifferentiated carcinoma.* There is little pat-

tern and marked variation in size of the cells, commonly with giant forms. Individual cells may show little evidence of a renal tubular origin.

4 *Oncocytic tumour*. This is a recently recognized entity of proximal renal tubular cell origin and consisting of large, eosinophilic, slightly granular cells of oncocytic appearance. Previously included in carcinomas of the kidney it is now known to be usually benign. Solid circumscribed and brown in colour with a central, pale, scar it may attain 15 cm or more in diameter.

Grade

Histological grading, in respect of the most poorly differentiated area seen, has an important prognostic significance:

Grade I (Low) 80 per cent 5-year survival.
Grade II (Average) 30 per cent 5-year survival.
Grade III (High) 10 per cent 5-year survival.

Spread

Direct. Renal parenchyma, renal pelvis and perinephric tissues.

Lymphatic. Para-aortic lymph nodes are invaded in 30 per cent of the cases; later, more distant groups of nodes.

Blood. Occurs early, with metastases commonly in the lungs, bone and brain. Sometimes, especially with low-grade tumours, the metastases may be few or even solitary.

Results

Low-grade tumours confined to the kidney substance and with no evidence of renal vein invasion carry a good prognosis.

All cases after nephrectomy:

Eighty per cent 1-year survival.

Forty per cent 5-year survival (nearly all Grade I).

Twenty per cent 10-year survival (all Grade I).

When the renal vein is invaded there is a 36 per cent survival at 3 years and 20 per cent at 5 years.

WILMS' TUMOUR – NEPHROBLASTOMA – EMBRYOMA OF KIDNEY – ADENOMYOSARCOMA – EMBRYONAL ADENOSARCOMA

Incidence

A rare tumour forming only 8 per cent of all malignant renal tumours; about 20 per cent of malignant tumours in childhood; 3.5 per cent are bilateral.

Sex

M:F equal.

Age

The average is 3 years; very rarely occur beyond the age of 7 years.

Nature

Probably arise from residual, embryonic, mesodermal, nephrogenic tissue.

Macroscopical

A solitary, rapidly growing, demarcated mass which is firm and usually homogeneous grey or white on section. At first, the renal tissue is only distorted but is later invaded by the tumour. The renal pelvis is seldom invaded so that haematuria is a late symptom and the tumour usually presents as an abdominal mass. Direct invasion of perinephric tissues is frequently seen.

Microscopical

There is a mixed picture of an abundant, embryonic, spindle cell stroma surrounding epithelial tubules of variable size and shape sometimes showing a rosette arrangement. Abortive glomerulus formation is occasionally seen together with smooth or striated muscle fibres.

Spread

Direct. Renal parenchyma and perinephric tissues.

Lymphatic. Regional lymph nodes are commobly invaded by the time of presentation.

Blood. Common, especially in the lungs, brain and liver.

Results

Until recently, 5-year survival was only 5 per cent, most of these being in children in whom the tumour was surgically removed before 1 year of age. Some improvement in prognosis now seems likely with aggressive combined cytotoxic chemotherapy.

SARCOMA

These are very rare renal tumours but occasional examples of fibrosarcoma, liposarcoma and leiomyosarcoma are seen. Most probably these arise in pre-existing hamartomas.

SECONDARY TUMOURS

Involvement of the renal parenchyma is seen in 50 per cent of cases of lymphoma. Secondary carcinoma occurs in about 8 per cent of all cases of malignant disease, i.e. a comparatively uncommon site for metastases.

Tumours of the renal pelvis and ureter

Incidence
These form approximately 12 per cent of all malignant renal tumours.

Age
50–70 years.

Sex
M:F 3:1.

Site
The right and left sides are equally involved and most tumours arise in the pelvis. They are multiple in 50 per cent but bilateral tumours are exceptionally rare.

Predisposing factors
1 *Industrial*. Aniline dye workers.
2 *Calculi*.
3 *Analgesic abuse*. There is a much enhanced incidence in patients with papillary necrosis and other changes of chronic analgesic overdosage.

Macroscopical
Three types:
1 Papillary with no infiltration.
2 Papillary with infiltration of adjacent tissues, e.g. kidney substance or peri-ureteric tissues.
3 Infiltrative or solid – this produces a pale, irregular, firm thickening of the pelvis or calyces with diffuse infiltration of the renal substance.

Microscopical
Two types:
1 *Transitional cell* – 80 *per cent*. These are papillary or anaplastic tumours of urothelial origin and ranging from the regular papillary differentiated non-infiltrating type, still regarded by a minority as papillomas, through more irregular solid and papillary transitional cell forms to the solid anaplastic highly invasive tumours.
2 *Squamous cell carcinoma* – 20 *per cent*. Rather more than 30 per cent are associated with calculi and presumably arise as a result of chronic irritation followed by squamous metaplasia. They are usually poorly differentiated and highly invasive.

Spread
Direct. Involve the renal substance and perinephric tissues. Forty-six per cent of papillary renal pelvic tumours develop further tumours in the ureter or bladder. It is disputed whether this represents:
1 Multiple primary tumours, *or*
2 Seedling deposits by implantation, *or*
3 Spread in peri-ureteric lymphatics.
Lymphatic. Common, with invasion of the para-aortic lymph nodes.
Blood. Metastases in lungs and other sites are common in the infiltrative types, although unlike adenocarcinoma of the kidney, demonstrable venous invasion in the primary tumour is rare.

Effects
1 Hydronephrosis due to the urinary obstruction.
2 Ulceration with haematuria.
3 Infection of the kidney.

Results
Following nephro-ureterectomy:
1 Tumour confined to the renal pelvis – 50 per cent 5-year survival.
2 Tumour not confined to the renal pelvis – 50 per cent 1-year survival, but very few survivors at 5 years.
3 Squamous cell carcinoma – 35 per cent 1-year survival, but nil at 5 years.

Haematuria

Causes
1 *'Pre-Renal'*. Less than 10 per cent – mostly haemorrhagic diatheses including:
(*a*) Purpura – thrombocytopenic or non-thrombocytopenic.
(*b*) Leukaemia – usually acute.
(*c*) Aplastic anaemia.

(*d*) Scurvy.

(*e*) Hypoprothrombinaemia – e.g. anticoagulant therapy.

Also occurs in systemic bacterial infections, e.g. septicaemia, especially meningococcal, and in rickettsial diseases.

2 *Renal*

(*a*) Glomerular disease – Nephritic syndrome.

(*b*) Vascular disease – Accelerated hypertension; polyarteritis nodosa; lupus erythematosus; infarction.

(*c*) Tubular disease – Acute tubular necrosis.

(*d*) Congenital polycystic disease.

(*e*) Pyelonephritis.

(*f*) Tuberculosis.

(*g*) Tumours – Adenocarcinoma with invasion of the renal pelvis; tumours of the renal pelvis; haemangioma.

(*h*) Calculi.

3 *'Post-renal'*

(*a*) Cystitis – Non-specific or tuberculous.

(*b*) Calculi and foreign bodies.

(*c*) Trauma.

(*d*) Tumours – Ureters; bladder; prostate; urethra.

(*e*) Diseases of neighbouring organs – with secondary involvement of the urinary tract, e.g. inflammations of the Fallopian tube, appendix and large intestine.

Tumours of the prostate, cervix, corpus uteri and rectum.

Secondary tumours in the peritoneum or lymph nodes.

Chapter 68
Genito-Urinary System – Bladder:
Congenital: Mechanical: Inflammations

DEVELOPMENT

The primitive cloaca, which is the terminal segment of the endodermal tube, is connected to the allantois by the elongated urachus. A septum divides the cloaca into the posterior portion – the rectum, and an anterior chamber which connects with the ureters and forms the bladder and urethra. A downgrowth of mesoderm invests the endodermal mucosa with a musculature. At birth, the urachus becomes obliterated.

STRUCTURE

MUCOSA

Transitional epithelium – urothelium.

TUNICA PROPRIA

A dense layer of connective tissue upon which the mucosa rests.

MUSCULARIS

Large bundles of smooth muscle which run in all directions and condense around the ureteric orifices and internal urethral meatus to form functioning, but anatomically poorly defined, sphincters.

SEROSA

The bladder is extraperitoneal except for the dome which is covered by peritoneum.

FUNCTION

Storage of urine with subsequent voluntary voiding. The adult capacity is 200–300 ml.

Congenital

ECTOPIA VESICAE – EXSTROPHY

Incidence
One in 50 000 births.

Sex
M:F 7:1.

Origin
Probably due to failure of union of the urogenital cleft.

Appearances
Absence of the anterior wall of the bladder and anterior abdominal wall, with eversion of the posterior bladder wall. The bladder, therefore, lies as an open sac on the lower surface of the abdomen or, in less severe cases, communicates with the external surface through a large defect in the suprapubic region. Urine is discharged on to the skin surface and the mucosa is exposed. In the complete lesion there is absence of the symphyis pubis and there may be other associated malformations, e.g. epispadias.

Effects
1 *Infection*. The bladder mucosa is subjected to repeated attacks of infection with ulceration, eventually leading to a granulation tissue lining. Marginal areas may show squamous metaplasia in which carcinoma may sometimes develop.
2 *Pyelonephritis*. Following infection of the bladder, possibly by direct ascent up the ureters.
3 *Hydronephrosis*. Due to ureteric obstruction.

Results
Fifty per cent die before the age of 10, due to renal failure from infection and hydronephrosis.

Seventy per cent die before the age of 20, for similar reasons.

A small proportion survive to adult life. Surgical correction, by transplantation of the ureters and excision of the bladder with closure of the abdominal wall defect, may be technically possible and prevent the complications.

PERSISTENT URACHUS

Types
1 Persistence as a closed fibrous cord.
2 Patency of the urachus in part or whole:
(*a*) When fully patent, a fistula connects the bladder with the umbilicus.
(*b*) When the lower portion is obliterated, a sequestrated umbilical rest with cyst formation may occur – urachal cyst.
(*c*) When the lower portion remains patent – urachal diverticulum from the bladder.

Effects
1 *Fistula*. Vesico-umbilical.
2 *Infection*.
3 *Carcinoma*. Adenocarcinoma occasionally develops.

DIVERTICULA

Nature
Pouch-like eversions or evaginations of the bladder wall.

Types
1 *Congenital*. Focal failure of muscular development with resulting herniation. The wall contains all layers, although the muscle may be thin. This type is frequently single or few in number.
2 *Acquired*. Associated with obstruction to urinary outflow; they form between the interlacing muscular bundles.

Incidence

Found in 5–10 per cent of males above the age of 50. Females are less frequently affected. The acquired type is much more common than those of congenital origin.

Formation

Sequence in the formation of the acquired type:
1 Obstruction to urinary outflow.
2 Hypertrophy of bladder muscle with trabeculation of the wall.
3 Formation of sacculations between the muscle bundles.

Effects

Predisposes to infection of residual static urine.

Appearances

The wall contains little muscle as it becomes replaced by fibrous tissue, especially when associated with infection. They are commonly multiple.

MISCELLANEOUS CONGENITAL CONDITIONS

1 Absence of the bladder.
2 Marked hypoplasia of the bladder
3 Transverse septum with 'hour-glass' deformity.
4 Congenital vesico-vaginal, vesico-rectal, vesico-uterine fistulae.

Rupture of the bladder

Causes

1 *Trauma*
(a) Crushing injuries to the pelvis.
(b) Suprapubic trauma associated with a full bladder.
2 *Spontaneous*. Associated with over-distension.

Effects

There is escape of urine into the extraperitoneal tissues and sometimes into the peritoneal cavity if the dome is involved.

Neurogenic bladder – cord bladder

Nature

Disturbance of normal vesical function due to interference or interruption of controlling nerve pathways.

Normally two sets of pathways operate:
1 Voluntary micturition is controlled by the brain.
2 Automatic conditioned emptying reflex – autonomic nerve impulses actuated through a spinal reflex arc.

Causes

1 *Severance of brain connections*. This leads to loss of volitional control and thus to totally automatic function. The main causes are, therefore, spinal lesions above the level of the reflex arc which may be traumatic, neoplastic, inflammatory or degenerative.
2 *Interruption of the reflex arc*. Injuries or lesions of the cauda equina, sacral plexus or peripheral nerves may lead to abolition of the reflex and evacuation then occurs only by overflow – *autonomic neurogenic bladder*.

Results

The neurogenic bladder is very vulnerable to infection and many cases of disease or injury to the spine die from renal failure secondary to chronic infection of the urinary tract and kidneys.

Calculi

Origin

1 From the kidney (see p. 371).
2 Form primarily in the bladder – primary bladder stones.

Age

Adults over 40 years of age.

Sex

M:F 20:1.

Aetiological factors

These are similar to those described for renal calculi, in particular, retention of urine due to incomplete emptying and infection, is important (see p. 390).

Types

Usually of mixed composition, containing calcium, ammonium and magnesium salts, phosphates, carbonates, oxalates and urates.

1 *Inflammatory type.* Predominantly phosphates – these are mostly formed in the bladder.
2 *Non-inflammatory.* Urates, oxalates, xanthine, cystine – mostly of renal origin, commonly with phosphatic encrustation acquired in the bladder.

Size
Single or multiple, varying from small stones forming gravel to very large – average 2–3 cm dia.

Effects
1 None.
2 Persistent cystitis; sometimes with squamous metaplasia.
3 Haematuria.
4 Obstruction at the bladder neck.
5 Spontaneous passage *per urethram.*

Foreign bodies

A most extraordinary assortment of foreign bodies have at various times been found in the bladder, usually self-introduced, but sometimes iatrogenic.

Effects
1 Chronic cystitis.
2 Form a central nidus for encrustation and calculus formation.
3 Obstruction of urinary flow.
4 Perforation of the bladder.

Inflammations

NON-SPECIFIC CYSTITIS

The normal bladder is very resistant to infection due to the mechanical barriers of the sphincters and to the frequent flushing of the mucosa by urine each time the bladder is emptied. The lining is smooth and there are no glands. Infection, therefore, usually complicates some local abnormality or is introduced from without.

ACUTE CYSTITIS

Incidence
Very common.

Sex
More common in females due to the shortness of the urethra.

Routes of infection
1 *Urethral.* Introduced from outside, especially by catheterization or by extension of urethral infection.
2 *Renal.* Descending infection.
3 *Haematogenous.* Occasionally.
4 *Lymphatic.* Probably rare.
5 *Direct.* From adjacent organs, e.g. diverticulitis coli.

Predisposing factors
1 *Urinary retention or stasis.* Obstruction, bladder paralysis, bladder diverticula, calculi, foreign bodies, tumours, uterine prolapse.
2 *Infection of adjacent structures.* Prostatitis, pyelonephritis, urethritis, vesiculitis, diverticular disease of colon.
3 *Chronic debilitating diseases.*
4 *Diabetes mellitus.*
5 *Pregnancy.*
6 *Trauma.* Especially catheterization.

Agents
1 *Bacteria.* Coliforms, staphylococci, *Streptococcus faecalis*, *Pseudomonas aeruginosa*, *Bacillus proteus*, gonococci, etc.
2 *Chemical irritants.* Heavy metals, including lead, arsenic, mercury.
3 *Mechanical irritants.* Catheters, calculi, foreign bodies.
4 *Parasites.* Schistosoma *haematobium* – bilharziasis.
5 *Fungi.* Monilia.

Macroscopical
The mucosa is hyperaemic with oedema, haemorrhagic discoloration and thickening of the wall. Later, the mucosa may become friable, granular and ulcerated.
   There are several descriptive types:
1 *Haemorrhagic.*
2 *Suppurative.* Marked exudation.
3 *Ulcerative.* Large areas of ulceration.
4 *Diphtheritic or pseudo-membranous.*
5 *Gangrenous.* Usually involves the mucosa only but occasionally the whole thickness of the wall.

Microscopical
The infection is usually limited to the mucosa and tunica propria with oedema, congestion and a polymorph infiltration. There are variable amounts of haemorrhage, fibrin and surface encrustation by phosphates.

Results
1 Resolution – usually occurs if the predisposing cause is removed.
2 Chronic cystitis.
3 Necrosis, gangrene and extension to surrounding structures rarely occur.

CHRONIC CYSTITIS

Origin
1 Following acute cystitis with persistence of the predisposing factor.
2 Low grade virulence of the infecting organism.

Macroscopical
The bladder is small and in severe cases markedly contracted. The muscular layer is fibrotic, thickened and inelastic.

Microscopical
Infiltration by chronic inflammatory cells and fibrosis of all layers of the wall which may extend into the paravesical tissues.

Results
A very small fibrous bladder of low urinary capacity which results in marked frequency of micturition and disability.

SPECIAL TYPES OF CYSTITIS

ENCRUSTED CYSTITIS

Grey-white granular deposits of precipitated urinary salts, associated with alkalinity of the urine due to urea-splitting organisms. The deposits may be focal or diffuse.

BULLOUS CYSTITIS

Large vesicles of submucosal oedema fluid seen as smooth, rounded projections from the surface.

They are usually seen in the acute stages of cystitis due to virulent organisms.

INTERSTITIAL CYSTITIS – HUNNER'S ULCER

Occurs almost exclusively in middle-aged women in whom an area of the bladder is thickened and usually ulcerated. Histologically, the epithelium is thinned or absent and there is oedema. Lymphocytic infiltration and later fibrosis of the submucosa, tunica propria and eventually the muscular layers. The bladder may eventually become very contracted with a capacity of only 60–90 ml of urine. The aetiology is not known but it may be due to lymphatic spread of infection through the bladder with obstruction of lymphatic drainage. However, endocrine or vascular factors at the time of the menopause may be contributory.

IRRADIATION CYSTITIS

Irradiation to the bladder, cervix or uterus may produce cystitis. Congestive hyperaemia may be followed by haemorrhagic cystitis, vascular thrombosis and ulceration with marked oedema. Later, the entire thickness of the wall may become fibrotic or even necrotic, with sloughing of the mucosal surface, perforation, secondary infection and fistula formation. Frequently telangiectases on the inner surface may develop and cause severe haematuria.

CYSTITIS CYSTICA

In chronic cystitis some cases show small cystic mucosal invaginations which grossly are seen as smooth irregularities of the lining. Microscopically, they contain albuminous fluid and are lined by flattened cuboidal epithelium. They arise from downgrowths of the surface transitional epithelium, which later become separated from the surface. Uncommonly this epithelium may undergo metaplastic change.

CYSTITIS GLANDULARIS

Most commonly arises in chronic cystitis by metaplastic change in epithelial downgrowths. These are usually formed in the trigonal region as cystic or gland-like spaces in the tunica propria which may or may not communicate with the bladder lumen. The epithelial lining of these spaces is usually columnar and mucus-secreting but may be cuboidal.

MALAKOPLAKIA – SOFT PLAQUE

Present as yellow-grey or brown, circumscribed, slightly elevated, soft plaques of a few millimetres to several centimetres in diameter. The edges are overhanging but sharply demarcated and separated by zones of inflamed but otherwise normal mucosa. Microscopically, the plaques are formed by massive submucosal aggregates of large macrophages, lymphocytes, occasional plasma cells and foreign body giant cells. Some cells contain basophilic laminated inclusions – *von Hansemann bodies*. The aetiology is unknown, although various agents have been indicted, including coliforms, parasites, tuberculosis and sarcoidosis.

FOLLICULAR CYSTITIS

Numerous, tiny, grey, elevated nodules which may be surrounded by a reddish zone and frequently occur in the trigonal area. This variant of chronic cystitis microscopically shows the nodules to be composed of lymph follicles in the mucosa and submucosa.

Chapter 69
Genito-Urinary System – Bladder:
Specific Infections: Tumours: Fistulae

TUBERCULOSIS

Origin
Almost always secondary to renal tuberculosis, possibly by extension down the ureter. Sixty per cent of cases of renal tuberculosis develop bladder involvement.

Macroscopical
The trigonal area, especially around the ureteric orifices, but later the entire bladder is affected.
Early. Tubercles are seen as very small, pin-head, mucosal elevations.
Later. These coalesce to form caseous nodules which ulcerate with the formation of ragged, slightly undermined edges, a base of yellowish tuberculous granulation tissue and dense fibrosis of the surrounding wall.
Late. The ureteric orifice often becomes widely dilated due to fibrotic contraction of the bladder wall – 'golf-hole' ureter.

Microscopical
Typical tuberculous caseating giant cell systems.

Results
1 Marked irritation and contraction of the bladder with severe and distressing urinary symptoms.
2 Healing with some fibrous scarring following appropriate antituberculous chemotherapy.
3 Fistula formation.

387

4 Extension to other organs, e.g. seminal vesicles and epididymis.

SCHISTOSOMIASIS – BILHARZIASIS

Organism – *Schistosoma haematobium*

Source and life cycle
See p. 72.

Geographical distribution
Mainly in Africa with minor foci in the Middle East, Portugal, Greece and Cyprus. In some of these countries, the disease is extremely common, e.g. Nile delta.

Pathogenesis
The worms attain maturity in the liver and thence travel against the venous blood flow to tributaries of the portal vein. *S. haematobium* has a tropism for pelvic plexuses, particularly vesical. The eggs, 20–30 for each pair of worms, are deposited in the small vessels of the bladder submucosa and then extrude to the mucosa and into the lumen where they appear in the urine 1–3 months after infestation. Many eggs are retained within the wall where they instigate a dense inflammatory reaction.

Macroscopical
The trigone is first affected but later the whole organ is involved. The mucosa is initially congested and shows yellow nodules up to 2 mm in diameter, which later become elevated brown-yellow areas. These coalesce and extend. Two or more years later, there is extensive fibrosis and muscular hypertrophy with mucosal thickening and bladder contraction. Similar changes are seen in the lower portions of the ureters.

Microscopical
  Early. Intense eosinophilia around the eggs in the submucosa.
  Later. Pseudo-tubercles form around the eggs which subsequently calcify and there is marked surrounding fibrosis which ultimately extends to all coats. Epithelial overgrowth and areas of squamous metaplasia develop at the trigone and may extend over the whole mucosa.

Effects
1 Contraction of the bladder.
2 Calculus formation around the eggs.
3 Ureteric obstruction leading to hydronephrosis.
4 Fistula formation.
5 Carcinoma may occur and in endemic areas bladder carcinoma is extremely common, e.g. Egypt.

Tumours

Virtually all bladder tumours are epithelial in origin.

CARCINOMA OF THE BLADDER

Incidence
Three per cent of deaths from malignant disease; the incidence is increasing.

Sex
M:F 3:1.

Age
A wide range, but usually between 60 and 70 years of age.

Predisposing factors
1 *Ectopia vesicae*.
2 *Cystitis glandularis*. Adenocarcinoma.
3 *Cystitis cystica*. Transitional cell or adenocarcinoma.
4 *Leukoplakia*. Associated with squamous cell carcinoma, although leukoplakia in the bladder is not necessarily pre-cancerous.
5 *Schistosomiasis*.
6 *Bladder diverticula*. Tumour complicates about 3 per cent of diverticula, and is commonly of squamous cell type.
7 *Chemical substances*. Particularly in aniline dye and synthetic rubber workers. Chemical substances implicated include β-naphthylamine, benzidine and xenylamine.
    There is much experimental and biochemical evidence to suggest that bladder tumours may be induced by chemical substances in the urine bathing the entire urinary tract; stasis from any urinary obstruction renders these carcinogenic substances more effective. Tryptophane and its aminophenol metabolites are of importance in this respect.

Sites

Mostly at the base, particularly the trigone and around the ureteric orifices.

Macroscopical

Multiple in 20–30 per cent, but these are probably multifocal tumours rather than tumour implants. The tumours may be:

1 *Papillary.* Growing into the lumen as fronded masses with little or no invasion of the wall. This is the more common form.
2 *Solid.* Growing into the wall with little projection into the lumen and often ulcerated or encrusted.

The adjacent mucosa is frequently abnormal, showing areas of irregular hyperplasia, oedema, cystitis cystica, leukoplakia or carcinoma *in situ*. Cystitis is a frequent accompaniment.

Microscopical

1 *Papilloma.* A fine vascular connective tissue core with fronds covered by regular transitional epithelium three to four cells thick. There is a tendency to local recurrence following removal, but there is no invasion of the stalk or the wall. This is a very uncommon type as a truly benign tumour and many authorities do not accept its separate existence from 2 below.
2 *Differentiated transitional cell carcinoma-urothelial.* A papillary structure with little invasive tendency, but the fronds are more stumpy and the cells show increased irregularity and greater thickness, with up to ten or more layers of cells covering the fronds.
3 *Undifferentiated transitional cell carcinoma-urothelial.* Usually solid, the origin from transitional epithelium is not clearly recognizable due to the undifferentiated nature of the cells, which show marked irregularity and numerous mitoses. Invasion is prominent and is usually extensive.
4 *Squamous cell carcinoma.* A bulky, widely invasive tumour of keratinizing squamous cell type arising in metaplastic epithelium.
5 *Adenocarcinoma.* Uncommon but is found at the base of the bladder arising from cystitis glandularis or in the dome of the bladder from urachal remnants. Mostly they are mucus-secreting and may be entirely submucosal in situation.

Spread

1 *Direct.*
Stage PTis. – No evidence of invasion, flat.

Stage PTa – Non-invasive, papillary.
Stage 1 – Invasion confined within the mucosa.
Stage 2 – Extension into muscle.
Stage 3 – Extension into perivesical tissues.
Stage 4 – Pelvic fixation.
2 *Lymphatic.* Occurs in at least 30 per cent of fatal cases and usually involves the iliac and para-aortic groups of nodes.
3 *Blood.* Occurs also in 30 per cent of fatal cases, but is usually late. Metastases may occur in the liver, lungs, bones and other organs.
4 *Implantation.* After cystotomy or partial cystectomy, tumour cell implantation may occur. The common sites of implantation recurrence are the prostatic bed, urethra, and in scars in the bladder or abdominal walls.

Effects

1 *Infection.* Cystitis and pyelonephritis.
2 *Ureteric obstruction.* Hydronephrosis and pyonephrosis.
3 *Urethral obstruction.* Retention of urine.
4 *Extension to neighbouring organs.* Fistula formation.
5 *Haematuria.*

Results

Much depends on the type of tumour, e.g.

Papillary differentiated carcinoma – 70 per cent 5-year survival.

Solid undifferentiated carcinoma – 30 per cent 5-year survival.

Death is due to renal failure in many cases.

OTHER TUMOURS

SARCOMA

These are rare, only accounting for approximately 0.5 per cent of bladder tumours. However, the following types have been reported; leiomyosarcoma; rhabdomyosarcoma; fibrosarcoma; Hodgkin's and non-Hodgkin's lymphomas.

BENIGN CONNECTIVE TISSUE TUMOURS

These are all uncommon but leiomyomas, fibromas, angriomas, etc., do occur at this site.

SECONDARY TUMOURS

Direct spread
The bladder is often invaded by carcinomas of the cervix, prostate, rectum, colon or ovary.

Metastatic
Uncommon, but occurs from primary carcinomas of the breast and stomach and from malignant melanoma.

Changes in bladder size and form

DILATATION

Causes
1 Stricture of the urethra.
2 Obstruction at the bladder neck, e.g. prostatic enlargement, uterine cancer, calculi, foreign bodies.
3 Neurogenic dysfunction – cord bladder.
When of long duration, hypertrophy of the bladder wall follows.

HYPERTROPHY

Causes
1 *Irritation*
(*a*) Inflammation.
(*b*) Calculi.
(*c*) Foreign bodies.
2 *Obstruction*. To outflow of urine.

DIVERTICULA (see p. 382)

HERNIATION

Inclusion of part of the bladder wall in the sac of an inguinal or femoral hernia. This usually occurs in elderly patients with direct inguinal hernias.

CYSTOCOELE

Protrusion of the bladder into the vagina forming a dependent pouch below the level of the urethra. This is due to relaxation of pelvic supports and is associated with uterine prolapse.

PROLAPSE OF THE BLADDER

This is rare and occurs only in females when it usually follows a difficult labour during which raised intra-abdominal pressure causes inversion of the dome of the bladder; this then passes through the urethra. Gangrene of the bladder rapidly develops due to vascular obstruction.

STENOSIS – MARION'S DISEASE

Congenital
An incomplete diaphragm of muscle and fibrous tissue obstructing the proximal end of the urethra.

Acquired
Occurs in males only and is associated with scarring due to prostatitis.

Fistulae

VESICO-VAGINAL

The commonest type
Causes
1 Obstetric injuries and pelvic operations.
2 Irradiation injury.
3 Inflammation.
4 Neoplasms of the bladder, cervix and vagina.

VESICO-ENTERIC AND
VESICO-RECTAL

Causes
1 Trauma.
2 Cystitis.
3 Diverticular disease of colon.
4 Irradiation injury.
5 Calculus.
6 Neoplasms of the bladder and intestine, e.g. rectum and colon.

VESICO-UTERINE

Less common than the other types.

Causes
Usually malignant disease or radionecrosis.

EFFECTS OF FISTULAE

Severe cystitis inevitably complicates these fistulous communications. Gas from the intestines may produce pneumaturia.

Chapter 70
Genito-Urinary System – Urethra : Prostate

Urethra

INFLAMMATIONS

NON-SPECIFIC URETHRITIS

Nature
Inflammation of non-gonococcal origin, caused by a large variety of agents and leading to urethral discharge.

Aetiology
Trauma, chemical irritants, redundant foreskin and pin-hole meatus are local factors. The infection may also be associated with pyelonephritis, cystitis, prostatitis or seminal vesiculitis.

The disease is usually classified as venereal infection in that the infective agent may be transmitted during sexual intercourse.

Bacteriology
Organisms may be profuse, scanty or absent; the

common bacteria found are staphylococci, streptococci and coliforms. An important aetiological agent was held to be organisms of the pleuropneumonia group but this view is no longer acceptable. Chlamydial infection is more likely.

Clinical

The urethritis has a very variable course. There may be an acute onset of urethral discharge which may be eliminated spontaneously or become chronic with recurrent acute exacerbations. The infection may be of low-grade virulence from the start and become chronic; when this occurs the disease is more difficult to cure completely.

Smears

The discharge is seldom profuse and cytological examination of smears shows variable proportions of pus cells and epithelial cells, commonly 70 per cent pus and 30 per cent epithelial cells.

REITER'S DISEASE – ABACTERIAL URETHRITIS

Clinical

Urethritis associated with conjunctivitis and arthritis.

Aetiology

This is probably an organism of the chlamydial group (see p. 43).

Results

There may be a spontaneous recovery but frequently there is a long history with many clinical exacerbations. In severe cases, there is ulceration of the buccal mucosa, skin of the feet, glans penis, urethra and bladder. Iritis and keratitis may complicate the conjunctivitis.

GONOCOCCAL URETHRITIS

Incidence

This is still a common disease in many parts of the world, the incidence being directly related to the promiscuity of the population.

Aetiology

Infection is almost invariably acquired during sexual intercourse. The gonococci multiply on the intact mucosa of the anterior urethra and subsequently invade the peri-urethral glands with an ensuing bacteraemia and lymphatic involvement.

Macroscopical

Acute inflammation of the urethral mucosa with a purulent exudate on the surface; ulceration of the mucosa may occur.

Discharge

Develops 3–8 days following the infection and is viscid, yellow and profuse. Smears show large numbers of pus cells (100 per cent), many containing the engulfed intracellular Gram-negative diplococci.

Course

1 May resolve in 2–4 weeks, either as a result of treatment or sometimes spontaneously.
2 Becomes chronic.

Complications

1 Posterior urethritis, prostatitis, vesiculitis, epididymitis and cystitis.
2 Peri-urethral abscess.
3 Systemic spread – suppurative arthritis or tenosynovitis are infrequently seen in neglected cases whilst endocarditis may occur very rarely.

URETHRAL STRICTURE

Aetiology

1 Mostly post-inflammatory – particularly gonococcal.
2 Trauma, (*a*) instrumentation, (*b*) obstetrical complications.

Sites

Any portion of the urethra may be involved but usually the bulbous or bulbo-membranous parts.

Macroscopical

Thickening and induration, with fibrosis of the urethral wall and narrowing of the lumen. A short or long segment may be involved.

Effects

Obstruction to the urinary outflow with difficulty of micturition leading to retention. There is also the increased hazard of false passage formation during therapeutic instrumentation, which, when followed by local infection may result in a urinary fistula.

URETHRAL CARUNCLE

Nature
A circumscribed prolapse of the urethral mucosa in females.

Aetiology
Unknown, but the lesion is non-neoplastic. Trichomonal infestation is commonly present.

Macroscopical
A small, 1–2 cm diameter, red, painful protuberance of tissue just outside or just within the external urethral meatus; it commonly ulcerates and bleeds.

Microscopical
A highly vascular connective tissue with a variable inflammatory infiltrate completely or partially covered by epithelium. This is commonly both transitional or squamous in type and shows epithelial ingrowths which form squamous or transitional cell-lined clefts.

Results
Rarely grow larger than 2 cm; surgical excision leads to a complete cure.

URETHRAL CARCINOMA

Incidence
Rare

Age
Sixty-five years and over.

Sites
1 Most commonly adjacent to the external urethral meatus.
2 Occasionally arises elsewhere in the urethra.

Macroscopical
Those at the external meatus are commonly papillary at first but later show ulceration and may fungate. The tumours elsewhere along the urethra are usually invasive and ulcerate from their onset.

Microscopical
1 Mostly squamous cell carcinomas, sometimes with transitional cell areas.
2 Rarely, adenocarcinomas arising from the peri-urethral glands.

Spread
1 *Direct*. Ulceration of the surrounding tissues with destruction.
2 *Lymphatic*. Occurs early and is often present at the time of the first presentation:
　　Male. Inguinal glands.
　　Female. Inguinal and iliac glands.

Results
The prognosis is very poor due to the early lymphatic spread.

Prostate

Normal
The normal adult gland weighs 20 g. This retroperitoneal organ encircles the bladder neck and the posterior urethra. It is sometimes divided into two lateral lobes and one median lobe but these are not anatomically distinct and are only apparent in enlarged prostate glands.

Microscopically, it is a compound tubulo-alveolar gland with a low columnar epithelium in an abundant fibro-muscular stroma. The gland is endocrine dependent but the mechanisms of its control remain unknown.

Changes occur with increasing age, so that, after the age of 40, irregular atrophy of muscle occurs with an increase in the fibrous tissue – presenile change. There may also be superimposed hyperplasia of the inner portions of the prostatic glands. The normal epithelium of the prostate elaborates small quantities of acid phosphatase.

INFLAMMATIONS

NON-SPECIFIC – ACUTE AND CHRONIC PROSTATITIS

Organisms
Staphylococci, streptococci, gonococci, coliforms.

Routes
Usually by direct extension from infection of the

posterior urethra or bladder, commonly associated with local surgical procedures.

Occasionally, infection may arise from distant foci by blood or lymphatic spread.

ACUTE PROSTATITIS

Macroscopical
Small multiple abscesses, or large areas of coalescent necrosis, or a diffuse boggy suppuration of the entire gland. The gland is usually enlarged.

Results
1 Complete resolution when mild.
2 Incomplete resolution with fibrous scarring.
3 Chronic prostatitis.
4 Prominent suppuration producing a large prostatic abscess.

CHRONIC PROSTATITIS

Macroscopical
The gland is irregular and firm or hard with areas of fibrous scarring. There may be thickening of the surrounding tissues.

Microscopical
Fibrous scarring around areas of lymphocytic and plasma cell infiltration. Dilated ducts frequently contain inspissated secretions or calculi.

Results
The resulting hard gland may clinically mimic carcinoma, and when calculi are present, recurrent, more acute exacerbations of infection are extremely troublesome – *calculous prostatitis*.

GRANULOMATOUS PROSTATITIS

Non-specific
May occur following acute or chronic prostatitis in which localized areas of inflammation cause obstruction of the prostatic ducts with inspissation of their secretion and a granulomatous reaction with foreign body giant cells.

Tuberculous
This is secondary to tuberculosis in some other regions of the renal tract, especially the kidney. However, the prostate may rarely be the site of

miliary spread. The gland may be considerably enlarged and firm, with extensive areas of caseation; the infection frequently also involves the seminal vesicles.

BENIGN PROSTATIC ENLARGEMENT – BENIGN PROSTATIC HYPERTRPHY – NODULAR HYPERPLASIA

Incidence
Extremely common over the age of 50, the incidence increasing with age so that 80 per cent of men over the age of 80 years are affected.

Nature
Nodular enlargement as a result of hyperplasia affecting all the tissue elements of the gland.

Aetiology
Endocrine imbalance with advancing age appears the most important factor. The likely mechanism appears to be a progressive decrease in testicular hormone output, particularly androgens. Thus, there is a relative hyperoestrogenic state, largely adrenal in origin, which causes the hyperplasia.

Macroscopical
The degree of prostatic enlargement is variable but usually the gland weighs between 60–100 g and seldom more than 200 g. The enlargement usually involves the lateral lobes and the median lobe (posterior to the urethra) but not in the posterior lobe. The gland is nodular, firm and rubbery. On section, two types of discrete nodules may be found, each appearing encapsulated:
1 Soft, yellow-pink tissue with a honeycomb appearance and containing milky fluid – predominantly glandular hyperplasia.
2 Tough, solid, glistening, grey nodules with no fluid – predominantly fibro-muscular tissue.

Microscopical
All three elements, epithelium, muscle and fibrous tissue, are involved by the hyperplasia in variable proportions from one case to another and from one part of the gland to another. This overgrowth is regular in focal areas but uneven in distribution, thus producing nodules surrounded by compressed gland tissue. Cystic dilatation due to retention of

secretions, infarction and secondary infection, are also common.

Effects

1 *Urethra*
Deformity of the prostatic urethra, frequently associated with obstruction due to median lobe enlargement, results eventually in urinary retention.

2 *Bladder*
(*a*) Obstruction leads to an hypertrophied and trabeculated bladder wall.
(*b*) Bladder diverticula.
(*c*) Acute or chronic cystitis following urinary stasis.
(*d*) Predisposes to calculus formation.

3 *Ureter*. Hydroureter.

4 *Kidneys*. Hydronephrosis; pyelonephritis; pyonephrosis; renal failure.

Carcinoma

Incidence

A common site of malignancy, accounting for 3.7 per cent of all deaths from malignant disease. However, the disease is more common than the above figure would indicate:

1 *Clinical*. This accounts for 7 per cent of all clinically overt cancers in males.

2 *Microscopical*. In many more cases there is no clinical evidence of prostatic disease but microscopic cancers are found on detailed histological examination of the prostate – '*latent*' *cancer*. These microscopic cancers are found:

Aged 80 to 90–80 per cent of prostates contain carcinoma.

Aged 70 to 80–50–60 per cent of prostates contain carcinoma.

Aged 60 to 70–30–40 per cent of prostates contain carcinoma.

Aged 50 to 60–15–30 per cent of prostates contain carcinoma.

However, there is no known method of determining which of these tumours would have progressed had the patient lived or the prostate not been removed, to produce eventually clinical evidence of prostatic carcinoma or metastases.

Age

Increasing frequency with age; the disease is rare below 50 years.

Site

Eighty per cent or more arise in the posterior lobe of the gland and 95 per cent of these arise adjacent to the capsule.

Aetiology

The important aetiological factor is probably an oestrogen–androgen imbalance with an excess of androgens. These tumours are hormone-dependent and their growth is inhibited by antagonism of the stimulating androgens. This can be produced by removing the sources of the stimulating androgens, e.g. by castration, or by the administration of oestrogens.

Inflammation and pre-existing benign enlargements are frequently found in carcinomatous prostate glands but these appear to be of little aetiological significance.

Macroscopical

Many of the cases show concomitant benign enlargement involving both lateral lobes and frequently the median lobe. However, carcinoma shows as a small, hard, pale area in the posterior lobe, posterior to the urethra, or in the posterolateral aspect of the gland in the subcapsular area, i.e. in areas not involved by benign enlargement. Frequently, the firm tumour tissue has spread through the capsule to invade the adjacent fatty tissue.

Microscopical

Adenocarcinoma. Ninety-six per cent – most have a well-defined tubular pattern but sometimes they are of the less well-differentiated spheroidal cell type. The cells are usually uniform in size and cuboidal in shape with a small central nucleus and a clear or vacuolated cytoplasm. Anaplastic tumours are uncommon.

The regularity and differentiation of some tumours is very pronounced and may lead to histological difficulties in diagnosis. Invasion of blood vessels or perineural lymphatics may, however, be seen and confirms the diagnosis of carcinoma as does penetration of the capsule, which may also be apparent.

Squamous cell carcinoma. Four per cent – these tumours arise in prostatic ducts following squamous metaplasia.

Spread

1 *Direct*. Invasion of the gland, especially poster-

iorly through the capsule to involve the periprostatic tissues, followed by invasion of the seminal vesicles, rectum or bladder.

2 *Lymphatic*. This is common and involves the iliac, aortic and sometimes mediastinal, lymph nodes.

3 *Blood*. Seventy per cent of cases show bony metastases which are often the presenting clinical feature. The spine is particularly involved by spread from the prostatic venous plexus into Batson's vertebral venous plexus. There is usually considerable new bone formation at the sites of these metastases – *osteosclerotic*. The liver and lungs may also be invaded.

Diagnosis

1 *Acid phosphatase*. Serum levels of greater than 6 i.u./l are very suggestive of prostatic carcinoma. This enzyme is produced by the epithelial cells and is partly a reflection of tumour differentiation and partly of the amount of tumour present. The levels are usually high, 15 i.u./l or more, when metastases are present but in many cases of established disease normal levels are found.

2 *Prostatic smears*. Smears made from material expressed by prostatic massage may show malignant cells before there is any clinical evidence of the disease.

3 *Biopsy*. Although this is usually satisfactory, sampling errors are common and in well-differentiated tumours the histological diagnosis may be very difficult. If the tumour is small and confined to the periphery of the gland, a trans-urethral biopsy will miss the carcinoma and biopsy through the perineum may then be necessary.

Effects

Local effects are not usually severe, obstruction to the urethra being less common than with benign hyperplasia. Most of the important effects result from the metastases.

Hormonal control

This can usually be obtained by oestrogen administration or castration or both. There is a marked decrease in the size of the tumour and frequently of the metastases. This oestrogenic effect may be visualized histologically as vacuolation of the tumour cells, disruption of cell membranes, pyknosis of nuclei and fibrosis of the tumour area. However, after a variable period of time, the tumour 'escapes' from hormonal control and renewed growth and extension occurs.

Results

Surgical removal is only rarely possible; in these circumstances the carcinoma is usually a chance finding in a gland removed for benign enlargement.

Overall 5-year survival – 25 per cent.

Where metastases are obvious at the time of clinical presentation, the 5-year survival figure of treated cases is approximately 20 per cent.

In older age groups (over 70 years) control by hormone therapy can usually be achieved for long periods but, in younger persons, 'escape' from treatment at an earlier stage causes a much poorer prognosis.

Chapter 71
Genito-Urinary System – Testis
and Epididymis

Congenital

CRYPTORCHIDISM
Nature
Site
Incidence
Effects

MISCELLANEOUS

Atrophy
Causes
Macroscopical
Microscopical

Lesions of the tunica vaginalis

HYDROCOELE
Nature
Incidence
Causes
Appearances
Fluid
Effects

HAEMATOCOELE

CHYLOCOELE

OTHER CYSTIC SCROTAL SWELLINGS
Spermatocoele
Varicocoele

Inflammations

NON-SPECIFIC
EPIDIDYMO-ORCHITIS
Origin
Organisms
Macroscopical
Microscopical
Results

GONOCOCCAL
EPIDIDYMO-ORCHITIS

MUMPS ORCHITIS

TUBERCULOUS EPIDIDYMITIS
Origin
Site
Macroscopical
Results

SYPHILITIC ORCHITIS
Site
Appearances
Results

GRANULOMATOUS ORCHITIS

MISCELLANEOUS

Torsion of the testis
Nature
Predisposing
Appearances
Results

Tumours
Incidence
Geographical and racial
Age
Side
Cryptorchidism

SEMINOMA
Incidence
Age
Macroscopical
Microscopical
Spread
Prognosis

TERATOMA
Definition
Incidence
Age
Macroscopical
Microscopical
Spread
Prognosis

COMBINED TUMOUR
Nature
Incidence
Age
Prognosis

OTHER TUMOURS
Interstitial cell
Sertoli cell
Yolk-sac
Malignant lymphoma
Adenomatoid
Others

SECONDARY TUMOURS

Diseases of seminal vesicles

Congenital

CRYPTORCHIDISM – MALDESCENDED OR UNDESCENDED TESTES

Nature
Failure of the testes to descend into the scrotal sac from their embryonic intra-abdominal position.

Site
Unilateral or bilateral. The testes may be found anywhere between the lumbar region of the posterior abdominal wall and the scrotal sac, but are most commonly in the inguinal canal.

Incidence
It is not uncommon for testes to be retracted in young boys, but true cryptorchidism is relatively uncommon.

Effects
1 Atrophy with fibrosis occurs after puberty, accompanied by hyperplasia of the interstitial cells.
2 Sterility when bilateral.
3 There is a high incidence of malignancy in cryptorchid testes, particularly when intra-abdominal in position.

MISCELLANEOUS

These are all uncommon.

ABSENCE OF ONE OR BOTH TESTES

FUSION

Synorchidism.

CYSTS

PATENT PROCESSUS VAGINALIS

With hydrocoele, due to the accumulation of peritoneal fluid in the directly communicating sac.

Atrophy

Causes
1 Increasing age – the male 'menopause'.
2 Following previous orchitis, particularly mumps (see 42).
3 Secondary to gonadotrophin deficiency.
(*a*) Disease of hypothalamus or pituitary.
(*b*) Drugs, e.g oestrogens, cyproterone acetate.
4 Irradiation.
5 Malnutrition and cachexia.
6 Cirrhosis of the liver.
7 Chronic alcoholism or opiate addiction.
8 Congenital – Klinefelter's syndrome (see p. 409).

Macroscopical
Small and firm with dense white fibrous tissue visible on the cut surface. The tubules cannot be 'teased out' as in the normal organ.

Microscopical
Increased interstitial tissue with atrophy and fibrous replacement of the tubules. The effects on the interstitial cells vary according to the cause of the atrophy and the aetiology may also be histologically apparent.

Lesions of the tunica vaginalis

HYDROCOELE

Nature
Accumulation of serous fluid in the tunica vaginalis.

Incidence
Common.

Causes
1 *Congenital*. Patent processus vaginalis.
2 *Infantile*. Incomplete obliteration of the processus vaginalis with development of a hydrocoele in infancy.
3 *Secondary*. Inflammations or neoplasms of the testes.
4 *Trauma*.

Appearances
The sac is single or loculated and has a smooth wall. Later, adhesions occur, together with fibrous thickening of the lining.

Fluid

Viscid, straw-coloured, relative density 1.025, 6 per cent protein. Microscopically, the fluid contains scanty mesothelial cells and lymphocytes.

Effects

1 *Infection*. Fluid may be infected due to extension of inflammation from adjacent structures or complicate aspiration.

2 *Testicular atrophy*. Occurs in longstanding cases due to pressure effects of the fluid.

HAEMATOCOELE

Nature

Presence of blood in the tunica vaginalis.

Incidence

Uncommon.

Causes

1 Trauma.
2 Torsion of the testis.
3 Haemorrhagic diatheses.
4 Tumours extending through the tunica albuginea.
5 Due to haemorrhage into a pre-existing hydrocoele.

Appearances

Distension of the sac by blood and blood clot with a thick fibrinous lining, later becoming organized to a fibrous wall.

CHYLOCOELE

Accumulation of lymph in the tunica, due to lymphatic obstruction, e.g. in elephantiasis.

OTHER CYSTIC SWELLINGS IN THE SCROTUM

SPERMATOCOELE

Cystic accumulation of semen in the spermatic cord due to dilatation of the ducts in the head of the epididymis.

VARICOCOELE

A cystic varix of the veins of the pampiniform plexus in the spermatic cord.

Inflammations

NON-SPECIFIC EPIDIDYMO-ORCHITIS

Origin

Most cases are related to infections elsewhere in the urinary tract, e.g. cystitis, prostatitis, urethritis. Organisms reach the epididymis and thence the testes via the vas deferens or spermatic cord lymphatics. Rarely, the infection may be haematogenous.

Organisms

Coliforms, streptococci, staphylococci are the most common.

Macroscopical

The epididymis is involved firstly with subsequent extension to the testis. Both epididymis and testis become swollen and congested with markedly increased tension of the tunica albuginea. The infection may progress to abscess formation or suppurative necrosis of the entire epididymis with involvement of the scrotal skin and sinus formation.

Microscopical

Acute inflammation, initially involving the interstitial tissue and later the epithelium of the tubules, with desquamation and destruction.

Results

1 Resolution – usually with some scarring.
2 Suppuration – uncommon.
3 Chronic infection – leading to fibrosis and atrophy.
4 Sterility – due to
(*a*) pressure atrophy,
(*b*) blockage of excretory ducts by fibrosis.

GONOCOCCAL EPIDIDYMO-ORCHITIS

The gonococci usually spread along the lumen of the vas from the posterior urethra via the prostate and seminal vesicles to the epididymis. It usually results in extensive destruction and in neglected cases proceeds to suppurative orchitis (see p. 399).

MUMPS ORCHITIS

Incidence
Twenty to twenty-five per cent of cases of mumps in adults develop orchitis about 7 days following the swelling of the salivary glands (see p. 42).

Appearances
Intense interstitial oedema with a patchy infiltration of lymphocytes and plasma cells. Occasionally suppuration may occur but more commonly the infection subsides with fibrosis. In severe cases, atrophy of the germinal epithelium follows which, when bilateral, may result in sterility.

TUBERCULOUS EPIDIDYMITIS

Origin
Nearly always secondary to tuberculosis of the kidneys or lungs.

When the primary disease is in the lungs there is a presumed haematogenous spread, whereas when renal in origin, a direct extension via the natural passages seems more likely. It is probable that in virtually every case of tuberculous epididymitis there is a renal focus although this may not always be clinically apparent.

Site
Epididymis; the testes are only involved in the later stages by direct extension to areas adjacent to the epididymis.

Macroscopical
Thickening of the epididymis leading to the formation of caseous masses which may replace the whole organ.

Results
1 Healing with fibrosis and often with calcification.
2 Secondary hydrocoele.
3 Skin involvement with sinus formation in the scrotum.
4 Extension into the testes.

SYPHILITIC ORCHITIS

Site
The testes are affected in both congenital and acquired syphilis. The epididymis is only rarely involved, usually at a late stage.

Appearances
1 *Gumma*. Nodular, painless enlargement of the testis with dense fibrosis surrounding foci of yellow-white structured necrosis.
2 *Diffuse*. Interstitial inflammation with endarteritis obliterans and perivascular cuffing by plasma cells and lymphocytes. This causes diffuse indurated swelling of the organ.

Results
Progressive fibrosis leading to atrophy and sterility. Interstitial cells are at first spared, but later may be destroyed with resulting loss of libido and secondary sex characteristics.

GRANULOMATOUS ORCHITIS

This uncommon condition causes firm swelling of the testis simulating a tumour. The organ is a pale homogeneous appearance on section and histologically shows loss of seminiferous tubules and replacement by granulomatous inflammation which may bear a superficial resemblance to tuberculosis. Of somewhat similar nature is *sperm granuloma of the epididymis* which may involve the testis. One or more firm nodules are present. Both conditions are probably unusual reactions to infection by non-specific organisms. In sperm granuloma, an immunological reaction to spermatozoa which have escaped from tubules is the aetiological factor but a similar mechanism has not been shown in granulomatous orchitis.

MISCELLANEOUS

The testes may be involved by haematogenous dissemination of many infective diseases, e.g. leprosy, typhoid, brucellosis and fungal diseases.

Torsion of the testis

Nature
Vascular disturbances due to twisting of the spermatic cord.

Predisposing factors

1 Violent movement or trauma.
2 Abnormalities of situation or of attachment of the epididymis, a long spermatic cord or abnormal mobility associated with testicular atrophy.

Appearances

Usually the venous drainage is impaired without arterial occlusion. Intense haemorrhagic engorgement and venous infarction rapidly follows the rotation. In a fairly longstanding example, the testis is markedly enlarged and converted by necrosis into a sac of soft, haemorrhagic, structureless material.

Results

Unless the twist can be reduced almost immediately, infarction occurs and destruction of the testis will lead to complete loss of function. The other testis commonly suffers the same fate at a subsequent date, unless anchored, if similar anatomical predisposing abnormalities are present.

Tumours

Differing, competing classifications of testicular tumours are numerous but, in recent years, the U.K. Testicular Tumour Panel and WHO classifications have become widely accepted.

Incidence

Rare: 0.5 per cent of male cancer deaths, 1–2 per cent of cases of male malignancy.

Geographical and racial

Testicular tumours are more common in white races than coloured even within the same geographical areas. Denmark has a particularly high incidence with a very high rate in Copenhagen and a much lower figure for rural areas.

Age

Age incidence is bimodal with peaks at 20–40 years and in the elderly.

Side

Right:Left 5:4. Bilateral in 3 per cent, mostly lymphoma.

Cryptorchidism

The risk of a cryptorchid developing a testicular tumour is 35 times greater than in a person with normally descended testes. Most tumours arising in maldescended testes are seminomas.

SEMINOMA

Incidence

Forty per cent of testicular tumours.

Age

Range 7–87 years; mean 41 years. Eighty per cent are under 50 years.

Macroscopical

The testis is enlarged, usually symmetrically, and replaced to a variable extent by homogeneous, firm, pale, pinkish-grey tumour. The tumour is usually well demarcated and invasion of the tunica albuginea is very rare. Foci of necrosis may be seen but haemorrhagic areas are rare.

Microscopical

This carcinoma of seminiferous epithelium is very uniform with rounded or polygonal cells, vacuolated glycogen-rich cytoplasm and small central nuclei. Fibrous septa divide the sheets and columns of cells into lobules but tubule formation is not seen. There is a variable lymphocytic infiltrate. Tumour giant cells are present in about 5 per cent. A distinctive sub-type is the *spermatocytic seminoma* seen in about 3–4 per cent, and more frequently found in the older age groups. Tumour cells are in sheets and not columns with darker non-vacuolated cytoplasm. Cells are very variable in size, mitoses are numerous and giant cells with 3–4 large nuclei usually present.

Spread

1 *Direct*. Common to the epididymis and spermatic cord but rare through the tunica.
2 *Lymphatic*. Para-aortic lymph node invasion is seen in most fatal cases.
3 *Blood*. Usually a later manifestation with metastases in the lungs and liver.

Prognosis

Standard treatment is orchidectomy and post-operative radiation to the para-aortic lymph nodes. As most patients who die from the disease do so in the first 3 years after orchidectomy, the 3-year corrected survival rate is acceptable and is 85–90 per cent. Good prognostic factors are:

(a) Absence of evidence of metastases at time of presentation 93 per cent, c.f. 55 per cent with metastases.

(b) Confinement of tumour to testis – 93 per cent, c.f. 80 per cent when upper cord invaded.

(c) Considerable lymphocytic infiltration – 95 per cent, c.f. 72 per cent with no lymphocytes.

(d) Absence of tumour giant cells.

(e) Spermatocytic type – fatalities from the tumour have not been recorded.

TERATOMA

Definition
A testicular tumour composed of multiple tissues foreign to the normal organ and showing variable degrees of cell differentiation. It is probable that teratomas arise from germ cells.

Incidence
Thirty-two per cent of all testicular tumours. The incidence is rising in many countries.

Age
Range 3 months–75 years, mean 30 years: 48 per cent occur in the 20–29 decade.

Macroscopical
Variable degrees of enlargement of the testis occur, sometimes very slight and often asymmetrical with a nodular surface. On section the tumour is, usually, part solid, part cystic and haemorrhagic: necrotic and yellowish foci are commonly found. The tunica is rarely penetrated.

Microscopical
There is an extremely wide range of appearances on which basic types are identified.

1 *Teratoma differentiated* (T.D). *Teratoma mature* (WHO). This comprises only fully differentiated or organoid structures.

2 *Malignant teratoma intermediate* (M.T.I.) Containing both differentiated and obviously malignant areas. The presence of any differentiated structures at all, however scanty, places tumours in this group rather than in 3 below.

3 *Embryonal carcinoma* (WHO). *Malignant teratoma undifferentiated* (M.T.U.) Complete absence of organoid or differentiated tissues with a generally carcinomatous appearance often dominated by adenocarcinoma.

4 *Malignant teratoma trophoblastic* (M.T.T.) Syncytiotrophoblast, cytotrophoblast and a papillary arrangement must be identifiable.

Spread
Blood spread, to lungs and liver particularly, is more commonly seen in teratoma than with seminoma. Para-aortic lymph node invasion is less common.

Prognosis
Orchidectomy and post-operative irradiation to the para-aortic region are standard treatments.

The 3-year corrected survival rate (C.S.R.) overall is 47 per cent; only a few die subsequently from this disease.

	3-year C.S.R.	
T.D.		92 per cent
M.T.I.		52 per cent
M.T.U.		38 per cent
M.T.T.		19 per cent

The prognosis is bad in all those who have demonstrable HCG in tumour cells.

COMBINED TUMOUR

Nature
Tumours with both teratomatous and seminomatous components. The tumours may be separate or intermingled. The teratomatous element is subdivided as above.

Incidence
M.T.I. + S 50 per cent
M.T.U. + S 40 per cent
T.D. + S }
M.T.T. + S } 10 per cent

Age
Range 17–76 years. Mean age 35 years.

Prognosis

	3YR C.S.R.	
T.D. + S		100 per cent
M.T.I. + S		67 per cent
M.T.U. + S		40 per cent
M.T.T. + S		15 per cent

i.e. much better than teratoma alone, particularly for M.T.I. + S.

OTHER TUMOURS

INTERSTITIAL CELL TUMOUR – LEYDIG CELL

Usually small circumscribed brown tumour in the testicular substance, forming about 2 per cent of testicular tumours. Mostly present in age range 20–60 years, but occasionally in childhood when they may cause precocious puberty. In adults gynaecomastia may be the presenting feature. The histological appearances are very typical with rounded or slightly elongated eosinophilic granular cells containing lipid and lipofuschin. The cells are usually in sheets. Less than 10 per cent behave in a malignant manner.

SERTOLI CELL TUMOUR – ANDROBLASTOMA

Tubule-forming tumours of cells resembling Sertoli cells form 1 per cent of testicular tumours. Variable amounts of mesenchymal stroma are also present. Approximately 20 per cent behave in a malignant manner.

YOLK-SAC TUMOUR – ORCHIOBLASTOMA – ENDODERMAL SINUS TUMOUR

A tubular or papillary mucus-secreting germ cell adenocarcinoma of infancy and childhood forming 2 per cent of testicular tumours and of similar appearance to tumours occasionally found in ovary, mediastinum and pineal gland (see p. 439); α-fetoprotein is commonly demonstrated in tumour cells and serum. The 3-year corrected survival rate is 64 per cent.

MALIGNANT LYMPHOMA OF TESTIS

Although it is not uncommon for malignant lymphomas presenting elsewhere in the body to involve the testes at a late stage of disseminated disease, some 6–7 per cent of testicular tumours are malignant lymphomas presenting in this site. It is thus accepted as a primary testicular tumour. They have a peak age incidence between 60 and 80 years but a range of 1–90 years. Synchronous or successive bilateral involvement occurs in 20 per cent. The tumour is usually large, creamy, homogeneous and ill-defined. Histologically, the lymphoma is of non-Hodgkin's lymphocytic type often poorly differentiated (see p. 582).

The prognosis is poor with 60 per cent dead in 2 years and only occasional long-term survivors.

ADENOMATOID TUMOUR

A benign tumour of Müllerian vestige origin composed of irregular clefts and spaces lined by flattened cuboidal cells in a fibro-muscular stoma. In the male the tumour, which is always benign, is predominantly epididymal rather than testicular. The same tumour occurs in females along the course of the Müllerian duct remnants, most commonly in the fallopian tube.

OTHER TUMOURS

Benign and malignant connective tissue tumours are rare, the most common being rhabdomyosarcoma and embryonal sarcoma. Mesothelioma of the tunica vaginalis is a further rare tumour.

SECONDARY TUMOURS

Secondary tumours in the testes are uncommon and are mostly deposits of leukaemia or lymphoma. However, presentation of primary tumours of other organs as testicular metastatic swellings does occur and may create diagnostic problems.

Diseases of the seminal vesicles

With the exception of inflammations, diseases of the seminal vesicles are rare. Infections of nonspecific, gonococcal or tuberculous aetiology, usually reach the organ by spread from the posterior urethra. When infection occurs in this anatomically folded and diverticular structure, it is usually very chronic.

Chapter 72
Genito-Urinary System – Penis: Scrotum: Hermaphroditism

Penis

CONGENITAL

Malformations of urethral canal
Hypospadias
Epispadias
Effects

Phimosis
Nature
Origin
Effects

Other congenital lesions

INFLAMMATIONS

Balanoposthitis

Syphilis – primary chancre

Chancroid (soft sore)
Organism
Geographical
Transmission
Site
Appearances
Course

Granuloma inguinale
Organism
Geographical
Transmission
Appearances
Diagnosis
Course

Lymphogranuloma venereum
Nature
Site
Geographical
Stages
Appearances
　Genital lesions
　Lymph nodes
Microscopical
Course
Diagnosis

'PRE-MALIGNANT' CONDITIONS
Nature

Leukoplakia

Erythroplasia of Queyrat

Bowen's disease

CARCINOMA
Incidence
Age
Aetiological factors
Macroscopical
Microscopical
Spread
Results

Scrotum
General

Carcinoma
Incidence
Age
Aetiological factors
Macroscopical
Microscopical
Spread
Results

Hermaphroditism and intersex

DEFINITIONS

Sex of the individual
　Genetic sex
　Gonadal sex
　Phenotypic sex
　Sex of upbringing
　Behavioural sex

Hermaphroditism
　True hermaphroditism
　Male pseudohermaphro-
　　ditism
　Female pseudohermaphro-
　　ditism

NORMAL SEXUAL DEVELOPMENT

ABNORMALITIES OF SEXUAL
DEVELOPMENT

Abnormalities of genetic sex
Turner's syndrome
Klinefelter's syndrome
True hermaphroditism
XYY syndrome

Abnormalities of phenotypic sex
Male pseudohermaphroditism
Other abnormalities
Female
　pseudohermaphroditism

Penis

CONGENITAL

MALFORMATIONS OF THE URETHRAL GROOVE AND CANAL

HYPOSPADIAS

The urethra opens on to the ventral surface of the penis.

EPISPADIAS

The urethra opens on to the dorsal surface of the penis.

Both are commonly associated with maldescent of the testes or other more severe congenital anomalies.

Effects
1 *Infection.* Particularly near the base of the penis.
2 *Sterility.*
3 *Obstruction.* When the orifice becomes stenosed.

PHIMOSIS

Nature
The orifice of the prepuce is too small to permit its retraction.

Origin
May be congenital, or acquired following inflammatory scarring.

Effects
1 Prevents the cleansing of the glans with accumulation of secretions in the prepuce; this predisposes to infection.
2 Forcible retraction of a phimotic prepuce over the glans penis may result in constriction and swelling so that it cannot be replaced – *paraphimosis.* This may cause urethral obstruction and urinary retention.

OTHER CONGENITAL LESIONS

Rare lesions include absence, hypoplasia, hyperplasia and duplication.

INFLAMMATIONS

BALANOPOSTHITIS

Nature
Non-specific inflammation of glans and prepuce.

Organisms
Staphylococci, streptococci, coliforms, gonococci, candid and chlamydia.

Aetiological factors
Usually associated with phimosis or a large redundant prepuce, venereal infection and coital trauma.

Appearances
Marked congestion and oedema with exudate on the surface of the glans. If neglected, ulceration occurs and if persistent and chronic, scarring occurs with aggravation of the underlying condition.

Diagnosis
Gonococci can be readily distinguished by examination of smears; other organisms can be identified by culture.

SYPHILIS – PRIMARY CHANCRE

This is by far the commonest site for a chancre in the male, particularly the glans and the inner side of the prepuce, but occasionally on the shaft.

Appearances
Begins as a solitary, slightly elevated, firm papule. Later there is superficial ulceration to form a shallow, clean-based depression, with extensive surrounding induration and inguinal lymphadenopathy.

Course
Healing with re-epithelialization in about 2 months occurs spontaneously, or more rapidly with treatment; slight scarring usually remains.

CHANCROID – SOFT SORE

Organism
Haemophilus ducreyi

Geographical distribution
Particularly common in the Orient, West Indies

and North Africa. Uncommon in Europe and North America.

Transmission
By sexual intercourse, inoculation occurring through abrasions of the surface.

Site
Usually the glans.

Appearances
A macule becomes a papule and thence a pustule which ulcerates. The ulcer is at first shallow and up to 1 cm in diameter but later deepens with necrotic purulent slough in the base and enlarges to 2–3 cm in diameter. It is soft with little or no surrounding induration. Inguinal lymphadenopathy usually follows in 1–2 weeks, is markedly painful and suppurates with discharge on the skin surface – '*bubo*'.

Course
Spontaneous or therapeutic healing with residual scarring, usually within 1 month.

GRANULOMA INGUINALE

Organism
Donovania granulomatis
An encapsulated cocco-bacillary organism found in the lesions within mononuclear cells – *Donovan bodies*.

Geographical distribution
World-wide but uncommon.

Transmission
Believed to be venereal, but infectivity and invasiveness of the organism are low. The incubation period varies from 3 days to several months.

Appearances
A papule may appear anywhere in the perineal or peri-anal regions or on the penis. The papule ulcerates and spreads, with a necrotic centre and raised red and exuberant inflammatory margins. Satellite lesions may occur along involved lymphatics. It is usually relatively painless but inguinal lymphadenopathy with suppurative necrosis occurs, leading to sinus formation. Extensive fibrosis occurs in this very chronic condition.

Diagnosis
Smears or tissue biopsies show the large vacuolated macrophages containing the Gram-negative Donovan bodies.

Course
Very chronic, with extensive local destruction and distortion of the affected site.

LYMPHOGRANULOMA VENEREUM – LYMPHOGRANULOMA INGUINALE – LYMPHOPATHIA VENEREUM

Nature
A venereal disease caused by a chlamydial organism.

Site
Glans, prepuce, urethra or perineal skin.

Geographical distribution
World-wide but uncommon.

Stages
1 *Invasive*. Usually a few days after inoculation.
2 *Genital or ano-rectal lesion*. The primary lesion at the site of inoculation is usually small, transient and inapparent.
3 *Lymphadenopathy*. One to two weeks later.
4 *Late complications*. Elephantiasis, or rectal stricture in females, may develop at a later date due to lymphatic obstruction (see p. 278).

Appearances
1 *Genital lesion*. A small vesicle ruptures to form a shallow ulcer which rapidly heals.
2 *Lymph nodes*. Progressive painful swelling. These nodes are at first discrete, but later coalesce, with necrosis and sinus formation on to the skin surface.

Microscopical
Characteristic granulomatous lesions of central, irregular, stellate abscesses containing polymorphs and ringed by radially arranged fibroblasts, epithelioid cells and histiocytes. Occasional giant cells of Langhans' type may be present. There is a surrounding zone of plasma cells and lymphocytes.

Course
Chronic, varying from weeks to months. Healing

with fibrosis occurs, producing distortion and lymphatic blockage which may lead to elephantiasis of the external genitalia or, when the pararectal lymph nodes are involved, rectal stricture.

In females, the primary lesion is frequently in the cervix and escapes notice. It is followed by pelvic lymph node inflammation and when healing occurs, the scarring commonly produces rectal stricture or *esthiomene* (see p. 424).

Diagnosis
1   *Frei test*. Intradermal inoculation of material from an infected case. This test is not entirely specific.
2   *Complement fixation test*. Specific for the disease.

PREMALIGNANT CONDITIONS

Nature
A group of dysplastic epithelial changes which occur on the penis and are of potential importance in the development of carcinoma.

LEUKOPLAKIA

Similar to the condition in other regions (see p. 171). Plaques of pearly-white mucosal thickening occur, associated with chronic irritation. There is hyperkeratosis, atypical squamous downgrowths, epithelial dysplasia and fibrosis, with chronic inflammatory cell infiltration in the subepithelial tissues.

ERYTHROPLASIA OF QUEYRAT

Single or multiple, flat, red crusting patches of the prepuce or the glans. There is marked keratosis, dysplasia and gross epidermal thickening and atypicality. The microscopic appearances are similar to 'carcinoma *in situ*' in other sites and must be regarded as established, but not yet invasive, carcinoma.

BOWEN'S DISEASE

Although distinguished from the above clinically, the histological changes are essentially similar.

CARCINOMA

Incidence
Infrequent, causing 0.5–1 per cent of cancer deaths in males in Europe and America. It is, however, more common in India and other Eastern countries where it causes as many as 10 per cent of male cancer deaths.

Age
Fifty to seventy years of age.

Aetiological Factors
1   *Circumcision*. Carcinoma of the penis is virtually unknown in Jews and very rare in Mohammedans; both are ritually circumcised. There is a high incidence in Hindus who are never circumcised. This is probably associated with chronic irritation due to retained smegma.
2   *Pre-malignant conditions*. As described above, these dysplastic lesions commonly proceed to invasive carcinoma.

Macroscopical
1   *Papillary*. Single or multiple papillary growths on the glans.
2   *Ulcerative*. Ulcerating, infiltrating tumours on the outer aspect of the glans or the inner side of the prepuce with leukoplakia commonly visible at the periphery. This is the more common type.

Microscopical
Squamous cell carcinomas; mostly well differentiated.

Spread
1   *Direct*. Proximal spread along the shaft with destruction, distortion and commonly urinary fistula formation.
2   *Lymphatic*. Thirty per cent of cases have inguinal lymph node metastases when first seen.
3   *Blood*. Rare and late.

Results
Surgical amputation, with block dissection of the groins if indicated, results in a 5-year survival of 50–70 per cent.

Scrotum

General
Disease in the scrotum is most commonly the result

of secondary involvement by diseases of the testes or epididymis. Skin lesions occur on the scrotum as in other sites of the body, but carcinoma, although of typical appearance, is of aetiological and historical interest (Pott).

CARCINOMA

Incidence
Rare; forming less than 0.25 per cent of male cancer deaths. It virtually occurs only in industrialized communities.

Age
Maximum 50–70 years.

Aetiological factors;
1 *Occupational.* Exposure to a variety of petroleum and coal tar derivatives. The tumours used to be very common in chimney sweeps at the time when the sweeper went up the chimney in addition to his brush and thus his clothing and skin became impregnated with coal tar derivatives in the soot – *'chimney sweep's cancer'.*
2 *Hygienic.* The carcinoma is also commonly associated with a low standard of personal hygiene.

Macroscopical
Single or multiple irregular ulcers with raised rolled edges; occasionally the tumour is in the form of low warty plaques.

Microscopical
Well-differentiated squamous cell carcinomas.

Spread
Slow direct extension may involve the testes. Inguinal lymph nodes are invaded in 20 per cent of cases, but blood spread is extremely rare.

Results
In the absence of extension to the testes, results following operative removal are good. When the testes are invaded, spread to abdominal lymph nodes may occur and the prognosis is then poor.

Hermaphroditism and intersex

DEFINITIONS

SEX OF THE INDIVIDUAL

The sex of the individual depends upon the context in which the term is applied. It may mean:
1 *Genetic sex.* The presence of a Y chromosome normally implies masculinity.
2 *Gonadal sex.* Presence of either ovaries or testes.
3 *Phenotypic sex.* Dependent upon the appearance of the external genitalia.
4 *Sex of upbringing.* Usually dependent upon phenotypic sex.
5 *Behavioural sex.* Although usually determined by sex of upbringing exceptions are common:
(*a*) Transvestism, homosexuality – for which there is no known physiological basis.
(*b*) In some cases of androgen resistance, genotypic males reared as females appear to develop an unequivocal masculine outlook by the time of puberty.

HERMAPHRODITISM

True hermaphroditism. The occurrence of both ovarian and testicular tissue in the same individual. This is presumed to be the result of a genetic mosaic, although sometimes only one genetic type is demonstrable.

Male pseudohermaphroditism. A genotypic male, with testes, who has ambiguous or female external genitalia and body habitus.

Female pseudohermaphroditism. A genotypic female, with ovaries, fallopian tubes and uterus, with varying degrees of masculinization of the external genitalia, and of body habitus.

NORMAL SEXUAL DEVELOPMENT

1 Genetic sex is determined at the time of fertilization when, normally, an ovum containing one X chromosome is fertilized by a spermatozoon containing either one X (female infant) or one Y (male infant) chromosome.
2 As a result of the genetic sex of the individual the primitive gonad differentiates in the eighth to tenth week of intra-uterine life. The primitive testis causes unilateral regression of the Müllerian system

by the release of a non-hormonal, unidentified factor – Müllerian inhibitory factor.

3 Testicular androgens. In males testosterone stimulates the development of the Wolffian system: epididymis, vas, seminal vesicles and dihydrosterone leads to the development of the external genitalia. In the absence of androgens, or in syndromes of androgen resistance, the Wolffian system does not develop, or develops only partially, and the phenotypic sex is female.

ABNORMALITIES OF SEXUAL DEVELOPMENT

ABNORMALITIES OF GENETIC SEX

May arise at the time of fertilization, or from subsequent aberrant meiosis (see p. 9).

1 *Turner's syndrome (XO) – gonadal dysgenesis.* Absence of the second sex chromosome leads to failure of gonadal development ('streak ovaries') and the individual is phenotypically female (see p. 14). Because of the absence of gonadal Müllerian inhibitory factor and of androgens, the Müllerian system is preserved, while the Wolffian system does not develop. There are associated abnormalities in other systems: small stature, shield-shaped chest, web neck, cubitus valgus and predisposition to abnormalities of the cardiovascular system, especially coarctation of the aorta. There are several variants of Turner's syndrome.

2 *Klinefelter's syndrome (XXY).* The presence of a Y chromosome leads to testicular development, Wolffian duct stimulation and Müllerian duct regression. The patient has unambiguous external genitalia and is reared as a male (see p. 14). The testis, however, is not capable of full maturation and remains small. Failure of the seminiferous tubules to develop normally leads to infertility, while variable failure of the interstitial cells leads to under-androgenization: eunuchoid habitus (failure of epiphyseal fusion), obesity, gynaecomastia, female distribution of body hair. Some patients are well-virilized and of normal habitus and the presenting symptom may be infertility. In these cases the only clinical abnormality is the presence of rather small testes.

3 *True hermaphroditism (XX/XY, and variants).* The presence of a mixed population of cells with different chromosomal content may lead to the development of both ovary and testis, or of combined ovo-testis, with consequently ambiguous development of internal and external genitalia.

4 *XYY syndrome.* These patients are phenotypically male, but are distinguishable, as a group, by a tendency to tall stature, and to reduced intelligence combined with antisocial behaviour.

ABNORMALITIES OF PHENOTYPIC SEX

1 *Male pseudohermaphroditism.* The subject is genetically male but phenotypically female. The gonads are testes and despite the presence of androgens in the plasma, target organs do not respond – syndromes of *androgen resistance* or *testicular feminization.* There are several different types with differing degrees of under-androgenization. The patient may be phenotypically female, although with absent body hair, and with only a short, blind vagina if the resistance is complete, or may be partially virilized with ambiguous external genitalia. In all cases, however, the presence of a testis leads to regression of the Müllerian system: uterus and fallopian tubes are absent.

2 *Other abnormalities of development of male external genitalia.* Micropenis, hypospadias. Most cases have no determined cause.

3 *Female pseudohermaphroditism.* A genotypic female with female internal genitalia who has varying virilization of external genitalia and of the rest of the body.

a Congenital adrenal hyperplasia.

b Administration of virilizing compounds to the mother during pregnancy, e.g. some progestogens.

Although the polycystic ovary syndrome and other endocrine diseases of later life cause varying degrees of virilization and may be accompanied by clitoromegaly, there is never any ambiguity over the sex of the patient and these conditions should not be referred to as intersexes.

Chapter 73
Genito-Urinary System – Uterus: Endometrium: Myometrium

NORMAL DEVELOPMENT

The uterus, cervix and vagina are formed by fusion of the paired Müllerian ducts. The Fallopian tubes arise from the unfused upper portions of these ducts.

CONGENITAL ABNORMALITIES

The common congenital abnormalities result from anomalies of fusion of the Müllerian ducts (see Fig. 41).

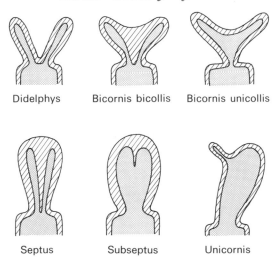

Didelphys   Bicornis bicollis   Bicornis unicollis

Septus   Subseptus   Unicornis

Fig. 41. Congenital abnormalities of the uterus.

If one Müllerian duct fails to develop the uterus is *unicornis*.

The uterus is only rarely totally absent; a lesser degree of developmental failure produces an hypoplastic organ. Canalization may be incomplete and may result in atresia in any part of the tract, usually in the cervical canal.

NORMAL MENSTRUAL CYCLE

A menstrual cycle is timed from the commencement of one period of menstrual loss to the commencement of the next and averages 28 days. Individual variations from 24 to 30 days are not uncommon, but if outside this range are usually regarded as abnormal.

In a 28-day cycle the changes, illustrated in Fig. 42 are as follows.

Menstruation
Lasts for 3–6 days.

Follicular phase
The follicle is maturing within the ovary and this phase is associated with oestrogen production.
(*a*) *Resting phase*. Following menstruation only the basal endometrial layers remain.
(*b*) *Proliferative phase*. This lasts until ovulation at the fourteenth day. Proliferative activity occurs in both endometrial tubules and stroma result-ing in progressive thickening of the endometrium by simple, straight, regular, endometrial tubular glands in a cellular stroma.

Ovulation
The follicle ruptures on the fourteenth day.

Luteal phase
Immediately following ovulation, the ruptured follicle develops into a corpus luteum and there is associated production of progesterone.

(*a*) *Early secretory phase*. This lasts for 2–3 days (fourteenth to seventeenth day) immediately following ovulation. There is subnuclear vacuolation of the epithelial cell cytoplasm with progressive displacement of nuclei towards the lumen. The glands become less straight.

(*b*) *Mid-secretory phase*. In the next 7–9 days (seventeenth to twenty-sixth day) the endometrium continues to increase in depth with increasing tortuosity of the glands. The nuclei resume their basal position and the luminal border becomes less well defined with intraluminal secretion. The stromal cells become plumper and less active.

(*c*) *Pre-menstrual phase*. In the 2–3 days preceding menstruation (twenty-sixth to twenty-eighth day) characteristic changes occur in the stromal cells which become plump – *decidual cells*. The glands are complex and very tortuous with a 'saw tooth' appearance and are filled with secreted material. As menstruation approaches, there is a polymorph infiltration and haemorrhages into the stroma of the superficial layers.

(*d*) *Menstruation*. Twenty-eighth day. All but the basal layers of the endometrium are shed.

PREGNANCY

If the ovum is fertilized, the corpus luteum persists and secretes progesterone. The secretory changes are therefore continued in the tubules and the decidual cells of the stroma persist, becoming the decidua of pregnancy.

ABNORMALITIES OF THE MENSTRUAL CYCLE

Abnormalities of menstrual bleeding are extremely common. The following features may be seen on histological examination of currettings.

Chapter 73

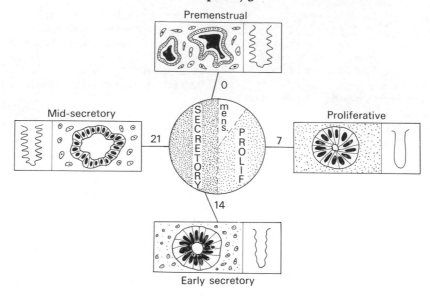

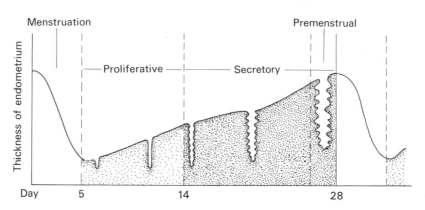

Fig. 42. Endometrial changes in the menstrual cycle.

Anovulatory cycle

Menstruation can occur without ovulation; thus there are no secretory changes and the endometrium remains proliferative throughout the cycle.

Delayed secretion

Ovulation may be delayed and thus the changes of early secretory endometrium do not appear until later in the cycle than normal. The cycle usually remains of normal length so that the time available for conception is shortened and infertility may result.

Reduced or absent proliferation

Endocrinological and other abnormalities may result in insufficient oestrogen production and the proliferative changes are reduced in degree or are absent. The result is oligomenorrhoea or amenorrhoea.

Excessive proliferation

Hyperplastic proliferative changes with a shortened or absent secretory phase are manifestations of oestrogen excess and are commonly found where there is hormonal imbalance, especially near the menopause. Similar changes are also induced by oestrogen therapy.

Effects of hormone therapy

In recent years, oral therapy with oestrogens and progestogens, alone or in combination, has rapidly increased. This is particularly so in respect of administration of oral contraceptives. Administration of these preparations causes marked changes in samples of endometrium removed by curettage and ignorance of the therapy may lead to difficulties in interpretation.

The commonest histological appearance is that associated with contraceptive pills where the endometrium is scanty, with gross reduction in the tubules which are inactive and non-secretory whereas the stroma is rather oedematous and may show a pseudo-decidual reaction.

Oestrogen therapy produces non-secretory hyperplasia similar to metropathia (see below) and progestogens give rise to secretory hyperplasia and decidual reaction in the stroma which may sometimes mimic the decidual reaction of pregnancy.

CYSTIC HYPERPLASIA – METROPATHIA HAEMORRHAGICA

Nature

An hyperplastic condition of the endometrium resulting from excessive oestrogen secretion of the ovaries and causing menorrhagia. The condition may occur at any time during the reproductive period but is most commonly seen at about the time of the menopause.

Macroscopical

The endometrium is thickened, vascular and polypoid; curettings are haemorrhagic and bulky.

Microscopical

The endometrium shows an hyperplastic, vascular, non-secretory appearance, the hyperplasia being prominent in both the tubules and the stroma. In addition, the tubules vary in size sometimes with areas of cystic dilatation – *cystic hyperplasia*. Atypical foci may be present which can cause difficulty in interpretation from well differentiated endometrial carcinoma.

Ovaries

The ovaries contain follicular cysts and corpora

lutea do not form; thus, the endometrium remains under the influence of oestrogens.

Results

1 Menorrhagia may result in anaemia of severe degree.
2 Irregularity of the menstrual cycle.
3 Sterility.
4 The condition shows a definite predisposition for subsequent development of endometrial carcinoma.

Inflammations

PUERPERAL SEPSIS

Nature

Puerperal sepsis is one cause of puerperal fever, which is defined as any febrile condition occurring within 21 days after childbirth or miscarriage in which a temperature of 38°C (100.4°F) or more is sustained for 24 hours. Infection of the genital tract following delivery or abortion is now an uncommon disease in its florid form, but less severe cases are still frequently encountered.

Organisms

Any pathogenic bacterium but most frequently β-haemolytic and anaerobic streptococci, clostridia, staphylococci, coliforms and *P. pyocyaneus*.

Sources of infection

1 Medical or nursing attendants.
2 Hands or instruments.
3 Skin of the perineum or from the vagina.
4 Auto-infection from the skin, mouth, respiratory tract.

Predisposing factors

1 Prolonged labour with laceration, trauma and bruising of tissues.
2 Retained placenta requiring manual removal.
3 Residual products of conception.
4 Instrumentation.

Site of entry

From the raw surface of the placental site or the lacerated cervix.

Macroscopical

The uterus is large and soft and the endometrium is

covered by a ragged slough bathed in foul smelling lochia, which may become frankly purulent.

Microscopical
Acute suppurative inflammation of the endometrium with extensive necrosis.

Spread
1 *Extension to myometrium.* Myometritis.
2 *Through the myometrium.* Pelvic peritonitis.
3 *Lymphatic.* Pelvic cellulitis.
4 *Fallopian tubes.* Acute salpingitis, and through the ostia – peritonitis.
5 *Uterine veins.* Septic thrombophlebitis which may produce septic emboli, septic infarcts and abscesses in the lungs, brain, etc.
6 *Blood.* Septicaemia or pyaemia.

Results
Early therapy with the appropriate antibiotic usually leads to resolution of the endometritis before spread had occurred and there are no significant sequelae as the endometrium regenerates from residual islands. In neglected cases, particularly those associated with induced abortion and infections with clostridia, death may occur from septicaemia and toxaemia.

ACUTE ENDOMETRITIS

The commonest cause of acute suppurative endometritis is puerperal sepsis. Acute gonococcal endometritis may occur but is usually overshadowed by the changes in the cervix, urethra and Fallopian tubes (see p. 426). Other causes include infection proximal to obstructive lesions of the cervical canal; the *pyometra* which results commonly accompanies carcinomas of the cervix or the body of the uterus. In all cases of suspected acute endometritis the histological finding of polymorphs in the endometrium is not by itself sufficient to substantiate the diagnosis since these cells are a normal feature of endometrium in the pre-menstrual phase.

CHRONIC ENDOMETRITIS

This is a very rare and doubtful entity. Chronic inflammation only rarely becomes established in the endometrium as this is shed each month. There is, however, a condition in which the endometrium shows infiltration by lymphocytes and plasma cells associated with an enlarged fibrotic uterus. This is probably an endocrine disturbance and is more accurately described as subinvolution of the uterus or alternatively fibrosis uteri.

A mild inflammatory reaction may be seen in patients with intra-uterine contraceptive devices.

TUBERCULOUS ENDOMETRITIS

Origin
Occurs secondarily to tuberculosis of the Fallopian tubes (see p. 426).

As with tuberculosis elsewhere it has become a less important disease and is now an uncommon cause of infertility.

Macroscopical
The endometrial cavity in advanced cases is lined by thickened, irregular, pale granulation tissue. In less severe cases, the endometrium appears grossly normal.

Microscopical
The endometrium is often non-secretory and contains typical tubercles if the sample is taken in the pre-menstrual phase. When the menstrual cycle continues these are incompletely formed as there is insufficient time for caseation to occur; Z.N. staining, or preferably culture of curettings, is necessary to confirm the diagnosis.

Results
Active tuberculosis is commonly associated with amenorrhoea. Even if the menstrual cycle continues, the patient is sterile, but following treatment a few cases may subsequently conceive, although this is dependent also on the fate of the tuberculous salpingitis and ectopic gestation is quite a common sequel.

Adenomyosis uteri

Nature
Endometrium which penetrates deeply into the uterine wall. The cause of this downgrowth remains obscure.

Macroscopical
The uterus is moderately enlarged either generally

or locally. On section, the myometrium is thickened and haemorrhagic or cystic foci may be visible. In the localized form, a poorly demarcated circular or oval mass reminiscent of a fibroid may be present in the wall – *adenomyoma*.

Microscopical

There are multiple foci of endometrial tissue deep within the myometrium and usually associated with muscular overgrowth. Sometimes, there is stroma but no endometrial tubules are present – *stromal endometriosis*. The misplaced endometrium usually does not show cyclical changes.

Results

Adenomyosis may be asymptomatic or be associated with menorrhagia, dyspareunia or pre-menstrual pain.

Endometriosis

Nature

Endometrial tissue outside the uterine wall.

Sites

Ovaries, round ligaments, Fallopian tubes, recto-vaginal septum, pelvic peritoneum, intestinal wall, abdominal wall, umbilicus, laparotomy scars, lymph nodes, lung, pleura.

Macroscopical

At any of these sites, there is an haemorrhagic or cystic focus of variable size. The endometrial tissue in this type of endometriosis is almost always under hormonal control and thus its size alters during the menstrual cycle. Menstruation occurs and produces 'chocolate cysts' which are especially common in the ovaries.

Microscopical

The presence of endometrial tubules, stroma and blood pigment are diagnostic but in the older lesions the repeated shedding of the endometrium may produce diagnostic difficulties. At a late stage, fibrous tissue is produced in the area with only scanty endometrial elements but profuse haemosiderin pigmentation remains. In areas containing smooth muscle, e.g. intestine and Fallopian tube, the muscle becomes hypertrophied.

Results

The condition may be asymptomatic or produce a painful mass in the area. Adhesions from the fibrous reaction may result in complications, e.g. intestinal obstruction.

Pathogenesis

No single hypothesis can explain the presence of endometrial tissue in all extra-uterine sites but theories include the following.

(a) *Implantation*. Reflux of shed menstrual endometrium via the Fallopian tubes and thence into the peritoneum to be implanted on the peritoneum or on any pelvic or abdominal organ. This method admirably explains peritoneal endometriosis but does not satisfactorily account for foci outside the peritonal cavity.

(b) *Metaplastic*. The uterus is formed from the Müllerian ducts which are derived from the lining of the coelomic cavity. Peritoneum has a similar origin and it is suggested that the serosal tissues are capable of metaplastic change into endometrial tissues. This is the most acceptable explanation of endometriosis in most sites.

(c) *Lymphatic or vascular emboli*. It has been suggested that endometrium may spread in emboli via lymphatic or blood vessels. Such a mechanism is necessary to explain the occurrence in distant sites, e.g. lung.

Tumours

ENDOMETRIAL POLYP

Macroscopical

Single or multiple polyps arising from the endometrium, particularly near the fundus.

Microscopical

The histological changes are variable. If there is a solitary polyp or only a few polyps, they show hyperplastic non-secretory epithelium with cystic tubules in a stroma of variable cellularity covered by a single layer of epithelium. The remaining portions of the endometrium are normal and show cyclical changes.

In other cases there are multiple polyps and no intervening normal endometrial tissue. In such examples, the polyps are also formed by non-secretory hyperplastic endometrium which is more cellular and may show atypical areas. The basement membranes, however, remain intact. This condition is sometimes known as *adenomatous hyperplasia* and may be hormonally induced.

LEIOMYOMA – FIBROID

Nature
Tumours composed of fibrous tissue and smooth muscle which are variously known as leiomyomas, myomas, fibromyomas or fibroids.

Incidence
These are the commonest tumours of females and practically every uterus contains at least one, although it may be very small.

Age
Commonly arise at a young age but usually do not produce symptoms until later – 30 to 40 years or above.

Origin
Arise within the myometrium from the uterine muscle or from the uterine blood vessels and are dependent upon the presence of oestrogens for continued growth.

Macroscopical
Firm, white, whorled, encapsulated, round or oval-shaped tumours which occur as subserosal, intramural or submucosal nodules. The subserosal and submucosal types frequently become pedunculated and the latter may present as fibroid polyps distending the endometrial cavity or cervical canal.

Microscopical
Composed of elongated muscle fibres in an abundant fibrous stroma. They are commonly cellular, with giant cells and pleomorphism. The presence of mitotic figures is the most important criterion in respect of sarcomatous change.

Degenerations
Fibroids are extremely susceptible to many forms of degeneration, including the following.
1 Simple atrophy.
2 Hyaline degeneration.
3 Cystic degeneration.
4 Mucoid degeneration.
5 Red degeneration.
6 Fatty degeneration.
7 Calcification.
8 Ossification.
9 Sarcomatous change.

These degenerative processes have all been previously described with the exception of red degeneration – *necrobiosis*. This produces a red colour in the fibroid, is often associated with pregnancy or progestogen therapy and is probably due to infarction.

Sarcomatous change is very infrequent and occurs in less than 0.1 per cent of all fibroids.

Results
They frequently cause no symptoms, cease to enlarge and often atrophy after the menopause. Many symptoms, however, may be caused by fibroids, especially menorrhagia, and these benign tumours are responsible for a high percentage of gynaecological hospital admissions.

CARCINOMA CORPUS UTERI – ENDOMETRIAL CARCINOMA

Incidence
About 1000 deaths annually in England and Wales – approximately 1 per cent of all deaths from malignant disease.

There is clear evidence of a 10–15 per cent increase in incidence in many countries in the last decade.

Age
A later age group than carcinoma of the cervix – average 55 years.

Predisposing factors
Endometrial hyperplasia is a known predisposing factor and it is thought that many of the remaining cases may be due to hormonal imbalance, especially oestrogen stimulation, e.g. granulosa cell tumours of the ovary (see p. 436) and oestrogen therapy by some synthetic compounds given over a prolonged time usually for menopausal symptoms.

Obesity and diabetes are also factors related to increased incidence.

Marital state
Predominates in unmarried and childless women; of the married patients, approximately 50 per cent are nulliparous.

Macroscopical

Frequently arises in the fundus as a papillary or solid tumour filling a dilated endometrial cavity or as a solid tumour invading deeply into the wall. Secondary infection with pyometra, areas of necrosis and haemorrhage are common.

Microscopical

Solid or papillary adenocarcinomas, the majority being well differentiated. Approximately 15 per cent show areas of benign squamous metaplasia and the tumour is then sometimes called *adeno-acanthoma*. This has a particularly good prognosis, unlike the *adeno-squamous carcinoma*, a variant of very high malignancy in which the squamous element is also malignant.

Spread

Direct. The well differentiated tumours commonly show little myometrial invasion but may spread along the surface to involve the Fallopian tubes, ovaries or cervix. The poorly differentiated and anaplastic carcinomas invade the myometrium deeply and may erupt through the serosal surface to invade adjacent structures, e.g. bladder, rectum, small intestine.

Lymphatic. Metastases to pelvic lymph nodes occur in the less well differentiated types.

Blood. Usually a late manifestation except with anaplastic tumours. Lungs are the commonest site of these metastases.

Prognosis

Eighty per cent 5-year survival following extended hysterectomy. The majority of the fatal cases occur with anaplastic and adeno-squamous tumours.

UTERINE SARCOMA

Nature

As noted on p. 416 sarcomatous change may rarely occur in a previously benign fibroid. Sarcomas may also arise *de novo* from the muscle – *leiomyosarcoma* – or fibrous tissue of the myometrium – *fibrosarcoma* – or from the endometrial stroma – *stromal sarcoma*. Sarcomatous elements both homologous and heterologous are also present in carcinosarcomas, particularly in *malignant mixed Müllerian tumours*, which may arise from the endometrium, usually fundal (see p. 421). All, however, are rare.

Macroscopical

The tumour is usually large and pale, with haemorrhagic areas and extensive necrosis. Remnants of a pre-existing fibroid may be apparent. Widespread local invasion is usually seen.

Microscopical

The tumour is basically a spindle cell sarcoma with bizarre cellular forms, mitoses and giant cells, but recognizable smooth muscle or collagen fibres may enable identification as leiomyosarcoma or fibrosarcoma to be made. The borderline between cellular fibroid and low grade sarcoma is difficult, the determining factor is the number of mitoses.

Prognosis

Long-term survival is rare. Almost half the patients die within the first year.

Chapter 74
Genito-Urinary System – Cervix Uteri: Vagina

Cervix

CONGENITAL ABNORMALITIES

The cervix is frequently involved by congenital abnormalities arising from faulty fusion of the Müllerian ducts (see p. 411). There may also be atresia of the cervical canal resulting in retention of secretions and of menstrual blood – *haematometra*.

INFLAMMATIONS

Extremely common and yet only a small proportion are of clinical significance.

ACUTE CERVICITIS

Aetiology
The vaginal flora contains a variable number of different organisms including Döederlein's bacillus, coliforms, non-haemolytic streptococci, and it is these 'commensal' organisms which are isolated from some cases of acute cervicitis. In addition, an acute cervicitis may result from gonococcal infection and in the puerperal infections with more virulent bacteria (see p. 413).

Predisposing factors
The main predisposing circumstances are cervical trauma and laceration in labour.

Macroscopical

Swelling, redness and laceration of endo- or ecto-cervix.

Microscopical

There is an intense acute inflammatory cell infiltration in the cervical tissues especially related to lacerations and around mucous glands.

Results

The infection may resolve and the cervix return to normal or progression to chronic cervicitis may occur.

CERVICAL EVERSION

Nature

A reddish patch on the portio vaginalis surrounding or beside the external os, due to displacement of the normal squamous epithelium by descent of the cervical wall and replacement of columnar epithelium. This is *cervical eversion*, a term which replaces that of the inaccurate 'cervical erosion'.

Pathogenesis

The descent is largely oestrogen-induced. The vaginal acidity induces catarrhal outpouring of mucus and inflammatory changes with 'healing' by proliferation of reserve or basal cells causing *squamous metaplasia*. These cells replace the columnar epithelium producing a *transitional* or *transformation* zone.

　　Gland ducts obstructed by metaplastic squamous epithelium dilate to produce cystic *Nabothian follicles*.

　　The accompanying inflammatory cell infiltrate has been previously designated *chronic cervicitis* but this is not an infective lesion and the term is better abandoned.

MICROGLANDULAR HYPERPLASIA

Cervical mucous glands undergo proliferation under hormonal influences particularly with oral contraceptive therapy. The resulting microtubular pattern can be mistaken by the unwary for adenocarcinoma.

MATERNAL OESTROGEN-INDUCED CHANGES

High dosage di-ethyl stilboestrol therapy during pregnancy has been subsequently associated with adolescent development in female offspring of cervical and upper vaginal lesions of a characteristic clear cell type including vaginal *adenosis* and *clear cell adenocarcinoma*.

CERVICAL TUMOURS

CERVICAL POLYP

Origin

Arises from the endocervical columnar epithelium. They are extremely common.

Macroscopical

Single or multiple polyps arising in and dilating the endocervical canal. If large enough, they may present through the external os. On section they are soft and frequently show haemorrhagic areas with surface ulceration and cystic gelatinous centres.

Microscopical

There is an oedematous, fibrous stroma in which there are many dilated or cystic, hypertrophic, endocervical mucous glands. There may be surface ulceration and associated inflammatory reaction, whilst some examples show extensive squamous metaplasia of the columnar epithelium. This appearance may mimic squamous cell carcinoma, but there is no association with malignant change. Removal is curative.

CERVICAL WARTS – CONDYLOMA ACUMINATUM

Nature

These squamous-cell papillary lesions are virus warts and may be venereal, i.e. sexually transmitted, in origin. Often multiple, friable and vulval as well as ectocervical. Histologically they are regular benign proliferative squamous cell masses of characteristic folded configuration. Inclusion bodies may be obvious.

　　They do not become malignant but have to be

differentiated from a rare type of *verrucous* squamous cell carcinoma.

A true *papilloma* is very rare indeed in this site.

CARCINOMA OF THE CERVIX

Incidence
Uterine cancer causes approximately 4 per cent of all deaths from malignant disease: cervical cancer is still responsible for 2.5 per cent, almost 2500 deaths annually in England and Wales.

The disease is unknown in virgins, of very low incidence in Jews, intermediate in frequency in Moslems and high in Caucasian and African races.

Age
Average 48 years but with a wide range from early 20's to 80 years. There is recent evidence of increase in younger persons in some countries.

Predisposing factors
It is now firmly identified that this is related to sexual activity with four primary factors.

1 Early age of first intercourse.
2 Early age of first pregnancy.
3 Multiparity.
4 Short interval between pregnancies.
  Co-variables which are also sexually related are:
 (*a*) Promiscuity – particularly multiple partners, e.g. prostitutes.
 (*b*) Low social class and poor hygiene.
 (*c*) Contraceptive techniques – 'barrier' methods appear to have slightly lower risk.
 (*d*) Race and religion – differences in social attitudes and codes of behaviour.

These factors readily explain the geographical variations in incidence and the recent increase in younger women in those countries where greater sexual activity at earlier age has become established due to change of social attitudes.

Pathogenetic factors
1 Herpes simplex virus infection (HSV2) and human papilloma virus (HPV). Serum antibody levels to specific strains are high in patients with cervical epithelial abnormalities. The infection is spread by intercourse.
2 Contact of sperm DNA with cervical epithelial cells. It is postulated that fusion with the cell nucleus may initiate mutational changes.

Evidence so far, in respect of these factors as causative mechanisms, is inconclusive.

Natural history
Abundant evidence that most, if not all, invasive carcinomas of cervix arise from a progressive range of pre-malignant epithelial changes which on average spans about 25 years.

This can be shown diagramatically as follows:

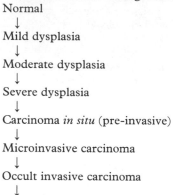

Normal
↓
Mild dysplasia
↓
Moderate dysplasia
↓
Severe dysplasia
↓
Carcinoma *in situ* (pre-invasive)
↓
Microinvasive carcinoma
↓
Occult invasive carcinoma
↓
Symptomatic invasive carcinoma

It is recognized that dysplasia is a potentially spontaneously reversible lesion but that once the stage of carcinoma *in situ* has been reached, either this persists or progression occurs through the remaining stages.

The process is accelerated in some cases; 5 per cent take less than 3 years.

Diagnosis of the presymptomatic invasive stage is normally made initially by abnormalities detected in routine cervical smears (see p. 162) and confirmed by histological examination.

Clinical stages
The internationally accepted FIGO staging is:

Stage 0 Carcinoma *in situ*.
Stage 1a Microinvasive carcinoma (invasion not more than 0.5 cm and only histologically diagnosable).
Stage 1b Confined to cervix.
Stage 2 Direct spread to involve extra-cervical tissues but not as far as pelvic side wall or lower one-third of vagina.
Stage 3 Direct spread to involve either pelvic side wall or lower one-third of vagina.
Stage 4 Direct spread to involve bladder and/or rectum or beyond true pelvis.
N.B. This is a clinical assessment and does *not* include lymphatic spread.

Macroscopical
The anterior lip of the cervix is more commonly

involved and may show enlargement with hardness and surface irregularity – *endophytic type* or be polypoid, ulcerated, necrotic with extension clinically apparent into vagina and other adjacent structures – *exophytic.*

Microscopical
Invasive. More than 95 per cent of invasive tumours are squamous cell carcinomas, mostly poorly differentiated and non-keratinizing. About 5 per cent are columnar cell adenocarcinomas arising from endocervical epithelium.

Carcinoma in situ. The squamous cells show absence of maturation, loss of polarity, pleomorphism, increased mitotic activity, presence of abnormal mitoses and disorderly growth pattern, but the basement membrane is intact. Extension into cervical gland ducts should not be mistaken for invasion.

Dysplasia. There is a varying degree of loss of orderly maturation of cells from basal layer to surface depending on the severity of the dysplasia which is classified as mild, moderate or severe. The borderline between severe dysplasia and carcinoma *in situ* is indistinct but, in dysplasia, some progressive maturation of cells remains.

Cervical epithelial neoplasia (CIN)
This recent concept is favoured by clinicians and colposcopists and is relevant to treatment decisions.

Very mild dysplasia ⎫
Mild dysplasia ⎬ = CIN Grade 1.
Moderate dysplasia = CIN Grade 2.
Severe dysplasia ⎫
Carcinoma *in situ* ⎬ = CIN Grade 3.

MANAGEMENT

(*a*) *Invasive carcinoma.* Treatment is usually by one or more forms of irradiation: sometimes radical surgery is utilized either primarily or after radiotherapy.

(*b*) *Pre-invasive lesions.* It is reasonable to assume that adequate treatment of these abnormalities will prevent development of invasive carcinoma and could lead to its elimination.

Initial diagnosis by the presence of abnormal cells in cervical cytological preparations (see p. 162) is followed either by:
1 Colposcopy and biopsy, or
2 Cone biopsy.

If histological appearances are of CIN 3, i.e.

carcinoma *in situ* or severe dysplasia, then cone biopsy is usually curative though long-term follow-up is essential.

For lesser grades of dysplastic abnormality (CIN 1 or 2), more conservative methods may be appropriate, e.g. diathermy, cryosurgery or laser therapy. This is particularly so in young patients who may wish to retain full fertility.

RESULTS

Stage 1a   99.5% 5 years, 99.0% 10 years.
Stage 1b   75%.
Stage 2   50%.
Stage 3   25%.
Stage 4   5%.
All stages   40% 5 years, 30% 10 years.

Death is commonly from local pelvic disease rather than blood-borne metastases. In particular, involvement of urinary tract by direct spread or lymph node invasion leads to obstructive renal failure.

Terminal stages are often very distressing with pain and vesico-vaginal or recto-vaginal fistulae frequent.

MALIGNANT MIXED MÜLLERIAN TUMOUR—SARCOMA BOTRYOIDES

Nature
A rare tumour in the genital tract derived from tissues of Müllerian duct origin.

Age
Occurs in the very young and the elderly.

Sites
May arise from the fundus of the uterus (see p. 417), the cervix or the vagina and also occurs in the ovary (see p. 435).

Macroscopical
A bulky and polypoid tumour frequently producing grape-like fronds, hence 'sarcoma botryoides'. On section, the tumour is gelatinous with haemorrhagic and solid areas.

Microscopical
A spindle cell sarcomatous stroma in which there are usually scanty adenocarcinomatous elements, i.e. 'carcino-sarcoma'.

The connective tissue elements may be homologous, e.g. smooth muscle, fibroblasts or heterologous, e.g. bone, cartilage, rhabdomyoblasts.

Prognosis

This is a rapidly growing, highly malignant tumour with an almost invariably fatal outcome within a year of diagnosis due to extensive direct, lymphatic and blood spread.

Vagina

CONGENITAL ABNORMALITIES

The vagina may be involved with the uterus in a failure of fusion of the Müllerian ducts and thus be septate, whilst atresia or even absence of the whole vagina occurs rarely. Vestigial remnants of the Wolffian ducts – Gärtner's ducts – lie in the lateral walls of the vagina and are occasionally the site of cyst formation. They are small fluid-filled cysts with a cuboidal epithelial lining.

INFLAMMATIONS

The vagina is extremely resistant to infection but may be involved secondarily from vulval inflammation.

GONOCOCCAL VULVO-VAGINITIS OF CHILDREN

This is now a rare infection in which the genital area is infected by gonococcal cross-infection from the mother.

TRICHOMONAS VAGINALIS INFECTION

Aetiology

The flagellate protozoon, *Trichomonas vaginalis*, measuring up to 30 μm long.

Macroscopical

A frothy, watery, yellow, vaginal discharge associated with a brilliant red vaginal mucosa.

Microscopical

The protozoa are readily identifiable in wet preparations and even more commonly in cervical smears by the Ayre scrape (see p. 161). The inflamed areas show an intense polymorph infiltration with somewhat irregular thickening of the squamous epithelium.

MONILIAL VAGINITIS

Surface infection with *Candida albicans* may cause a vaginal discharge (see p. 58).

CHLAMYDIAL INFECTION

These small gram-negative, obligate intracellular parasites are a relatively common cause of vaginitis and cervicitis.

SENILE VAGINITIS

Physiological oestrogen-deficient post-menopausal atrophy of the vaginal epithelium predisposes to low grade infection and inflammation.

TUMOURS

Benign connective tumours, e.g. fibromyoma, haemangioma, etc., occur but are rare and show no special features in this site.

MALIGNANT TUMOURS

Primary malignant tumours of the vagina are very rare but include the following.

Squamous cell carcinoma
This has to be differentiated from vaginal invasion by a primary carcinoma of the cervix.

Malignant mixed Müllerian tumour
See p. 421.

Tumours of Gärtner's duct
This very rare tumour is a columnar cell adenocarcinoma arising in Gärtner's duct remnant.

Chapter 75
Genito-Urinary System – Vulva: Fallopian Tube: Abnormalities of Gestation

Vulva

CONGENITAL

The vulva may be absent or hypoplastic, usually associated with an hypoplastic uterus and a deficiency of secondary sexual characteristics. There may be duplication of the vulva associated with a double vagina or a septate uterus. The most common congenital abnormality is an imperforate hymen, which may escape notice until the onset of menstruation occurs to produce *haematocolpos* (vagina), *haematometra* (uterus), or even *haematasalpinx* (tubes) due to the progressive accumulation of menstrual blood.

INFLAMMATIONS

NON-SPECIFIC INFECTIONS

Non-specific infections of the vulva are frequent, especially when associated with a vaginal discharge, vaginitis or with pruritus vulvae from any cause.

SYPHILIS

The vulva and cervix are the commonest female sites of the primary chancre of syphilis (see p. 53).

OTHER INFECTIONS

As described on p. 406, granuloma inguinale and lymphogranuloma venereum may affect the vulva. Granuloma inguinale produces gross deformity of the area by the locally destructive process. Lymphogranuloma venereum, draining in the female to the perirectal and pelvic lymph nodes, produces lymphatic obstruction and results in esthiomene of the vulva at a later stage.

VULVAL DYSTROPHY

Nature
White lesions of vulval skin which formerly had a confused and no longer acceptable nomenclature, including such terms as 'leukoplakia' and 'kraurosis vulvae'. Many lesions are not degenerative and have no pre-malignant potential.

Classification
The international classification widely accepted is:
Hyperplastic:
  No atypia.
  Atypia – mild, moderate, severe.
Lichen sclerosus.
Mixed:
  No atypia.
  Atypia–mild, moderate, severe.

Hyperplastic dystrophy
A condition which, in the absence of atypia does not proceed to pre-malignancy and is characterized by elongation, widening, clubbing or confluency of the rete ridges of epidermis, often with hyperkeratosis. Cells are regular and there is a dermal inflammatory cell infiltrate.

Lichen sclerosus
There is blunting and loss of rete ridges with concomitant homogeneous eosinophilic subepithelial layer in the dermis. There is decrease in the number of layers of epithelial cells and the basal layer is hydropic. There is no significant malignant potential.

Mixed
Ten to 15 per cent of dystrophies show a variable combination of the two above types.

Atypia
Variable grades largely correspond to degrees of dysplasia seen in the uterine cervix (see p. 420). Mild involves only the lower third, moderate a half to two-thirds and severe more than two-thirds of the thickness of the epithelium.

Less than 10 per cent progress to invasive cancer and the pre-malignant potential of atypia is not so well documented on the vulva as on the cervix. Cases regress spontaneously or with therapy, but require follow-up.

BARTHOLIN'S CYST

Nature
A retention cyst of Bartholin's gland in the labia minora.

Macroscopical
A mucus-containing cyst at the site of Bartholin's

gland. Frequently there is superimposed infection – Bartholin's abscess.

Microscopical

The cyst is lined by cuboidal or columnar epithelium with mucous glands in the fibro-muscular wall. The epithelial lining is destroyed by infection so that the cyst commonly contains inflammatory material and is lined by granulation tissue. However, some mucous glands remain in the fibrous wall which enable recognition of the tissue of origin.

TUMOURS

VIRUS WARTS – CONDYLOMA

These common virus induced squamous cell papillary lesions are usually sexually-transmitted, multiple and benign (see p. 729).

SQUAMOUS CELL CARCINOMA

This tumour is responsible for approximately 1 per cent of malignant disease. Most vulval carcinomas are preceded by vulval dystrophy and this is usually visible at the periphery of the tumour. The majority (65 per cent) have evidence of metastases to the inguinal or pelvic lymph nodes at the time of diagnosis. Although blood spread is unusual, the prognosis is poor, with an approximate 30 per cent 5-year survival.

OTHER TUMOURS

The vulva is a relatively common site for malignant melanoma, basal cell carcinoma and sweat gland tumours, particularly the benign *hidradenoma*. It is also the site of the uncommon condition of *Paget's disease of the vulva*. This is due to a carcinoma of the underlying apocrine glands with malignant Paget's cells in the overlying epidermis. The condition is thus similar to Paget's disease of the nipple (see p. 230).

Fallopian tube

CONGENITAL

Abnormalities of the Müllerian ducts may result in absence, reduplication or atresia of one or both Fallopian tubes. These abnormalities are, however, all rare.

INFLAMMATIONS

ACUTE SALPINGITIS

Aetiology

The commonest organisms are gonococci, with streptococci, staphylococci, coliforms and pneumococci being much less frequent.

Mode of infection

The usual route of infection is via the lumen of the uterus and commonly complicates gonococcal or post-partum infections. The tubes may also be infected via the blood stream, from the peritoneum, or from contact with adjacent and inflamed structures, e.g. appendicitis.

Macroscopical

The tube is tense, red and swollen, the lumen contains pus, and there is a peritoneal exudate.

Microscopical

An acute pyogenic inflammatory reaction in all coats of the wall with pus in the lumen. Culture is necessary to identify the causal organism.

Results

1 *Resolution*. With early and effective treatment the condition may resolve and the tubes return to normal. However, this is unusual.

2 *Pyosalpinx*. The tubes become more and more distended by pus, especially if the fimbrial end seals. The dilated tubes then become characteristically 'retort-shaped'.

3 *Tubo-ovarian abscess*. The fimbriae may become adherent to the adjacent ovaries with the production of oophoritis. Eventually, both the tubes and ovaries form an inflammatory suppurating mass – tubo-ovarian abscess.

4 *Subacute salpingitis*. The inflammation may not resolve but pass into a subacute stage with persistence of the inflammation and an intense plasma cell infiltration of all coats of the wall, associated with increased fibrosis. This is a relatively common occurrence.

5 *Chronic salpingitis*. The inflammation may become chronic with gross fibrous thickening of the

wall of the tube, in which there is a chronic inflammatory cell infiltration of lymphocytes and scanty plasma cells.

A variant is *salpingitis isthmica nodosa* in which epithelial sinuses grow from the lumen into the muscle wall to produce glandular spaces and a beaded nodularity of the wall at the isthmus. The condition is almost certainly inflammatory in origin.

The infection may die out and the pus be converted over a period of time to a thin watery fluid distending the fibrotic and occluded tubes – *hydrosalpinx*. In other cases, the distension may be due to mucoid material – *mucocoele*.

Effects

Unless complete resolution occurs there is a high incidence of subsequent sterility. Should conception occur, there is an increased hazard of tubal pregnancy due to delay in passage of the fertilized ovum down the tube.

GONOCOCCAL SALPINGITIS

Aetiology

A venereal infection due to *Neisseria gonorrhoeae*.

Macroscopical

Four or more days following the infection, an inflammatory reaction is visible in the urethral (Skene's) glands, Bartholin's gland, the anterior urethra and the cervix, but the stratified squamous epithelium of the vulva and vagina is resistant to the infection.

Microscopical

There is an intense polymorph infiltration in the affected areas and a purulent discharge in which the gram-negative intracellular diplococci can be identified.

Spread

In untreated or inadequately treated cases, the disease spreads along the lumen of the cervix producing a cervicitis and through the endometrial cavity, almost always sparing the endometrium, to the Fallopian tubes, where an acute salpingitis results. This may spread via the fimbrial end to the ovaries – acute salpingo-oophoritis. As a result of formation of fimbrial adhesions, a closed cavity is formed resulting in a pyosalpinx, but later this may become sterile and converted into a hydrosalpinx with the typical 'retort-shaped' tubes. There is then permanent sterility.

TUBERCULOUS SALPINGITIS

Aetiology

This is usually an example of single organ tuberculosis of the genital tract due to blood spread from a pulmonary focus. Rarely it may occur secondary to a tuberculous peritonitis.

Macroscopical

The tubes are swollen and firm with multiple tubercles on the serosal coat. The wall is thickened and there may be caseous material present within the lumen.

Microscopical

The wall contains multiple caseating tubercles.

Results

Unless actively treated, the tube will become progressively disorganized by fibrous tissue and sterility will result. In the active stages, the tubercle bacilli pass from the tube into the endometrium where they commonly cause a tuberculous endometritis (see p. 414).

TALC GRANULOMA

Aetiology

Talc powder, introduced into the peritoneal cavity at operation on surgical gloves, may gravitate to the Fallopian tubes and cause a granulomatous reaction.

Macroscopical

The tubes are thickened and the external surface is granular.

Microscopical

There is increased fibrosis of the wall which contains multiple foci of inflammatory cells and foreign body giant cells surrounding or containing doubly-refractile crystalline talc particles.

Results

In exuberant examples, sterility may follow due to fibrous obliteration of the lumen.

CYSTS

Small cysts at the fimbrial end of the tube – *fimbrial cysts* – are extremely common. They are small, unilocular and benign with clear fluid contents.

Cysts of Morgagni occur adjacent to the tube near the fimbrial end and are presumed to be derived from remnants of the Wolffian duct.

CARCINOMA OF THE FALLOPIAN TUBE

Incidence

This is a rare tumour. Its classical presentation is by watery vaginal discharge.

Macroscopical

The tube is grossly thickened with an intact 'skin' so that it resembles a 'sausage'. The tubal tumour may be visible sprouting through the fimbrial end. On section, the tube is distended and invaded by a solid or papillary tumour.

Microscopical

Adenocarcinomas of varying grades of differentiation.

Spread

Transcoelomic spread via the fimbrial end results in multiple peritoneal tumour nodules and a very poor prognosis.

SECONDARY CARCINOMA IN THE FALLOPIAN TUBE

This is much more common than the primary carcinoma and occurs by invasion from a carcinoma of the ovary or as a result of extension from a primary carcinoma of the uterus.

Abnormalities of gestation

ABORTIONS

Spontaneous abortion is of common occurrence and has been estimated as terminating one of every four pregnancies. Frequently, some residual products of conception remain within the uterus – *incomplete abortion*. This may be attended by haemorrhage of varying severity and duration, sometimes responsible for a considerable degree of anaemia. The presence of the dead and degenerate chorionic and decidual tissue predisposes to uterine and pelvic infection (see p. 413).

CARNEOUS MOLE

Nature

Haemorrhage in and around the implanted gestation sac resulting in the death of the foetus.

Macroscopical

A nodule of brown-coloured tissue at the placental site within the uterus. The sac is usually recognizable but the dead foetus is absorbed.

Microscopical

Haemorrhage of variable age with death and disappearance of the embryo. The placental tissues are degenerate.

Results

The involved area may become organized or passed *per vaginam*.

PLACENTAL POLYP

Nature

A portion of retained placental tissue may remain viable and produce a polypoid mass.

Macroscopical

A polyp of variable size with an haemorrhagic appearance, attached to the uterine wall.

Microscopical

The polyp is composed of placental tissue, i.e. chorionic villi and decidua together with fibrous tissue.

Results

Severe uterine haemorrhage, discharge, or infection, may occur.

ECTOPIC PREGNANCY

Nature

This implies implantation of a fertilized ovum outside the endometrial cavity.

TUBAL PREGNANCY
(95 per cent)

Predisposing factors
The ovum is normally fertilized within the lumen of the tube and any delay in its passage to the uterus, e.g. by previous salpingitis, increases the risk of tubal implantation. There is also increased risk in patients with intrauterine contraceptive devices (IUCD).

Sites
The ovum may implant at the fimbrial end, in the mid-portion or in the interstitial portion.

Incidence
Approximately one in every 150 pregnancies.

Macroscopical
The tube is distended by an haemorrhagic mass in the centre of which is the gestation sac containing the foetus; this is the commonest cause of haemato-salpinx. The wall is thickened and haemorrhagic but in areas becomes thinned by chorionic action and rupture is extremely common.

Microscopical
Blood clot containing chorionic villi and decidual cells. In addition, there is a decidual reaction in the mucosa of the whole tube and sometimes on the serosal surface. The uterine endometrium also shows a decidual stromal reaction which is shed as a decidual cast when the ectopic pregnancy terminates.

Results
1 *Tubal mole*. The embryo may die and form a tubal mole similar to a carneous mole in the uterus.
2 *Tubal rupture*. If the foetus continues to grow the tube wall will rupture. This is almost always followed by severe intraperitoneal haemorrhage and death of the foetus. On very rare occasions, the placenta may reimplant within the abdomen – *abdominal pregnancy*. The foetus may alternatively be extruded from the tube into the peritoneal cavity and become mummified – *lithopaedion*.

OTHER ECTOPIC SITES
(5 per cent)

The embryo may be implanted on the ovary,

probably following the rare event of fertilization at the time of rupture of the ovarian follicle – *ovarian pregnancy*. Abdominal pregnancy may follow tubal ectopic pregnancy or be primary, due to extrusion of the ovum from the fimbrial end with implantation on to the peritoneal surface. In this manner, placenta, membranes and the foetus develop within the peritoneal cavity and this has very occasionally resulted in the operative recovery of a live foetus.

TOXAEMIA OF PREGNANCY – ECLAMPSIA

Nature
A disease occurring in pregnancy, usually in the later stages and manifest by proteinuria, hypertension and oedema. Convulsions may occur in severe cases – eclampsia. Some degree of generalized oedema occurs in 75 per cent of pregnant women; it is only when associated with albuminuria or hypertension that it becomes significant.

Aetiology
This remains unknown but the disease usually regresses dramatically after the uterus is emptied of the foetus and placenta. This suggests the important factor is either of foetal, or more probably, placental origin. Predisposing factors include inadequate diet, excessive weight gain in pregnancy, elderly mothers and pre-existing hypertension.

Organ changes

KIDNEY
Macroscopical. Slight or moderate swelling with small petechial haemorrhages in the cortex.
Microscopical. There is a specific diffuse glomerular lesion.
  Mild cases. Swelling of all the glomeruli, primarily due to swelling of the endothelial cells of the capillary loops.
  Severe cases. The swelling is more pronounced and affects endothelial cells, epithelial cells and basement membranes. Arterioles show swelling and oedema of the media and intima, most marked in the eclamptic cases.

LIVER
Macroscopical. In 50 per cent of cases the liver is affected. It is enlarged, soft and yellow with subcapsular and parenchymal haemorrhages. In severe

cases, the appearance are those of acute massive necrosis with haemorrhages a prominent feature (see p. 552).

Microscopical. There is zonal necrosis usually affecting the peripheral zone of the lobules but of variable and patchy distribution throughout the liver. Extravasated red cells are usually seen and in these haemorrhagic areas abundant fibrin is a notable feature.

PLACENTA

Macroscopical. The placenta is bulky and excess intervillous fibrin and infarcts are prominent.

Microscopical. There is degeneration of the syncytiotrophoblast signifying premature ageing of the chorionic villi. The more severe the toxaemia the greater the number of villi show this change, so that in eclamptic cases 90–100 per cent are affected.

Results

1 Labour, at term in mild cases, or induced early in severe cases, leads to a dramatic regression of the clinical signs. Most cases show no subsequent evidence of hepatic or renal dysfunction.
2 In severe cases, the foetus may die *in utero* and require removal, following which the clinical condition regresses. The foetal mortality rate is high.
3 In a few cases, the liver lesions progress to acute massive necrosis with death from liver cell failure.
4 In cases with pre-existing hypertension, the progression of the vascular disease may be accelerated, the speed of progression being related to the severity of the glomerular lesions seen in renal biopsy specimens. In the absence of pre-existing hypertension, however, the renal lesions do not appear to produce permanent hypertension nor subsequent impairment of renal function.

Abruptio placentae

Nature

Premature separation of the normally implanted placenta occurring after 20 weeks' duration.

Types

Marginal – causing revealed accidental ante-partum haemorrhage.
Central – causing concealed haemorrhage which may dissect into the myometrium to produce a large, boggy, bluish uterus – *Couvelaire uterus.*

Aetiology

There is a significantly high incidence in patients with pre-eclamptic toxaemia but not with pre-existing essential hypertension. However there is no antecedent history in at least 30 per cent of cases.

Effects

1 Haemorrhage – ante-partum or immediately post-partum.
2 Foetal death – from anoxia when placental separation is extensive.
3 Premature labour.
4 Disseminated intravascular coagulation – placental abruption is an important and often fatal cause of this consumptive coagulopathy (see p. 531).

HYDATIDIFORM MOLE

Nature

A disorder of chorionic tissue.

Incidence

About one in every 1500–2000 pregnancies in Caucasians, but about one in 300 in Middle Eastern races and one in 100 in the Philippines and Formosa.

Age

During reproductive life only.

Macroscopical

The majority occur within the uterus, although the placenta at the site of ectopic pregnancies may rarely be affected. The uterus is larger than normal for the stated duration of the pregnancy and the cavity is filled with thin-walled, cystic, grape-like, chorionic villi. No foetus remains although sometimes a small amniotic sac can be seen. The ovaries frequently contain simple luteal cysts.

Microscopical

The chorionic villi are composed of completely or comparatively avascular, oedematous and myxomatous tissue to produce the 'bunch of grapes' appearance. They are covered with trophoblastic epithelium which may be normally arranged in its double layer of cells but show varying degrees of hyperplasia.

Results

1 Spontaneous or assisted evacuation of the mole

with follow-up H.C.G. studies for 1 year but no sequelae.

2 Evacuation followed by bleeding and persistence of H.C.G. urine level may be due to *persistent mole* in the myometrium. This may be variably aggressive and can sometimes produce difficulties of management – *invasive mole*.

3 Subsequent development of chorion carcinoma.

Clinical effects

The hydatidiform mole produces uterine enlargement greater than that expected for the duration of the pregnancy and is associated with high levels of human chorionic gonadotrophin (H.C.G.) in the urine. The majority behave in a completely benign manner and only about 10 per cent are sufficiently atypical to suggest the possibility of malignancy, with only about 2 per cent progressing to chorion carcinoma.

CHORION CARCINOMA

Nature

A malignant tumour of the chorionic trophoblast.

Incidence

An extremely rare tumour which occurs once every 30,000–40,000 pregnancies in Caucasian peoples but more frequently in other races corresponding to the relative incidence of hydatidiform mole (see p. 429).

Age

During child-bearing age.

Predisposing factors

Fifty per cent arise in hydatidiform moles, 25 per cent in abortions and about 22 per cent in normal pregnancies. The remaining 3 per cent arise in ectopic pregnancies or in malignant teratomas, e.g. teratoma of the testis (see p. 402).

Macroscopical

The uterus is bulky and is occupied by an haemorrhagic tumour which extensively invades the myometrium and frequently extends to the serosal surface. Secondary deposits may be visible in the tubes, ovaries and vagina.

Microscopical

There are sheets of irregular, large, polyhedral cells and giant cells invading and destroying the myometrium. These cells are mostly from the Langhans' layer of cytotrophoblast and areas of necrosis and haemorrhage are usually present in adjacent myometrium. Chorionic villi are not seen.

Spread

Early blood spread is extremely common with secondary deposits in the lungs and other viscera, in addition to local spread to the vulva, vagina and broad ligaments.

Prognosis

Prior to the advent of chemotherapy by methotrexate this was almost invariably rapidly fatal, but a few authenticated cases have been cured by hysterectomy. It is also substantiated that, in a very few cases, established secondary tumours have regressed following removal of the primary. It should be noted that many cases of invasive mole are overdiagnosed as chorion carcinomas; these tend to be locally invasive and chemotherapy or local resection is curative. Microscopically, the invasive moles show chorionic villi in addition to the atypical trophoblastic epithelium. The histological diagnosis of chorion carcinoma, however, may be extremely difficult. Most cases of the disease can now be controlled by use of methotrexate even when metastases are clinically apparent.

Hormonal effects

This tumour also secretes gonadotrophic hormones similar to those produced by a normal placenta and produces luteal cysts in the ovaries. H.C.G. is therefore present in the urine, which is useful diagnostically and in the 'follow up' period after treatment. N.B. Radioimmunoassay methods for estimation of titres are necessary rather than the less sensitive methods used in pregnancy testing.

Chapter 76
Genito-Urinary System – Ovary

Development of ovary

The early development is characterized by four main phases.

1 Primordial germ cells, probably of yolk-sac origin, migrate to the genital ridges which are bilateral coelomic epithelial thickenings ventral to the mesonephros.
2 Proliferation of coelomic epithelium and underlying mesenchyme.
3 Gonadal division into cortex and medulla.
4 Cortical development and medullary involution in the female and the reverse in the male.

Subsequent to this the primitive germ cells – *oogonia*, proliferate by mitosis and then subsequently by meiosis (see p. 9) forming *oocytes*.

Developmental abnormalities

1 *Streak gonads*. The uterus and tubes are small and the gonads form small streaks of tissue, normally situated. Surface epithelium covers the largely fibrous tissue centre resembling ovarian stroma. Hilar cells can often be found but germ cells are absent by the time the individual reaches puberty. Most of these patients have identifiable chromosomal abnormalities usually 45 XO – *Turner's syndrome* (see p. 14).
2 *Hermaphroditism*. True hermaphrodites with recognizable ovarian and testicular tissue, either as ovotestes or differing types of gonads on different sides, are very rare (see p. 408).
3 *Heterotopia*. Misplaced nodules of adrenal tissue may be juxta-ovarian but not within the ovarian tissue.

Inflammations

Primary inflammation of the ovary is extremely rare but the ovary is frequently involved by infections of the Fallopian tube (see p. 425). Mumps infection and, occasionally, other viruses may cause oophoritis with resulting fibrosis and sterility.

Torsion of the ovary

Predisposing factors
It is rare for torsion to occur with a normal ovary but common when the ovary is enlarged by a cyst or tumour.

Macroscopical
The ovary is enlarged, plum-coloured and congested with thrombosis of veins and, later, the artery in the twisted pedicle.

Microscopical
Extreme haemorrhagic congestion is followed by infarction. This may be so complete as to pose problems of identification or possible malignancy when the torted ovary is the seat of a tumour.

Endometriosis

The ovary is the most frequent site of endometriosis with resulting 'chocolate cysts' (see p. 415). Cysts containing altered blood may give identical gross appearances when due to haemorrhage into cystic follicles or corpora lutea.

Simple cysts

The most frequent cause of enlargement of the ovaries is the presence of solitary or multiple retention type cysts related to Graafian follicles. They are of two types:
1 *Follicular*. Containing clear or blood-stained

fluid and lined by several layers of epithelial cells of the follicle. They seldom are more than 10 cm in diameter and more commonly are 1–3 cm.

2 *Luteal.* Contents more commonly blood-stained and with a lining of flattened luteinized cells. Usually solitary or few in number and seldom more than 5 cm in diameter.

These simple cysts form over 95 per cent of ovarian swellings less than 5 cm in diameter.

Tumours of the ovary

Incidence
Ovarian tumours cause the deaths of approximately 3000 women each year in England and Wales, about 3 per cent of deaths from malignant disease. Their incidence is increasing in many Western countries with a corresponding rise in mortality, indicating a lack of success with therapy. The incidence is much greater in whites than in coloured races.

Classification
The World Health Organization (1973) classification has become widely and internationally accepted and is used in this book.

COMMON EPITHELIAL TUMOURS

Origin
It seems likely that all the tumours in this group have a common origin from surface ovarian mesothelium.

Types
These most numerous of the ovarian tumours are subdivided by histological characteristics.
1 Serous.
2 Mucinous.
3 Endometrioid.
4 Clear cell (Mesonephroid).
5 Brenner.
6 Mixed (of above).
7 Undifferentiated carcinoma.
8 Unclassified.

SEROUS TUMOURS

Incidence
Serous tumours form about 40 per cent of ovarian neoplasms.

Age
Benign – most are in the 20–50 age groups. Mean 38 years.
Malignant – most are in the 30–60 age group. Mean 45 years.

Origin
Surface mesothelium with a strong resemblance to Fallopian tube epithelium. Psammoma bodies and some extracellular mucin are commonly seen and ciliated cells are usually found.

Macroscopical
Benign tumours. There are three basic patterns, each of which can occur separately or in combination.
1 *Cystic-Serous cystoma.* A thin-walled usually unilocular cyst with clear watery content and variable in size from a few cm to 30 cm in diameter. The lining and serosal surfaces are both smooth.
2 *Papillary cystadenoma and surface papilloma.* The papillary areas are usually present in part of a cyst wall lining or on the cyst outer surface – *surface papilloma*. They are more frequently bilateral than cystomas and may be associated with ascites and implantation of tumour on the serosa of other intra-peritonal organs, though without subsequent malignant behaviour.
3 *Cystadenofibroma and adenofibroma.* Solid, pale, whorled fibrous areas up to several cm. in diameter can occur in the wall of a serous cyst – *cystadenofibroma* or, less commonly, with only a minor cystic component – *adenofibroma*.
Malignant tumours. Usually large and bilateral in 60 per cent or more. They may be largely cystic (25 per cent), semi-solid (65 per cent) or entirely solid (10 per cent). The solid areas can be partly papillary lining cysts but more often there is pale, solid tissue invading the wall. Areas of haemorrhage and necrosis are common.

Microscopical
Benign. Cuboidal or columnar epithelium, some ciliated, some secretory and vacuolated in a single regular but often crowded layer.
Malignant. The epithelial cells are dedifferentiated to a variable degree and arranged in papillary, acinar or solid pattern. Cytological characteristics of malignancy are evident and there is invasion of the supportive stroma or the whole thickness of the wall.
Borderline. In some serous tumours cytological

features of malignancy are seen but there is no stromal invasion. These are classified as of 'borderline malignancy', and are prognostically important.

MUCINOUS TUMOURS

Incidence
Mucinous tumours form about 35 per cent of ovarian tumours but mucinous carcinomas are 3–4 times less common than their serous counterparts.

Age
Benign-mean 40 years.
Malignant-mean 45 years.

Origin
Surface mesothelium but largely composed of mucin-filled cells resembling endocervical or intestinal epithelium. Occasionally, argentaffin and Paneth cells may be seen.

Macroscopical
Benign tumours. Ten per cent are bilateral with wide variation in size but commonly very large – 30 cm in diameter, or more. The outer surface is smooth and glistening and on section numerous loculi are usually present of varying size and containing thick tenacious mucus. Less commonly there is one large cyst often with more serous content and a cluster of small daughter cysts of frankly mucinous appearance in the wall. Leakage or frank rupture of a benign mucinous cystadenoma may result in peritoneal seedlings – *myxoma peritonei*, in about 2 per cent of cases (see p. 221).

Malignant tumours. Mucinous cystadenocarcinomas are bilateral in about 30 per cent. They may show obvious solid areas with penetration of the wall and adhesion to other organs. Necrotic and haemorrhagic areas are frequent. Entirely solid tumours are infrequent.

Microscopical
Benign. Remarkably uniform, tall, single-layered columnar cells with basal nuclei and basophilic mucin-containing cytoplasm, together with shorter goblet cells.

Malignant. Multilayered epithelium of variable degrees of dedifferentiation and of irregularity in size and shape of microloculi. Stromal or frank invasion of the wall is seen.

Borderline. As with serous tumours so the mucinous neoplasms show a proportion of cases with cytological features of malignancy but without evidence of invasion.

ASSOCIATION WITH OTHER OVARIAN TUMOURS

Both serous and mucinous tumours may be associated with the presence of a teratoma, fibroma or Brenner tumour. Dimorphic cystic tumours of distinctive serous and mucinous parts are found in 5–10 per cent of cystadenomas and less commonly when malignant.

SPREAD OF OVARIAN CARCINOMAS

1 *Direct.* To adjacent organs in the pelvis.
2 *Peritoneal.* Transcoelomic spread is common causing ascites and frequently intestinal obstruction.
3 *Lymphatic.* To iliac and para-aortic nodes.
4 *Blood.* To lungs and liver, but relatively uncommon.

Prognosis
5-year survival—serous carcinomas 35 per cent;
5-year survival—mucinous carcinomas 50 per cent.

Stage I malignant tumours, confined within the serosal coat, have a 5-year survival of about 80–90 per cent. The prognosis is less favourable for serous tumours than for mucinous.

ENDOMETRIOID TUMOURS

Definition
Primary ovarian neoplasms which, histologically, closely resemble uterine endometrial tumours (see p. 416). Endometrioid tumours can develop from pre-existing ovarian endometriosis (see p. 415) or from the surface epithelium through Müllerian metaplasia along endometrial lines.

ENDOMETRIOID ADENOCARCINOMA

Incidence
Probably about 30 per cent of ovarian adenocarcinomas.

Age
Average 53 years.

Macroscopical

No distinguishing features: solid, partly cystic or cystic, often papillary.

Microscopical

Columnar cells in a tubular or acinar pattern usually multilayered and often in a lobulated papillary form. Cytological features of malignancy are usually evident but a relatively high proportion are well differentiated. Squamous metaplasia is common and of regular appearance: it may be dominant and resemble closely the *adenoacanthoma* of the uterus. Vacuolated or clear cytoplasm is seen in areas of most of those tumours and may be a dominant feature needing differentiation from clear-cell carcinoma (see below). Both mucin and glycogen are demonstrable in areas within endometrioid adenocarcinomas.

Associated features

1 *Ovary.* Accompanying endometriosis is only found in about 10 per cent.
2 *Endometrium.* Up to 30 per cent may have a concomitant carcinoma of the endometrium, and endometrial hyperplasia is seen in 15 per cent.

Prognosis

5-year survivals 40–50 per cent;
10-year survivals 30–35 per cent;
5-year survivals 75 per cent of Stage I tumours only.

The presence of squamous foci is of good prognostic significance.

OTHER ENDOMETRIOID TUMOURS

Malignant mixed Müllerian tumours (mixed mesodermal) carcinosarcomas of similar appearance to those arising in the endometrium, are rare (see p. 421).

CLEAR-CELL MESONEPHROID TUMOURS

Definition

Tumours composed of glycogen-containing clear cells resembling those of a renal adenocarcinoma or with small cysts and tubules lined by peg-shaped

and hobnail cells. Alternative names formerly used include mesonephroma, hypernephroid, mesometanephric and clear-cell tumour.

Origin

Probably from ovarian mesothelium which has retained its mesonephric competence.

Incidence

About 2 per cent of ovarian neoplasms and less than 10 per cent of common malignant epithelial tumours.

Age

Most occur between 50 and 70 years.

Macroscopical

Usually unilateral and markedly variable in size. They are mostly not distinguishable on gross appearance from other partly or wholly cystic tumours.

Microscopical

Tubular and cystic structures surrounded by fibrous stroma and lined by cells with large, dark nuclei which protrude into the lumen – *hobnail cells*. Other areas may show papillary structures of glomeruloid appearance and numerous cytoplasmic vacuoles which stain for glycogen and traces of mucin and lipids are very common. Fibrous areas and foci of transformation from epithelial to stromal type cells may be seen.

Prognosis

5-year survival 45 per cent;
5-year survival 65 per cent.
Stage I tumours only.

BRENNER TUMOURS

Definition

An ovarian tumour characterized by well-demarcated nests and columns of epithelial cells in a fibrous stroma.

Incidence

One to two per cent of ovarian tumours.

Origin

This is debatable and the precise histogenesis is uncertain. Similarities of the epithelial cells with urothelium suggests a possible origin from surface epithelium or hilar tissues via urothelial metaplasia.

Age
Rare in childhood and adolescents. Mean 45 years.

Macroscopical
Many are microscopic in size and about 30 per cent are less than 0.5 cm in diameter. Relatively few are more than 10 cm. About 5 per cent are bilateral. Circumscribed hard or gritty, whorled tumours either solid pale or yellowish or, in 20 per cent, occurring as pale nodules in the wall of a cyst. Finely cystic areas are not uncommon.

Microscopical
Variable proportions of fibroblastic stroma and circumscribed islands of polygonal transitional type epithelial cells of regular appearance. Central cyst formation in these islands is quite common and 10 per cent show mucinous metaplasia. Stromal calcification is common. Associated cysts may be mucinous, usually benign but occasionally malignant, or serous or as an element of a benign cystic teratoma (see p. 439). Slight cystic hyperplasia of the endometrium occurs in about 10 per cent of cases but oestrogen production by these tumours is unproved.

Results
The vast majority of Brenner tumours are benign but malignant change in the epithelial element can rarely occur. The prognosis of malignant examples is very poor. The *proliferating Brenner tumour* is benign, rare and shows very active epithelial elements.

OTHER COMMON EPITHELIAL TUMOURS

Mixed
Mixtures of two, or rarely more, of the previously described types of epithelial tumours are not particularly rare. This is understandable when the common origin is considered.

Undifferentiated
This carcinoma shows no differentiating features and is usually solid or, if cystic, degenerate. These tumours are highly malignant.

Unclassified
Occasional epithelial tumours show some differentiating features but insufficient for classification.

SEX CORD STROMAL TUMOURS

GRANULOSA – STROMAL CELL TUMOURS

GRANULOSA CELL TUMOUR

Definition and histogenesis
Tumours composed of cells resembling the granulosa cell layer of ovarian follicles. It is probable that the tumour develops due to stimulation, in some unknown way, of the latent competence of the tissue anlage from which granulosa cells originate. Granulosa cells differentiate from primitive sex cords in the indifferent gonad but it is uncertain whether these are mesenchymal or coelomic epithelial in origin.

Incidence
One to two per cent of ovarian tumours. Mean age 48 years but wide range from infancy to the elderly.

Macroscopical
Only 5 per cent are bilateral. Very variable in size from microscopic to huge; also variably solid, part cystic or largely cystic. Distinguishing gross features are not found.

Microscopical
The cells are characteristically small, round or spindle-shaped with scanty cytoplasm and a large rather characteristic nucleus. Patterns of arrangement of these epithelial cells are variably trabecular, insular, follicular or cystic. Microfollicles with a central core of eosinophilic material containing nuclear fragments are commonly found – *Call–Exner bodies*. True tubular arrangements are not found. A fibrous stroma separates the epithelial cell conglomerates. Small lipid droplets are present within cytoplasm and luteinization with increase in fat content may also be seen.

Associated features
These tumours produce oestrogen and endometrial

hyperplasia is therefore usually found. The incidence of endometrial adenocarcinoma at about 6 per cent is higher than coincidence would allow.

Prognosis
This is notoriously difficult to predict and histological features are unreliable in assessing malignancy. Approximately 50 per cent will die from the tumour if follow-up is continued for 20 years. Poor prognostic features include: aged over 40, palpable mass, tumour more than 15 cm in diameter, bilaterality, extra-ovarian spread, solid tumour and numerous mitoses.

THECOMA

Definition and histogenesis
Oestrogen-producing tumours of probable origin from ovarian mesenchyme and possibly developing on a basis of cortical stromal hyperplasia.

Incidence
Less than 1 per cent of ovarian tumours. Average age 53 years – rare prepubertally and most common post-menopausally.

Macroscopical
Usually unilateral of wide range of size but seldom above 8 cm in diameter. Well demarcated, firm or hard and usually solid with, occasionally, foci of central cystic degeneration. The cut surface is usually pale yellow in areas and whorled.

Microscopical
Plump, pale spindle cells in bundles with intervening fibrous tissue of less cellular appearance. Lipid is constantly demonstrable in the cells and, from the practical viewpoint, determines the differentiation from fibromas which may appear otherwise largely indistinguishable.

Associated features
The oestrogen produced by thecomas usually causes endometrial hyperplasia and there is associated hyperplasia of the ovarian stroma in the same and in the contralateral ovary. Coexistent endometrial adenocarcinoma is even more common than with granulosa cell tumours.

Behaviour
Only very rare examples of malignant thecoma have been identified.

GRANULOSA CELL–THECOMA MIXED

Mixtures of variable amounts of granulosa cell tissue and thecomatous tumour are quite common. Even when the granulosa cell component is small the likely behaviour is related to its presence.

FIBROMA

Definition
Fibroblastic tumours of stromal mesenchymal origin.

Incidence
Four to five per cent of ovarian tumours. Most common in 50–60 age group and rare in prepubertal girls.

Macroscopical
Commonly bilateral, variably sized, circumscribed, nodular, hard, pale, whorled tumours.

Microscopical
Bundles of fibroblastic cells, variably cellular in appearance but regular. Collagen production may be prominent. Cells of thecal type must be absent to differentiate from thecomas and fat stains are negative.

Effects
These are invariably benign inactive tumours which not infrequently undergo torsion (see p. 432). Ascites is found in association in 20–30 per cent of fibromata, usually when they are large. In 1–2 per cent of cases pleural hydrothorax is also present – *Meigs' syndrome*.

ANDROBLASTOMA

Definition
Neoplasms composed of Sertoli cells, Leydig cells, or the precursors of either, alone or in any combination. The former name of *arrhenoblastoma* implied inevitable virilization, which is incorrect.

Histogenesis
This is not agreed. One theory accepts homology between granulosa cells and Sertoli cells by being derived by stimulation of latent bisexual competence of either gonadal mesenchyme or epithelial sex cords. Subsequent development along male lines will produce androblastoma. A contrasting

theory suggests that 'male' cells are derived from mesonephric mesenchyme via the medulla of the primitive gonad, i.e. that androblastomas would arise by stimulation of latent competency of residual medullary tissue in the ovarian hilum.

Incidence

This group of tumours is very uncommon, forming about 0.1 per cent of ovarian neoplasms. Age incidence varies with the differing types.

Types

1 Well-differentiated tumours.
(a) Sertoli cell.
(b) Leydig Cell.
(c) Mixed Sertoli–Leydig cell.
2 Intermediate differentiation. Both types of cells present.
3 Minimal differentiation. Largely undifferentiated but recognizable Leydig or Sertoli cells present.

Many of these tumours are androgenic but a proportion are non-endocrinologically active and some, including the differentiated Sertoli cell tumour, may be oestrogenic. Most are small and the majority benign in behaviour.

GYNANDROBLASTOMA

Nature

A very rare tumour in which both granulosa–theca and Sertoli–Leydig cell types are present and are intermingled. Origin is either from gonadal mesenchyme or epithelial sex cords which have retained their potential for differentiation along bisexual lines. Reported tumours are small unilateral and with variable endocrinologically active secretions. Some produce both androgen and oestrogen, some solely one or the other. They are benign.

LIPOID CELL TUMOURS

These rare tumours were originally described on the basis of demonstrable lipid content but are now generally agreed to be mesenchymal endocrine tumours without thecal cells. There are three types.
1 *Leydig cell tumours.* Also included under androblastoma (see p. 403).
2 *Adrenal-like tumours.* Morphologically resembling adrenal cortical tissue of zona glomerulosa or fasciculata-type (see p. 289). These tumours are virilizing and some are malignant.
3 *Luteoma.*
(a) *Luteoma of pregnancy.* This is not a true neoplasm and regresses post-partum. Bilateral in 50 per cent of cases and of average size 8 cm. They bear superficial resemblance only to corpora lutea of pregnancy and do not secrete progestogens. When any endocrine effects are identified they are usually virilizing.
(b) *Stromal luteoma.* Small, intra-ovarian benign collections of luteinized cells of probable stromal origin. Some oestrogen or progestogen production is usually identifiable.

GERM CELL TUMOURS

DYSGERMINOMA

Definition

This ovarian homologue of seminoma of the testis (see p. 401) is thought to arise from primitive germ cells which have migrated from the yolk sac to the gonadal ridge.

Incidence

One to two per cent of ovarian neoplasms in Caucasian races but more common in India and Japan. Most common in 20–40 age group but the age range is 1–80 years.

Macroscopical

Usually large tumours, bilateral in 15 per cent. Lobulated, firm, rubbery and solid, the cut surface shows a slightly pinkish-grey homogeneous appearance.

Microscopical

Uniform polyhedral and rather large cells with sharply defined borders and often vacuolated or granular cytoplasm rich in glycogen. Degenerate foci are common as are granulomas and, sometimes, multinucleate cells resembling syncytiotrophoblast. As in the testicular seminoma lymphocytic infiltration is frequently seen (see p. 401).

Associated conditions

Other types of germ cell tumours are commonly associated, particularly teratoma, endodermal sinus tumour and choriocarcinoma. Some patients have developmental genital tract abnormalities or dysgenetic gonads.

Spread

1 *Local*. Extension to extra-ovarian tissues is found at the time of operation in 25 per cent.
2 *Contralateral ovary*. Common but often only as a small focus of tumour cells.
3 *Lymphatic*. Retroperitoneal and paraortic.
4 *Blood*. In 90 per cent of fatal cases, particularly lungs and liver.

Prognosis

Very radiosensitive even when metastases have occurred at the time of operation:
5 year survival – 90 to 95 per cent;
10 year survival – 85 per cent.
If metastases present at time of operation 33 per cent at 5 years.

YOLK-SAC TUMOUR– ENDODERMAL SINUS TUMOUR

Nature

A rare highly malignant tumour of yolk-sac origin occurring in the young.

Characteristic histological features include, the presence of a loose vacuolated network of cells and microcysts, glomerulus-like perivascular formations – Schiller-Duval bodies, cystic structures with lining of flattened cells, aggregate of undifferentiated 'embryonal' cells and PAS-positive hyaline globules. They often occur associated with other germ cell tumours. Most examples produce α-fetoprotein. The ovarian tumours of this type are identical to those of similar histological features in the testis of infants (see p. 403), the anterior mediastinum and the pineal gland.

Results

Average survival is 6 months with only a few long-term survivors reported.

CHORIOCARCINOMA

A very rare highly malignant tumour either gestational with a primary ovarian or tubal or intrauterine pregnancy or non-gestational. Most of the latter are associated with a teratoma or other germ cell tumour (see below).

TERATOMA

These are tumours showing differentiation along embryonic lines.

BENIGN CYSTIC TERATOMA – OVARIAN DERMOID CYST

Nature

A benign cystic tumour composed of fully differentiated tissues, usually predominantly ectodermal but with variable mixtures of tissues of mesodermal and endodermal origin.

Incidence

Approximately 20 per cent of ovarian neoplasms. This type forms more than 97 per cent of ovarian teratomas.

Age

Wide range from infancy to the eighth decade, but most occur in the reproductive age groups. Mean 35 years.

Macroscopical

Bilateral in 10 per cent or more and variably sized but only occasionally large. Predominantly cystic with one or more of the cysts usually containing hair and sebaceous material which gives the tumour a characteristic doughy feel. In the wall there is a protuberance or tubercle from which the hairs sprout. Usually adjacent to this structure more solid tissues are present of widely variable type but commonly containing bone, teeth or brain.

Microscopical

Skin and appendage structures can nearly always be found, usually lining the main cystic cavity. Beyond this, combinations of a very wide range of adult type tissues may be found, most commonly neural tissue, bone and teeth.

Complications

1 *Torsion*. This is common (see p. 432).
2 *Rupture*. Uncommon but may further complicate torsion or infection.
3 *Infection*. Rare but dangerous.
4 *Malignant change*. This is relatively rare occurring in about 1–2 per cent of previously benign teratomas. Most of these are squamous cell carcinomas, less commonly adenocarcinomas or carcinoids and, rarely, other malignant tumours.

SOLID TERATOMA

Nature
Totally or mostly solid, unilateral, usually large, rare ovarian tumours. Mean age 16 years. About 1 per cent of ovarian teratomas. A wide range of tissues may be present of variable differentiation. A proportion contain only fully differentiated tissues and pursue a benign course but the remainder have embryonal tissue present and are aggressively malignant.

MONOPHYLETIC TERATOMA

These very rare tumours are thought to arise from pre-existing teratomas or from germ cells which differentiate only along one tissue line. They may either occur as a localized tumour mass in a benign, cystic teratoma or may grow to obliterate evidence of previous teratomatous tissues and appear to be pure primary tumours. Types described include:
1 *Carcinoid tumour.* Similar to the intestinal tumours (see p. 212) and occasionally hormonally active producing the carcinoid syndrome.
2 *Struma ovarii.* Most or all of the tissue is of thyroid gland usually normal but occasionally hyperplastic and thyrotoxic. Occasional thyroid carcinomas develop.
3 *Malignant melanoma.* A very rare primary ovarian tumour. Secondary deposits in the ovaries from primary melanomas of skin, eye or other sites are much more common.
4 *Mucinous ovarian tumours.* It has been argued that these common ovarian tumours described on p. 434 are monophyletic teratomas of gastrointestinal tract derivation. From all practical viewpoints however they must be separately identified.

GONADOBLASTOMA

Nature
A very rare tumour composed of germ cells, sex cord derivatives of immature granulosa or Sertoli cell type and, usually, stromal elements of luteal or Leydig cell appearance. They are usually small or microscopic and histologically show germ cells, usually in a dysgerminomatous pattern patchily mixed with epithelial cells of granulosa cell or Sertoli cell type. Calcification is almost always present. The course is benign unless true dysgerminoma develops.

Gonadoblastoma nearly always develops in a previously abnormal gonadal individual. Most of the patients have a Y chromosome, many are mosaics. They have either pure gonadal dysgenesis with bilateral streak gonads or mixed gonadal dysgenesis with one streak gonad and a contralateral dysgenetic testis. A few have occurred in male pseudohermaphrodites but very rarely in patients with somatic features of Turner's syndrome.

SOFT TISSUE TUMOURS NOT SPECIFIC FOR OVARY

These include haemangioma, lymphangioma, neurofibroma, leiomyoma, oesteoma, fibroma and their malignant counterparts. Adenomatoid tumours (see p. 403) are also sometimes ovarian in position.

SECONDARY TUMOURS

Secondary deposits of carcinoma in the ovary are common, particularly from gastrointestinal tract and breast. A particular type is the *Krukenberg tumour* of characteristic histological appearance with signet-ring, mucus-secreting, adenocarcinoma cells in a cellular fibrous stroma. These arise from primary tumours in large intestine and stomach.

The ovaries may also be involved by malignant lymphoma either as part of disseminated disease, occasionally as an apparent primary site of origin and, in Burkitt's lymphoma, as a common presenting and clinically prominent feature (see p. 583).

Chapter 77
Haematology – Blood Cells and Their Formation

Bone marrow

Blood formation

IN THE FOETUS
In the foetus, blood is formed firstly in the yolk sac and then in the liver and spleen. After about 3 months of intra-uterine life, blood production commences in the bone marrow, and at birth this is the only site of formation of the red cells, granular cells and platelets.

IN THE CHILD
At birth, all the bones contain *red marrow*, i.e. active haematopoietic tissue. During childhood, this red marrow shrinks from the periphery to the centre of the body, so that by puberty, the limb bones, with the exception of the heads of the humeri and femora contain only fat – *yellow marrow*.

IN THE ADULT

The red marrow is confined to the skull, vertebrae, thoracic cage, pelvis, and the heads of the femora and humeri. Even this red marrow can be demonstrated to contain about 50 per cent of fat. Although some lymphocytes are formed in the bone marrow, the majority are produced in lymph nodes. Monocytes are formed in the spleen, lymphoid tissue and bone marrow.

Marrow reserve

In response to stimulus, the marrow output of the normal adult can be increased in three ways:

1 *Increase in the anatomical space occupied by the red marrow:*
(*a*) By eliminating the fat spaces within the red marrow.
(*b*) By extending the red marrow in the limb bones.

The volume of haematopoietically active marrow may thus be increased by about four times.

The anatomical reserve created by the presence of fat in the marrow space of the limb bones is not available to the young child. In the presence of severe chronic anaemia, e.g. thalassaemia major (see p. 502), the child can only increase the marrow space by eliminating the fat content of the normal red marrow and subsequently by enlarging the marrow cavity of the bones. The latter can be recognized on X-ray examination:

(*a*) Skull: the outer table of bone is eroded by the expanding marrow; the fine spicules of bone in the enlarged marrow space present a 'hair on end' appearance. A co-existent, enlargement of the zygomas may result in facial disfigurement – 'mongoloid' facies.
(*b*) Phalanges: the expansion of the marrow in the shaft converts the normal dumb-bell-shaped phalanges into rectangular-shaped bones.

2 *An alteration in the myeloid/erythroid ratio.* In a normal marrow the proportion of nucleated white cells to nucleated red cells – myeloid/erythroid ratio (M/E ratio) – lies between 2 : 1 and 5 : 1 (see p. 444).

A marrow biopsy taken when it is under stress would show that the proportion of the cell line in particular demand, e.g. the red cell in most types of anaemia or the granulocytes in pyogenic infection, will have specifically increased. The M/E ratio will be outside the normal limits.

3 *Rapid maturation of the percursors in the bone marrow.* Output of red cells and granular cells can also be increased by a reduction in the maturation time of their precursors within the bone marrow. An increase in the number of mitotic figures in the cell lines under stress can be identified.

In a case of severe chronic anaemia, combination of these three methods may lead to the output of red cells from the marrow being increased 13 times above the normal figure.

Myeloid metaplasia – extra-medullary haematopoiesis

In certain diseases, e.g. myelosclerosis (p. 460), the bone marrow may cease to produce blood; the spleen and, to a lesser extent, the liver, recommence haematopoiesis, thus resuming an embryonic role.

Bone-marrow biopsy

In many haematological disorders, a bone-marrow biopsy is very important to establish a diagnosis or to control treatment. Severe coagulation disorders, e.g. haemophilia, are a contra-indication to biopsy; it is permissible, however, in thrombocytopenia when excessive bleeding can be prevented by firm pressure to the biopsy site. Interpretation can only be relied upon when the sample is technically adequate. This requires expertise both in obtaining the sample and more particularly in making good films.

SITE OF BIOPSY

(*a*) Children: up to 2 years of age, from the shaft of the tibia, a little below the level of the tibial tubercle. In older children, the iliac crest is the site of choice.
(*b*) Adults: the site of choice is now the posterior part of the ilium, the patient being positioned as for a lumbar puncture and the needle being inserted perpendicularly about 1 cm below the posterior superior iliac crest. Alternative sites are the anterior iliac crest and the sternum.

ANAESTHESIA

After cleaning the skin, local anaesthetic is infiltrated into the tissues from the skin to the periosteum. This ensures that the obtaining of the biopsy should be virtually painless. To avoid psychological trauma, children should be sedated, or they may require a light general anaesthetic, especially if treatment demands repeated biopsies.

BIOPSY NEEDLE

A marrow biopsy needle is guarded, the position of the guard on the shaft being adjustable to allow for the depth of the patient's subcutaneous tissue at the chosen site.

In order to penetrate bone, a biopsy needle is strong and contains a stillette. To avoid overpenetration, the main physical effort, as with a bradawl, is put into rotation of the instrument, downward pressure being minimal and controlled. A sense of 'give' may be felt as the outer table of bone is penetrated and aspiration should be attempted as soon as the needle stands firmly upright. If the patient is osteoporotic, the needle may still have to be supported even if the tip is in the marrow cavity! Marrow tissue may then be aspirated from the cavity with a syringe which fits the needle and which allows strong suction. It is usual to aspirate 0.1–0.2 ml of marrow and this is commonly accompanied momentarily by 'suction' pain which confirms that the tip of the needle is in the marrow cavity. If the tap is dry, the stilette is replaced and the needle may then be cautiously inserted a little deeper.

THE MARROW SAMPLE

Aliquots of the marrow are spread without delay, and before clotting occurs, on 4–6 glass slides. If fragments are very plentiful, only a very small drop need be applied to the slide. If fragments are fewer a larger drop should be applied and the excess 'blood' sucked back before spreading the smear. The more swiftly the smear is spread, the less far the fragments will travel across the slide. The slides should contain marrow fragments which are recognized as translucent granules of tissue at the tips of the smear trails. They are dried rapidly by waving them in the air. Remaining marrow may be used for:

1 Fixation prior to histological processing and subsequent sectioning for marrow architecture, etc.
2 Microbiological cultures.

The slides are carefully transported in racks or trays and stained by both a Romanowsky stain, usually May–Grünwald–Giemsa, and also by Perls' Prussian blue stain; the latter to demonstrate iron stores (see p. 473). Additional cytochemical staining procedures may be occasionally employed.

Bone marrow trephine

Marrow biopsy may fail to yield a satisfactory sample, dry or blood only. This may be due to:

1 Faulty technique. Over-penetration is commoner than under-penetration.
2 Marrow pathology:
(*a*) Replacement by fat in aplasia.

(*b*) Infiltration by carcinoma or occasionally by leukaemic or myeloma cells, which resist aspiration by suction.
(*c*) Excessive fibrosis of the marrow in myelosclerosis, secondary carcinoma or tuberculosis.

A marrow trephine may be carried out by a number of cutting needles of varying size of which the Jamshedi needle gives satisfactory specimens with little or no distortion of structure and can also be used for aspiration during the same procedure. Iliac crest is the site of choice. If these methods fail an open wedge biopsy of iliac crest by an orthopaedic surgeon may be necessary.

Interpretation of bone marrow sample

Careful preliminary low power microscopic examination is followed by the identification of individual cells in the trails behind the fragments using either a cover slip and × 40 objective or oil immersion.

LEVEL OF MARROW ACTIVITY

The cellularity of the marrow fragments is assessed by the ratio of fat to cellular content. Occasionally, the marrow fragments may be solid and lack any fat spaces as in any condition where either leucopoiesis or erythropoiesis is grossly excessive, e.g. leukaemia (see p. 453), pernicious anaemia (see p. 483), polycythaemia rubra vera (see p. 458). Solid fragments are also found if there is infiltration with plasma cells in myelomatosis (see p. 470) or cells normally foreign to the marrow such as secondary carcinoma (see p. 444).

Conversely, in hypoplasia or aplasia, the cellular content of the marrow fragments may be reduced or almost absent.

Provided excessive dilution by blood has been avoided, the number of free marrow cells may also give a somewhat unreliable indication of marrow activity.

PROPORTIONS OF NORMAL MARROW CELLS

Megakaryocytes

It is important to estimate not only the number of megakaryocytes but also to establish normality of morphology and maturation with platelet production, i.e. have platelet material breaking from the edge of the cytoplasm.

Leucopoiesis

The developing and mature leucocytes, granular,

lymphocytic, and plasma cell series, are recognised and their proportions assessed.

Erythropoiesis
It is necessary not only to assess the number of nucleated red cell precursors but also to recognize the nuclear change of megaloblasts (see p. 483).

Myeloid/erythroid ratio (M/E ratio)
The numerical ratio of developing and mature white cells to nucleated red cell precursors is determined (see p. 442). Normally this myeloid/erythroid (M/E ratio) or leuco-erythroblastic ratio (L/E ratio) lies within the range of 2:1–i 5:1. By a combined assessment of the cellularity of the marrow fragments and the M/E ratio one can obtain a rough indication of the leucopoietic and erythropoietic activity of the marrow sample.

Examples:
 (i) Marrow fragments hypocellular.
    M/E ratio 1:1 = leucopoiesis depressed.
 (ii) Marrow fragments hypercellular.
    M/E ratio 1:1 = erythropoiesis increased.

RECOGNITION OF 'FOREIGN' CELLS, PARASITES AND ORGANISMS
The most commonly seen foreign cells are from metastatic deposits of carcinoma. These malignant cells are characteristically dark staining and clumped but may require confirmation by histology of the marrow fragments. On rarer occasions, diagnosis may depend upon the recognition of parasites, e.g. in kala azar (see p. 62); bacteria, e.g. tuberculosis, or the large pale cells characteristic of the lipoidoses (see p. 113).

ASSESSMENT OF IRON STORES
A Perls' Prussian blue preparation of normal marrow contains a small quantity of blue-staining iron as haemosiderin. Stainable iron is occasionally also demonstrated as granules in developing red cells – *sideroblasts* (see p. 479). On rare occasions, these blue-staining iron granules may be observed in ring formation around the nucleus of the red cell precursor – *'ring' sideroblast*. This is usually associated with marked iron overload.

Maturation of normal marrow cells

The authors would suggest that the developing marrow cells are best recognized through the microscope rather than by the study of photographs or the written word. For this reason, the following description of the marrow cells is kept to the minimum.

'STEM CELLS'

Difficult to distinguish morphologically according to any destined cell line. Approximately 1 per cent of cells in marrow smears are of this type. Usually about 16–20 μm with pale blue cytoplasm, large nuclei containing lightly staining chromatin and several nucleoli.

ERYTHROPOIESIS

The maturation of the red cell is achieved by three simultaneous processes.

DIMINUTION IN CELL SIZE

The most primitive recognizable red cell precursor – pronormoblast – is 12–20 μm in diameter whereas the mature erythrocyte is about 7.2 μm.

MATURATION OF THE NUCLEUS

The primitive nucleus is large, the chromatin pattern is fine and nucleoli are present. With maturation, the nucleoli disappear and the chromatin pattern becomes coarser until, at the stage of the orthochromatic normoblast, a small, pyknotic nuclear remnant is expelled. The pronormoblast has a high nuclear/cytoplasmic (N/C) ratio, the cytoplasm being merely a dark-blue halo around the large finely stippled nucleus. As the nucleus shrinks during red cell maturation, the N/C ratio reduces.

DEVELOPMENT OF HAEMOGLOBIN

The cytoplasm of the pronormoblast and basophilic normoblast is dark blue with a Romanowsky stain. Haemoglobin is first identified in the polychromatic normoblast when the cytoplasm begins to develop a greyish colour.

	Old units	S.I. units
Haemoglobin, male	13.0–18.0 g/100 ml	13.0–18.0 g/dl
female	11.5–16.5 g/100 ml	11.5–16.5 g/dl
MCHC	32–36%	32–36 g/dl
MCH	27–31 $\mu\mu$g	27–31 pg
MCV	75–99 μm^3	75–99 fl
PCV, male	40–54%	0.40–0.54
female	37–47%	0.37–0.47
Red cell count, male	4.4–6.1 m/mm^3	4.4–6.1 $\times$ 10^{12}/l
female	4.2–5.4 m/mm^3	4.2–5.4 $\times$ 10^{12}/l
Total white cell count, adults	4000–11 000/mm^3	4.0–11.0 $\times$ 10^9/l
infants 1 year	6000–18 000/mm^3	6.0–18.0 $\times$ 10^9/l
infants 1 day	10 000–26 000/mm^3	10.0–26.0 $\times$ 10^9/l
Neutrophils, adults	2500–7500/mm^3	2.5–7.5 $\times$ 10^9/l
children 1 year	2500–6000/mm^3	2.5–6.0 $\times$ 10^9/l
Lymphocytes, adults	1500–4000/mm^3	1.5–4.0 $\times$ 10^9/l
children 1 year	5000–8500/mm^3	5.0–8.5 $\times$ 10^9/l
Platelets	150 000–400 000/mm^3	150–400 $\times$ 10^9/l
Serum iron, adult males	70–180 μg/100 ml	13–32 μmol/l
females 15–45 years	56–160 μg/100 ml	10–29 μmol/l
TIBC	250–400 μg/100 ml	47–70 μmol/l
Serum B$_{12}$	160–925 pg/ml	160–925 ng/l
Serum folate	3–20 ng/ml	3–20 μg/l
Red cell folate	160–640 ng/ml	160–640 μg/l

These values vary slightly from laboratory to laboratory

Fig. 43. Normal haematological values.

Pronormoblast

A large cell, 12–20 μm in diameter, consisting of a large, finely chromatin patterned nucleus bearing nucleoli and surrounded by a halo of dark-blue cytoplasm.

Basophilic normoblast

This cell is basically similar to a pronormoblast but without nucleoli. Some shrinkage in cell size and some coarsening of the nuclear chromatin pattern is discernible.

Polychromatic normoblast

Haemoglobin is recognized in the cytoplasm by its grey polychromatic colour. The nuclear size has diminished and the chromatin pattern is coarser. The cell diameter is 8–14 μm.

Orthochromatic normoblast

The fully haemoglobinized cytoplasm now stains entirely pink and the nuclear remnant has become a shrunken coarsely stranded or condensed pyknotic lump.

Reticulocyte

The nuclear remnant has been expelled.

With Romanowsky stains, the reticulocyte appears slightly larger than the mature erythrocyte, and also has a polychromatic cytoplasm due to the presence of RNA remnants which can be demonstrated only by vital staining.

GRANULOPOIESIS

Usually only mature forms are present in the peripheral blood.

Granulocytes

So-called because of the granules in their cytoplasm with a Romanowsky stain – neutrophils, eosinophils and basophils. They are also known as *polymorphonuclear* cells because of their multilobed nuclei. Their main function is to engulf and eliminate micro-organisms by phagocytosis (see p. 23).

ORIGIN AND DEVELOPMENT – GRANULOPOIESIS

Myeloblast

The earliest precursor and present in small numbers only in the bone marrow. About 12–18 μm in size with a small amount of basophilic cytoplasm and a large round or slightly oval nucleus containing 3–5 nucleoli. With further development the nucleoli become more vestigial, the cytoplasm increases and specific granules begin to appear – *promyelocyte*.

Myelocyte

This cell is smaller, about 12 μm, but with relatively more pink-staining cytoplasm and containing prominent granules. The nucleus has lost its nucleoli and is more coarsely structured.

Up to this stage mitotic division can occur, but subsequent cells appear by maturation only with progressive indentation of the nucleus.

Metamyelocyte

At first reniform in appearance, the nucleus then becomes thinner and horseshoe-shaped in the later 'band' form and finally becomes lobulated to form the mature granulocyte.

Mature granulocyte

About 10 μm in diameter with coarse granules and a nucleus consisting usually of about 3–4 segments each joined by a thin strand of chromatin. In normal women, 3 per cent of the neutrophils have a sex chromatin *drumstick appendage*, a dense chromatin fragment attached to a lobe by a narrow stalk. Mature neutrophils contain a variable quantity of *alkaline phosphatase*. It can be detected as a brown granularity by applying a histochemical technique to a freshly made blood film. This can be roughly quantitated by scoring each of 100 cells 0–4 according to the intensity of staining – a normal score is 20–80.

Eosinophils

Recognized by their nucleus, which is almost always only bi-lobed even when mature, and the characteristic large orange granules in the cytoplasm. Their function is associated with defence against foreign substances (see p. 448).

Basophils

Present in small numbers in the peripheral blood and readily recognized by their very coarse purple-black granules which fill the cytoplasm and often obscure the nucleus. Functionally they release histamine, heparin-like substances and SRS-A (see p. 92). They may be responsible for delaying coagulation at the site of inflammatory lesions.

OTHER LEUCOCYTES

Monocyte

These cells of the lymphoreticular system (previously reticulo-endothelial system – see p. 90) are about 14–20 μm and are released from the marrow where they develop rapidly. Their precursor, the *monoblast*, is difficult to distinguish from the myeloblast. An intermediate stage of maturation, the *promonocyte* is recognized which has vestigial nucleoli and an in-folded nucleus. The mature cell has a rather eccentric nucleus which may be oval, horseshoe-shaped or convoluted and has a rather delicate structure. The cytoplasm is pale grey-blue in colour and contains scattered fine pink granules.

The *function* of the monocyte is not well understood but it is phagocytic and develops into the tissue macrophage; having migrated from the blood to an inflammatory lesion it appears to proliferate there, and interact with the lymphocytes (see p. 23).

Lymphocyte

These cells comprise almost half the leucocyte population in the peripheral blood. They are mostly small, about 10 μm, consisting almost entirely of nucleus, with a thin rim of blue cytoplasm containing occasional scattered azurophilic granules. About 10 per cent of the lymphocyte series are larger – 15 μm; the nucleus may contain nucleoli and the cytoplasm is more extensive with more pronounced granules. Lymphocytes are mostly found in lymph nodes, spleen, bone marrow and thymus and are of two main types: 'T' and 'B' (see p. 89). Little is known about the lymphocyte precursor but they are unlikely to be identified with the lymphoblasts seen in lymphoblastic leukaemia.

Lymphocyte *function* is primarily concerned with immune defence mechanisms (see p. 89).

(i) Cellular immunity. Delayed hypersensitivity, graft versus host reactivity and graft rejection. Most of the circulating lymphocytes are of this 'T' cell type – 70 per cent.

(ii) Production of humoral antibody and immunoglobulins. After being produced in the bone marrow, these 'B' cells occupy the germinal centres and the peripheral zone of lymph nodes.

Immunoglobulins (IgG, IgA, IgM and IgD) are produced by:

(i) Plasma cells in the germinal centres, bone marrow and intestinal mucosa.

(ii) Small lymphocytes of the germinal centres.

Plasma cell

These arise from 'B' lymphocytes in lymphoid tissue and are not normally seen in the peripheral blood. They are present in the bone marrow, but form only about 2 per cent of the nucleated cells. Typically, they are variable in size, up to 20 μm with an eccentric nucleus and deep blue cytoplasm. Condensation of chromatin of 'cart-wheel' type can be seen in the nucleus and there are usually a few 'pinkish' granules in the cytoplasm which is rich in RNA as shown by methyl green pyronin stain (MGP).

NORMAL VALUES

These are given in Fig. 43 on p. 445.

The control of marrow output

Some factors controlling erythropoiesis are understood but there is still very little knowledge about the mechanisms which stabilize the numbers of leucocytes and platelets.

THE CONTROL OF ERYTHROPOIESIS-ERYTHROPOIETIN

The output of red cells from the marrow is stimulated by a glycoprotein produced mainly in the kidney. A renal erythropoietic factor is secreted into the blood stream as a response to renal tissue anoxia where it combines with a plasma protein probably produced by the liver, to become erythropoietin. Under normal circumstances, the red cell mass is controlled by a 'feed-back' mechanism.

Erythropoietin production will be stimulated by any factor which predisposes to renal tissue anoxia.

1 A reduction in the haemoglobin level – anaemia.

2 Incomplete oxygenation of the arterial haemoglobin as in residence at high altitude, pulmonary emphysema or congenital heart disease with arteriovenous shunts.

3 Reduction in blood flow to nephrons – renal ischaemia (see p. 367).

4 An abnormal haemoglobin with a high oxygen affinity (see p. 458).

It is self evident that for effective oxygenation of the renal tissue, haemoglobin in the capillaries must be present in adequate concentration and also be well oxygenated. It is less obvious but equally important that the affinity of the haemoglobin for oxygen should be so adjusted that it will effectively release its oxygen during the passage of the red cell through the renal capillaries. An abnormal haemoglobin which is so avid for oxygen that it will remain fully oxygenated during its passage through tissue cannot contribute to tissue oxygenation (see p. 458). In these circumstances a patient may have a haemoglobin level of 16 g/dl, but if half of his haemoglobin is so avid for oxygen that it is incapable of releasing oxygen, he will have an *effective* haemoglobin level of only 8 g/dl. Consequently erythropoietin production will be stimulated and the patient will present with a pathologically raised haemoglobin level – polycythaemia.

The opposite situation, i.e. reduced erythropoietin production due to a circulating haemoglobin with a reduced oxygen affinity which releases more oxygen to the tissues than normal.

Pathological (uncontrolled) production of erythropoietin

In certain circumstances, the feed-back mechanism governing the control of erythropoietin production breaks down. Such patients, with excessive quantities of plasma erythropoietin production, will have an increased number of circulating red cells, i.e. will have polycythaemia. This statement necessarily implies that the erythropoietic tissue in the marrow is capable of responding to erythropoietin by increasing red cell production. However, in many aplastic anaemias (see p. 452), the renal erythropoietin production is raised, but the anaemia persists because the marrow cannot respond to the challenge.

The quantitation of erythropoietin

The quantitation of erythropoietin is time consuming but can be measured by ^{59}Fe uptake following the injection of the urine or plasma in mice or rats rendered polycythaemic in order to depress their own erythropoietin production.

LEUCOCYTOSIS

An increase in leucocytes, usually neutrophils, in the peripheral blood.

Main causes of neutrophil leucocytosis
  (i) Acute bacterial infections.
 (ii) Neoplastic conditions, e.g. rapidly growing tumours, Hodgkin's disease.
(iii) Chronic granulocytic leukaemia.
 (iv) Following acute haemorrhage or haemolysis.
  (v) Myelofibrosis.
 (vi) Polycythaemia rubra vera.
(vii) Tissue damage, e.g. burns, infarcts, surgical operations.

Main causes of eosinophil leucocytosis
  (i) Parasitic infestation, especially when tissues are involved, e.g. helminths and schistosomiasis.
 (ii) Allergic conditions, e.g. asthma, hay fever, various drug reactions.
(iii) Malignant conditions with metastasis; Hodgkin's disease (in about 5 per cent of cases), carcinomatosis.
 (iv) Skin conditions of generalized distribution, e.g. dermatitis herpetiformis, eczema, pemphigus.
  (v) Polyarteritis nodosa.
 (vi) Miscellaneous, including: familial eosinophilia and pulmonary eosinophilia (Loeffler's syndrome).

Main causes of basophil leucocytosis
 (i) Most often found in association with chronic granulocytic leukaemia.
(ii) Myeloproliferative disorders, e.g. polycythaemia rubra vera, myelosclerosis.

LYMPHOCYTOSIS

It is important to distinguish a *relative* lymphocytosis which is due to reduction of neutrophils from a real increase in lymphocytes – *absolute* lymphocytosis.

Main causes
  (i) Acute virus and bacterial infections, e.g. infectious mononucleosis, whooping cough, mumps, rubella.
 (ii) Chronic infections, e.g. tuberculosis, brucellosis.
(iii) Chronic lymphocytic leukaemia.
 (iv) Lymphoma with 'spill-over' into the peripheral blood.

MONOCYTOSIS

Main causes
  (i) Infections, e.g. tuberculosis, typhoid, brucellosis.
 (ii) Neoplastic conditions, e.g. Hodgkin's disease and carcinoma.
(iii) Protozoal infections, e.g. trypanosomiasis, kala-azar, malaria.
 (iv) Leukaemia – monocytic and myelomonocytic.

LEUKAEMOID REACTIONS

In some conditions, leucocyte production is so marked in response to an inflammatory or neoplastic lesion, that the picture mimics a leukaemic state. In the more common granulocytic type, myelocytes, metamyelocytes and even a few 'blast' cells, may be present in the blood so that diagnosis may be difficult. The mature granulocytes, however, frequently show toxic granulation and the neutrophil alkaline phosphatase is typically much increased (c.f. p. 446).

Causes
  (i) Acute infections especially in childhood or when overwhelming: granulocytic, e.g. septicaemia, pneumonia, meningococcal. Lymphocytic, e.g. whooping cough, infectious mononucleosis.
 (ii) Neoplasia, e.g. carcinoma with multiple metastases in bone.
(iii) Toxic, e.g. extensive burns, fulminating ulcerative colitis.

LEUCO-ERYTHROBLASTOSIS

When immature cells of both red cells (normoblasts) and granulocyte (myelocytes, metamyelocytes, myeloblasts) type appear in the blood together with anaemia, the condition is termed leuco-erythroblastic. The cause is usually either metastasic malignant disease in bone or a myeloproliferative disorder, e.g. myelofibrosis (see p. 459).

INFECTIOUS MONONUCLEOSIS – GLANDULAR FEVER

Nature
World-wide in distribution and affecting predominantly young adults. It is probably caused by the Epstein–Barr (EB) virus, which was originally isolated from Burkitt's lymphoma in Africa (see p. 583). Most often sporadic in occurrence and as such is not contagious, but there is evidence that it may be transmitted by intimate mouth to mouth contact. The clinical features usually last for 3–4 weeks but changes in blood film, serology and residual debility may last for months.

Clinical
1 *Fever.* Often mild but may reach 40°C with malaise and marked debility.
2 *Pharyngitis.* Severely inflamed pharynx and fauces with hyperplasia of tonsils. Oedema of soft palate with membranous exudate which does not bleed when separated.
3 *Lymphadenopathy.* Almost invariably present. Symmetrical, bilateral and tender, particularly in the cervical and supraclavicular groups: firm, discrete and unattached.
4 *Splenomegaly.* Occurs in over 50 per cent of cases. Usually moderate to about 4 cm below the costal margin. Splenic rupture occurs rarely.
5 *Hepatic involvement.* Liver palpable in 30 per cent cases with abnormal enzyme tests in almost all patients. Jaundice is a feature in about 8 per cent.
6 *Rash.* Usually on the trunk. May mimic other exanthemata – especially scarlet fever and rubella.
7 *Haemorrhage.* Epistaxes, bleeding gums or haemoptysis: rarely gastro-intestinal. Purpura may occur but thrombocytopenia is not usually marked.
8 *Central nervous system.* Neurological symptoms in about 2 per cent including headache, blurring of vision and meningism. Rarely spinal cord involvement with respiratory paralysis and peripheral and cranial nerve palsies.
9 *Gastro-intestinal.* Nausea, vomiting and central abdominal pain may be troublesome.

Blood changes
1 Anaemia is usually absent unless complicated by haemolysis (see p. 486).
2 The total white cell count is commonly 12 to 18×10^9/l.
3 The 'glandular fever' cell. The leucocytosis is due to the presence of mononuclear cells of an abnormal or 'atypical' variety. These are large (12–18 μm) with a nucleus which has condensations of chromatin but which only rarely contains nucleoli (i.e. *not* a typical leukaemic cell). The cytoplasm is abundant, grey-blue in colour and often foamy and fenestrated. The cytoplasm stains notably more intensely at the periphery where it is indented by adjacent red cells.
4 Thrombocytopenia is uncommon but occasionally severe.

Bone marrow
This is only examined if the diagnosis is in doubt. There are no specific changes.

Histology
The lymph nodes are hyperplastic but show preservation of normal architecture (see p. 43). The liver may show an active hepatitis (see p. 551).

Serology
Patients with infectious mononucleosis have serum agglutinins against sheep red cells – *heterophile antibodies* – because they appear to react against antigenic material different from the antigen that stimulated their production. A titre higher than 1:112 is definitely significant though high titres may also be found in certain other lymphoproliferative diseases, e.g. leukaemia, lymphoma and in polycythaemia, serum sickness and after immunization with blood group substances. 'Forssman' antibodies which also agglutinate sheep red cells are found in healthy subjects. All these antibodies react with other animal tissues including guinea-pig kidney. The differential absorption test depends on the fact that the heterophile antibodies of infectious mononucleosis are not absorbed (or only partially) by guinea-pig kidney but completely by ox red cells. *Cold agglutinins* appear in a number of cases, most often IgM in type with anti-i specificity: rarely they may cause overt haemolytic anaemia.

Diagnosis
Infectious mononucleosis may simulate many diseases: pharyngitis due to streptococci, Vincent's

angina and diphtheria, Liver dysfunction must be distinguished from infective hepatitis and the serum examined for HB_sAg (see p. 551).

General infectious diseases, e.g. influenza, brucellosis, thyroid, rubella and other exanthemata, may need exclusion.

Acute lymphoblastic or monocytic leukaemia can be excluded by a bone marrow examination if necessary.

Malignant lymphoma, e.g. Hodgkin's disease, is distinguished by a lymph node biopsy when diagnosis is particularly difficult.

All the abnormalites may not be present simultaneously and tests may be carried out after serology or blood abnormalities have returned to normal.

Treatment

No specific therapy available.

1 Supportive treatment – corticosteroid therapy if prostration severe or where liver involvement is marked.

2 Acquired haemolytic anaemia and thrombocytopenia are indications for corticosteroid therapy.

Antibiotics are valueless except when there is secondary infection.

Chapter 78
Haematology – Marrow Failure, Spleen, Myeloproliferative Disorders

Normal blood cell production

Types of marrow failure
Functional
Aplastic
  Definition
    Pancytopenia
    Aplastic anaemia

Causes of aplastic marrow failure
Familial
Acquired
Familial aplasia
  Fanconi's anaemia
  Diamond–Blackfan anaemia
Acquired aplasia
  Acute
  Chronic
    Idiopathic
    Thymoma-associated
    Drugs and chemicals
    X- and gamma-irradiation
    Secondary anaemias
    With P.N.H.
    Pre-leukaemic state
Laboratory findings
  Blood count
  Blood film
  Marrow
  Haemoglobin analysis
  Serum iron and T.I.B.C.
  Ferrokinetics
  Cytogenetics
Treatment
  Supportive
  Steroids
  Splenectomy
  Marrow transplant
Prognosis

Spleen
Functions
  Haemopoiesis
    Foetal
    Adult
  Cell modification
    Pitting
    Culling
  Cell sequestration
  Cell destruction
  Role in iron metabolism
  Immunoprotection
    Antibody formation
    Phagocytosis
  Control of plasma volume
Effects of splenectomy
Hypersplenism
Causes of splenomegaly
  Infections
  Congestion
  Myeloproliferative disorders
  Lymphoproliferative disorders
  Lipid storage and associated diseases
  Systemic diseases
  Haemolytic anaemias
Investigation of splenic function

Chronic myeloproliferative syndromes
Definition
Types

Polycythaemia
Definition
Classification
  Primary
  Secondary

Polycythaemia vera
Age
Sex
Clinical
Blood findings
Bone marrow
Other investigations
  Red cell volume
  Plasma uric acid
Diagnosis
Prognosis
Treatment

Myelosclerosis – myelofibrosis
Definition
Age and sex
Clinical
  Splenomegaly
  Hepatomegaly
  Other clinical features
Blood findings
Bone marrow
Other laboratory investigations
Radiological features
Isotope studies
Diagnosis
Prognosis
Treatment

Essential thrombocythaemia
Definition
Clinical picture
Haematology
Bone marrow
Treatment
Results

Normal blood cell production

In the normal adult, approximately $2\frac{1}{2}$ million red cells are made and destroyed every minute. This corresponds to about 2×10^{11} cells – which is about 20 ml – every day. As 1 ml of red cells contains very nearly 1 mg of iron there must be an effective turnover of 20 mg of iron every day in the red cells of normal adults. This is about two-thirds of the total body iron turnover as radioactively measured.

More precisely, adult men produce about $2\cdot9 \times 10^9$ red cells per kilogram body weight per day (or $0\cdot25$ ml red cells); and women $2\cdot5 \times 10^9$ ($0\cdot21$ ml red cells).

The production of white cells and platelets is more difficult to assess. Some lymphocytes are very long-lived, while granulocytes and platelets are turned over very rapidly as they only survive in the circulation for a few days.

Under normal conditions, the numbers of cells made and destroyed are equal – i.e. the turnover, is constant. Whenever destruction exceeds production, anaemia will develop and will only stop progressing when production once again equals destruction at a lower equilibrium.

Excessive destruction with normal or increased production is characteristic of haemolytic states. Diminished production with normal destruction is characteristic of the anaemias of bone marrow failure.

Types of marrow failure

Functional
The bone marrow may contain many cells, which are dividing and metabolizing very actively, but which are unable to produce enough viable mature cells. This *'ineffective haemopoiesis'*, or *'ineffective erythropoiesis'* if only the red cells are affected, is characteristic of the megaloblastic anaemias, thalassaemia major and the leukaemias.

Aplastic
Cell production declines because of a decrease in absolute numbers of the precursor or stem cells. If very early stem cells are affected, all the cellular elements will be diminished in the blood – complete pancytopenia.

However, only some cell lines may be affected, leaving others intact. This depends on the level of stem cell affected (Fig. 44). In myelogenous (marrow-producing) pancytopenia, in which the lymphoid stem cell line is intact, only the myelogenous line is diminished. If just one of the later stem cells of the myelogenous line is affected, e.g. erythroblasts, there will be a specific lack of one cell line – in this case *pure red cell aplasia*.

DEFINITION

Pancytopenia
Reduced cell production will be reflected by a pancytopenia in the blood and may accompany either an ineffective or an aplastic marrow.

Aplastic anaemia
Pancytopenia, caused by an aplastic marrow, can only be diagnosed by a bone-marrow biopsy which shows diminished or absent haemopoiesis.

Causes of aplastic marrow failure

Familial
1 Fanconi's anaemia – all cell types.
2 Diamond–Blackfan anaemia – red cells only.

Acquired
1 *Acute*:
(a) Transient infections.
(b) Episodic in hyperactive marrows.
2 *Chronic*:
(a) Idiopathic.
(b) Thymoma-associated red cell aplasia.
(c) Drugs and chemicals:
  (i) Dose dependent.
  (ii) Idiosyncratic.
(d) X-irradiation.
(e) Secondary to other disorders – the anaemias of chronic disorders:
  (i) Chronic inflammatory states.
  (ii) Renal insufficiency.
  (iii) Neoplastic diseases.
(f) Accompanying paroxysmal nocturnal haemoglobinuria (P.N.H.).
(g) The 'pre-leukaemic' state.

Familial aplasia

FANCONI'S ANAEMIA
Rare; also affects skeleton and gonads. Full disorder characterized by:
1 Pancytopenia.

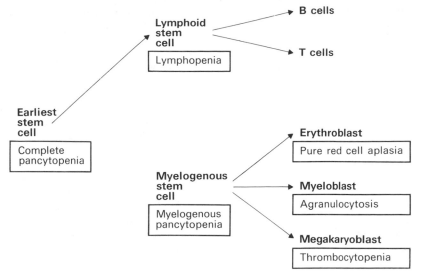

Fig. 44. How the blood is affected by aplasia according to the stem-cell level affected.

2 Marrow aplasia – sometimes patchy.

3 Skin hyperpigmentation.

4 Skeletal malformations, especially of wrist and thumb.

5 Small stature.

6 Hypogonadism.

7 Familial occurrence.

8 Additionally, there may be mental retardation and renal abnormalities.

An individual may show only a few of these features.

DIAMOND–BLACKFAN ANAEMIA

Rare; sole defect is the pure red cell aplasia. Can be severe, becoming manifest any time after birth, and requiring life-saving blood transfusions. There are occasional periods of remission in some cases.

Acquired aplasia

ACUTE

May accompany many viral infections, particularly RNA viruses; e.g. rubella, influenza, mumps, hepatitis. Is usually transient.

Hyperactive marrows such as those in chronic haemolytic states are particularly liable to episodes of aplasia after viral infections.

CHRONIC

Idiopathic

Usually, an intensive enquiry into the drug or environmental history, or sometimes further investigation, elicits a cause. The diagnosis of idiopathic aplasia is therefore one of exclusion.

Thymoma-associated

Very rare cases of pure red cell aplasia associated with a thymoma, and sometimes with myasthenia gravis, have been reported. Removal of the thymoma usually, but not always, cures the anaemia.

Drugs and chemicals

These constitute the majority of cases of aplasia. Reactions are of two types:

(i) Drugs which always cause aplasia, the degree being dependent on the dose received. This is mostly confined to drugs used in cancer chemotherapy and in immunosuppression, which are unavoidably toxic to all dividing cells.

(ii) In certain individuals only, due to an idiosyncrasy to the drug. 'High risk' preparations include those which only infrequently produce aplasia but are used widely – such as chloramphenicol in some parts of the world – and those used less widely but which have a greater incidence – such as gold. Other preparations produce aplasia only very infrequently, but the aplasia can be lethal. Such drugs should be regarded as having a 'moderate' but definite risk. Some, such as chlorothiazide are particularly notable for just producing agranulocytosis.

It should be remembered that many drugs have been incriminated in sporadic cases of aplasia, and comprehensive lists are difficult to compile and always incomplete. This list is therefore intended merely to show the more common examples:

(i) *Dose dependent*
   Azathioprine
   Busulphan
   Cytosine arabinoside
   Daunorubicin
   Mercaptopurine
   Methotrexate
   Mustine and derivatives
   Procarbazine
   Vinblastine
   Vincristine.
(ii) *By idiosyncrasy*
   High risk
   Arsenicals
   Benzene
   Chloramphenicol
   Colchicine
   Gold
   Mesantoin and related drugs
   Phenylbutazone
   Tolbutamide
   Moderate but definite risk
   Chlorothiazide
   Chlorpromazine
   Indomethacin
   Isoniazid
   Nitrofurantoin
   Para-amino salicylate
   Penicillin
   Quinidine
   Sulphonamides
   Tetracycline

Exposure to X- and gamma-irradiation
Causes complete pancytopenia. The radiosensitive lymphocytes disappear rapidly, but anaemia develops only slowly as the red cells reach the end of their life span. Reticulocytopenia is found after the first day; and agranulocytosis and thrombocytopenia after 3 or 4 days.

Secondary anaemias
The anaemias of chronic disorders. Marrow failure characterizes many chronic disorders which are otherwise unrelated (see p. 509). The anaemia is part of the systemic manifestation of the disease and can only be relieved after effective treatment of the original disorder. Erythropoiesis becomes hypoplastic, the release of iron stores to the developing red cells is reduced and both the serum iron and the T.I.B.C. are low. The E.S.R. is often very high as a reflection of the primary disorder.

(i) Chronic inflammatory states. This includes both infective and non-infective conditions. Osteomyelitis, bacterial endocarditis, rheumatoid disease, S.L.E. and the other connective tissue diseases all have similar effects on the marrow.

(ii) Renal insufficiency. Untreated chronic renal failure produces marrow failure by the accumulation of toxic metabolites. Many cases (except polycystic disease and some adenocarcinomas) also have reduced erythropoietin production (see p. 511) so that removal of the metabolites by haemodialysis fails to relieve the anaemia.

Haemoglobin levels of 5 g/dl are usual in patients on chronic dialysis: they are mostly well compensated for the anaemia, and their marrow samples usually show normal numbers of red cell precursors indicating that the marrow-suppressive effects of the metabolites have been removed. However, inspection of the cells show a ragged appearance betraying their ineffectiveness. These patients are frequently venesected for numerous tests and it is wise to prevent iron deficiency by prophylactic iron therapy.

(iii) Neoplastic states. Debilitating carcinomatosis is usually accompanied by anaemia even in the absence of haemorrhage. The leukaemias and lymphomas are considered separately (see p. 462) and modern therapy has complicated the issue of anaemia in these disorders. Anaemia is unusual even in advanced Hodgkin's disease at presentation, but may occur, particularly at the terminal stages.

Aplasia accompanying paroxysmal nocturnal haemoglobinuria – P.N.H.
P.N.H. is caused by a somatic mutation in the myeloid cell line and affects red cells, granulocytes and platelets. The most common manifestation is haemolysis (see p. 491) but about 20 per cent of

cases develop marrow aplasia. The hallmark of P.N.H. is the acidified serum lysis test – *Ham's test* – which demonstrates the increased sensitivity of the red cell membrane to complement.

There have been several documented cases of temporary or permanent aplastic anaemia following a well recognized cause such as a drug, which have subsequently developed a positive Ham's test. Such cases are usually regarded as genuine P.N.H. following aplasia even if a period of recovery has preceded the development of the positive Ham's test. In such cases, the drug may have induced a mutation.

Aplasia and the pre-leukaemic state
There is an increased incidence of leukaemia developing in aplastic anaemia, particularly in idiopathic forms. P.N.H. is also associated with an increased incidence of leukaemia.

In *Subleukaemic leukaemia* there is pancytopenia, but the marrow is hypercellular and the majority of cells are leukaemic blasts. Careful inspection of the blood film will often reveal a few of these blast cells.

It is important, therefore, to follow by blood film as examination all patients with aplastic anaemia in order to anticipate the possible onset of leukaemia.

Laboratory findings in marrow aplasia

BLOOD COUNT
Anaemia with decrease of relevant cell lines. Cell indices (MCH, MCV, MCHC) usually normal. Reticulocyte count low – less than 0·2 per cent (2×10^6/l).

BLOOD FILM
Normocytic normochromic red cells.
White cells and platelets diminished according to lines affected. Morphology unremarkable.

MARROW
Aspirate – hypocellular or acellular fragments with hypocellular trails. May be a dry or blood tap.
Biopsy – confirms hypocellularity.

Sometimes the sample may show normal cellularity, but when repeated in another site the aplasia is revealed. This indicates that the disorder may be patchy.

HAEMOGLOBIN ANALYSIS
There is often a rise in foetal haemoglobin level, shown both by electrophoretic and alkali-resistant analysis. Usually up to 5–10 per cent of total; occasionally reaching over 50 per cent.

SERUM IRON AND T.I.B.C.
In the untreated *anaemias of chronic disorders* both may be low, with a normal percentage of transferrin saturation. In idiopathic aplasia, the serum iron may be high, particularly if the patient has received blood transfusions.

FERROKINETICS
In normal persons, radioactive iron injected intravenously can be traced to the marrow within an hour or two, and subsequently in blood cells after several days. In aplastic anaemia, the marrow uptake is impaired, confirming the lack of red cell production.

CYTOGENETICS
Usually normal. However, inconstant chromosome breakages may be found in Fanconi's anaemia and after exposure to X-rays and some chemicals such as benzene.

Treatment

SUPPORTIVE
The anaemia may be relieved by blood transfusions but it is important to minimize the onset of iron overload.

Platelet transfusions may be necessary to control bleeding episodes and neutrophil transfusions – which can be prepared using modern cell-separating equipment – have been advocated in the control of infections. However, it may be important to minimize contact with incompatible HLA if bone marrow transplantation is to be considered. For this reason, it may be wise to use white-cell poor red cells, i.e. washed red cells, for the anaemia.

Vigorous antibiotic therapy is indicated in infections, but there is probably no place for prophylactic antibiotics.

STEROIDS
Corticosteroid therapy may be helpful in thrombocytopenia (see p. 517). However, they do not have any marrow-stimulating effect and they also induce lymphopenia.

Anabolic steroids increase haemopoiesis, particularly erythropoiesis, in normal marrow. Opinion is divided on their effect in aplastic marrows, but high doses of oxymetholone or a related drug may be beneficial. Unfortunately hepatotoxic and androgenic side effects are common at the doses required, and remission may not occur for 2–3 months.

SPLENECTOMY

Occasionally, particularly after many transfusions, the spleen becomes enlarged and transfusion requirements increase – i.e. hypersplenism has developed (see p. 457). In these circumstances, splenectomy may be beneficial, but it has no place in the routine management of aplastic anaemia.

MARROW TRANSPLANT

There are reports of success, when marrow from a well-matched histocompatible donor is used. Myeloid antigen systems, other than the major HLA system, may cause rejection of the donor cells unless immunosuppressive treatment is given to the recipient. Unfortunately, this does not eradicate the donor lymphocytes, which are able to override present immunosuppressive drugs, and induce a 'graft-versus-host' reaction because they recognize the recipient as being foreign. This is the main complication of marrow transplants at present.

Prognosis

Acute episodes of aplasia are usually self-limiting although supportive therapy may be required when the pancytopenia is most profound.

Chronic aplasia is more difficult. Wherever possible, the cause must be removed, but unfortunately, especially after some drug exposures, the aplasia may persist. Supportive therapy must always be given in the hope of a remission developing. Profound thrombocytopenia is an unfavourable sign and, unless it resolves, is usually fatal. Unfortunately, thrombocytopenia is resistant to anabolic steroid therapy. The success rate of allogeneic transplantation (matched sibling) is now 60–70 per cent long-term survival.

Spleen

In effect, the spleen is a large contained mass of lymphoid tissue connected to the systemic blood circulation. Normal weight 150-200g.

Functions

HAEMOPOIESIS

Foetal
Granulopoiesis and platelet production in early life. Erythropoiesis in mid-uterine life.

Adult
Monocyte and lymphocyte production only except:
(i) Myeloid metaplasia, e.g. in myelofibrosis (see p. 459) when all lines of cells may be produced in the spleen.
(ii) Congenital haemolytic anaemia, e.g. thalassaemia – persistent erythropoiesis in the spleen post-natally.

CELL MODIFICATION

Pitting
Removal of iron particles from siderocytes by phagocytic cells.

Culling
Removal of nuclear remnants – *Howell–Jolly bodies*, from red cells.

CELL SEQUESTRATION – POOLING

A reservoir function, not affecting red cells in healthy humans. There is a pool of neutrophils and at least one-third of the body's platelets in the spleen.

CELL DESTRUCTION

Red cells are removed by the spleen towards the end of their life-span where they become spherocytic and are then destroyed. Some neutrophils are destroyed in the spleen and most platelets.

ROLE IN IRON METABOLISM

Iron released from 'haem' in the spleen is more effectively transported to marrow iron stores than from other sites, and is then re-utilized for red cell haemoglobin.

IMMUNOPROTECTION

Antibody formation
In early childhood a serious hazard following splenectomy is vulnerability to infection. Less serious in later life.

Phagocytosis
By cells of the phagocytic cell system in the pulp (see below).

CONTROL OF PLASMA VOLUME
Spleen possibly plays a role – plasma volume varies with splenic enlargement (see p. 460).

Effects of splenectomy
(i) *Thrombocythaemia*. Platelet count may rise to over $1000 \times 10^9/l$.
(ii) *Neutrophilia*. Granulocytes may rise to 15–$20 \times 10^6/l$.
(iii) *Alteration of red cell morphology*. The inclusion bodies remain in the red cells so that siderocytes and Howell–Jolly bodies are present in significant numbers.
(iv) *Lack of 'damping'*. Of marrow haemopoietic response after challenge, e.g. haemorrhage.

Hypersplenism
A reduction of one or more of the cellular elements of the circulating blood and correctable by splenectomy.
It results in:
(i) Destruction of red cells, neutrophils and/or platelets which can be demonstrated as a shortening of their life-span.
(ii) Possibly decreased marrow production of blood cells due to production of a splenic hormone.
(iii) Pooling or sequestration within the spleen.
(iv) Increase in plasma volume.
Enlarged spleens are usually but not necessarily accompanied by hypersplenism. Conversely not all spleens which produce hypersplenism are clinically palpable.

Causes of splenomegaly

INFECTIONS
Acute, e.g. bacterial endocarditis, glandular fever, typhoid, septicaemia.
Chronic, e.g. tuberculosis, syphilis, brucellosis.
Tropical, e.g. malaria, kala-azar.

CONGESTION
Cirrhosis of liver with portal venous hypertension or thrombosis, Banti's syndrome.

MYELOPROLIFERATIVE DISORDERS
Chronic granulocytic leukaemia, myelofibrosis, essential thrombocythaemia (megakaryocytic myelosis), polycythaemia rubra vera.

LYMPHOPROLIFERATIVE DISORDERS
Chronic lymphocytic leukaemia, malignant lymphomas, 'non-tropical splenomegaly'.

LIPID STORAGE AND ASSOCIATED DISEASES
Gaucher's disease, Neimann–Pick disease, histiocytosis X.

SYSTEMIC DISEASES
Sarcoidosis, systemic lupus erythematosus, rheumatoid arthritis (Felty's syndrome and Still's disease), amyloidosis.

HAEMOLYTIC ANAEMIAS
Splenic enlargement secondary to abnormality of the red cells.
Congenital, e.g. hereditary spherocytosis, hereditary elliptocytosis, pyruvate–kinase deficiency, thalassaemia, abnormal haemoglobins (e.g. sickle cell disease in children and S-C disease).
Acquired, e.g. auto-immune haemolytic anaemia, paroxysmal nocturnal haemoglobinuria, haemolytic disease of the newborn.

Investigation of splenic function
Labelling of patient's red cells with radioactive chromium; ^{51}Cr, as hexavalent anions of sodium chromate diffuse into red cells where reduction occurs to trivalent cations which bind to the β chains of the haemoglobin molecule. The 'labelled' cells can then be re-injected in saline suspension.
1 *Sequestration or pooling of red cells*. Can be demonstrated by placing a surface counter over the spleen. Normally, equilibration of the rate of production over the organ takes place in 90 s, but with sequestration the counts increase gradually over many minutes.
Counts are compared with those produced from the sites of the liver and the heart (as a measure of circulating radioactivity) at intervals over several days, thus providing evidence of whether the spleen and/or the liver are organs of excess red cell destruction.
2 *Plasma volume expansion*. May be measured by using radioactivated human serum albumin which is injected into one arm and a venous sample taken 10 min later from the other arm. The ^{131}I-labelled

plasma is separated from the blood by centrifuging. The plasma volume is calculated from the formula:

$$\frac{\text{Counts per millilitre per minute injected} \times \text{volume injected}}{\text{Counts per millilitre per minute in 10 min sample}}$$

Chronic myeloproliferative syndromes

Definition
A group of disorders arising from a proliferative process involving one or more cell elements of the bone marrow. The liver and spleen are also frequently involved.

Types
It is reasonable to consider the pathogenesis of these conditions by reference to the development of haemopoietic tissue from a common multipotential stem cell.

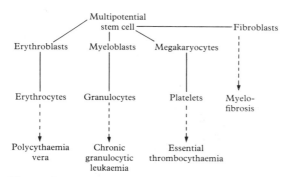

Fig. 45. The pathogenesis of myeloproliferative syndromes.

Thus the chronic syndromes are:
1. Chronic granulocytic leukaemia (see p. 466).
2. Polycythaemia vera.
3. Myelofibrosis.
4. Essential thrombocythaemia.

Because of the common origin of these cell lines, there is often considerable overlap in the type of proliferation. Thus in polycythaemia there is usually a marked increase in the platelet and granulocyte series and in myelofibrosis, thrombocythaemia occurs in addition to increased granulopoiesis. Chronic granulocytic leukaemia is frequently accompanied by considerable increase in platelets in the early stages.

All these conditions may terminate in an acute myeloblastic transformation.

Because of the increased cellular turnover in these disorders there is often excessive breakdown of nucleo-protein with release of uric acid. Hyperuricaemia is a frequent complication which may produce secondary gout or uric acid calculi in the urinary tract (see p. 460).

Polycythaemia

Definition
An absolute increase in red cell volume.

Classification

PRIMARY
Myeloproliferative – polycythaemia vera.

SECONDARY
Associated disease or abnormal stimulus to erythropoiesis including:
  (i) Reduced oxygen saturation of the blood, e.g. pulmonary diseases, congenital heart disease and living at high altitudes.
 (ii) Renal lesions, e.g. carcinoma of the kidney, polycystic disease.
(iii) Other tumours, e.g. uterine fibroids, liver tumours, infratentorial brain tumours.
(iv) Acquired abnormal haemoglobin, e.g. methaemoglobinaemia.
 (v) Congenitally abnormal haemoglobins with high oxygen affinity, e.g. haemoglobin Chesapeake.

In cases of (ii) and (iii) there is inappropriate increase in erythropoietin.

Polycythaemia vera

AGE
Commonly older age groups with a peak around 50.

SEX
Male > females.

CLINICAL
Usually due to increased blood volume with thrombotic or occasionally haemorrhagic tendencies. Onset may be insidious but sometimes presents as acute cerebrovascular accident, myocardial infarction or limb gangrene.

Symptoms commonly include headache and vertigo, generalized pruritis especially in bed and bath and increased redness or cyanosis of face with suffused conjunctivae. The spleen is moderately enlarged in about 75 per cent of cases and often there is associated hepatomegaly.

Blood findings

Haemoglobin, P.C.V. and red cell counts are increased. The red cells are mostly hypochromic due to chronic blood loss. The total leucocyte count is moderately increased to $15-20 \times 10^9/l$ with neutrophilia. Neutrophil alkaline phosphatase score is high in most cases.

Platelet count is increased above $500 \times 10^9/l$ in about half the patients. The ESR is characteristically reduced to 0 or 1 mm per hour.

Bone marrow

Characteristically an increase in cellularity with reduction or total lack of fat spaces. All cell types increased with megakaryocytes particularly numerous. Staining for iron shows stores reduced or absent.

Other laboratory investigations

RED CELL VOLUME

Estimation using a radio-isotope label – usually ^{51}Cr, is the only certain way of establishing the diagnosis; the plasma volume is variable and the P.C.V. value may not therefore reflect the increase in red cell mass. Values are raised in both polycythaemia vera and secondary polycythaemia.

PLASMA URIC ACID

This is usually markedly raised.

Diagnosis

Some cases of polycythaemia vera are associated with hypertension – Gaisbock's syndrome.

Differentiation from secondary polycythaemia depends upon exclusion, e.g. by searching for tumours by pyelography, gynaecological examination etc., or by assessing lung function and arterial oxygen saturation.

The spleen is usually not enlarged in these secondary causes and the ESR is usually elevated.

The 'pseudopolycythaemia' of stress associated with an anxiety state may be confused with the myeloproliferative condition but is distinguished by a lack of cyanotic plethoric features and the absence of splenomegaly. There is only a moderate rise in red cell values and no leucocytosis or thrombocytosis. The red cell volume also is normal.

Prognosis

Episodes of vascular thrombosis may be incapacitating or fatal, otherwise terminal myelosclerosis (see below) or myeloblastic leukaemia follow. Only 50 per cent of untreated cases survive more than 2 years.

Treatment

(i) *Venesection*. Rapidly lowers the P.C.V. but does not control white cell and platelet counts. It does not, therefore, prevent vascular complications. Only increases 50 per cent survival to $3\frac{1}{2}$ years when used alone.

(ii) *Chemotherapy*. Busulphan suppresses erythropoiesis but other marrow elements are also suppressed and more markedly, with danger of thrombocytopenia. Frequent monitoring by blood counts is necessary. It is usual to combine use of this drug with intermittent venesection.

(iii) *Radiotherapy*. In the form of a single dose of radioactive phosphorus – ^{32}P, given intravenously. The advantages of this choice of therapy are the ease of administration, without the necessity for frequent blood counts and the absence of side effects. The possibility that it increases the likelihood of acute leukaemia ultimately complicating the disease has been suggested and seems likely.

The preferred treatment is a combination of venesection or removal of red cells by a cell separator to control red cell mass with ^{32}P to control the platelet count. With this regime the 50 per cent survival is about 12 years.

Busulphan is better reserved for later, more sinister myeloproliferative stages.

Myelosclerosis – Myelofibrosis

Definition

Replacement of the bone marrow by cancellous bone and/or collagen. This may follow another myeloproliferative disorder.

Age and sex

Fifty to 70 years. M:F equal.

Clinical

Patients typically present with symptoms of anaemia and gross splenic enlargement, i.e. weakness, dyspnoea and abdominal pain either 'dragging' or acute episodic.

SPLENOMEGALY
Usually extends well below the umbilicus. Splenic infarcts produce acute pain with localized tenderness and friction rubs.

HEPATOMEGALY
Is commonly present and portal hypertension may occur.

OTHER CLINICAL FEATURES
Weight loss and wasting, particularly terminally. Purpura and epistaxes due to a qualitative platelet deficiency especially with thrombocythaemia or, in thrombocytopenia in the later stages of the disease.

Blood findings
Typically a leuco-erythroblastic anaemia of variable degree. Normochromic or hypochromic red cells with marked anisocytosis and poikilocytosis. The anaemia is due to diminished red cell production and haemolysis. In the later stages 'pooling' of red cells in the spleen and increased plasma volume contribute to the reduction in haemoglobin values.

Total white cell count is often moderately increased up to 50×10^9/l.

Platelets are normal or increased but may be abnormally large and are often reduced later.

Nucleated red cells and immature granulocytes are seen in the film, the latter usually myelocytes and metamyelocytes but occasionally a few 'blast' cells are present. 'Blast' cells become numerous in the later stages of leukaemic transformation.

Bone marrow
Typically difficult to obtain due to the areas of sclerotic tissue. Aspiration of one of the intervening areas of haemopoietic tissue may show markedly increased cellularity.

Trephine bone biopsy is usually necessary and demonstrates the typical histological picture ranging from early abnormally distributed increase of reticulin with fibroblastic proliferation and increase in megakaryocytes to later collagenization of marrow spaces and increase in thickness of bone trabeculae.

Other laboratory investigations
A raised neutrophil alkaline phosphatase in most cases.

The plasma uric acid is frequently raised and may be symptomatic.

The serum folate is usually reduced, presumably due to considerably increased turnover of myeloid cells.

Radiological features
In about half the cases, typical signs of coarsening of trabeculae with mottling are seen. Most frequently this affects the upper ends of femora and humeri but may also be seen in bones of pelvis, spine and ribs.

Radioisotope studies
A moderate shortening of red cell life span to a mean cell life of 30–40 days is demonstrated by ^{51}Cr survival studies. The spleen increases the plasma volume and 'pools' red cells out of the circulation together with active destruction to a minor degree. Radioactive iron studies demonstrate that red cell utilization is decreased and that much of the erythropoiesis is ineffective. Extramedullary erythropoiesis in the spleen takes place in about 75 per cent of cases with myeloid metaplasia also commonly present in liver and lymph nodes.

Diagnosis
Chronic granulocytic leukaemia is the condition most likely to be confused with myelosclerosis because of the very large spleen and immature granulocytes in the peripheral blood in both conditions. Differentiating features are

	Myelosclerosis	Chronic granulocytic leukaemia
Lymph node enlargement	Less common	More common
Total white count	Moderately raised	Often over 100×10^9/l
Neutrophil alkaline phosphatase	Markedly raised	Reduced or nil
Platelets	Abnormal giant forms	Usually normal in size
Red cell poikilocytosis	Marked	Slight if present
Ph′ chromosome	Negative	Positive

The differential diagnosis must also include tuberculosis and other causes of leuco-erythroblastic anaemia (see p. 448).

Prognosis
Average life expectancy is about 7 years, usually

with termination by pancytopenia or acute myelo-blastic transformation.

Treatment

(i) *Supportive therapy*. Blood transfusion is the main form of therapy available.

(ii) *Bone marrow stimulus*. Anabolic steroids, e.g. oxymethalone, may help: corticosteroids are doubtfully effective.

(iii) *Folic acid supplements*. May partially rectify the anaemia.

(iv) *Cytotoxic therapy*. By ^{32}P or Busulphan if leucocyte and platelet counts are high, but used with caution.

(v) *Splenectomy*. May be indicated if isotope studies indicate marked red cell destruction and 'pooling' in the spleen. Splenic irradiation may occasionally be helpful.

(vi) *Hyperuricaemia*. Should be anticipated and treated with allopurinol.

Essential thrombocythaemia

Definition

A sustained rise in platelet count which is usually as high as $1000 \times 10^9/l$ or more. It is often difficult to distinguish from other myeloproliferative disorders except for the particularly excessive platelet production.

Clinical picture

Typically a middle aged or elderly person with a recent history of spontaneous haemorrhage, e.g. gastro-intestinal or urinary with bruising. Spleno-megaly is marked and hepatomegaly is also commonly found.

Haematology

Massive increase in platelets, verified in the blood film where frequent abnormal giant forms are usually seen. They may be poorly functional. There may be an associated leucocytosis, red cells usually normal in appearance may be increased in number.

Bone marrow

Increase proliferation of all cell elements with megakaryocytes particularly abundant.

Treatment

Cytotoxic therapy with either ^{32}P or Busulphan. For the reasons mentioned previously (see p. 459) radioactive phosphorus is usually preferable.

Results

Poor: death usually from haemorrhage associated with poor function of the enormous numbers of platelets.

Chapter 79
Haematology – Leukaemia, Lymphoma, Myeloma

The leukaemias

Nature

Conditions resulting from neoplastic proliferation of leucocytes. In the more common varieties either lymphoid cells or myelogenous cells are involved. When the proliferation affects the early, immature cells the disease is recognized to be acute leukae-mia – commonly *lymphoblastic* or *myeloblastic*. In the more slowly progressive states, predominantly mature cells are present in excess – *chronic lymphocytic* and *chronic granulocytic leukaemia*. Much less commonly, the monocytic series is involved. Chronic monocytic leukaemia is very rare.

In all forms of leukaemia, the abnormal proliferating cells affect the bone marrow. Normal haemo-

poiesis is disorganized and therefore these conditions, sooner or later, produce:
1 Anaemia.
2 Neutropenia – resulting in severe infections.
3 Thrombocytopenia – resulting in spontaneous haemorrhages.
    Ultimately – total failure of marrow function.

Aetiology
The following factors have been related:
1 Association with congenital disorders, e.g. Down's syndrome (see p. 13).
2 Exposure to ionizing radiation, e.g. X-rays, nuclear fission products (see p. 75).
3 Benzene poisoning.
4 Virus infections, oncorna types.

Age incidence
Chronic leukaemias especially lymphocytic are more common in the older age groups. Acute leukaemia has a higher incidence in childhood where it is lymphoblastic in type and another peak in the 40–60-year-old subjects when it is more often myeloblastic.

Acute leukaemia

Types
1 *Lymphoblastic (ALL)* – variants:
Common – non-T, non-B.
Thy-ALL.
B-cell ALL.
2 *Myeloblastic (AML)* – variants:
Poorly differentiated
Well differentiated
Promyelocytic

Nature
A neoplastic proliferation of primitive 'blast' cells in the bone marrow. Infiltration of the liver and spleen also occurs and, in lymphoblastic leukaemia, there is prominent involvement of the lymph nodes. Other tissues affected may be the central nervous system, kidneys, skin and lungs.

Clinical
The patient typically presents with symptoms of anaemia, fever, infection and spontaneous bruising or bleeding from mucous membranes, particularly the gums.
    There is enlargement of liver, spleen and lymph nodes – the latter especially in the lymphoblastic type. Oral ulceration with white leukaemic deposits at the gum margins is very common.
    Pain and tenderness in bones especially in children is common.

Blood
Typically
    Anaemia. Moderate to severe with Hb level of from 7 to 9 g/dl.
    Platelet count usually very low—about 30×10^9/l.
    Total white count much increased up to 200×10^9/l.
    Blood film and differential white cell count – platelets scanty, red cells normochromic. The predominant white cell is the 'blast' cell with only a few scattered mature neutrophils and lymphocytes.
    The 'blast' cell. This is a large cell similar to the earliest granulocyte precursor which is seen in small numbers in the normal bone marrow (see p. 446). About 16 μm in size, with basophilic cytoplasm and prominent nucleoli. In acute myeloblastic leukaemia the blast cells may contain Auer rods.
    In 'subleukaemic' cases a normal or reduced total white count is found and, in the blood film, 'blast' cells may be present in only small numbers or even totally absent.

Bone marrow
Marked hypercellularity due to great increase in 'blast' cells. Consequently, normal granulopoiesis and erythropoiesis is excluded and much reduced. Occasionally erythropoiesis is megaloblastic due to the rival demands on available folate by the proliferating 'blast' cells.

Diagnosis
1 Lymphoblastic or myeloblastic? (See Fig. 46. p. 464.)
    Immunological markers and enzyme assays. These also help to differentiate acute lymphoblastic (ALL) and acute myeloblastic leukaemias (AML). They are very helpful in recognizing the individual variants – common (non-B, non-T), Thy-ALL and the rare B-ALL. The enzyme terminal deoxynucleotidyl-transferase (TdT) is increased in ALL and normal in AML blasts.
2 Subleukaemic leukaemia. May be confused with aplastic anaemia (see p. 452) because in both conditions there is:
 (i) Pancytopenia – often without immature leucocytes.
(ii) Hepatosplenomegaly is not usually found.

		Lymphoblastic	Myeloblastic
Age		Children	Usually 30–60
Lymphadenmopathy		Usually	Uncommonly
Bone marrow	Blast cells	Nucleoli 1 or 2	Nucleoli 3–5
	Promyelocytes	Few	Increased
Peripheral blood	Immature granulocytes	Few	Increased
	Neut. alk. phosphatase	Increased	Reduced
Cytoplasmic special stains	(i) Periodic acid Schiff	Coarse clumps	Faintly diffuse
	(ii) Sudan black	Negative	Positive granules

Fig. 46. Salient features of lymphoblastic and myeloblastic leukaemias.

Bone marrow examination is, however, diagnostic as, even at this stage, numerous blasts are present.

3 Purpura – both thrombocytopenic and non-thrombocytopenic (see p. 516).

4 Fever and lymphadenopathy, e.g. infectious mononucleosis (see p. 449).

5 Bone pain, e.g. osteomyelitis. Radiology should help.

6 Throat infection, e.g. acute tonsillitis. Microbiology assists.

Treatment

1 *Supportive*

  (i) Prevent infection by antibiotic therapy and barrier nursing or isolation.

 (ii) Blood transfusion to relieve anaemia.

(iii) Platelet transfusion to control haemorrhage.

(iv) Allopurinol to reduce plasma uric acid released from leukaemic cells.

 (v) In the promyelocytic variant of AML, disseminated intravascular coagulation (DIC) is likely and heparin and vigorous platelet support are required.

2 *Specific anti-leukaemic therapy*

(i) Combination chemotherapy by cytotoxic drugs (see p. 465). A wide range of such substances are available and new agents and differing mixtures are constantly being tried. The objectives of any mixture should be:

(a) Reduce the development of resistance to the therapy which tends to happen when a single agent is used.

(b) Enhance their effectiveness synergistically.

The situation is thus analogous to combined therapy used in bacterial infection.

(c) Smaller doses so that their individual unwanted toxic effects, e.g. marrow depression or neurotoxicity, are reduced but their combined antitumour action is sustained.

(ii) X-ray therapy when central nervous system is affected in acute lymphoblastic leukaemia. Applied to brain and/or spinal cord, supplemented with intrathecal methotrexate. Also used prophylactically after the first remission and in continuation therapy.

Courses of combined therapy are always given at planned intervals so that the drugs will attack the neoplastic dividing cells but then allow sufficient time for the normal cells, especially those of the bone marrow, to recover during the rest periods.

In the treatment of acute leukaemia the principles pursued are sequentially:

1 To produce a remission.

2 To reduce the total number of malignant cells as low as possible.

3 Continuation therapy to maintain remission. Usually in the form of further combination therapy and, in the case of myeloblastic leukaemia, immunotherapy with BCG and infusions of killed leukaemic cells.

4 Bone-marrow transplantation. Allogeneic marrow from an HLA-compatible sibling is used in some centres following first remission in patients under 40 years with AML and in ALL patients after a second successful remission. Intensive chemotherapy and irradiation is first given to remove all residual leukaemic cells.

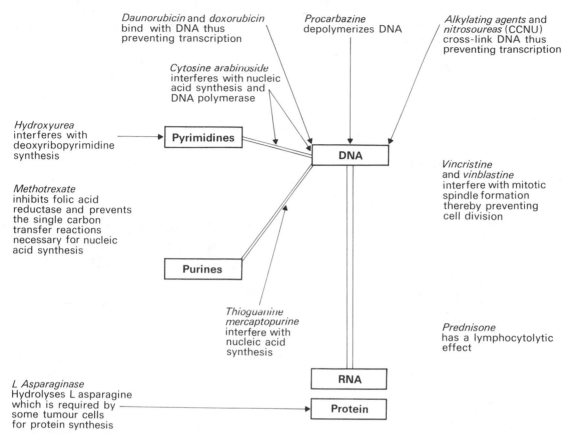

Daunorubicin and *doxorubicin*
bind with DNA thus
preventing transcription

Procarbazine
depolymerizes DNA

Alkylating agents and
nitrosoureas (CCNU)
cross-link DNA thus
preventing transcription

Cytosine arabinoside
interferes with nucleic
acid synthesis and
DNA polymerase

Hydroxyurea
interferes with
deoxyribopyrimidine
synthesis

Pyrimidines

DNA

Vincristine
and *vinblastine*
interfere with mitotic
spindle formation
thereby preventing
cell division

Methotrexate
inhibits folic acid
reductase and prevents
the single carbon
transfer reactions
necessary for nucleic
acid synthesis

Purines

Thioguanine
mercaptopurine
interfere with
nucleic acid
synthesis

Prednisone
has a lymphocytolytic
effect

L Asparaginase
Hydrolyses L asparagine
which is required by
some tumour cells
for protein synthesis

RNA

Protein

Fig. 47. Some important chemotherapeutic mechanisms.

Prognosis

A variable course with occasional spontaneous remissions but which untreated is invariably fatal, usually from haemorrhage or infection.

With careful treatment methods currently available, the 50 per cent median survival in lymphoblastic leukaemia is 5 years and in myeloblastic cases, 16 months. Between 30 and 50 per cent of children with common ALL (non-B, non-T) can expect to be alive and off all treatment 5 years from presentation. There is a less favourable prognosis in the rare B-ALL, and Thy-ALL (20 per cent of all cases) carries a high relapse rate.

Chronic lymphocytic leukaemia

Incidence
Commonly aged 50–70; M:F 2:1.

Clinical

Usually symptomless and discovered accidentally. Otherwise typically:

1 Splenomegaly. Sensation of increasing fullness and prominence of the abdomen. Sometimes with attacks of acute left hypochondrial pain due to splenic infarcts.

2 Anaemia. Due to reduced erythropoiesis and/or acquired haemolytic anaemia (see p. 504).

3 Lymphadenopathy. Neck, axillae and groins.

4 Other features:

(a) *Anorexia and fever* – usually late onset.

(b) *Bruising* and other haemorrhagic features are uncommon initially but are more likely later when the bone marrow becomes severely involved.

(c) *Infections*. Due to lack of mature neutrophils and/or reduced production of immunoglobulins.

Blood

1   Anaemia. Variable intensity and normochromic: Hb may be normal at onset.

2   Reticulocytosis. If acquired haemolytic anaemia is present, usually with positive direct antiglobulin test.

3   Total leucocyte count. Typically as high as 300×10^9/l.

4   Blood film. Almost all leucocytes present are lymphocytes. Usually many bare broken nuclei – *smear* cells, are seen.

5   Platelets. Normal initially, reduced later.

6   Bone marrow. Cellularity is increased due to the dense infiltration with lymphocytes, both large and small. In the later stages erythropoiesis and megakaryocytes are reduced by exclusion.

Treatment

The disease has been classified into five stages (Rai) with decreasing length of expected survival

   o   Absolute lymphocytosis $> 15 \times 10^9$/l.

   I   As stage o with enlarged lymph nodes.

   II   As stage o with enlarged liver and spleen ± enlarged lymph nodes.

   III   As stage o with anaemia (Hb < 11 g/dl) ± enlarged lymph nodes; ± enlarged liver and spleen.

   IV   As stage o with thrombocytopenia (platelets $< 100 \times 10^9$/l) ± enlarged lymph nodes; ± enlarged spleen

There is no need to treat Stage o. Other stages need treatment if there is symptomatic involvement due to lymph node enlargement, symptoms of splenic enlargement, reduced haemopoiesis due to bone marrow involvement or secondary auto-immune haemolysis.

1   *Chemotherapy.* Either by Chlorambucil or Cyclophosphamide (see p. 465). Both drugs also depress the leucocyte and platelet counts, so that regular monitoring of blood is required.

2   *Radiotherapy.* May be effective in reducing degree of splenomegaly and this can result in general clinical improvement. Local treatment to large superficial lymph node masses or for relief of obstruction due to deeper groups of nodes may be very beneficial.

3   *Corticosteroids.* Valuable for treatment of associated acquired haemolytic anaemia and may help to maintain platelet count if thrombocytopenia develops. Has some effect in reducing lymphocyte production.

4   γ-Globulin. These patients tend to be more

vulnerable to infection, especially respiratory, due to hypo-γ-globulinaemia. Therapeutic γ-globulin may be indicated.

Prognosis

This condition is commonly non-progressive and such patients lead a normal life requiring no treatment but with regular blood counts 3 or 4 times a year. However, at any time, the disease may become more aggressive, in which case the measures listed above become necessary either singly or in combination. Sometimes the condition is more progressive from the time of diagnosis.

Chronic granulocytic leukaemia (Syn. chronic myeloid or myelogenous leukaemia)

Incidence

Highest incidence 40–50 years. Rare below 20. M:F equal.

Clinical

1   Presenting symptoms insidious and include anaemia, loss of weight and abdominal discomfort from splenomegaly. Occasionally there is bruising and disturbance of vision.

2   Examination shows hepatosplenomegaly and wasting, but lymph node enlargement is not significant until late stages.

Blood

1   *Anaemia.* Normochromic with Hb moderately reduced to about 9 g/dl.

2   *White cells.* Usually very high – 100–400 $\times 10^9$/l.

3   *Platelets.* Initially shares in the myeloproliferation and is usually moderately raised to about 500–600 $\times 10^9$/l but becomes reduced later.

4   *Blood film.* The predominant cells are granulocytes and their precursors. Most are segmented polymorphs with many metamyelocytes, some myelocytes and about 5 per cent blast cells. Basophils are usually abnormally prominent. Occasional nucleated red cells present. Platelets increased in number and often also in size.

5   *Neutrophil alkaline phosphatase.* Characteristically very low.

6   *Bone marrow.* Aspiration produces hypercellular fragments. Most of the cells are myelocytes with

increase in mature forms and of blast cells. There may be some megaloblastic erythropoiesis due to folate deprivation by the proliferating cells.

7 *Philadephia (Ph') chromosome*. In most cases chromosome 22 has a considerable part of its long arm deleted and translocated to chromosome 9. This change is present in erythroid, granulocytic and megakaryocytic series of cells and persists after effective treatment.

Diagnosis

The condition may be confused with:

1 Leukaemoid reaction. In these cases splenomegaly is usually absent and the neutrophil alkaline phosphatase is high (see p. 446).

2 *Myelofibrosis*. Splenomegaly is marked in this disease and granulocytes are often considerably increased but not usually to such high levels (see p. 460). The neutrophil alkaline phosphatase is typically very high.

Marrow aspiration produces 'dry' tap with no fragments and the Ph' chromosome is negative.

Treatment

Remission is not yet possible, so therapy is palliative and is aimed at controlling the disease to effect the longest comfortable life.

1 *Chemotherapy*. Busulphan is the drug of choice. After about 3 weeks there is a progressive fall in the white count with reduction in spleen size. Progress must be monitored by regular blood counts to avoid excessive bone-marrow depression with resulting neutropenia and thrombocytopenia. If this occurs, treatment must be stopped immediately. Hydroxyurea is an alternative drug, especially when resistance to Busulphan has developed.

2 *Irradiation of the spleen*. Frequent applications, e.g. alternate days, of small doses of X-rays can reduce the white count by about one-third each week until level reaches about $15 \times 10^9/l$. This usually takes about a month by which time the spleen is considerably reduced or impalpable and is accompanied by relief of symptoms, and subsequent rise in haemoglobin. This is particularly valuable when resistance to chemotherapy develops.

Both forms of treatment need to be repeated at intervals.

3 *Supportive*

(a) Blood transfusion. May be required at the commencement of treatment or in the later stages when response to treatment is no longer effective.

(b) Antibiotic treatment. To combat infections.

(c) Allopurinol. To prevent hyperuricaemia.

4 *Blast-cell metamorphosis*. Usually evidenced by onset of resistance to the above methods of treatment and is then managed as for myeloblastic leukaemia (see p. 464).

Prognosis

Median survival time from diagnosis is usually about 3 years but can be as long as 10–12 years. Usually terminates as myeloblastic phase with clinical features previously described on p. 463. The blood film shows replacement of the more mature cells of the chronic stage by 'blasts' which constitute up to 90 per cent of the marrow cells. Thrombocytopenia becomes evident and progressively severe anaemia develops.

Monocytic leukaemias

ACUTE MONOCYTIC LEUKAEMIA

Two types are recognized.

'Schilling' type
Regarded as the true monoblastic variety. Blasts, many of them indistinguishable from lymphoblasts and myeloblasts are accompanied by a variable number of more mature monocytes. Some of the immature cells promonocytes, have an unfolded lobulated nucleus with abundant pale blue cytoplasm. This variety is rare and typically follows a rapidly progressive course.

'Naegeli' type
Really a form of acute myeloblastic leukaemia. The blood film contains frequent 'monocytoid' cells together with 'blast' cells. The bone marrow reveals the true character of the condition where the leukaemic cells are usually more obviously myeloblasts. This is not a true monocytic leukaemia and is more accurately termed *acute myelomonocytic leukaemia*. Usually pursues a slightly less aggressive course.

CHRONIC MONOCYTIC LEUKAEMIA

This condition exists but is very rare.

Other uncommon forms of leukaemia

Erythraemic myelosis – di Guglielmo's disease

A neoplastic proliferation of erythroblasts and characterized by numerous nucleated red cells in the peripheral blood and a gross erythroid hyperplasia in the bone marrow. Morphologically they have typically a bizarre megaloblastic appearance. In the later stages a myeloblastic type of leukaemia is superimposed.

Eosinophilic and basophilic leukaemias

These are usually examples of chronic granulocytic leukaemia in which these particular types of granulocytes are for some reason more prominent. However, rare cases of true eosinophilic leukaemia have been described.

Hairy-cell leukaemia

An uncommon form of leukaemia presenting usually age 40–60 more often in males, with moderate enlargement of the spleen and pancytopenia. The typical abnormal cell in the peripheral blood is a B-lymphocyte with an irregular 'hairy' outline to the cytoplasm. These cells are also found to be infiltrating the bone marrow, liver and spleen. The serum may contain a paraprotein. Splenectomy can often alleviate the pancytopenia. Otherwise no specific therapy is usually indicated and the disease pursues a fairly chronic course.

Malignant lymphomas

Though the subject of much dispute in respect of details of classification, etc., this important group of primary tumours of the lymphoreticular system are divisible into:
1　Hodgkin's lymphoma.
2　Non-Hodgkin's lymphoma.
Further discussion is contained in Chapter 95 on page 578.

Hodgkin's lymphoma

Clinical

Presenting symptoms may be:
1　*Due to lymph node, splenic, hepatic enlargement.*
Superficial: giving rise to swelling in neck, axillae and groins. Deep, e.g. mediastinum, retroperitoneal, producing local pressure symptoms. The nodes are typically discrete in the early stages, non-tender and 'rubbery' in consistency. Later, extracapsular extension of the disease produces matting of the node masses and fixation. The spleen is sometimes enlarged but this does not necessarily indicate that it contains tumour. Conversely an involved spleen may not be palpable. Liver may be enlarged in advanced stages.
2　*Constitutional.*Including fever, heavy sweats, pruritis, weight loss, lassitude, anorexia and malaise. Fever particularly occurs if abdominal tissues are involved. It typically follows an undulating pattern of 7-day cycles of up to about 40°C.
3　*Involvement of other tissues*, e.g. lung, skin and bone, may produce respiratory symptoms, rashes or bone pain.
4　*Anaemia*, occasionally.

Blood

The blood picture is not distinctive.

　Anaemia. A slight normochromic normocytic anaemia of about 10 g/dl in the later stages due to:
(*a*) Anaemia of chronic disorders (see p. 454).
(*b*) Progressive infiltration of bone marrow.
(*c*) Acquired (auto-immune) haemolytic anaemia (see p. 505).

　Total white count. Increased during active episodes of the disease to about 15–$20 \times 10^9/l$ due to neutrophil leucocytosis. Extensive marrow involvement in later stages may cause leucopenia. Eosinophilia occurs in about 10 per cent of cases, especially when skin and intestine are infiltrated.

　Neutrophil alkaline phosphatase. Usually moderately increased.

　Platelet count. May be increased unless marrow is replaced by tumour.

Bone marrow

Not usually diagnostic. Tumour tissue rarely found except in the late stages when infiltration may be extensive. Areas of involvement often indicated by local bone tenderness which are likely to be the most rewarding sites for aspiration. Often a moderate increase in 'reticulum cells' is the only feature. Rarely Reed–Sternberg cells (see p. 581) can be distinguished. Histological section of marrow trephine tissue of aspirated fragments will be more informative.

Diagnosis

Lymph node biopsy. This provides the most reliable evidence (see p. 581). Usually it is possible to excise a superficial node but inguinal nodes are best avoided. In order to plan the best possible treatment and management for each case, it is essential to assess the extent of the disease as accurately as possible.

Clinical staging

Management and prognosis are based on recognized clinical stages which are given in Chapter 95 on p. 581.

Important aids to clinical staging are:

1 *Radiology:*
 (i) X-ray of chest to demonstrate mediastinal lymph node enlargement and lung involvement.
 (ii) Lymphangiography to demonstrate enlargement of retroperitoneal lymph nodes and usually accompanied by pyelography.

2 *Bone marrow trephine biopsy*. Although ordinary marrow aspirate films are rarely diagnostic, valuable information may be obtained by histological section of marrow tissue obtained with a trephine biopsy.

3 *Laparotomy*. A staging laparotomy may be necessary for accurate assessment of involvement with biopsy of deep abdominal lymph nodes, spleen and liver.

Treatment

Localized disease – stages I and II. X-ray therapy.

Generalized disease – stages III and IV. Combination chemotherapy administered in regular 'pulsed' courses has been demonstrated to be the most effective form of therapy currently available (see p. 464). At the present time the combination most used is mustine hydrochloride or cyclophosphamide with prednisolone, procarbazine and vinblastine.

The inhibitory effect of the drugs on the patient's normal haemopoietic tissue must be monitored by regular leucocyte and platelet counts.

Supportive therapy. In the later stages, anaemia may require blood transfusion and intercurrent infection needs swift antibiotic treatment. X-ray treatment may help bone pain. Hyperuricaemia may occur, especially during active cytotoxic therapy and prophylaxis with allopurinol is recommended.

Prognosis

This is considered on p. 582.

Non-Hodgkin's lymphoma

Classification

The classification is currently much in dispute but simplistically can be identified as given in more detail on p. 582 (old terminology, etc., in brackets).

1 Good prognosis group:
(a) Follicular lymphoma.
(b) Diffuse lymphoma, lymphocytic small cell type (lymphocytic lymphosarcoma).
(c) Small follicle centred cell.

2 Poor prognosis group – all diffuse:
(a) Lymphocytic large cell (lymphoblastic lymphosarcoma).
(b) Undifferentiated (reticulum cell sarcoma).
(c) Burkitt's lymphoma.
(d) Histiocytic.

Chronic lymphocytic leukaemia (p. 465) is a variant of diffuse small cell lymphocytic lymphoma.

Clinical

Slight male preponderance with increasing incidence over 40 years.

(a) *Lymph node enlargement*, splenomegaly or proliferation of other lymphoid tissue, e.g. nasopharynx and bowel. Often multifocal and may present extranodally.
(b) *Auto-immune haemolytic anaemia*. May precede lymphoma by several years (see p. 506).
(c) *Organ transplant recipients*. Immunosuppressed patients who have transplanted kidneys, etc., have an increased incidence.

Blood

Anaemia is common in the poor prognosis group and is usually normocytic, normochromic or haemolytic. Chronic lymphocytic leukaemia (p. 465) is usually obvious. In some cases abnormal lymphoid cells 'spill over' into the peripheral blood – *leucosarcoma*.

Marrow

This can assess whether haemopoiesis is normal and whether there is tumour infiltration.

Diagnosis

Lymph node biopsy. This provides the most important means of definitive diagnosis.

Lymphangiography. Or scanning to assess intra-abdominal lymph node involvement.

Liver biopsy. Occasionally helpful.

Splenectomy and laparotomy. Sometimes indicated.

It is usually possible to apply the same staging criteria as that used for Hodgkin's disease (p. 581) though with less significance for management and prognosis.

Treatment

Cytotoxic therapy with alkylating agents and corticosteroids is the main form of management for lymphocytic small cell lymphoma, together with local irradiation of large lymph node masses. The poor prognosis group tumours require intensive local radiotherapy. Metastatic disease needs aggressive combined chemotherapy as described for Hodgkin's disease (see p. 469) administered in full dosage as short courses at regular intervals. Treatment needs to be continued long after clinical remission.

Prognosis

This is discussed on p. 582. As suggested by the nomenclature, treatment of the poor prognosis group patients is predominantly symptomatic but is more effective and potentially curative in those with good prognosis types of the disease.

Myelomatosis – multiple myeloma

Nature

A malignant proliferative disease of plasma cells. These cells are the manufacturers of immunoglobulins (see p. 91) and thus a significant feature of myelomatosis is the presence of high levels of a monoclonal paraprotein in plasma.

These consist of a heavy chain, usually IgG, less commonly IgA, others only rarely, and a light chain mostly κ or λ (see p. 471).

Age and sex

Peak 60–70 years but it is known that the cells proliferate relatively slowly and that the disease has already been present for many years prior to diagnosis.

M:F equal.

Sites

1 *Bones*. Active marrow sites, e.g. spine, skull, ribs, pelvis, upper ends of femur, humerus.
2 *Spleen, liver, lymph nodes*. Uncommonly.
3 *'Solitary plasmacytoma'*. A rare single tumour of soft tissues or bone which may pursue a benign course but usually later develops into disseminated myelomatosis.

Macroscopical

Clear circumscribed deposits of pink, soft or gelatinous tumour tissue destroying bone and often producing a characteristic 'punched-out' radiolucent appearance. Small lesions may not be demonstrable radiologically. Pathological fractures are common.

Microscopical

The tumour is composed of sheets of typical and atypical plasma cells. The latter are often larger and may contain a solitary nucleolus. The basophilic cytoplasm is very strongly pyroninophilic with the MGP stain. Occasionally the tumour cells are so atypical as to be difficult to recognize as plasmacytic in origin.

Clinical

Main presenting features are bone pain, anaemia, infection, e.g. pneumonia, renal failure or symptoms secondary to amyloidosis.

Blood

(*a*) *Anaemia*. Normocytic normochromic, usually not severe initially – 10 g/dl or so.
(*b*) *Neutropenia and thrombocytopenia*. When advanced.
(*c*) *Leucoerythroblastosis*. In about 10 per cent of cases (see p. 448).
(*d*) *Plasma cells*. 'Spill' of myeloma cells into the peripheral blood: only rarely are they numerous – *plasma cell leukaemia*.
(*e*) *Sedimentation rate*. This is usually very high – in excess of 100 mm in 1 hour.

Marrow

The findings are variable. Sometimes aspiration will achieve almost pure plasma cells but more commonly there is an increase in normal plasma cells and the presence of abnormal forms.

Biochemistry

(*a*) *Paraprotein*. In nearly all cases there is a high

level of monoclonal paraprotein in blood and urine most frequently IgG, κ or λ. Total serum proteins may be within the normal range though the normal immunoglobulins are depressed. Blood albumin levels are usually low.

(b) *Bence-Jones protein.* In 65 per cent of cases this substance is produced by synthesis of monoclonal light chains and is present in blood and urine where it is readily detected by its physical characteristic of precipitation at 50–60°C with resolubility above 70°C.

(c) *Hypercalcaemia.* Commonly present.

(d) *Renal failure.* Precipitation of the abnormal protein in renal tubules is associated with the presence of 'hard casts', a syncytial histiocytic reaction and renal failure in a high proportion of cases – *myeloma kidney* (see p. 366).

(e) *Cryoglobulinaemia.* This may be associated.

Other effects

(a) *Amyloidosis.* This develops in about 10 per cent of cases.

(b) *Hyperviscosity syndrome.* If the level of paraprotein rises above 18 g/l, blood viscosity may increase to such a degree that problems of flow develop.

Diagnosis

Two of the following three features are necessary:

(a) Characteristic radiological appearances in bones.

(b) Excess and abnormal plasma cells in the marrow.

(c) Monoclonal paraprotein in plasma or urine or both.

Treatment

(a) *Chemotherapy.* With alkylating agents, melphalan or cyclophosphamide and cortico-steroids. Usually given as 5-day courses every 4 weeks indefinitely unless side effects on marrow function intervene.

(b) *X-ray therapy.* May be useful for symptomatic relief of bone pain and to promote healing of pathological features.

(c) *Supportive.* Dialysis may be necessary for renal failure and hypercalcaemia. Blood transfusion will relieve anaemia if severe. Orthopaedic measures may be required for spinal support, pinning of fractures etc.

(d) *Plasmapheresis.* This may be useful to remove gross excess of the abnormal protein and thus reduce hyperviscosity and renal complications.

Prognosis

Treatment is largely symptomatic and there is, as yet, no good evidence that it prolongs life.

The disease is invariably fatal, usually within 3 years of diagnosis.

Waldenström's macroglobulinaemia

Nature

Characterized by the presence of high molecular weight IgM protein in the plasma and the presence in bone marrow of abnormal lymphocytes, many of which have plasmacytoid features.

Clinical

Occurs in elderly patients and usually presents with mental confusion, myopathy or neuropathy, visual disturbances, skin haemorrhages, bleeding from gastro-intestinal and genito-urinary tracts. The spleen is usually moderately enlarged and lymphadenopathy may be found.

Blood

(a) *Serum proteins.* The symptoms are largely due to hyperviscosity of the plasma which contains IgM paraprotein (MW 1 million) at a concentration of 25 g/l or higher. A cryoglobulin may also be present. The levels of normal IgG and IgM are usually low.

(b) *Bence-Jones proteinuria.* May be present in very small amounts.

(c) *Erythrocyte sedimentation rate.* Very high – often more than 100 mm in 1 hour.

(d) *Peripheral blood.* Marked rouleaux formation due to the high protein content. This may be visible as a bluish-staining background to the cells. Plasmacytoid lymphocytes may be present: neutrophils and platelets are often decreased.

Marrow

Abnormal infiltration of pleomorphic lymphocytes, some with pyronin-positive plasmacytoid appearance, mast cells and histiocytes. These abnormal lymphocytes are probably responsible for manufacture of the IgM.

Lymph nodes
Infiltration by abnormal plasmacytoid lymphocytes, plasma cells, mast cells and histiocytes,
usually with loss of follicular pattern.

Treatment
(*a*) *Chemotherapy*. A combination of alkylating
agents such as chlorambucil or cyclophosphamide with prednisolone on a continuous basis,
monitored by peripheral blood counts.
(*b*) *Plasmapheresis*. To reduce blood viscosity may
be required urgently and repeated until chemotherapy takes effect.
(*c*) *Penicillamine*. Breaks up the macroglobulin by
disrupting the internal disulphide bonds.
Works *in vitro* but now largely discontinued as a
form of therapy because the effective dose *in
vivo* is too toxic.

(*d*) *Blood transfusion*. Haemorrhagic features are
due to both thrombocytopenia and qualitative
dysfunction associated with coating of the
platelets with macroglobulin (see p. 517). Thus
transfusions of whole blood or platelet-rich
preparations are more useful after plasmapheresis.

Prognosis
The course is often protracted and benign but, in
untreated cases particularly, death may occur from
complications of hyperviscosity and haemorrhage
in particular. A more aggressive picture may
develop after many years from extensive marrow
infiltration.

Chapter 80
Haematology – Iron Deficiency and Excess: Sideroblastic Anaemia

Iron metabolism

A normal 70 kg man contains 4 g of iron, about equivalent in quantity to a 5 cm nail; this amount is fixed by controlling the absorption of iron through the small intestine. Failure to maintain this delicate balance results in either:
1 Iron deficiency–common.
2 Iron overload–rare.
   Both these situations are debilitating and in extreme cases may be fatal.

Distribution of body iron

The body iron is distributed as follows:
1 Circulating haemoglobin 70 per cent.
2 Body stores 20 per cent.
3 Tissue iron (myoglobin and respiratory enzymes) 10 per cent.
4 Transferrin. A small quantity of iron (4 mg or 0.1 per cent of the body iron) is bound to the plasma protein transferrin.

Circulating haemoglobin
The iron of blood, 3 g, is contained in the haem of haemoglobin. The adult blood volume is 5 l, so each litre of blood contains 600 mg of iron.

Body stores
Iron is normally stored in the phagocytic cells of the liver, spleen and bone marrow both as haemosiderin and ferritin. Only when the body is overloaded with iron will it be found in any quantity within the parenchymal cells of, for example, the liver.
1 *Haemosiderin.* An insoluble iron-protein complex staining blue with Perls' Prussian Blue stain. Staining of marrow fragments for iron by this method gives an indication of the patient's iron stores.
2 *Ferritin.* A soluble complex of iron with the protein apoferritin. Being soluble, the iron in ferritin does not stain by Perls' method.
   When iron stores are normal, ferritin forms 60 per cent and haemosiderin 40 per cent. When iron stores increase, the proportion of haemosiderin

473

greatly increases. During the development of an
iron deficiency these iron stores are at first utilized
to maintain the haemoglobin level, anaemia occurring only when the stores have been depleted.

Tissue iron
The iron contained in myoglobin – 5 per cent,
cytochrome and the tissue respiratory enzymes, e.g.
catalase, is essential to cellular function and is not
available to correct an iron deficiency.

Transferrin
Iron travels in the blood, bound to the plasma
protein transferrin. Each molecule of transferrin is
capable of binding with two ferric iron atoms.
Normally, only 1/3 of the circulating transferrin is
combined with iron, the total iron-binding capacity
(TIBC) of normal plasma or serum being therefore,
33 per cent saturated.

TRANSFERRIN LEVELS IN HEALTH AND DISEASE
Serum iron   20 μmol/l
Total iron binding capacity (TIBC)   60 μmol/l
Percentage saturation   33 per cent
Unsaturated iron binding capacity
(UIBC)   67 per cent.

The alterations in the serum iron, unsaturated
iron-binding capacity and total iron-binding capacity in various disorders of iron metabolism, are of
diagnostic value and summarized in Fig. 48 on p.
475.

FUNCTIONS OF TRANSFERRIN
1   Transport of iron.
2   Biochemical control of iron absorption.

At the end of its life the normal red cell is
engulfed by a phagocytic system cell. The iron of
the haemoglobin is bound to transferrin and transported to the bone marrow for reutilization.

Iron is absorbed from the bowel lumen into the
upper small intestinal epithelial cells. The passage
of the iron from these cells into the plasma is
probably controlled by the saturation per cent of
the plasma transferrin.

N.B. Iron absorption is increased by:
1   Increased erythropoietic activity of the bone
marrow.
2   Low iron stores.

Unwanted iron that has been absorbed into the
intestinal cells is bound to apoferritin to form
ferritin. An intestinal cell in which all apoferritin
has been saturated with iron will not absorb further

iron from the intestine. Indeed, the unwanted iron
that has already been absorbed will be lost when
that cell ultimately dies and is shed into the lumen
of the intestine.

In the presence of increased erythropoietic activity, e.g. a chronic haemolytic anaemia, iron may
continue to be over-absorbed even if the stores are
overloaded. Such iron overload will especially
occur if the patient is mistakenly given iron therapy
in an attempt to increase the haemoglobin level, e.g.
in β-thalassaemia minor (see p. 502).

Iron balance

In order to maintain iron balance the small obligatory loss of iron common to all humans must be
replaced. In addition, the increased demands of
growth in children and of menstrual loss and
pregnancy in women must be met. The role of
transferrin in the biochemical control of iron
absorption has already been considered (see above).

Iron requirements

Obligatory
One mg of iron is lost each day, mainly due to the
desquamation of cells from the bowel, skin and
urine.

Additional physiological iron loss

FEMALE OF REPRODUCTIVE AGE
1   Menstruation. Up to 30 mg of iron loss for each
normal cycle.
2   Pregnancy. Up to 500 mg of iron for each
pregnancy.

However, due to the cessation of menstruation,
the net loss of pregnancy is reduced to about 250 mg
iron.

Increased physiological iron demand – growth
The foetus contains 250 mg of iron: the 4 g body
store of the adult is acquired during growth. The
lower Hb of 10–12 g/dl, accepted as 'normal' in the
young child, may result from iron deficiency.

Balancing intake requirements
To maintain iron balance, the following quantities
iron must be *absorbed*.

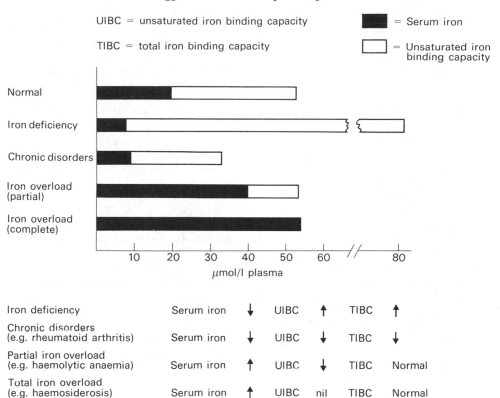

Fig. 48. The serum iron, unsaturated iron-binding capacity and total iron-binding capacity in disorders of iron metabolism.

1　Males – 1 mg of iron per day.
2　Females of reproductive age and growing children – 2 mg of iron per day.

Thus women and children are more susceptible to iron deficiency.

Factors influencing the absorption of dietary iron

A good diet contains 20 mg of iron/day. Meat, fish, eggs and green vegetables are rich sources but are more expensive. The low iron content of flour is sometimes supplemented by the addition of inorganic iron.

Factors increasing iron absorption
1　Iron-rich diet.
2　Acid pH. Post-gastrectomy states and atrophic gastritis with achlorhydria are often associated with iron deficiency. Increase of gastric HCl promotes absorption.
3　Ferrous iron is absorbed more easily than ferric iron. Reducing agents, e.g. ascorbic acid in fruit and vegetables and sulphydryl (-SH) groups in meat protein, convert ferric to ferrous iron and increase absorption. In particular, the presence of meat greatly increases the percentage absorption of the total dietary iron as well as increasing the amount of iron in the diet.

Factors decreasing iron absorption
1　Iron-poor diet, e.g. the bread and jam diet of the elderly or poor.
2　Phytic acid, present in cereal, and forms insoluble iron phytates.
3　Phosphates, present in cereal, form insoluble ferric phosphate.
4　Intestinal malfunction. Iron is optimally absorbed in the duodenum and jejunum. Steatorr-

hoea may result in malabsorption of iron as with other haematinics (see p. 209).

Iron deficiency

Causes
Iron deficiency occurs in two consecutive stages.
1 Utilization of iron stores – symptomless.
2 Reduction of circulating haemoglobin – anaemia.

Precipitating factors may include:
1 *Increased physiological demand.*
2 *Reduced iron absorption.*
3 *Pathological blood loss – chronic haemorrhage.*
(*a*) Uterine abnormalities.
(*b*) Gastro-intestinal tract bleeding.

It is especially important to exclude a gastro-intestinal bleed, e.g. peptic ulcer, large bowel neoplasm, haemorrhoids, etc., as the cause of unexplained iron-deficiency anaemia in men and post-menopausal women. Intestinal parasites, especially hookworms, are a very common cause of iron deficiency in the tropics.
4 *Malabsorption*
Factors identified on p. 482.

Clinical

GENERAL SYMPTOMS OF CHRONIC ANAEMIA
These include fatigue, dyspnoea on exertion, palpitations, pallor, headaches and dizziness.

The general symptoms of chronic anaemia are similar whatever the aetiology and are dependent on the extent and rate of the drop in Hb, the slower the rate of fall, the better the anaemia is tolerated. By contrast, the symptomatology of acute anaemia is mainly caused by a fall in blood volume and not by the reduced Hb level. Older patients with pre-existing cardiovascular disease are especially intolerant of anaemia, which may precipitate attacks of angina or intermittent claudication. 'Compensated' anaemia, where the haemoglobin is less avid for oxygen and the patient is 'protected' from a low level of circulating haemoglobin, is considered in Fig. 50 on p. 492.

SPECIFIC
A small proportion of patients with chronic iron deficiency develop epithelial changes. With the earlier recognition of iron deficiency, these changes are now less commonly seen.

1 *Nails.* Thin, brittle and classically spoon-shaped – *koilonychia.*
2 *Tongue.* Smooth, shiny and free of fur with soreness – *glossitis.*
3 *Mouth.* Cracking of the angles of the mouth – *cheilosis or angular stomatitis.*
4 *Hair.* Dry and brittle.
5 *Gastrointestinal*
(*a*) Post-cricoid webs may cause dysphagia. Carcinoma of the pharynx and oesophagus may follow (see p. 184).
(*b*) Atrophic gastritis and achlorhydria is commonly associated with iron deficiency (see p. 187).
6 *Plummer – Vinson – Kelly – Paterson syndrome.* This is the association of chronic iron-deficiency anaemia, dysphagia and glossitis (see p. 183).

Blood
1 *Haemoglobin.* Reduced according to the severity of the anaemia.
2 *Blood film.* Hypochromic, microcytic, with poikilocytosis and polychromasia when due to chronic blood loss.
3 *Red cell indices.* MCV↓ MCHC↓ MCH↓
4 *Serum iron.* Reduced with increase in TIBC.
5 *Marrow*
(*a*) Normoblasts show ragged cytoplasmic edges.
(*b*) Perls' Prussian Blue stain of marrow fragments negative for iron.

Treatment
The aim of therapy is:
1 Correct the cause.
2 Raise haemoglobin to normal range.
3 Replenish iron stores.
4 Prevent recurrence of anaemia.

ORAL IRON THERAPY
One ferrous sulphate tablet daily (63 mg elemental iron). Higher oral intakes of iron, e.g. 3 FeSO4 tablets daily, give an increased incidence of gastrointestinal side-effects and results in defaulting in therapy without any significant increase in efficacy. A daily oral intake of 63 mg elemental iron is most unlikely to give rise to any adverse side-effects. At such doses there is little evidence that one type of iron preparation is better tolerated than another. Meat increases iron absorption, and an attempt should be made to give a dietary increase of this protein as well.

PARENTERAL IRON THERAPY

There are a few indications for intramuscular, e.g. 'Jectofer' – iron sorbital citric acid, or intravenous, e.g. 'Astrafer' – iron dextran, iron preparations. Allergic reactions may occur and, in addition, sarcoma at the injection site has been reported following long-term administration of intramuscular iron dextran in animals. Oral iron should always be given if clinically practicable.

Indications for parenteral iron

1 *Patient not taking iron tablets.* Some 30 per cent of antenatal patients fail to take oral iron and default in therapy is probably as common in other groups of patients. If this is suspected, and the faeces are negative for inorganic iron, a course of parenteral iron may avoid a blood transfusion.

2 *Malabsorption syndrome.* It may not be possible to achieve a satisfactory response to oral iron in this situation.

3 *Necessity for a rapid therapeutic response.* The therapeutic response to parenteral iron is only marginally faster than oral iron. In fact only the total dose therapy with iron dextran is capable of speeding the response.

Note: In estimating the amount of parenteral iron required it is important to remember to replenish the iron stores of 1–1.5 g, as well as to correct the anaemia.

Response to treatment

CLINICAL

1 The general symptoms of anaemia rapidly abate as the haemoglobin rises.

2 The epithelial changes respond more slowly, and dysphagia may be persistently troublesome.

HAEMATOLOGICAL

1 The expected rise of haemoglobin level in response to iron therapy is 0.1–0.2 g/dl/day.

2 Blood film. Polychromasia is followed by the appearance of well-haemoglobinized normal cells, which contrast with the residual hypochromic, microcytic cells to give a *dimorphic* appearance.

3 The reticulocyte count does not exceed 15 per cent even with the most severe anaemias, c.f. therapeutic response of an equivalent anaemia of megaloblastic type to vitamin B_{12} or folic acid (see p. 484).

FAILURE OF RESPONSE

Causes include

1 Failure to take iron tablets→parenteral iron.

2 Continued blood loss.

3 Malabsorption of iron→parenteral iron.

4 Incorrect diagnosis. Iron deficiency is not the only cause of hypochromic anaemia. A similar blood picture may be given by:

(a) Defective globin synthesis, e.g. thalassaemia minor (see p. 502).

(b) Inability to utilize iron in the anaemias of chronic disease (see p. 508) or in sideroblastic anaemias (see p. 478).

Iron overload

Chronic iron overload

On rare occasions the total body iron may exceed the normal 4 g. Such excess iron is usually stored harmlessly as haemosiderin in the lymphoreticular system in the liver, spleen and bone marrow. However, if the iron stores become really excessive, e.g. over 10 g, iron may also be deposited in the parenchymal cells of the liver, pancreas, skin and heart, where it may cause damage.

NOMENCLATURE

Conditions with excessive iron stored as haemosiderin in the phagocytic cell system used to be called haemosiderosis, whereas excessive haemosiderin in parenchymal cells was labelled *haemochromatosis* (see p. 478). As excessive iron may be deposited simultaneously in both these types of cells, this classification is not satisfactory.

It is perhaps reasonable to classify all examples of iron overload as haemosiderosis or siderosis and, for historical reasons, to retain the term haemochromatosis for the inherited rare disease caused by over-absorption of iron which results in massive deposits of haemosiderin in the parenchymal cells (see p. 562).

In the sideroblastic anaemias (see p. 478) the primary lesion is an inability of the developing red cell to utilize iron to make haemoglobin and excess iron accumulation in sideroblasts in the marrow and in phagocytic cells and sometimes parenchymal cells of liver etc., occurs.

AETIOLOGY

The excessive iron may enter the body because of

increased intestinal absorption or because of excessive parenteral intake, e.g. blood transfusion.

1 Excessive dietary iron. By inappropriate long-term iron therapy or gross dietary excess.

2 Excessive absorption of iron. In idiopathic haemochromatosis or secondary to chronic increased erythropoietic activity of the marrow, e.g. chronic haemolytic anaemia (see p. 489).

The organ changes and pathogenetic factors of haemochromatosis are discussed on p. 562.

Acute iron overload – iron poisoning

Accidental iron poisoning amongst young children is relatively common. This is because iron tablets for routine prophylaxis are dispensed in antenatal clinics and are therefore available in homes that frequently contain young children. The fact that, in addition, many of the tablets look like sweets is especially unfortunate.

In adults, iron poisoning is rare and is likely to be the result of a suicide attempt.

CLINICAL

Acute iron poisoning presents in a manner similar to other acute heavy metal poisonings.

1 *Gastro-intestinal.* Vomiting, abdominal pain and diarrhoea.

2 *Quiescent period.* Even in ultimately fatal cases some apparent clinical recovery may follow the initial phase.

3 *Shock and collapse.* The patient's condition rapidly deteriorates and death may follow.

4 *Gastro-intestinal tract obstruction.* Due to scarring, recovery may be followed some weeks later by intestinal obstruction.

TREATMENT

Iron poisoning in children carries a high mortality. In the young child death has been reported following the swallowing of as few as 15 ferrous sulphate tablets. Urgent treatment is therefore called for if either the clinical picture or a tablet count suggests that, in a young child, more than five tablets have been taken.

1 Desferrioxamine 2 g, intramuscularly. This may be repeated, but no more than 6 g should be given in 24 hours.

2 Give an emetic or stomach lavage with 1 per cent sodium bicarbonate. A laparotomy with gastro-intestinal washout has been advocated if a massive overdose is known to have been taken.

3 Give 5–12 g desferrioxamine in 100 ml water either swallowed or down the lavage tube.

4 In event of shock, set up an intravenous drip and give desferrioxamine 15 mg/kilo/hr into the drip. No more than 80 mg/kilo should be given over a 24-hour period.

Transfusion siderosis

Patients requiring repeated transfusions to maintain a satisfactory haemoglobin level receive 0.25 g of iron in each unit of blood transfused. If patients receiving multiple transfusions have an erythropoietically active marrow, e.g. in chronic haemolytic anaemia, they will, in addition, overabsorb dietary iron from the bowel. Such patients suffer from iron overload faster than patients requiring transfusions with an inactive marrow, e.g. aplastic anaemia.

Treatment of iron overload

Cases of moderate iron overload without clinical symptoms require no treatment. However, primary haemochromatosis and transfusion haemosiderosis are two clinical situations where, in most cases, an attempt must be made to reduce iron stores.

1 Without anaemia, i.e. primary haemochromatosis

Recurrent, weekly, venesections of one unit of blood until evidence of iron deficiency is recognized by development of a hypochromic anaemia with low serum iron.

A low iron diet to ensure a simultaneous reduction of iron absorption, is impracticable.

2 With anaemia, i.e. in aplastic anaemia etc.

Many patients with severe chronic anaemias require a long-term blood transfusion regime to maintain a tolerable Hb level. It is apparent that patients with chronic anaemia and iron overload caused by multiple transfusions cannot be submitted simultaneously to therapeutic venesections. Iron-chelating agents, e.g. desferrioxamine, combine with iron and increase urinary and biliary iron excretion. The therapeutic effect is increased if ascorbic acid is given as well. Iron-chelating agents are worth adding to each bottle of blood transfused, but the value of additional daily injections is more problematical.

Sideroblastic anaemias

Chemistry

The protoporphyrin ring of haem is manufactured

in the red-cell precursor through a number of intermediate compounds, the rate-limiting step being the condensation of a succinyl Co A and glycine to form δ-aminolaevulinic acid (ALA). The enzyme responsible, ALA synthetase, requires pyridoxal phosphate as a coenzyme.

Iron is donated to the developing red cell by transferrin where it combines with protoporphyrin to make haem which subsequently combines with globin to form haemoglobin. When, through any cause, there is an excess of iron relative to either protoporphyrin or globin, then the nett unutilized iron will accumulate in the developing red cell in the form of granules which can be demonstrated with Perls' Prussian Blue stain. This situation may come about through a depression of either protoporhyrin or globin manufacture. Alternatively, even in the presence of a plentiful supply of protoprophyrin and globin, non-haem iron may accumulate if it is taken up to excess by the developing red cell or if it cannot be utilized effectively in the manufacture of haem.

Definition

SIDEROBLAST
A nucleated red-cell precursor in the marrow containing one or more iron – siderotic granules which, on rare occasions, may be clustered in the form of a ring around the nucleus – *'ring' sideroblasts*.

A normal marrow may demonstrate small, barely discernible siderotic granules in the occasional normoblast.

SIDEROCYTE
A mature non-nucleated red cell in the peripheral blood containing one or more siderotic granules. With Romanowsky stains these are black and are called *Pappenheimer bodies*. Siderocytes are commonly seen post-splenectomy, probably because the spleen normally removes any iron granules as the red cell circulates through that organ (see Heinz bodies p. 456).

Nature of sideroblastic anaemias
These are a rare group of erythropoietic disorders in which sideroblasts become demonstrable in the bone marrow. Aetiologically they are divided into primary and secondary. For the most part, 'ring' sideroblasts are found only in the primary type, with siderotic granules randomly scattered in the

cytoplasm in the secondary type. There are exceptions to this differentiation, e.g. 'ring' sideroblasts may be found in secondary sideroblastic anaemia due to β-thalassaemia major (see p. 502) where there is gross depression of globin production combined with iron overload resulting from repeated transfusions.

PRIMARY SIDEROBLASTIC ANAEMIA
The peripheral blood film shows a dimorphic blood picture with a variable proportion of normochromic and hypochromic cells. The marrow shows 'ring' sideroblasts with, usually, grossly excessive iron deposits in the marrow fragments.

Congenital
This rare condition is inherited in a sex-linked pattern presenting as an anaemia in boys, females being virtually unaffected. The foetal haemoglobin is normal, distinguishing this condition from β-thalassaemia major (see p. 502).

Acquired
A progressive disease affecting middle-aged or elderly people. The severity of the anaemia may require the use of transfusion therapy which, as with aplastic anaemia (see p. 455), worsens the iron overload.

A number of cases respond to pyridoxine and a small number of pyridoxine-resistant patients may respond to pyridoxal phosphate. The doses required for a therapeutic effect, up to 500 mg daily, are much larger than needed merely to correct a dietary deficiency. A simple dietary deficiency of Vitamin B_6 (pyridoxal phosphate) must not be presumed, even in responsive cases.

SECONDARY SIDEROBLASTIC ANAEMIA

Vitamin B_6 – pyridoxine, deficiency
Dietary deficiency of Vitamin B_6 in experimental animals gives rise to iron overload and non-ring sideroblasts in the marrow. The role of dietary deficiency in man is uncertain. Vitamin B_6 antagonists, e.g. isoniazid, may occasionally give rise to sideroblastic anaemia.

Interference with haem formation
1 Lead poisoning is known to interfere with haem formation and may give a sideroblastic marrow picture.

2 Chloramphenicol depresses mitochondrial function – the site of haem formation, and sideroblasts may result.

3 Erythropoietic porphyria (see p. 479) may give rise to sideroblasts in the marrow.

Other haematological disorders

Sideroblasts have been found in a number of marrow disorders including anaemias of megaloblastic and haemolytic types, leukaemias and myeloproliferative disorders.

Chapter 81
Haematology – Megaloblastic Anaemias

Megaloblastic anaemias

Nature
Megaloblastic anaemias are almost always caused by a deficiency of vitamin B$_{12}$ and/or folate – the lack of either vitamin produces a similar defect in red cell maturation. Macrocytes appear in the peripheral blood and an abnormal red cell precursor – the *megaloblast*, can be demonstrated in the marrow. The clinical recognition of megaloblastic anaemias is important because of their excellent therapeutic response.

VITAMIN B$_{12}$
The term vitamin B$_{12}$ covers a related group of cobalt-containing chemicals collectively called *cobalamins.*

Source
Food of animal origin, particularly liver, meat and, to a lesser extent, eggs and milk.

Requirement
1 μg per day.

Absorption
Vitamin B$_{12}$ present in food must be combined with intrinsic factor, a glycoprotein secreted by the parietal cells of the fundus and body of the stomach, before it can be absorbed by the terminal ileum.

Although vitamin B$_{12}$ is produced in considerable quantities by the bacterial flora of the colon this source is unavailable to the host as its absorption cannot take place from the large bowel.

Body stores
Normal liver stores are sufficient for about 3–5 years, i.e. about 1000 μg.

CAUSES OF VITAMIN B$_{12}$ DEFICIENCY
In Northern Europe pernicious anaemia occurs in about one in a thousand of the population and is the

most important cause of vitamin B_{12} deficiency. This disease is uncommon in the Negro and Asian and an inadequate dietary intake due to malnutrition is the most common cause of vitamin B_{12} deficiency in developing countries.

DIMINISHED DIETARY INTAKE

Malnutrition – inadequacy of food of animal origin and including volitional vegetarian diet.

DIMINISHED ABSORPTION

1 *Loss of intrinsic factor*
(a) Pernicious anaemia.
(b) Postgastrectomy.
2 *Malabsorption syndromes.* Folic acid deficiency is likely to be of greater clinical significance, although vitamin B_{12} and iron may also be malabsorbed (see p. 209).
3 *Anatomical intestinal lesions.* Lesions such as a gastro-colic fistula may bypass the small intestine where optimal absorption occurs. Alternatively, the formation of blind loops may permit the overgrowth of bacteria which compete with the host for the available vitamin B_{12}.
4 *Fish tape-worm – diphyllobothrium latum.* This intestinal parasite, occurring in Finland, competes with the host for the available vitamin B_{12}.

Pernicious anaemia – Addison's anaemia

Pathogenesis
Mucosal atrophy in the body and fundus of the stomach results in a diminished secretion of intrinsic factor and, therefore, of vitamin B_{12} absorption.
1 *Hereditary factors.* Relatives of patients with pernicious anaemia show both an increased incidence of impaired absorption of vitamin B_{12} and of gastric and thyroid autoantibody formation and concomitant autoimmune disease.
2 *Autoantibodies.* The great majority of patients have gastric autoantibodies. The antibody may be active against either intrinsic factor or the gastric parietal cells, which also secrete hydrochloric acid or, on occasions, against both. The exact significance of these antibodies is uncertain but it is of interest that 50 per cent also have thyroid antibodies.

Clinical
The classical patient is elderly, has blue eyes and prematurely grey hair. The onset of the disease is insidious, the anaemia, and therefore the pallor, at times being extreme at the time of diagnosis. Slight jaundice may be noticeable. Occasionally there is a fever.
1 *Anaemia.* Symptoms and signs include weakness, fatigue, dyspnoea and pallor. Angina of effort and congestive cardiac failure may be precipitated. Slight hepatosplenomegaly is usual.
2 *Neurological.* Degenerative changes with demyelination may occur throughout the nervous system and in the advanced case some degree of neurological abnormality is commonly present.
(a) *Cerebral.* Mental disturbance varying from personality difficulties to major psychoses.
(b) *Spinal.* Subacute combined degeneration of the cord. This demyelination predominantly affects the dorsal columns, though the lateral columns may be affected also. (see p. 618).
(c) *Peripheral neuritis.* The lesion produced is symmetrical and peripheral. The presence of a lower motor neurone lesion will result in peripheral muscular weakness with diminished reflexes, and peripheral sensory loss with paraesthesia.
3 *Glossitis.* About half the patients complain of a sore tongue. On examination it will be without fur, smooth and, on occasions, looks red and raw – '*beefsteak*'.
4 *Gastrointestinal.* Patients may also present with some weight loss and gastrointestinal symptoms such as dyspepsia and diarrhoea. It is also important to remember that carcinoma of the stomach occurs with increased frequency in this condition (see p. 190).

Diagnosis
Laboratory tests permit early diagnosis.
1 *Blood.* A megaloblastic marrow not only produces an inadequate number of circulating red cells, but those that are produced have a shortened life span. This haemolytic element is demonstrated by the slightly raised plasma bilirubin. Although the characteristic feature is a macrocytic anaemia, there is in fact a pancytopenia.
(a) *Red cells.* The degree of anaemia is commonly severe, haemoglobin levels between 3–7 g/dl

being usual. The diagnostic features in the blood film are the presence of normochromic oval macrocytes with markedly raised M.C.V. and normal M.C.H. and tear-drop poikilocytes.

Although a lack of vitamin B_{12} or folic acid characteristically gives rise to a macrocytic anaemia, a hypochromic normocytic or microcytic picture results when there is a co-existent iron deficiency.

The presence of macrocytes in the peripheral blood does not necessarily imply a megaloblastic marrow. Normoblastic macrocytic anaemias are sometimes found in marrow depression, leukaemia, liver disease and alcoholism together with conditions causing a reticulocytosis.

(b) *White cells.* The coexistent defect in white cell maturation may give rise to neutropenia, the nuclei of the polymorphonuclear leucocytes being hypersegmented, so that many of them have more than the usual 3–4 lobes.

(c) *Platelets.* Due to diminished production there may be a thrombocytopenia, but seldom to a degree that causes spontaneous haemorrhage.

2 *Marrow.* There is marked erythroid hyperplasia with active marrow extension in long bones, and a marked diminution in fat content. The stained fragments appear solid with plentiful free cells, mostly megaloblasts. Iron content of the fragments is usually increased.

During normal (normoblastic) red-cell maturation the nuclear material coarsens, shrinks and is eventually expelled. Simultaneously, the cytoplasm develops haemoglobin, changing with Romanowsky stain, from dark blue to a polychromatic, grey colour, with the first appearance of haemoglobin. With subsequent full haemoglobinization the bright orange/pink colour of the mature red cell is achieved. At the stage of early haemoglobinization the normal nucleus should appear after staining as a small, black, coarsely striated or solid lump. In contrast, the larger megaloblast has an immature nuclear pattern which is still finely stippled, although the cell is sufficiently developed to have pink-staining haemoglobin demonstrable in the cytoplasm – nuclear-cytoplasmic dissociation. In addition, rounded nuclear fragments – *Howell–Jolly bodies,* may be found lying in the cytoplasm of the megaloblast. White cell maturation is also affected, giving rise to giant metamyelocytes. Megakaryocytic maturation may also be reduced.

3 *Vitamin B_{12} assay.* A pretreatment blood sample is mandatory but therapy does not have to await the result.

(a) *Microbiological assay.* This technique depends upon the selection of an organism which requires vitamin B_{12} for growth, e.g. Euglena gracilis or Lactobacillus leishmanii.

(b) *Radioimmunoassay.* This technique is now preferred in some centres. Normal range is 160–925 ng/l.

4 *Radioactive vitamin B_{12} absorption.* This test permits a diagnosis of pernicious anaemia to be established, even if vitamin B_{12} has been previously administered.

5 *Histamine-fast achlorhydria.* This can be demonstrated by an augmented histamine test meal or by use of pentagastrin. It is rarely necessary when the above tests are available.

6 *Satisfactory response to vitamin B_{12} therapy.* A good clinical response with rapid reticulocytosis usually confirms the diagnosis.

Treatment

To overcome an absorption defect vitamin B_{12} is administered intramuscularly, although the oral route is permissible in deficiency due to malnutrition. Folic acid must never be given as an alternative to a patient with vitamin B_{12} deficiency, because the neurological manifestations may become rapidly exacerbated.

SPECIFIC TREATMENT

Intramuscular injection of 1000 μg of vitamin B_{12} (cyanocobalamin), repeated daily for 5 days. Because injections must subsequently be given monthly for the rest of the patient's life every attempt must be made to establish a firm diagnosis, preferably before treatment is commenced. Hydroxocobalamin is excreted much less readily in the urine and it is sufficient to maintain the patient with 2000 μg i.m. of this preparation every 2 months.

GENERAL TREATMENT

Bed rest may be required and complications such as infections and congestive cardiac failure are treated. Whole blood transfusion is generally contraindicated because of the danger of circulatory overload, though an infusion of 'packed' red cells may be life-saving, particularly if an i.v. quick acting diuretic is given.

CLINICAL RESPONSE

The patient may feel better within a few hours of

the injection, and this is followed by rapid clinical improvement. Whilst the peripheral neuritis will disappear the neurological manifestations of the spinal cord lesion may well persist in part if they are of long standing.

HAEMATOLOGICAL RESPONSE

The megaloblastic changes in the marrow will disappear within a few hours. The response to therapy is measured by daily reticulocyte counts over a period of 7 days. The percentage of reticulocytes found, maximal usually on the fifth day, may be as high as 50 per cent if the initial Hb level was below 5 g/dl. The Hb level rises to normal over a few weeks. The therapeutic response will be slow in the presence of infections or renal failure and will be incomplete if iron deficiency is also present.

Prognosis

Untreated cases are invariably fatal. Treated cases do very well and all should respond. Associated conditions are however common, including myxoedema, diabetes and carcinoma of the stomach (see p. 190).

Juvenile pernicious anaemia

A rare form of pernicious anaemia due to a genetically determined lack of intrinsic factor may present in the first 2 years of life. There is no gastric atrophy, acid being normally secreted, and autoantibodies are absent.

Folate

The term folate is given to a group of related chemicals based on the parent molecule folic (pteroylglutamic) acid.

Source

The main source is green vegetables – 'foliage' and liver. An indifferent diet may contain little more than the minimal requirement and the majority of this may be lost in the water used for cooking, this being especially true in institutions.

Requirement

Normally about 100 μg a day.

Absorption

Naturally occurring folic acid has additional glutamic acid residues attached to the parent molecule and is thus a polyglutamate. All but one of these are removed during absorption through the duodenum and jejunum so that serum folate is in the monoglutamate form.

Body stores

Normal body stores, principally in the liver, are probably sufficient to last 3 months.

CAUSES OF FOLATE DEFICIENCY

The commonest cause of folate deficiency is nutritional. Since the widespread therapeutic introduction of prophylactic antenatal folic acid the severe manifestations presenting in pregnancy are now seldom seen in developed countries.

1 *Diminished dietary intake.* Whilst malnutrition may lead to folate deficiency at any age it is particularly prevalent in the old, in infants fed on dried milk and in alcoholic cirrhotics. Any patients with long-standing anorexia, especially if associated with chronic pyrexia, which increases the body requirements, are also at risk.

2 *Diminished absorption.*

(a) *Malabsorption syndromes.* Whilst these usually result in folate deficiency an associated deficiency of vitamin B_{12} and/or iron is sometimes found (see p. 482).

(b) *Antiepileptic drugs.* Patients taking long-term anti-epileptic drugs, e.g. phenytoin or primidone, may develop a megaloblastic anaemia. This may be due to malabsorption resulting from drug-induced inability to remove the excess glutamic residues attached to folic acid from natural sources.

3 *Increased demand*

(a) *Megaloblastic anaemia of pregnancy.* This disease presents in late pregnancy and the puerperium, being more common in multiparous women of lower social class on a poor diet. Because of the foetal requirements the maternal demand for folate more than doubles. When pregnancy is complicated by anorexia and vomiting an acute insufficiency rapidly occurs. The deficiency tends to be more severe in multiple pregnancies.

(b) *Megaloblastic anaemia in chronic haemolytic anaemia.* The increased erythropoiesis of the bone marrow necessary to compensate for shortened red cell life span results in an increased demand for folic acid. Patients with chronic haemolytic anaemia, e.g. sickle cell disease, require prophylactic folic acid and this is even more necessary if they become pregnant.

4. *Folic-acid antagonists.* Folic acid plays an essential role in the formation of DNA (see Fig. 47 on p. 465). Folic acid antagonists such as methotrexate are used in the treatment of acute leukaemia because of their ability to reduce cell division by purposely creating a folate-deficient state.

Clinical

The patient has a megaloblastic macrocytic anaemia and glossitis, but there are *no* neurological manifestations apart from personality disorder.

Diagnosis

1 *Blood.* Identical to pernicious anaemia. It is important to appreciate that all grades of folate deficiency occur and those with minimal deficiency may have normocytic red cells with minimal megaloblastic change in the marrow.

2 *Marrow.* Identical to pernicious anaemia.

3 *Folic acid assay.* An organism (lactobacillus casei) is selected, which is dependent upon folic acid for growth. In an otherwise complete nutrient medium, growth will depend upon the folic acid in the added serum. Normal range is above 3 ng/ml serum. Red cell folate levels are also measured and reflect a more accurate indication of the tissue-folate stores. The red cell folate level is usually low in vitamin B_{12} deficiency whereas the serum folate

will be normal or raised. Vitamin B_{12} assay may be more readily available, and if the result of this test is normal it gives presumptive evidence of folate deficiency in the presence of a megaloblastic anaemia.

4 *Satisfactory response to folic acid therapy*

Treatment

(*a*) *Specific.* Folate deficiency is treated by oral folic acid 15 mg daily, adequate quantities being absorbed at such high dosage even in malabsorption syndromes. Patients on antiepileptic drugs also respond to oral dosage because synthetic folic acid is not in the polyglutamate form and is, therefore, readily absorbed.

The usual prophylactic dose given in pregnancy or to patients with chronic haemolytic anaemia is one 5 mg tablet daily which is many times the normal daily requirement.

(*b*) *Other aspects.* The clinical and haematological response and general management are the same as for B_{12} deficiency.

ASCORBIC ACID DEFICIENCY

Ascorbic acid and folic acid occur in the same foodstuffs and a combined deficiency is common; the megaloblastic anaemia previously ascribed to scurvy probably being due to the coexistent folate deficiency. The usual haematological manifestation of ascorbic acid deficiency is that of iron deficiency due to both malabsorption of iron and haemorrhages (see p. 475).

Chapter 82
Haematology – Haemolytic Anaemias: Inherited

Haemolytic anaemias

Definition
The normal red cell survives 100–120 days. A haemolytic anaemia is the result of an increase in red cell destruction and shortening of the normal red cell life span. The wide range of disease states capable of causing a haemolytic anaemia have nothing in common except this tendency to destroy the circulating red cell prematurely.

A haemolytic process need not necessarily result in anaemia, when the excessive red cell loss may be totally compensated by increased production by the marrow – *compensated haemolytic anaemia*.

DIAGNOSIS OF HAEMOLYSIS

1 *Clinical.* A patient with haemolytic anaemia may give a history varying from, in severe cases, an episode of haemoglobinuria to, in more mild examples, pallor with periodic bouts of jaundice. Splenomegaly is usual.

2 *Laboratory.* A number of tests are commonly employed to establish the presence of increased haemolysis by recognizing:

(a) Increased red cell destruction.

(b) Increased marrow output of red cells.

Many of these tests are insensitive and may give negative results in mild haemolytic processes, e.g.

486

patients may not be jaundiced. A direct measurement of the red cell life span, using radioactive chromium (see below), is increasingly relied on firmly to establish the presence of a clinically equivocal haemolytic process.

EVIDENCE OF INCREASED RED CELL DESTRUCTION

DEMONSTRATION OF ABNORMAL RED CELLS IN THE PERIPHERAL BLOOD

Spherocytes can often be recognized by microscopy, their presence being an especially prominent feature in the blood film of a patient with hereditary spherocytosis (see p. 490). Unlike the normal biconcave red cell the spherical cell cannot expand further without rupturing. Their presence can therefore be confirmed by increased lysis when they are suspended in hypotonic saline during an osmotic fragility test. Target cells (see p. 501), sickle cells (see p. 499), red cell fragments (see p. 531), elliptocytes (see p. 491) and acanthocytes (see p. 499) may all be recognized in a peripheral blood film.

SITE OF RED CELL DESTRUCTION

Haemolysis may occur principally in the lymphoreticular system – *extravascular lysis*. Surface counting of ^{51}Cr over the liver and spleen, usually during the cell survival study, can be used to assess the most active sites of red cell destruction.

When destruction is for the most part *intravascular* there is also evidence of increased haemoglobin catabolism. Haemoglobin released into the plasma is rapidly bound to haptoglobin. Normally there is only sufficient to bind about 50–200 mg Hb/dl plasma, i.e. about 5–15 ml of red cells in the normal male plasma volume.

N.B. The haptoglobin content of serum may be increased in cases of malignancy including Hodgkin's disease, infections with tissue damage and S.L.E. Liver damage may deplete the haptoglobin without haemolysis.

Some of the remaining 'free' haemoglobin is broken down in the circulation to form methaemalbumin, the presence of which indicates a recent intravascular episode. Unchanged haemoglobin passes in the glomerular filtrate, some of which is degraded and can be detected as haemosiderinuria. The remainder can be identified in the urine as methaemoglobin and oxyhaemoglobin.

MEASUREMENT OF THE RED CELL LIFE SPAN

Radioactive chromium (^{51}Cr) will combine with the haemoglobin molecules within the red cells. The rate at which such labelled red cells subsequently disappear from the circulation can be assessed by periodic measurement of the radioactivity of the patient's blood. If surface counting demonstrates a rise in radioactivity over the spleen, suggesting red cell destruction in that organ, a splenectomy may restore normal red cell life span.

DEMONSTRATION OF FREE HAEMOGLOBIN IN THE PLASMA AND URINE

1   *Haemoglobinaemia.* Normal red cell destruction occurs mainly in the cells of the phagocytic system of the spleen, liver and bone-marrow and not in the bloodstream. Only if haemolysis is exceptionally severe, e.g. an incompatible transfusion, will free haemoglobin be recognized by the pink-coloured plasma.

2   *Haptoglobin.* Small quantities of free haemoglobin in the plasma can combine with the plasma protein haptoglobin (an $\alpha_2$globin) and form a molecular complex too large to pass through the glomerulus into the urine. This haemoglobin–haptoglobin complex is subsequently rapidly removed from the circulation by the phagocytic cell system. It follows that uncombined haptoglobin is usually decreased in a haemolytic process. Only when all the haptoglobin has become totally complexed with haemoglobin will the excess haemoglobin appear in the urine.

3   *Methaemalbumin.* During a moderately severe haemolytic process some free haem which has been released from haemoglobin becomes oxidized to haematin ($Fe^{++} \rightarrow Fe^{+++}$), and is then attached to plasma albumin as methaemabumin and is detectable by spectroscopy – *Schumm's test.*

4   *Haemoglobinuria.* If haemolysis is sufficiently severe to saturate the haptoglobin the size of the excess free and uncombined circulating haemoglobin molecule (M.W. 64 000) is small enough to pass through the glomerulus into the urine.

Haematuria may be differentiated from *haemoglobinuria* by demonstrating, in a centrifuged urine deposit, intact red cells in haematuria (see p. 379) but not in haemoglobinuria (see p. 506), e.g. 'Blackwater fever' in malaria (see p. 65).

5   *Haemosiderinuria.* Haemosiderin is deposited in the kidney tubule cells during an episode of hae-

moglobinuria. Because these kidney tubule cells are subsequently desquamated, haemosiderin will continue to be detectable in urinary deposit by a Perls' stain long after the haemolytic episode has ceased, e.g. paroxysmal nocturnal haemoglobinuria (see p. 491).

DEMONSTRATION OF INCREASED HAEMOGLOBIN CATABOLISM

When a red cell is digested by a phagocytic cell the haemoglobin molecule is catabolized.

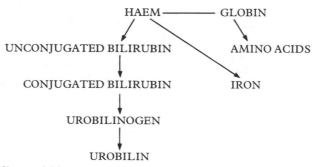

Fig. 49. The breakdown of haemoglobin.

Measurement of the excretion of the breakdown products of haem will indicate the rate of haemoglobin catabolism and therefore of haemolysis.

1   *Haem→Bilirubin*. The iron is released from the haem and the porphyrin ring then opens to become converted to bilirubin:

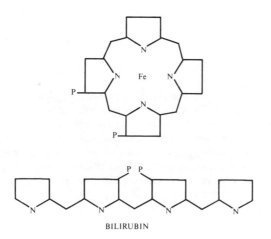

BILIRUBIN

The bilirubin is water-insoluble and is transported in the plasma linked with albumin, a molecule too large to pass through the glomerulus into the urine. In the liver the link with albumin is broken and the bilirubin is made water-soluble by being conjugated to glucuronic acid to form water-soluble bilirubin–glucuronide. In uncomplicated cases of haemolytic anaemia this conjugated water-soluble bilirubin is totally excreted in the bile into the intestine. However, if there is a superimposed biliary obstruction, e.g. gall stones, the level of conjugated bilirubin will rise in the plasma. Being water-soluble and unassociated with albumin this conjugated bilirubin–glucuronide will freely pass into the urine.

Van den Bergh reaction. Plasma bilirubin may be estimated by the van den Bergh test.

1   The first part of the test measures the water-soluble, conjugated bilirubin—bilirubin-glucuronide only – the '*direct acting*' fraction.

2   An organic solvent (alcohol) is now added and the total, water-soluble + water-insoluble bilirubin is measured. The difference between the total bilirubin and the 'direct acting' fraction gives the '*indirect acting*' bilirubin – the water-insoluble unconjugated fraction. The typical jaundice of haemolytic anaemia shows a raised 'indirect acting' bilirubin in the plasma.

2   *Bilirubin→urobilinogen→urobilin*. Bilirubin-glucuronide is converted in the intestine to urobilinogen. After excretion in the faeces urobilinogen is oxidized to urobilin. During its passage down the bowel a small amount of the faecal urobilinogen is absorbed through the intestine wall. Whilst the majority of this absorbed urobilinogen is re-excreted in the bile and thus reappears in the faeces,

a small quantity appears in the urine. After voiding, the colourless urinary urobilinogen is oxidized to brown urobilin.

N.B. In a haemolytic anaemia:

1 Jaundice is due to 'indirect acting' albumin-linked bilirubin.
2 There is no bilirubin in the urine – *'acholuric' jaundice.*
3 There is increased urobilinogen/urobilin in the urine.
4 There is increased urobilinogen/urobilin in the faeces.
5 The picture may be complicated by bile duct obstruction secondary to pigment stones formed in the gall bladder as a result of excess bilirubin in bile in chronic haemolytic states (see p. 490).

EVIDENCE OF INCREASED MARROW RED CELL OUTPUT

Blood
The reticulocyte count is raised and, in severe cases, nucleated red cells are seen in the peripheral blood – *erythroblastosis or erythroblastaemia.* In a chronic haemolytic anaemia the delicate balance between increased marrow output and haemolysis may well be disturbed. Infections are particularly liable either to depress marrow output – *aplastic crisis,* or increase haemolysis – *haemolytic crisis.* In both cases there may be a catastrophic fall in the Hb level with a low reticulocyte count in the former and a raised reticulocyte count in the latter.

In an acute haemolytic process, even when unassociated with infections, it is common also to find a polymorphonuclear leucocytosis.

Marrow
1 *Macroscopical.* There is an increase in erythropoietic marrow activity to compensate for the increased haemolysis with extension of red marrow in the limb bones of the adult (see p. 442). In a severe chronic haemolytic anaemia radiological abnormalities may be produced (see p. 442).
2 *Microscopical.* Loss of fat spaces due to erythroid hyperplasia and alteration in M:E ratio (see p. 444) from normal 4:1 to as much as 1:2. Initially normoblastic, but may later become megaloblastic due to excessive folic acid utilization.

RADIOACTIVE IRON (^{59}FE) STUDIES

The quantity of iron transported from the site of red-cell destruction in phagocytic cells to the erythropoietic tissue in the marrow – *plasma iron turnover,* can be measured by radioactive iron studies, and is increased in haemolytic anaemia.

After the radioactive iron has been taken up by the marrow, the majority will be utilized to make haemoglobin and will subsequently appear in the circulating red cells of the peripheral blood. If red cell life span is very short, e.g. β Thalassaemia major p. 502, many developing red cells are destroyed in the marrow before their release into the peripheral blood – *ineffective erythropoiesis.* This is demonstrated by an increased plasma iron turnover with poor utilization of the radioactive iron, i.e. little radioactive iron is subsequently demonstrable in the circulating red blood cells.

CAUSES OF HAEMOLYTIC ANAEMIA

There are two main groups:
1 An abnormality within the red cell – *corpuscular or intrinsic.*
2 An abnormal red-cell environment – *extracorpuscular or extrinsic.*

There is slight overlap, e.g. anti-malarial drugs (i.e. an extracorpuscular stress) which are harmless to the normal red cell, may precipitate a haemolytic episode in red cells deficient in the enzyme glucose-6-phosphate dehydrogenase (i.e. a corpuscular defect).

CORPUSCULAR (INTRINSIC)

With the exception of paroxysmal nocturnal haemoglobinuria, all the corpuscular causes of haemolysis are *inherited.* Clinically, therefore, symptoms may date from childhood and there is usually a well-defined family history.

Membrane abnormalities
1 *Congenital.*
(a) Hereditary spherocytosis.
(b) Hereditary elliptocytosis.
2 *Acquired.* Paroxysmal nocturnal haemoglobinuria.

Metabolic abnormalities – Enzymopathies

1 *Energy production failure* – Pyruvate kinase deficiency.
2 *Oxidation-reduction failure* – Glucose-6-phosphate dehydrogenase deficiency.

Haemoglobin production abnormalities – Haemoglobinopathies

1 *Abnormal haemoglobins.*
2 *Thalassaemia.*

EXTRACORPUSCULAR (EXTRINSIC)

Extracorpuscular (extrinsic) defects are almost exclusively *acquired* disorders. The rare exception to this statement are inherited abnormalities of plasma lipoprotein, which cause red-cell lysis by a secondary effect on the fat content of the red cell envelope. Extracorpuscular defects responsible for haemolysis are, therefore, commonly generally referred to as '*acquired haemolytic anaemias*'. They are considered in more detail in Chapter 84 but the main causes can be classified as follows:

Immune factors

1 *Auto-immune haemolytic anaemia.*
(*a*) Acute.
  (i) Primary.
  (ii) Secondary.
(*b*) Chronic.
  (i) Primary.
  (ii) Secondary.
(*c*) Paroxysmal cold haemoglobinuria.
2 *Immune response to drugs* – e.g. methyl dopa.
3 *Foetal–maternal incompatibility* – e.g. rhesus.
4 *Incompatible blood transfusion.*

Chemical injury

1 *Chemicals* – e.g. arsine.
2 *Haemolysins.*
(*a*) Bacterial haemolysins.
(*b*) Venoms.
3 *Plasma lipid abnormalities.*
(*a*) Inherited.
(*b*) Acquired – e.g. liver disease.

Physical injury

1 *Hypersplenism.*
2 *Fragmentation haemolytic anaemias.*
(*a*) Microangiopathic haemolytic anaemia.
(*b*) Heart valve replacements.

(*c*) March haemoglobinuria.
3 *Burns.*
4 *Intracorpuscular parasites* – malaria.

CORPUSCULAR DEFECT

Membrane abnormalities – (1) congenital

HEREDITARY SPHEROCYTOSIS

Pathogenesis
Due to a defect in the red-cell membrane the cells take on a spherocytic form and are selectively trapped in the spleen.

Inheritance
The condition is more common in Northern Europeans and is inherited as an autosomal dominant. Family studies commonly discover other cases who are often asymptomatic or only mildly affected, i.e. have a palpable spleen but no clinical history of haemolytic episodes.

Clinical
1 *Anaemia.* The haemoglobin is often only slightly reduced and may even be within the normal range. The course of the disease is interspersed with aplastic or haemolytic crises, which commonly follow infections (see p. 453). Folic acid deficiency may result in a complicating megaloblastic anaemia (see p. 484).
2 *Jaundice.* The findings are typical of a haemolytic anaemia (see p. 489). There is commonly an increased level of plasma bilirubin of the unconjugated type, without bilirubin in the urine. Excess urobilinogen/urobilin is present in both urine and faeces. Gallstones frequently occur in this disorder and complications such as biliary obstruction and cholecystitis are common (see p. 575).
3 *Splenomegaly.* A palpable spleen, of moderate size, is usually present.
4 *Leg ulcers.* Leg ulcers have been described in a number of chronic haemolytic aneamias including hereditary spherocytosis.

Blood
1 *Haemoglobin.* Hb 7–14 g/dl.
2 *Blood film.* Small dark-staining spherocytes together with polychromasia.
3 *Reticulocytes.* Raised.
4 *Osmotic fragility test.* Increased lysis of red cells suspended in hypotonic saline.

5 *Marrow:* Normoblastic erythroid hyperplasia.

Spleen
Moderately enlarged due to hyperplastic pulp crowded with red cells. Excess iron present, also in liver and kidney.

Treatment
Splenectomy is followed by a marked reduction in haemolysis although the red cell defect remains. The risk of gallstones and cholecystitis is thereby reduced.

HEREDITARY ELLIPTOCYTOSIS – OVALOCYTOSIS

Pathogenesis
Probably due to a fault in the red cell membrane, the red cells assume an oval shape.

Inheritance
The condition is inherited as an autosomal dominant defect. In some cases its inheritance has been found to be linked closely to the Rhesus blood group genes. Elliptocytosis is an uncommon condition described in most racial groups.

Types
Hereditary elliptocytosis trait – heterozygous
Such carriers are clinically well with either a mild haemolytic process or none at all.

Homozygous hereditary elliptocytosis
This very rare condition results in severe anaemia with up to 25 per cent abnormally shaped red cells in the peripheral blood. Splenectomy will lessen the haemolysis.

Membrane abnormalities – (2)
Acquired
PAROXYSMAL NOCTURNAL HAEMOGLOBINURIA (P.N.H.)

Nature
A rare form of acquired chronic haemolytic anaemia affecting adults. There is an abnormality of the red cell envelope which results in excessive sensitivity to complement and tendency to lysis.

Clinical
1 *Haemolysis.*
(a) Haemoglobinuria. More common in early morning urine samples.
(b) Haemosiderinuria is detected during remissions free from haemoglobinuria.
2 *Marrow failure.* Aplastic anaemia is commonly associated with PNH causing:
(a) Increasing anaemia.
(b) Thrombocytopenia leading to bruising and haemorrhage.
(c) Leucopenia which, if severe, may encourage chronic infections.
3 *Thrombosis.* Venous thrombosis may complicate the course of the disease and ultimately prove fatal.

Blood
1 *Haemoglobin.* The degree of anaemia depends upon both the severity of the haemolysis and the degree of marrow failure. Iron deficiency may be superimposed if haemoglobinuria is severe and prolonged.
2 *Reticulocytes.* The reticulocyte count is commonly raised but may, like the platelet and white count, be lowered in marrow failure.
3 *Tests detecting sensitivity to complement.*
(a) Acid serum lysis test – Ham's test. Red cells of PNH patients lyse when incubated in fresh, i.e. complement-containing, ABO compatible serum acidified to pH 6.5–7.
(b) Sucrose lysis. Isotonic sucrose solutions have low ionic strength. Red cells suspended in such media become coated with complement and in these conditions PNH cells lyse.
   N.B. Patient's serum complement may be deficient due to continuous utilization.
4 *Leucocyte alkaline phosphatase.* Low in uncomplicated PNH and is raised in aplastic anaemia unassociated with PNH

Treatment
Transfusions should be avoided unless the anaemia is life-threatening. Washed, complement-free red cells are then required. Splenectomy is contraindicated.

Results
This disease usually proves fatal although spontaneous remissions may occur.

Metabolic abnormalities – (1)
Defects of energy production
To maintain its structural integrity the mature red cell requires
1 Energy production.
2 Protection against oxidative stress.

Biochemistry

Ninety-five per cent of glucose is metabolized through the Embden–Meyerhof pathway: each molecule of glucose anaerobically converted to lactic acid yields energy in the form of two molecules of ATP. At the same time, NADH (reduced NAD^+) is produced which is utilized by the physiologically important variety of methaemoglobin reductase to reduce the ferric (Fe^{+++}) iron atom of methaemoglobin to the ferrous (Fe^{++}) iron atom of haemoglobin.

$$
\begin{array}{cc}
& \text{Methaemoglobin} \\
& \text{reductase} \\
\left.\begin{array}{l}\text{Methaemoglobin } Fe^{+++} \\ \text{Haemoglobin } Fe^{++}\end{array}\right) & \downarrow \quad \left(\begin{array}{l}NADH \\ NAD^+\end{array}\right.
\end{array}
$$

N.B: The Embden–Meyerhof pathway:

1 *Produces ATP.* A failure of energy (ATP) production prevents the 'sodium pump' removing excess sodium and water from the cell. As a result the red cell swells and eventually lyses.

2 *Produces NADH.*

3 *NADPH is not produced.*

PYRUVATE-KINASE DEFICIENCY

Nature

A number of rare, enzyme deficiencies have been described which impede one of the essential steps in energy production. Pyruvate-kinase (PK) deficiency decreases the conversion of glucose to lactic acid on the Embden–Meyerhof pathway by preventing the conversion of phosphoenolpyruvate to pyruvate (see Fig. 50).

Clinical

Patients present with the stigmata of a chronic haemolytic anaemia, i.e. anaemia, jaundice and splenomegaly.

Blood

1 *Haemoglobin.* Hb 4–10 g/dl.

2 *Blood film:* Polychromasia may be marked but spherocytes are not a prominent feature.

3 *Reticulocytes:* Raised.

4 *Pyruvate kinase enzyme assay:* Diminished activity.

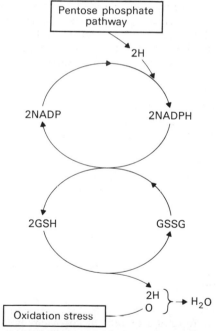

Fig. 51. The role of the Pentose phosphate pathway, NADPH and reduced glutathione in protecting the red cell from oxidation stress.

N.B. The Pentose phosphate pathway: produces NADPH. This maintains glutathione in the reduced form (GSH). Reduced glutathione protects the red-cell membrane from rupture and the haemoglobin molecule from denaturation (Heinz body formation).

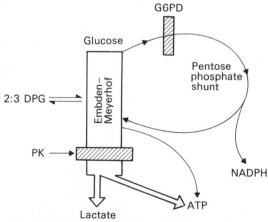

Fig. 50. Glucose metabolism in the mature red cell.

PF = Site of metabolic block due to pyruvate kinase deficiency.

G6PD = Site of metabolic block due to glucose-6-phosphate dehydrogenase deficiency.

2:3 DPG = 2:3 Diphosphoglycerate (decreases the affinity of the haemoglobin molecule for oxygen (see p. 476).

ATP = Adenosine 5′ triphosphate.

NADH = Reduced form of nicotinamide-adenine-dinucleotide.

NADPH = Reduced form of nicotinamide-adenine-dinucleotide-phosphate.

Treatment
Patients may be surprisingly symptom free but sometimes require transfusions. Splenectomy may be helpful.

Metabolic abnormalities – (2)
Defects of oxidation-reduction

Biochemistry
Both the red-cell membrane and the globin portion of the haemoglobin molecule require protection from oxidation and this is achieved by the release of hydrogen atoms through the conversion of reduced glutathione (GSH) to glutathione (GSSG) by the enzyme glutathione reductase.

Even in the presence of an oxidative stress, the red cell can still be protected from harmful oxidation provided that an adequate supply of reduced glutathione can be regenerated from glutathione. This is achieved by transferring the hydrogen atoms from NADPH which is generated by the pentose phosphate shunt. Failure to maintain an adequate quantity of intra-erythrocytic NADPH, and therefore of reduced glutathione, results in red cell fragmentation and the deposition of denatured haemoglobin as *Heinz bodies* within the red cell.

GLUCOSE-6-PHOSPHATE
DEHYDROGENASE – G6PD DEFICIENCY

Nature
G6PD is one of a number of enzymes in the pentose phosphate shunt. Under normal circumstances the mature red cell can survive reasonably well when G6PD activity is diminished. However, numerous drugs or their metabolites possess, like methylene blue, both an oxidized and reduced form, i.e. have redox potential and their presence within the red cell stresses the protective mechanism against oxidation and increases the demand for reduced glutathione. The normal red cell responds by increasing the activity of the pentose phosphate shunt but if, in G6PD deficiency, this is not possible, then reduced glutathione will diminish within the red cell and Heinz body formation and haemolysis results. Of the many varieties of abnormal G6PD described two only, affecting millions of people, warrant mention:
1 Mediterranean deficiency variant.
2 African deficiency (A type) variant.

The African variant possesses a little enzyme activity and its clinical manifestations are less severe than the virtually totally inactive Mediterranean enzyme deficiency.

It is possible that patients who are G6PD deficient also have some resistance to malaria.

Inheritance
The gene for G6PD is on the X chromosome and gives a sex-linked recessive pattern of inheritance. The male, possessing only one X chromosome, has either a normal or an abnormal gene. The female, having two X chromosomes, may have two normal genes or two abnormal genes or may be a carrier with both one normal and one abnormal gene.

One or the other of the two X chromosomes in every female cell are randomly inactivated during the development of the foetus (Lyon hypothesis). Depending upon which X chromosome was inactivated in the embryonic cells subsequently responsible for the erythropoietic tissue, an *individual* red cell in a female carrier will either possess full enzyme activity or be G6PD deficient. Whilst most female carriers have *in toto* about half the normal enzyme activity (i.e. half their red cells are fully active and half are deficient), a few have red cells which are almost all active and a few have red cells which are almost all deficient (see also p. 528).

Clinical
1 *Haemolytic crisis*
(*a*) *Drugs and chemicals.* Numerous drugs may precipitate a haemolytic crisis, i.e. the drug or its metabolite has redox potential. These include
   (i) Antimalarials, e.g. primaquine.
   (ii) Antibiotics, e.g. sulphonamides.
   (iii) Analgesics, e.g. phenacetin, acetylsalicylic acid.
   (iv) Vitamin-K analogues.
   (v) Chemicals used in the home, e.g. naphthalene mothballs, or in industry, may also cause haemolysis.
In a haemolytic crisis the older red cells, because of their diminished enzyme activity, are often specifically lysed. In contrast, the relatively young red cells with higher enzyme activity may persist in the circulation even if the provocative drug is continued at the same dose. If this situation occurs the patient's haemoglobin level may finally stabilize when the population of young red cells are established, thus limiting the severity of the haemolytic process.
(*b*) *Favism.* Some (not all) patients with the Medi-

terranean type of G6PD deficiency have a haemolytic crisis after eating the fava bean (broad bean). Even the inhalation of bean pollen may precipitate a crisis – *Baghdad spring fever*.

2 *Neonatal jaundice*. Jaundice in the newborn may be caused by G6PD deficiency and be sufficiently severe to result in kernicterus – bilirubin greater than 350 mmol/l. Routine administration of Vitamin-K analogues to newborn babies should be avoided in ethnic groups with G6PD deficiency.

3 *Chronic haemolytic anaemia*. Rarely, patients with G6PD deficiency may suffer from chronic haemolysis even in the absence of provocative drugs.

Blood

Betweeen attacks, the routine haematological findings are normal. During an acute haemolytic crisis haemoglobinuria and the other stigmata of acute haemolysis as described below may be found.

1 *Haemoglobin*. Reduced during the acute haemolytic crisis.

2 *Blood film*. Red cell fragments and polychromasia are found.

3 *Reticulocytes*. Raised.

4 *Heinz bodies*. May be demonstrated.

5 *Demonstration of diminished G6PD activity*.

(a) *Dye decolourization tests*. These depend upon the production of colour from substrates which rely on an intact pentose–phosphate shunt.

(b) *Cytochemical test*. A refined cytochemical technique which detects NADPH in individual red cells is able to demonstrate even a small proportion of enzymatically deficient red cells. This test is particularly valuable in recognizing female heterozygotes with unusually high G6PD activity, i.e. with relatively few G6PD-deficient cells.

Treatment

The numerous drugs and chemicals capable of precipitating a haemolytic crisis should be avoided. Patients with favism should not eat broad beans. If transfusions are required it is wise to screen the donor blood for G6PD activity, especially if relatives are used as donors, or G6PD deficiency is common in the area.

Chapter 83
Haematology—Haemoglobinopathies

Normal haemoglobins

Each haemoglobin molecule has four haem/polypeptide chain units combined in a tetrameric structure. There are four different polypeptide chains, alpha (α), beta (β), gamma (γ) and delta (δ), each with its own specific amino-acid sequence and each manufactured under the control of different structural genes. The three important physiological haemoglobins, adult haemoglobin, foetal haemoglobin and haemoglobin A_2 are constructed from the polypeptide chains on page 496.

N.B.: 1 During the first few months of life, foetal haemoglobin is almost completely replaced by adult haemoglobin.

2 All three haemoglobins, A, A_2 and F, contain α chains. An abnormality of α chain production will, therefore, affect all three haemoglobins.

3 Only HbA ($\alpha_2\beta_2$) contains β chains. An abnormality of β chain production, e.g. sickle cell anaemia or β thalassaemia major will affect only adult haemoglobin. The newborn child will be protected and will only be clinically affected after a few months when foetal haemoglobin production has diminished.

	Polypeptide chain	Proportion (adult) %
Normal adult haemoglobin (HbA)	$\alpha_2\beta_2$	97
Haemoglobin A$_2$	$\alpha_2\delta_2$	2
Foetal haemoglobin (HbF)	$\alpha_2\gamma_2$	1

		Proportion (newborn) %
Foetal haemoglobin (HbF)	$\alpha_2\gamma_2$	70
Adult haemoglobin (HbA)	$\alpha_2\beta_2$	30

Fig. 52. Normal haemoglobin components.

Types of haemoglobinopathies

1 *Abnormal haemoglobins*. A change in the DNA of the structural gene results in the production of a polypeptide chain with, commonly, a single amino-acid substitution. The important abnormal haemoglobins all have amino-acid substitutions in the β polypeptide chain, e.g. sickle cell haemoglobin (HbS) has a substitution of valine for glutamic acid in the sixth position of the β chain: the α polypeptide chains being normal:

$$HbS = \alpha^A{}_2\beta_2{}^6 \text{ glutamic acid} \rightarrow \text{valine.}$$

N.B. The rate of production of the abnormal polypeptide chain is normal, the end product is abnormal.

1 *Thalassaemias*. These are due to a reduction of the amount of a specific polypeptide chain, either α or β, produced. The small amount that is produced has a normal amino-acid structure. The important variety of thalassaemia – Mediterranean or Cooley's anaemia, has a severe depression of β polypeptide chain production – β thalassaemia major.

Inheritance of the haemoglobinopathies

Each individual has two β polypeptide chain genes situated on homologous (paired) chromosomes, one inherited from the mother and one from the father. It follows that there are four possible genetic situations.

1 *The normal homozygote*. Each parent has donated one normal β polypeptide chain gene to the offspring. The two β polypeptide chain genes of the offspring are both normal and, therefore, produce normal β polypeptide chains in normal quantity.

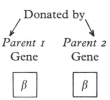

2 *The heterozygote*. One β polypeptide chain gene is normal and one is abnormal.

(*a*) *Sickle cell haemoglobin*:

Such a person is a carrier of sickle cell haemoglobin. Half the β polypeptide chains produced will carry the amino-acid substitution of sickle cell haemoglobin and the other half will be normal. It follows that roughly half the patient's haemoglobin will be sickle cell haemoglobin and the other half will be normal adult haemoglobin. Carriers of haemoglobin C, D or E also carry one abnormal gene and one normal gene, i.e. HbC carrier $= \beta \, \beta^C$ and, as in the case of a sickle cell carrier, carry normal and abnormal haemoglobin in approximately equal amounts.

(*b*) *Thalassaemia*:

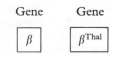

Such a person is a carrier of β thalassaemia, i.e. has β thalassaemia minor. There are little or no β polypeptide chains produced by the thalassaemic gene. However, in the carrier, the normal β polypeptide chain gene produces enough β chains to maintain the Hb level around 10–12 g/dl.

3 *The abnormal homozygote.* Both β chain genes are abnormal, each parent having contributed an abnormal gene to the offspring.

(*a*) *Sickle cell haemoglobin*:

Gene   Gene

$\boxed{\beta^S}$ $\boxed{\beta^S}$

Such a patient suffers from sickle cell anaemia with virtually all haemoglobin being sickle cell haemoglobin. There is no production of normal β polypeptide chains and, therefore, there is no normal adult haemoglobin ($\alpha_2\beta_2$). It is usual for a small quantity of foetal haemoglobin (5–10 per cent of the total) to continue to be produced even in the adult.

Patients with haemoglobin C disease, D disease and E disease are all homozygous for their specific abnormal gene, e.g. haemoglobin C disease $=\beta^C\,\beta^C$. As in the case of sickle cell anaemia, no normal haemoglobin is found, only HbC, HbD or HbE together with a small quantity of foetal haemoglobin.

(*b*) *Thalassaemia*:

Gene   Gene

$\boxed{\beta^{Thal}}$ $\boxed{\beta^{Thal}}$

Such a patient has β thalassaemia major. The quantity of β chains and therefore adult haemoglobin $\alpha_2\beta_2$, found on haematological examination, will depend on whether the thalassaemia genes are of the type which produces either a little β polypeptide chain or none at all. Some total haemoglobin is still produced.

4 *The doubly abnormal heterozygote.* It is possible for both β polypeptide chain genes to be abnormal, and yet the abnormality in one may be dissimilar to the abnormality in the other. Numerous genetic combinations are possible of which three only are sufficiently common to deserve mention.

(*a*) *Sickle cell haemoglobin C disease*:

Gene 1   Gene 2

$\boxed{\beta^S}$ $\boxed{\beta^C}$

The patient has one β polypeptide chain structural gene with the DNA abnormality producing the amino-acid substitution characteristic of the β^S polypeptide chain. The other β polypeptide chain structural gene carried by the patient has the DNA abnormality, producing the amino-acid substitution characteristic of the abnormal β polypeptide chain present in haemoglobin C (β^C). Such a patient produces sickle cell haemoglobin ($\alpha_2\beta_2{}^S$) and haemoglobin C($\alpha_2\beta_2{}^C$) only and has no normal adult haemoglobin because there is no normal β polypeptide chain gene.

(*b*) *Sickle cell β thalassaemia*:

Gene 1   Gene 2

$\boxed{\beta^S}$ $\boxed{\beta^{Thal}}$

One β polypeptide chain gene produces the sickle cell β polypeptide chain and the other gene, being a β thalassaemia, has little or no β polypeptide chain production. This patient would have a preponderance of sickle cell haemoglobin with a little foetal haemoglobin and, depending on whether the β thalassaemia gene produces few or no β polypeptide chain genes, a little or no normal adult haemoglobin will be present.

(*c*) *Haemoglobin E-β thalassaemia*:

Gene 1   Gene 2

$\boxed{\beta^E}$ $\boxed{\beta^{Thal}}$

The inheritance pattern is similar to that described for sickle cell β thalassaemia above. However, in this example, the abnormal β polypeptide chain gene produces the β polypeptide chain characteristic of haemoglobin E.

Genetic counselling

1 Sickle cell anaemia usually arises from a mating of two sickle cell trait carriers (Fig. 53).

2 β thalassaemia major usually arises from a mating of two carriers of β thalassaemia (β thalassaemia minor) (Fig. 54).

In the case of both sickle cell haemoglobin and β

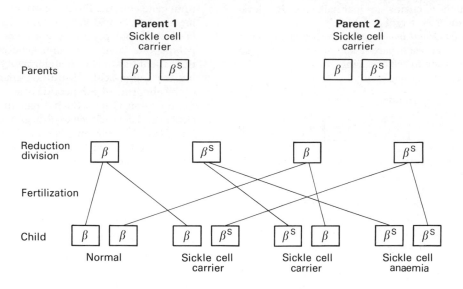

Fig. 53. Inheritance of sickle-cell anaemia.

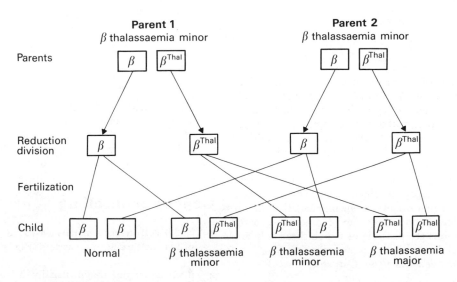

Fig. 54. Inheritance of thalassaemia.

thalassaemia the mating of two carriers has a one-in-four chance of producing a severely affected child, either sickle cell anaemia or β thalassaemia major. Genetic counselling is being increasingly requested to avoid such matings. Antenatal diagnosis by fetoscopy is becoming increasingly available.

Abnormal haemoglobins

There are four common abnormal haemoglobins, sickle-cell haemoglobin and haemoglobins C, D and E, of which the most important clinically is HbS.

GEOGRAPHICAL DISTRIBUTION OF THE ABNORMAL HAEMOGLOBINS

	Main reservoir
HbS (Sickle cell)	Central African and New World Negro
HbC	West African and New World Negro
HbD (Punjab)	Punjab
HbE	South-East Asia

SICKLE CELL HAEMOGLOBIN – HbS

When sickle cell haemoglobin is deoxygenated, it becomes insoluble and crystallizes out in the red cell. Such red cells take on a characteristic sickle shape and may obstruct blood flow and cause infarction. Infarction is a clinical complication unique to sickle cell haemoglobin and largely responsible for the high mortality of sickle cell anaemia compared with cases of haemoglobin C, D or E disease.

SICKLE CELL CARRIER

Clinical
Twenty per cent of Central African Negroes and 8 per cent of New World Negroes are sickle cell carriers. Such people are fit although they may suffer from episodes of infarction, especially in the spleen, if grossly deoxygenated by anaesthetic accidents or high-altitude flying in unpressurized aircraft.

Young children, who are sickle cell trait carriers,

have an increased resistance to malignant malaria (see p. 64).

Blood
1 *Haemoglobin.* Normal.
2 *Blood film.* Normal.
3 *Sickle cell haemoglobin may be recognized*:
(a) *Sickling test.* Red cells are suspended in a reducing solution and examined, under the microscope, to see if they '*Sickle*'.
(b) *Solubility test.* Red cells are lysed and, in the presence of a reducing agent and phosphate buffer, sickle cell haemoglobin will precipitate out of solution.
(c) *Electrophoresis.* The migration of haemoglobin is observed after a direct electric current has passed through a suitable supporting medium, e.g. paper, starch gel, cellulose acetate, to which the haemoglobin has been applied. Electrophoresis detects a charge change in the protein molecule caused by the amino-acid substitution. With electrophoresis the sickle cell trait carrier shows sickle cell haemoglobin and normal adult haemoglobin in approximately equal quantities.

Treatment
None is required.

SICKLE CELL ANAEMIA

Clinical
These patients suffer from chronic haemolytic anaemia and are often jaundiced. Leg ulcers or scars of leg ulcers are common around the ankles. Because of multiple splenic infarcts – 'autosplenectomy', splenomegaly is unusual after the age of 5. The 'steady state' of patients with sickle cell anaemia is interrupted by periodic crises which are commonly precipitated by infections and may prove fatal.
1 *Infarctive crisis.* Presents with painful attacks commonly in the bones, abdomen or chest. Bone infarcts may be followed by marrow embolism, pulmonary infarction and sometimes by death.
2 *Aplastic crisis.* Temporary reduction in red cell output may cause a dramatic lowering of the haemoglobin in patients whose red cell life span is commonly less than 20 days.
3 *Haemolytic crisis.* There may be an increase in the 'steady state' haemolytic rate.
4 *Sequestration crisis.* Sudden pooling of red cells

which commonly occurs in infants in the spleen, may fatally exacerbate the anaemia.

Blood

1 *Haemoglobin.* Hb 5–9 g/dl.
2 *Blood film.* Circulating sickle cells, target cells, polychromasia, sometimes erythroblasts.
3 *Sickling tests.* Positive.
4 *Electrophoresis.* HbS with small quantity HbF. No HbA.

N.B. Sickle cell tests and solubility tests are purely qualitative. They are positive in both the sickle cell carrier and in sickle cell anaemia and do not differentiate between them.

Treatment

Provided they are well cared for, many patients with sickle cell anaemia will survive into adult life and lead useful lives.

1 *General* – to prevent crisis.
(a) Good diet plus folic acid supplementation.
(b) Malarial prophylaxis.
(c) Prompt treatment of infections and infestations.
(d) Prevention of dehydration.
(e) Prevent exposure to cold.
(f) Long-term prophylactic oral sodium bicarbonate is recommended to prevent acidosis – an acid pH enhances sickling.
2 *Treatment of crises:*
(a) Aplastic, haemolytic and sequestration crises. Patients with sickle cell anaemia remain active at haemoglobin levels between 5 and 10 g/dl. Whilst transfusion may be required to preserve life in an aplastic, haemolytic or sequestration crisis, no attempt should be made to raise the haemoglobin level as high as that found in the normal person. 'Fresh' blood is desirable in order to provide red cells with a long life-span.
(b) Infarctive crisis. Every effort should be made to avoid crisis by the general measures outlined above. Once the crisis has occurred, the patient should be kept well hydrated and at an equable temperature. Oxygen is given if the arterial pO_2 is reduced. Analgesics may be required but care must be taken if the patient is also G6PD deficient (see p. 493). If the severity of the crisis is threatening life, an exchange transfusion may be beneficial.

SICKLE CELL HAEMOGLOBIN C DISEASE

Clinical

Patients with this condition, although often well, may yet have severe and sometimes fatal infarctive crises. Retinal infarction and post-partum maternal death are particularly associated with this condition. Splenomegaly is present in the majority of cases.

Blood

1 *Haemoglobin.* Hb 10–14 g per dl, i.e. in some cases may be within the normal range.
2 *Blood film.* Numerous target cells.
3 *Sickling tests.* Positive.
4 *Electrophoresis.* HbS and HbC.

Treatment

As for sickle cell anaemia.

SICKLE CELL THALASSAEMIA

The manifestations of this disease vary according to the percentage of normal adult haemoglobin HbA present in the patient. Depending upon the activity of the β thalassaemia gene (see p. 497) HbA will be at a level between 30 and 0 per cent of total haemoglobin production. High levels of HbA give mild clinical manifestations, i.e. a clinical and haematological picture similar to the sickle cell trait. Low levels of HbA may result in severe clinical and haematological manifestations resembling sickle cell anaemia.

HAEMOGLOBINS C, D AND E

THE CARRIER OF HAEMOGLOBINS C, D OR E

These are well with no abnormal haematological findings and haemoglobin C, D or E are present in equal quantities.

HAEMOGLOBIN C, D AND E DISEASE

Clinical

These patients usually have a mild or moderate anaemia, splenomegaly and jaundice.

Blood

1 *Haemoglobin.* Hb 10–14 g per dl.
2 *Blood film.* Numerous target cells.
3 *Electrophoresis.* HbC, HbD or HbE often with a small amount of HbF.

Treatment

Unless complicated by an aplastic or haemolytic crisis, which may follow infection, no special medical care is required. Folic acid is, however, desirable, especially in pregnancy.

HAEMOGLOBIN E
β THALASSAEMIA

Clinical

This condition is relatively common in South-East Asia, where HbE and β thalassaemia both occur. It presents as a moderate or severe haemolytic anaemia with splenomegaly and commonly jaundice.

Blood

1 *Haemoglobin.* Hb 5–10 g/dl.
2 *Blood film.* Target cells.
3 *Electrophoresis.* HbE plus some HbF. Unusually some HbA.

Treatment

As for HbE disease.

Unstable haemoglobins

Clinical and blood

Some amino acid substitutions result in distortion of the globin polypeptide chain and instability of the haemoglobin molecule. Such unstable haemoglobins may present with chronic haemolysis exacerbated by oxidant drugs, e.g. sulphonamides (see p. 493). Laboratory tests show the presence of intracellular denatured haemoglobin – *Heinz bodies*, as well as the usual findings of a chronic haemolytic anaemia. Unstable haemoglobins are particularly susceptible to heat denaturation, precipitating *in vitro* when blood is heated to 50°C – *heat denaturation test*.

Treatment

Some patients may require transfusions; they should avoid potential redox drugs.

M HAEMOGLOBINS

The haem group is deeply inserted into a water-repellant cleft in the globin – the haem pocket. The ferrous iron (Fe^{++}) atom of the haem is attached to the amino-acid histidine, situated one on either side of this pocket. Some abnormal haemoglobins have either an amino acid substitution replacing one of these histidines or another substitution which results in water molecules entering the haem pocket.

In either case the Fe^{++} ferrous iron atom of the haem is permanently converted into the Fe^{+++} ferric form, i.e. the haemoglobin has become methaemoglobin and the patient has methaemoglobinaemia. This type of methaemoglobinaemia does not clinically respond to the injection of either reducing agents, e.g. ascorbic acid or injections of methylene blue.

β Thalassaemia

The production of either the β polypeptide chains (β thalassaemia) or the α polypeptide chains (α thalassaemia) may be depressed. Both these conditions result in unbalanced polypeptide chain production – excess α chains are found in β thalassaemia and excess β and γ chains in α thalassaemia. These excess polypeptide chains precipitate within the red cell. Precipitated intra-erythrocytic globin, whether it occurs as either α or β polypeptide chains, or consists of unstable haemoglobin – Heinz bodies, damages the red-cell envelope and causes haemolysis.

β thalassaemia major is the most important variety of thalassaemia. The inheritance of this condition has already been discussed (see p. 497). β thalassaemia minor, the carrier state of β thalassaemia is extremely common but is not a debilitating condition.

β THALASSAEMIA –
MEDITERRANEAN ANAEMIA –
COOLEY'S ANAEMIA

Geographical

β Thalassaemia is widespread in the Mediterranean, Middle and Far East. It is uncommon in the African and New World Negro. Large populations have a carrier rate of almost 10 per cent.

β THALASSAEMIA MINOR

Foetal haemoglobin ($\alpha_2\gamma_2$) and haemoglobin $A_2(\alpha_2\delta_2)$ do not possess β chains. A depression of β polypeptide chain production may be accompanied by a compensatory increase in the output of foetal haemoglobin and haemoglobin A_2.

Clinical

Although suffering from a mild anaemia these people are usually well. They are usually only detected during routine haematological checks or during genetic counselling programmes.

Blood

1 *Haemoglobin.* Hb 10–14 g/dl.
2 *Blood film.* Hypochromia, which is therefore commonly mistaken for iron deficiency.
3 *Red cell indices.* The very numerous microcytic hypochromic red cells are reflected in the very low mean corpuscular haemoglobin (MCH) level. This is a useful distinguishing feature between β thalassaemia minor and iron deficiency.
4 *Serum iron.* Normal or raised – this feature also differentiates β thalassaemia minor from iron deficiency.
5 *Electrophoresis.* Demonstrates raised HbA_2.
6 *Foetal haemoglobin.* Half the cases of β thalassaemia minor will have a raised HbF ($\alpha_2\gamma_2$) recognizable either by a *Kleihauer stain* – staining of a blood film for HbF-containing cells, or by the resistance of foetal haemoglobin to alkali denaturation – *alkali denaturation test.*

Treatment

No treatment is indicated but folic acid may be beneficial especially in pregnancy. Iron should be avoided unless a complicating iron deficiency has been proved by a low serum iron and/or absent iron stores in bone marrow fragments.

N.B. Cases of β thalassaemia minor often present with hypochromic anaemia with a haemoglobin level of about 10 g/dl during pregnancy. They are commonly misdiagnosed as iron-deficiency anaemia and are presented to the haematologist only after they have failed to respond to a course of iron therapy.

β THALASSAEMIA MAJOR

Clinical

Children with this disorder are protected during their first 6 months of life by the production of HbF. Thereafter they develop increasing anaemia with massive splenomegaly, some hepatomegaly and radiological abnormalities in bones described on p. 442.

Blood

1 *Haemoglobin.* Hb 4–8 g/dl.
2 *Blood film.* Gross hypochromia with poikilocytosis, polychromasia and nucleated red cells.
3 *Other haemoglobins.* A small amount of HbA ($\alpha_2\beta_2$) may be present but commonly the majority of haemoglobin is HbF ($\alpha_2\beta_2$) demonstrated by alkali denaturation or a Kleihauer blood film HbA_2 ($\alpha_2\delta_2$) may be slightly raised.

Treatment

Transfusions are usually required to maintain life although some cases run a milder course. Chelating agents, which increase the urinary excretion of iron, may be given to reduce the consequent iron overload, which may eventually cause death in childhood or adolescence. Splenectomy is not usually beneficial.

α Thalassaemia

α Thalassaemia is geographically distributed in the same area as β thalassaemia, i.e. Mediterranean, Middle and Far East. In contrast with β thalassaemia, the carrier state of α thalassaemia appears common in Negroes although the severe manifestations of α thalassaemia are rare in that ethnic group.

Because they all contain α polypeptide chains (see p. 496), lack of α chain production reduces the output of haemoglobin A ($\alpha_2\beta_2$) haemoglobin F ($\alpha_2\gamma_2$) and haemoglobin A_2 ($\alpha_2\delta_2$). Some haemoglobin H (β_4) and haemoglobin Bart's (γ_4) are commonly found, thereby demonstrating the imbalance of chain production referred to on p. 501.

α THALASSAEMIA MAJOR

This condition has been frequently described in Asia. It is incompatible with life and presents with intra-uterine death as a hydrops foetalis (see p. 542) but without evidence of blood group incompatibility. The major haemoglobin is Hb Bart's (γ_4). There is no α polypeptide chain production, and therefore no HbF ($\alpha_2\gamma_2$) or HbA ($\alpha_2\beta_2$) present in the dead foetus.

HAEMOGLOBIN H DISEASE

In this uncommon condition, patients present with a moderate anaemia – Hb 8–12 g/dl and splenomegaly. The majority of the patient's haemoglobin is normal HbA ($\alpha_2\beta_2$) but 5–20 per cent of haemoglobin H (β_4) is produced. Haemoglobin H easily precipitates in the red cell, i.e. it is unstable. Haemoglobin H may be identified by:
1 Electrophoresis.
2 Heat denaturation test.
3 Demonstration of small intracellular red cell inclusions – *H bodies* consisting of denatured HbH (β_4). These appear after the red cells have been incubated with a suitable dye, e.g. methyl violet.

Patients with haemoglobin H disease should be given folic acid supplements especially during pregnancy. Redox drugs (see p. 493) should be avoided.

α THALASSAEMIA CARRIERS

Carriers of α thalassaemia are symptomless. They may be possible to detect in the laboratory by demonstrating the presence of very occasional red-cell inclusions – H bodies, in the blood smear. When born, such carriers of α thalassaemia have a raised level (greater than 1%) of Hb Bart's (γ_4) demonstrable on electrophoresis of a cord blood sample.

Chapter 84
Haematology – Haemolytic Anaemias: Acquired

Extracorpuscular

Immune factors

ANTIBODY TYPES
Heterologous
Isologous
Autologous

CHARACTERISTICS OF ANTIBODIES

AUTO-IMMUNE

Primary and secondary

Relation to blood groups

IDIOPATHIC WARM AIHA
Age
Sex
Clinical
Blood
Marrow

IDIOPATHIC COLD AIHA
Incidence
Age
Sex
Clinical

SECONDARY WARM AIHA
Other auto-immune disorders
Infections
Tumours
Drugs

SECONDARY COLD AIHA

PAROXYSMAL COLD
   HAEMOGLOBINURIA
Donath–Landsteiner test
Clinical

Isologous immune

Incompatible blood transfusion

Foeto–maternal incompatibility

Non-immune
Chemical and drugs

Physical factors

Abnormal vascular environment

Burns

Parasites

The acquired haemolytic anaemias

With the exception of paroxysmal noctural haemoglobinuria (PNH) (see p. 491), the remainder are caused by 'extra-corpuscular' factors. Although the red cells are intrinsically normal, they become destroyed by 'hostile' environmental factors. Classification is given in outline on p. 490.

The extracorpuscular factors are:
1 Immune factors – antibodies.
2 Chemicals, drugs and poisons.
3 Abnormal vascular environment.

Immune factors – antibodies

TYPES OF ANTIBODIES

Antibody reaction to red cells may be:
1 *Heterologous–Heterophile*. React with red cells of another species, e.g. the 'Paul Bunnell' antibody which arises in persons affected with infectious mononucleosis (see p. 449) and acts against sheep red cells.
2 Isologous. React with red cells from other individuals of the same species, e.g. the blood group antibodies.
3 *Autologous–auto-antibodies*. React to red cells from the same individual or, in laboratory animals, to an individual of identical genetic strain.

CHARACTERISTICS OF ANTIBODIES IN IMMUNE HAEMOLYTIC ANAEMIA

Each of the types 1, 2, 3 above are either *cold acting* – optimal temperature 4°C, or *warm acting* – optimal temperature 37°C.

Cold antibodies are usually IgM and produce 'complete' agglutination of sensitized cells visible macroscopically. Traces of autologous cold agglutinins are often found in normal persons and are of no pathological significance.

Warm antibodies are usually IgG and 'incomplete', sensitization of cells only being demonstrable by the *Coombs' anti-globulin test*. Autologous warm antibodies are always pathological.

AUTO-IMMUNE HAEMOLYTIC ANAEMIA (AIHA) CAUSED BY AUTOLOGOUS ANTIBODIES

PRIMARY AND SECONDARY

Secondary antibodies arise in association with certain drugs and disorders. If no such factor can be found, the cause is said to be *primary* or *idopathic*.

RELATIONSHIP OF AUTOLOGOUS ANTIBODIES TO BLOOD GROUPS

Autologous antibodies do not usually display blood group specificity although presumably their sites of attachment are discrete components of the red-cell membrane. This is particularly so for 'warm' antibodies, although when specificity is expressed it is usually directed in a general sense to the rhesus antigens, and occasionally to a specific antigen such as 'e'. (see p. 539). The non-pathological low titre 'cold' antibodies are similarly non-specific but the more active pathological cold agglutinins are often found to express reactivity towards the 'I' system (see p. 540). Secondary cold agglutinins of IgG class in paroxysmal cold haemoglobinuria are characteristically anti 'p' (see p. 506).

IDIOPATHIC WARM AIHA

Age
Bimodal distribution with peaks at 10–20 years and 40–60 years.

Sex
There may be a slight preponderance of females.

Clinical
Splenomegaly is usually marked.
Acute. Tends to afflict the younger persons. Is often severe, with haemoglobinuria, but is self-limiting.

Chronic. Tends to afflict the older persons. Is often difficult to treat and may develop pigment gallstones (see p. 489).

Blood
During active phases of both acute and chronic cases there is spherocytosis and reticulocytosis. Mechanical and osmotic fragility is increased but, in contrast with hereditary spherocytosis, the MCHC is not high and the direct antiglobulin (Coombs') test is positive.

Ingestion of erythrocytes by monocytes – *erythrophagocytosis*, particularly in buffy coat preparations, indicates active haemolysis. The white cell and platelet counts are variable. The biochemical features of '*acholuric jaundice*' (see p. 489) are also present.

Marrow
Typically hyperplastic with particularly intense erythropoiesis which may be megaloblastic if the marrow activity has depleted the body stores of folic acid. Iron stores are usually present unless the urinary iron loss in haemoglobin and haemosiderin is excessive. 'Aplastic crises' (see p. 489) may be accompanied by hypoplastic marrow.

IDIOPATHIC COLD AIHA – COLD AGGLUTININ DISEASE

Incidence
Less common than warm AIHA

Age
Very rare in children.

Sex
Probably equal.

Clinical
Chronic in type: splenomegaly is present but less marked than in warm AIHA. In cold weather, agglutination in the vessels of the extremities, e.g. hands, feet, nose, may cause Raynaud's phenomena (see p. 130). Subsequent lysis of the agglutinated cells produces haemoglobinuria and haemosiderinuria which, if prolonged, will lead to renal tubular siderosis.

SECONDARY WARM AIHA

Clinically very similar to idiopathic type, but an associated disorder is present. Recognized associated disorders include:

Other autoimmune disorders

S.L.E., rheumatoid disease, ulcerative colitis, thyroiditis, pernicious anaemia.

Thus detailed antoantibody screening is an essential investigation in all acquired immune haemolysis.

Infections

Viral – e.g. measles, herpes simplex, hepatitis. Bacterial – tuberculosis.

Tumours

Lymphomas – particularly chronic lymphocytic leukaemia. Carcinoma.

Drugs

1 Inducing antibodies by haptene action, e.g. penicillin.
2 Inducing antibodies not active against the drug itself, but to a structurally unrelated membrane component, e.g. methyl dopa, which generates anti-rhcsus antibodies, usually anti-E, in as many as 30 per cent of patients on prolonged therapy. Mefenamic acid (ponstan) has a similar effect.

SECONDARY COLD AIHA

Clinically similar to the idiopathic type. Most common cause is the atypical pneumonia caused by *Mycoplasma* (see p. 661). This nearly always produces anti-'i' which is active against nearly all donors, thus making transfusion therapy very difficult. Anti-'i' is often found in infectious mononucleosis, but rarely causes auto-haemolysis, unless the patient is of the very unusual blood group 'i' positive (see p. 540).

PAROXYSMAL COLD HAEMOGLOBINURIA – PCH

Although classifiable as a type of secondary cold AIHA, PCH deserves separate recognition due to its peculiar characteristics. The antibody is directed to the 'P' blood group system being 'anti-$P_1 + P_2$'. Although 'cold' it is an IgG. Its presence *in vitro* is demonstrable by *The Donath–Landsteiner* reaction –*D.-L*. On incubating sensitive cells to the antibody at 4°C, sensitization follows. On warming the suspension, complement becomes fixed and the antibody elutes off. On approaching 37°C the complement, if fresh, induces haemolysis.

Clinical

The condition is chronic and is characterized by bouts of severe haemolysis and haemoglobinuria, particularly in cold weather and accompanied by cramps, headaches and rigors. It is classically associated with late or congenital syphilis, although more recently other infections, usually viral, such as mumps, have been increasingly recognized. Not surprisingly, there is no clear clinical division between non-syphilitic PCH and primary or secondary cold AIHA. Indeed, typical D–L reactions may be given by other isologous or autologous cold antibodies.

ISOLOGOUS IMMUNE HAEMOLYTIC ANAEMIAS

INCOMPATIBLE BLOOD TRANSFUSION

Reactions due to cold antibodies such as anti-A tend to be worse than those due to warm antibodies such as anti-Rh. But fatalities have occurred with both (see p. 541).

FOETO–MATERNAL INCOMPATIBILITY–HAEMOLYTIC DISEASE OF NEWBORN

This is described on pages 541–543.

As only IgG can cross the placenta, is usually of the 'warm' type.

NON-IMMUNE ACQUIRED HAEMOLYTIC ANAEMIA – CHEMICALS AND DRUGS

Those substances causing direct haemolysis include:

Acetyl phenylhydrazine. Formerly used in polycythaemia to reduce the red cell mass.

Naphalene. 'Mothball' poisoning in children.

Arsine. In the recent case of the 'Asia Freighter' one of the eventual survivors had a haematocrit of zero, *all* his red cells having been rapidly destroyed. He survived on the oxygen-carrying capacity of his plasma, which because of the acute lysis, contained 10 g of haemoglobin/dl prior to exchange transfusion.

Biological haemolytic poisons. Usually 'detergent' in type, emulsifying membrane lipids, e.g. snake and insect venoms; bacterial lysins, e.g. streptolysin o, particularly in bacterial septicaemia.

HAEMOLYSIS DUE TO PHYSICAL FACTORS

ABNORMAL VASCULAR ENVIRONMENT

1 *Hyperplenism* (see p. 457).
2 *Intravascular deposition of fibrin.*
(*a*) Disseminated intravascular coagulopathy – D.I.C. (see p. 531).
(*b*) Local, often with microangiopathy – microangiopathic. haemolytic anaemia. Also found in cavernous haemangiomata.
3 *Excessive turbulence of flow*, e.g. around diseased or prosthetic heart valves.

4 *March haemoglobinuria.* 'March' refers to the military style of bipedal locomotion rather than a seasonal factor. Normal blood cells in otherwise healthy men are apparently lysed during marching, sometimes sufficiently to cause visible haemoglobinuria, although rarely with any other specific symptoms. The condition is alleviated by increasing the padding in the footwear!

BURNS

Red cells will lyse as a direct result of exposure to heat. Those less exposed may be damaged and lyse subsequently. Burns may also release 'toxic' factors inducing methaemoglobinaemia and lysis several days after the initial injury (see p. 74).

DIRECT INJURY BY PARASITES

Malaria, trypanosomes, etc.

Although it is tempting to regard such parasites as causing lysis solely by physically stressing the red cells, endothelial damage and complex immunological changes are now becoming apparent and may well be of equal importance aetiologically.

Chapter 85
Haematology – Anaemias of Chronic Disease and the Symptomatic or Secondary Anaemias

Main factors
Inability to incorporate iron
Marrow hypoplasia
Chronic haemolysis
Malnutrition

Causes of symptomatic anaemias

INFECTIONS
Acute
  Marrow hypoplasia
  Haemolysis
  Reaction to drug therapy
Chronic
Tuberculosis
Malaria

CONNECTIVE TISSUE DISEASES
Rheumatoid arthritis
Systemic lupus erythematosus
Polyarteritis nodosa

ENDOCRINE DISORDERS
Hypopituitarism
Thyroid disease
  Diminished tissue oxygen
    requirements
  Associated iron deficiency
  Autoimmune disease
  Dietary
  Thyrotoxicosis
Adrenal insufficiency
Hypogonadism

RENAL DISEASE
Haemolysis
Marrow depression and
  ineffective erythropoiesis

Reduced erythropoietin
  production
Haemorrhage
Nutritional
Renal dialysis

LIVER DISEASE
Chronic haemolysis
Marrow hypoplasia
Haemorrhage
Dietary deficiency
Hypersplenism

MALIGNANT DISEASE
Haemorrhage
Bone marrow depression
Acquired haemolytic anaemia
Infections and renal failure
Dietary
Malignant cachexia

Chronic disease and anaemia are historically associated: the waxen child dying of tuberculosis has become part of folklore immortalized by the Victorian novelist. In such anaemias the white cell and platelet counts are usually normal

There is usually a combination of causative factors in any anaemia due to chronic disease.

Main factors

An inability to incorporate iron into the developing red cell
Iron stores assessed by Perls' Prussian blue staining of the marrow fragments (see p. 473) may be demonstrated as adequate but this iron is not transferred to the developing red cell. The red cells in the peripheral blood are characteristically normochromic and normocytic, but, on occasions, may

be hypochromic and microcytic, in which case, the blood film will give an initial impression of iron deficiency. The reticulocyte count may be reduced, normal or raised depending upon whether there is a superimposed marrow hypoplasia or a haemolytic element.

The differentiation between the sideropenic, iron deficient, and non-sideropenic, *toxic*, hypochromic anaemias is important in assessing the likely response of a patient with a chronic disease, e.g. rheumatoid arthritis, to a course of iron therapy. Suspicion that a hypochromic anaemia may not be a simple iron deficiency anaemia may be first raised by the presence in chronic infections in the blood film of *excessive red cell rouleaux*. In addition, although the ESR rate may be somewhat raised in uncomplicated iron deficiency anaemia, it is commonly much higher in any chronic infection which is severe enough to cause an associated depression of iron incorporation and a resultant hypochromic anaemia. Although the serum iron in both conditions may be low, the total iron binding capacity is high in iron deficiency and low in the toxic, non-sideropenic hypochromic anaemias.

Marrow hypoplasia

The marrow is commonly hypoplastic and there appears to be poor erythropoietin production in response to the presence of anaemia (see p. 447). Erythropoietin production is diminished especially in destructive chronic renal disease. In other cases, the response to erythropoietin, either naturally occurring or parenterally administered, is impaired.

Chronic haemolysis

A moderate or minor reduction of the normal red cell life span is common in symptomatic anaemias: in some cases, e.g. virus infections or lymphomas, the presence of red cell antibodies may precipitate a more severe haemolytic crisis (see p. 506).

Malnutrition

Inadequate diet, perhaps associated with anorexia, may lead to deficiencies of essential haematinics, especially folate.

Causes of symptomatic anaemias

1 Infection $\begin{cases} \text{acute.} \\ \text{chronic.} \end{cases}$
2 Connective tissue diseases.
3 Endocrine disorders.
4 Renal disease.
5 Liver disease.
6 Malignant disease $\begin{cases} \text{carcinoma.} \\ \text{lymphoma.} \end{cases}$

INFECTIONS

Acute

MARROW HYPOPLASIA

Marrow activity may be reduced during an acute illness such as a viral pneumonia. This may be of critical importance if it occurs in a patient with chronic haemolytic anaemia (see p. 489).

HAEMOLYSIS

Acute haemolysis may be a feature of both bacterial, e.g. *Clostridium perfringens* septicaemia (see p. 131); viral disease, e.g. acute autoimmune haemolytic anaemia (see p. 506); or protozoal infections, e.g. malaria.

REACTION TO DRUG THERAPY

(a) Glucose-6-phosphate-dehydrogenase deficiency (see p. 493), may result in a haemolytic reaction to drug therapy.
(b) Marrow depression, may follow therapy with chloramphenicol (see p. 454.)
(c) Antibody formation to drugs or their metabolites (see p. 506).

An unusually high polymorphonuclear leucocyte count may be present – *leukaemoid reaction* – in any acute infection. The polymorphonuclear cells in acute infections have extremely granular cytoplasm, *toxic granulation* and a high alkaline phosphatase. The polymorphonuclear cells in leukaemia commonly have few granules in the cytoplasm and a low alkaline phosphatase content (see p. 466).

Chronic

With the advent of antibiotics, many chronic suppurating lesions, e.g. empyema and chronic osteomyelitis, are now uncommon in developed countries. Chronic gynaecological and renal infections still abound in medically sophisticated countries and should be sought for in unexplained anaemias.

Anaemia may result from:

1 Defective iron utilization.
2 Diminished erythropoietin production or response.
3 Malnutrition leading to folate, iron or Vitamin B_{12} deficiency.
4 Drug reactions (see above).

N.B. Although commonly there may be some marrow hypoplasia and some shortening of the red cell life span, these are seldom the major causative factors in the anaemia of chronic infection.

Tuberculosis

Tuberculosis may present in the most bizarre fashion and should be considered in the differential diagnosis of any obscure haematological disorder. It should also be remembered that active tuberculosis may be 'opportunistic' as a terminal feature in a haematological disease with an associated impaired immune response.

More closely allied manifestations of tuberculosis are:

1 Myelosclerosis (see p. 460).
2 Pancytopenia usually with splenomegaly, but sometimes without a palpable spleen.
3 Lymphocytic leukaemoid reaction.

Malaria

Chronic haemolysis is usual in malaria as a result of both destruction of the red cells by the parasite and hypersplenism. On occasions the haemolysis may become acute – blackwater fever (see p. 65). Antimalarial drugs may cause haemolysis in the presence of Glucose-6-phosphate-dehydrogenase deficiency (see p. 493).

CONNECTIVE TISSUE DISEASES

Rheumatoid arthritis

The causes of anaemia in rheumatoid arthritis are similar to those of the chronic infectious diseases already discussed. In addition, drugs used for treatment may depress the marrow, e.g. phenylbutazone, gold salts, or cause gastro-intestinal bleeding, e.g. aspirin.

Systemic lupus erythematosus (SLE)

This disease, most common in middle-aged women, may present clinically in a number of bizarre ways which include fever, arthritis, renal failure, pleural and pericardial effusions and psychiatric changes (see p. 281). A minority of cases have lymphadenopathy, hepato- and splenomegaly.

Haematological changes are common:

1 Autoimmune haemolytic anaemia (see p. 505).
2 Idiopathic thrombocytopenic purpura (see p. 517).
3 Leucopenia. Because of the commonly associated anaemia and thrombocytopenia, SLE is a significant cause of pancytopenia (see p. 452).
4 Raised ESR.
5 A false positive WR is occasionally found.
6 Presence of LE cell phenomenon.

LE CELLS

In cases of SLE, after incubation, the neutrophil leucocytes of the blood or marrow, will contain the digested remains of a previously ingested nucleus. On Romanowsky's staining (p. 281) the nuclear material will appear as a large circular pink/purple staining homogeneous body pushing the dark staining nucleus of the ingesting cell to one side. The LE cell phenomenon is caused by an IgG antibody (see p. 281) capable of lysing the nuclei of the patients own leucocytes, i.e. it is an autoantibody.

The 'LE cell' must be distinguished from a Tart cell where the ingested nucleus is intensely staining and has recognizable nuclear structure.

Polyarteritis nodosa

This collagen disease may present like SLE in a puzzling clinical manner. The patient commonly has anaemia and, usually, a polymorphonuclear leucocytosis and eosinophilia.

ENDOCRINE DISORDERS

Hypopituitarism

Pituitary failure causes a normochromic normocytic anaemia. Such an anaemia may be reversed by thyroid, adrenal and androgen substitution therapy.

Thyroid disease

The anaemia associated with myxoedema is usually only mild and its causes are, as yet, not clearly understood. Whilst usually normochromic, normocytic in type, occasionally the anaemia is of a macrocytic type.

DIMINISHED TISSUE OXYGEN REQUIREMENTS

In myxoedema it would be reasonable to assume that the lowering of the BMR would diminish tissue oxygen requirements. The resultant surfeit of oxygen would diminish erythropoietin production.

ASSOCIATED IRON DEFICIENCY

Iron deficiency may be dietary in origin, or aggravated by impaired absorption of iron if there is an associated achlorhydria (see p. 475). The increased blood loss of menorrhagia, a common complication of myxoedema, may also precipitate iron deficiency.

AUTOIMMUNE DISEASE

There is an association between pernicious anaemia and myxoedema and between the presence of gastric and thyroid antibodies in the sera of patients with these conditions.

DIETARY

Poor diet may result in iron, B_{12} and folate deficiency.

THYROTOXICOSIS
Contrary to expectations, the haemoglobin level in hyperthyroidism is usually normal, though an increased plasma volume may hide a real increase in the red cell mass.

Adrenal insufficiency
A mild or moderate anaemia may be found in Addison's disease and reflects a lack of the erythropoietic stimulating effect of adrenal cortical hormones (see p. 290). It should be remembered that there is a diminution in plasma volume which masks the true extent of the haemoglobin reduction. Such an anaemia can be rapidly manifested following therapeutic correction of the plasma volume.

Hypogonadism
Androgens are capable of stimulating red cell production and mainly explain the difference between the normal male (16 ± 2 g/dl) and female (14 ± 2 g/dl) haemoglobin levels. Androgens are widely used in an attempt to stimulate erythropoietic activity in marrow aplasias (see p. 455).

RENAL DISEASE

Chronic renal failure is accompanied by an anaemia which is characteristically normochromic and normocytic in type, and is often severe and progressive though well tolerated. The causes of this anaemia are multiple and are still only partially understood.

Haemolysis
There is usually a mild or moderate haemolytic element in chronic renal failure which may be manifested by the presence of *burr cells*. These are sufficiently characteristic to suggest renal failure in the presence of an otherwise unexplained anaemia.

Marrow depression and ineffective erythropoiesis
Normally functioning marrow would easily compensate for the modest extra load caused by the shortened red cell life-span in renal failure. On morphological examination, erythropoiesis may appear hypoplastic, normal or hyperplastic. In the latter case, the erythropoietic activity may well be ineffective – mature red cells failing to enter the blood stream.

Reduced erythropoietin production
Due to destruction of renal tissue, the level of production of erythropoietin may be reduced. The marrow also responds poorly to any erythropoietin produced at other sites.

Haemorrhage
Purpuric haemorrhages are commonly associated with renal failure and may result from poor platelet function. In addition blood loss may occur during dialysis.

Nutritional
Impaired appetite may lead to dietary deficiency of iron, B_{12} or folate.

Renal dialysis
Patients on maintenance dialysis remain anaemic when this is largely caused by decreased erythropoietin production.

Blood loss associated with the techniques may result in iron deficiency but is correctable by iron therapy.

Recently, planned small transfusions of whole blood have been found to be beneficial to renal tissue transplant recipients in respect of graft function. Transfusion is otherwise contra-indicated.

Some anaemic non-acidotic patients have raised $2:3$ DPG levels and decreased oxygen affinity of their haemoglobin – compensated anaemia (see p. 492). Such patients are clinically little incommoded by low haemoglobin levels.

LIVER DISEASE

The increase in plasma volume may give a false impression of the size of the red cell mass. Because of this dilution of the red cells, a peripheral haemoglobin level in hepatic failure may underestimate the size of the red cell mass.

The peripheral blood film characteristically shows target cells and sometimes macrocytes; anaemia, leucopenia and thrombocytopenia, i.e. a pancytopenia, may be a feature in the presence of associated hypersplenism.

Even in the absence of complications such as haemorrhage, dietary deficiency or hypersplenism, the majority of patients with cirrhosis of the liver have some degree of anaemia. Factors include:

Chronic haemolysis

This may become a marked feature in chronic active hepatitis. The presence of hyperlipidaemia may exacerbate the haemolysis by affecting the lipid content of the red cell envelope.

Marrow hypoplasia

In some cases.

Haemorrhage

(*a*) Oesophageal varices.
(*b*) Coagulation defect due to liver disease (see p. 525).
(*c*) Thrombocytopenia due to hypersplenism.

Dietary deficiency

Folic acid deficiency is common and may result in a frank megaloblastic anaemia; iron deficiency – in the absence of haemorrhage – and B_{12} deficiency are unusual. Indeed, iron overload, haemochromatosis, may be associated with concomitant chronic alcoholism.

Hypersplenism

Portal venous hypertension caused by cirrhosis will cause splenomegaly and this may give rise to hypersplenism and pancytopenia (see p. 457).

MALIGNANT DISEASE

Unless haemorrhage is a feature, e.g. gastro-intestinal tract carcinoma, anaemia is normally a feature of advanced rather than early malignancy. On occasions, malignant disease may cause a leukaemoid blood picture. Factors causing anaemia include the following.

Haemorrhage

Whilst spontaneous haemorrage is a presenting feature in some malignancies, in others it may be secondary to thrombocytopenia.

Bone-marrow depression

(*a*) Metastases to bone marrow are a feature especially of carcinoma of the stomach, lung, breast, kidney, thyroid and malignant melanoma. The peripheral blood picture is commonly that of a leucoerythroblastic anaemia, i.e. both nucleated red cells and immature granulocytes are present (see p. 448).
(*b*) Bone marrow depression commonly follows radiotherapy or cytotoxic chemotherapy.

Acquired haemolytic anaemia

Whilst this may occur in any malignancy, it is an especial feature of the lymphomas and chronic lymphocytic leukaemia (see p. 506).

Infections and renal failure

Anaemia developing as a result of infections or renal failure from obstruction are especially common in pelvic tumours.

Dietary

Lack of essential haematinics, Vitamin B_{12}, folate and iron, may occur especially if anorexia or nausea and vomiting are present over any length of time.

Malignant cachexia

This ill-understood wasting phenomenon of malignancy probably also contributes to anaemia (see p. 159).

Chapter 86
Haematology – Normal Haemostasis: Defects of Vascular and Platelet Function

Normal haemostasis

In healthy persons, the cessation of haemorrhage is brought about by:

(*a*) Vasospasm.

(*b*) Adhesion and aggregation of platelets – plug formation.

(*c*) The blood clot.

These constitute the three components of the haemostatic mechanism.

In normal persons, the spontaneous minor traumata of everyday life damage the small blood vessels. These are immediately plugged by platelets and deposits of fibrin. Platelets are essential to haemostasis because they contribute both to vascular function, by plugging microscopic haemorrhages, and to clot formation, by supplying essential clotting factors.

The blood vessels

The collagenous basement membrane of capillaries is lined by endothelial cells which normally promote a smooth blood flow by:

(*a*) Discouraging platelet adhesion largely by the production of prostacyclin (PGI_2).

(*b*) Secreting substances which lead to fibrin dissolution – fibrinolysis (see p. 531).

(*c*) Releasing heparin secreted from neighbouring mast cells.

Blood flow is regulated by the smooth muscle fibres of the terminal arterioles which respond to neurogenic or blood-borne vasodilators and constrictors.

The platelets

CHARACTERISTICS

1 Non-nucleated.

2   Derived from megakaryocyte cytoplasm.
3   Metabolize aerobically (with mitochondria).
4   Circulate for 7–11 days.
5   Are 'stickier' and larger when regenerating, e.g. after haemorrhage or temporary marrow hypoplasia.
6   Have vacuoles containing *'vasoactive'* amines (ADP, 5HT, adrenalin, etc.), and *'thromboplastic'* *phospholipids*, collectively called *platelet factor 3* (PF3).
7   Have contractile proteins – *thrombosthenin*, under the membrane and throughout the cytoplasm.
8   Mature platelets do not have an active endoplasmic reticulum and protein synthesis is low; however, a microtubular system and Golgi apparatus are present.
9   Have clotting factors V, VIII and fibrinogen in their substance.
10 Carry a heparin-neutralizing substance – *platelet factor 4* (PF4).

PLATELET REACTIONS IN HAEMOSTASIS
Platelets flowing past a recent injury undergo a series of reactions summarized below.
1   *Adhesion* to damaged endothelium and exposed collagen.
2   *Release* of vasoconstrictors, especially 5HT, to produce local vasospasm.
3   *Aggregate* to seal the site of injury – *platelet plug*.
4   *Release* PF3.
5   *Retract* the clot to form a *firm scab*.

The initial adhesion of a few platelets encourages those flowing nearby to join in the aggregate. Further aggregation is encouraged by the vasoactive amines and later by thrombin.

All these reactions are vital to the control of capillary haemorrhage and are tested by the *bleeding time* – see below.

The clotting proteins
The clotting process results from the interaction of plasma proteins at the site of blood loss giving rise to a controlled production of fibrin. This seals the site and provides a basis for permanent healing (see p. 33).

Tests of vascular and platelet function

Bleeding time
The skin is pricked or cut and the time taken for bleeding to stop is measured. There are several techniques differing in detail, all with a wide normal range, indicating the generally imprecise nature of these investigations. However, there is no other convenient direct measure of micro-vascular function. The test is contra-indicated in severe thrombocytopenia.

DUKE'S METHOD
Uses ear lobe, which must be clean, warm and dry. Pin-prick cut to 0.3 cm using sterile lancet. Touched (not blotted) every 30 s with absorbent paper. Normally bleeding stops within 4 min, occasionally persists 6–7 min.

'VENOSTASIS' METHODS, BASED ON IVY'S TECHNIQUE
Pneumatic cuff over upper arm inflated to precisely 40 mm Hg. This flushes the venules and capillaries of forearm skin but is low enough to avoid anoxic damage to vascular endothelium.

Standard technique – template bleeding time
Skin washed with warm soapy water and dabbed thoroughly dry.
N.B. Avoid cooling effects of ether or alcohol. Avoiding obvious venules make two parallel cuts, 1 cm long and 0.1 cm deep, through slits in a flat plate (template).

Issuing blood is touched with absorbent paper every 15 s. The mean of all end-points may be taken or just the longest of all three so long as it is not obviously different, e.g. if a venule is struck at one site, artefactually prolonged bleeding may follow which should be discounted.

Tends to leave scars if the bleeding time is prolonged, unless the cuts are washed afterwards and dressed with adhesive tapes.

With all venostasis methods, bleeding tends to be longer than Duke's method, particularly with the modifications. Bleeding with the standard technique usually stops within 6 min, but may go on as long as 9 min.

The template Ivy technique is recommended as a screening test.

Hess's test of capillary fragility
Number of petechial spots on forearm skin counted after inflating a pneumatic cuff over upper arm to 80 mm Hg for 5 min. Should be less than 19 in a circle 2.5 cm in diameter in the cubital fossa. Although of considerable bedside or outpatient convenience this

test is scarcely ever of any use and, in cases of severe platelet deficiency, may cause dangerous extravasation of blood into the tissues.

Tests of platelet function

1 *Light microscopy* of blood film – for platelet morphology and numerical assessment.

2 *Blood platelet count* – direct visual counting chamber or automated particle counts. Normal range 150–$450 \times 10^9/l$.

3 *Platelet adhesion* – platelet counts measured before and after exposure to a foreign surface, e.g. glass beads, cellophane dialysis membranes, etc.

4 *Platelet aggregation* – the response of platelets in citrated plasma to amines (ADP, Adrenaline, 5HT, etc.), thrombin and collagen particles. Samples of the platelet-rich plasma must be fresh and not refrigerated. Records traced by an 'aggregometer' reveal two stages of aggregation (see Fig. 51). The second stage is due to endogenous release of ADP from platelet vacuoles and is irreversible. This stage depends on prostaglandin synthesis and is inhibited by ATP, AMP, and drugs such as dipyridamole (persantin) and aspirin. Aggregating

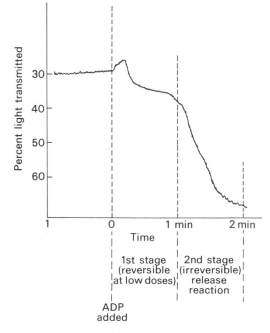

Fig. 55. Record of normal platelet aggregation. Suspension of platelets in plasma to which 5μmol ADP added as indicated. During aggregation the amount of light transmitted through the suspension increases.

agents which act directly on the platelet surface bypass this mechanism; such agents include bovine Factor VIII and ristocetin which are useful in the diagnosis of von Willebrand's disease (see p. 529) and certain rare platelet disorders, e.g. Bernard–Soulier syndrome.

5 *Tests of the availability of PF3.* Various clotting tests, particularly the KCCT or the RVV (see p. 524) which usually use platelet-poor plasma (PPP) from the patient may be adapted to use slowly sedimented plasma which is rich in platelets (PRP). The accelerated clotting in the PRP reflects PF3 availability.

6 *Clot retraction* – tests the activity of 'thrombosthenin'. Unanticoagulated blood is incubated in a glass test tube for 1 hour, and the degree of clot retraction measured.

Interpretation

1 The bleeding time is always prolonged, and hence contra-indicated, in severe thrombocytopenia.

2 Prolonged bleeding time with normal platelet count. There must be a deficiency either of vascular or of platelet function. Carry out the further platelet function tests.

N.B. Severe vitamin K deficiency, as in obstructive jaundice or with oral anticoagulants, prolongs Ivy's bleeding time.

3 Prolonged bleeding time with increased platelet count. Suggests platelet, rather than vascular disorder, particularly if platelet morphology is abnormal, e.g. in myeloproliferative disease (see p. 458). The platelet function tests may be abnormal.

4 Normal bleeding time with clear-cut clinical bleeding disorder. Characteristic of disorders of coagulation, e.g. haemophilia (see p. 526).

Defects of vascular and platelet function

These disorders predispose to *purpura*, which may take the form of petechiae—pin-point haemorrhages, or ecchymoses—larger extravasations of blood in the skin. Similar haemorrhages may occur in the gastro-intestinal mucosa and visceral tissues.

VASCULAR DEFECTS

Congenital

All are rare, are inherited autosomally and are not sex-linked.

HEREDITARY HAEMORRHAGIC TELANGIECTASIA – OSLER–WEBER–RENDU

Inherited tendency to microvascular dilatations in skin, mucosa and gastro-intestinal tract. Tend to bleed, especially from nose and gets worse with age. The telangiectasiae can be distinguished from purpura by pressing the skin with a glass slide: the telangiectasiae will disappear, but purpura remains.

EHLERS–DANHLOS DISEASE

Inherited mesenchymal defect, characterized by hyper-extensibility of joints. Large bleeds may occur into tissue spaces.

HEREDITARY CAPILLARY FRAGILITY

Some examples are probably cases of von Willebrand's disease (see p. 529), or of other platelet disorders (see below).

Acquired

HENOCH–SCHÖNLEIN PURPURA

This follows inflammatory conditions, sometimes streptococcal. The aetiology may be similar to acute nephritis and rheumatic fever, the vascular basement membrane being damaged by immune complexes (see p. 361).

INFECTIONS AND DRUGS

Less specific capillary damage accompanies many bacterial and viral infections, and certain drug rashes. Some of these are also accompanied by disordered platelet function or by thrombocytopenia.

MISCELLANEOUS

The integrity of the vessel wall is weakened in Cushing's syndrome and high doses of corticosteroids in debility, protein starvation, scurvy and old age. The accumulation of toxic metabolites in uraemia also has a deleterious effect (see p. 511).

PLATELET DEFECTS

Thrombocytopenia

EFFECTS OF LOW PLATELET COUNT

The bleeding tendency is roughly proportional to the degree of thrombocytopenia but not precisely, e.g. some cases of chronic thrombocytopenia bleed surprisingly little.

Below approximately $30 \times 10^9/l$ haemorrhages are spontaneous, or follow minor traumata.

Between $30 \times 10^9/l$ and $80 \times 10^9/l$, surgical and accidental traumata are followed by increased tendency to bleed persistently.

Between $80 \times 10^9/l$ and $150 \times 10^9/l$, haemostasis is virtually normal except to major trauma.

CAUSES

Reduced numbers of megakaryocytes
(a) After therapy with marrow-depressive drugs, e.g. cytotoxics, gold, chlorpropamide.
(b) Massive infiltration of marrow, e.g. carcinomatous metastases, acute leukaemia.
(c) Idiopathic marrow hypoplasia.
(d) Poisons.

Inhibition of megakaryocyte maturation
(a) Septicaemia.
(b) Viral infections such as influenza, hepatitis.
(c) Typhoid fever.
(d) Miliary tuberculosis.
(e) Renal failure.
(f) Ineffective haemopoiesis, e.g. megaloblastic anaemias.

Excessive destruction of circulating platelets
(a) Drugs, e.g. quinine, which in hypersensitive persons can induce production of antibodies to a *drug–platelet complex*.
(b) Hypersplenism (see p. 457).
(c) Immune thrombocytopenic purpura – *I.T.P.*
(d) Disseminated intravascular coagulation – *D.I.C.*
In these conditions, the numbers of megakaryocytes in the marrow may be increased in an attempt to compensate for the excessive platelet loss.

ABNORMALITIES OF PLATELET FUNCTION WITH NORMAL OR INCREASED CIRCULATING NUMBERS

Congenital

1 *Thrombasthenia* – Glanzmann's disease. An inborn error of membrane glycoprotein.
2 *Storage pool disease*. With reduced release of vasoactive amines.
   1 and 2 are autosomal recessive.
3 *Von Willebrand's disease* (see p. 529).

Acquired

DRUGS

(*a*) Cytotoxic therapy may generate defective platelets.

(*b*) Anticoagulants.

   (i) Vitamin K antagonists reduce platelet function.

   (ii) Specific *anti-platelet anticoagulants*, e.g. dipyridamole, which interfere with amine release.

(*c*) Anti-inflammatory drugs, especially aspirin, which stops prostaglandin synthesis.

NEOPLASTIC

(*a*) *Haemorrhagic thrombocythaemia – megakaryocytic myelosis* (see p. 461) and myelofibrosis (see p. 460). The first is the platelet equivalent of polycythaemia rubra vera. The neoplastic platelets may number over $1000 \times 10^9/l$ but most are defective in function, particularly in prostaglandin synthesis. Alternatively, if their function is normal, the increased number may predispose to thrombus formation.

(*b*) *Other myeloproliferative disorders*, e.g. chronic myeloid leukaemia; probably a similar biochemical defect to above.

(*c*) *Paraproteinaemias* – myeloma and macroglobulinaemia (see p. 470). Platelets fail to function as they are covered in a 'blanket' of paraprotein. The vascular endothelial cells may be similarly embarrassed.

METABOLIC

(*a*) Uraemia interferes with platelet function by accumulation of nitrogenous products.

(*b*) Diabetes and scurvy may interfere with platelet metabolism.

Treatment of vascular and platelet disorders

1   *Treat or remove predisposing cause*, e.g. drugs, scurvy, leukaemia, etc. Macroglobulins may be temporarily reduced in paraproteinaemias by plasma exchange.

2   *Platelet replacement*. Only if effective thrombopoiesis is reduced. Of no use in increased platelet destruction, e.g. I.T.P. or hypersplenism.

(*a*) Whole fresh blood.

(*b*) Platelet-rich donor plasma.

(*c*) Platelet concentrates.

   Both should be given within 12 hours of donation if possible and are no use after 48 hours.

3   *Corticosteroids*. May reduce any platelet antibody activity and hypersplenism by general suppression of immune-related activity. May increase thrombopoiesis.

   Once thought to stabilize vascular structures but probably not true, indeed prolonged therapy weakens these tissues, as in Cushingoid states (see p. 291).

Immune thrombocytopenic purpura (I.T.P.)

Nature

An autoimmune disease. Adult cases may be related to SLE and other immune disorders. Antibodies are demonstrable in about half the cases. The infantile form is usually acute and self-limiting but the adult form is more chronic and difficult to treat.

   Platelet life span is severely reduced, with excessive sequestration and destruction of platelets in the spleen.

Treatment

Corticosteroids. Particularly helpful in acute (juvenile) cases, although many paediatricians are now in favour of delaying therapy as the natural course of many cases is so short.

Splenectomy. Often helpful in chronic adult cases if corticosteroids fail but further steroid therapy may be needed after splenectomy. There is an unfortunate residuum of patients whose thrombocytopenia persists even after splenectomy and steroids.

Plasma exchange and cytotoxic therapy. May be indicated in some cases.

Chapter 87
Haematology – Blood Coagulation

Basic features

The process must be rapid yet localized.
1 *Rapidity*. This is achieved by a series of accelerating steps – *cascade*.
2 *Localization*. By self limiting mechanisms (see p. 524), inhibitors – antithrombins, fibrinolysis.
   Essentially consists of two paired systems (see Fig. 56),
(*a*) Clotting proteins and inhibitors of coagulation.
(*b*) Fibrinolysis and its inhibitors.
Of these four systems, the 'forwards' generation of the clot is the best understood and is the most accessible to study. Fibrinolysis will be discussed separately (see p. 531).

Clotting factors

The blood clot is the end result of a chain reaction between blood clotting factors. These factors are enzymes which circulate as inactive precursors. Activation occurs in stages in which a few active factor molecules can 'start up' many precursor molecules of the next stage – *amplifying cascade*.

The blood plasma supplies ionic calcium and 10 protein factors. These were known by several confusing names, so that the numbers I to XIII were given by an International Committee in 1959. Factor VI does not exist; and factor III, or 'thromboplastin', is not a single substance. The names are listed below:

  I Fibrinogen.
 II Prothrombin.
III 'Thromboplastin', 'thrombokinase',
     prothrombinase.
 IV Ionic calcium.
  V Pro-accelerin – labile factor.
 VI Accelerin; hypothetical and never
     substantiated.
VII Pre-convertin – stable factor.
VIII Anti-haemophilic globulin.
 IX Christmas factor; plasma thromboplastin
     component (P.T.C.).
  X Stuart–Prower factor.
 XI Plasma thromboplastin antecedent (P.T.A.).
XII Hageman factor.
XIII Fibrin stabilizing factor.

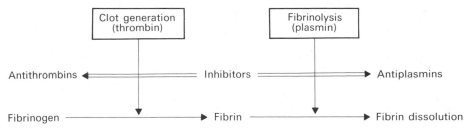

Fig. 56. Basic blood clotting systems.

The blood coagulation process

Although a continuous process, blood coagulation may be considered to pass through four stages:
1. Initiation.
2. Generation of prothrombinase.
3. Generation of thrombin.
4. Fibrin formation.

Coagulation tests have revealed two distinct but closely linked systems:
(a) *'Intrinsic'*, so-called as all required factors are present in normal circulating blood thus giving rise to the spontaneous clotting of shed blood.
(b) *'Extrinsic'*, so-called because an external source of tissue extract takes part.

Both systems finally result in activation of factor X to 'Xa'. Xa formation eventually results in fibrin production via two more cascading stages. N.B. The suffix 'a' is used throughout to denote the 'activated' type of factor.

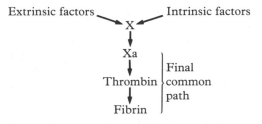

Fig. 57. Simplified scheme of blood coagulation.

INITIATION OF COAGULATION

Intrinsic system

ACTIVATION OF FACTOR XI
(a) *By platelets.* Platelets adhering to wounds convert factor XI into the active compound – 'XIa', directly. The detailed mechanism not clear but appears to be related to the altered platelet surface.
(b) *By 'contact activation'.* This involves Hageman factor – factor XII, and is the main initiator of coagulation by contact with glass surfaces *in vitro*. Factor XII is closely related to the kinin, plasmin and complement systems and, indeed, at least two intermediate stages, involving kininogen and kallikrein are known to be concerned in the activation of XI by contact-activated XII.

ACTIVATION OF FACTOR IX
Factor IX, inactive precursor of IXa, is activated directly by the enzymic action of XIa. Many molecules of IXa are produced by only a few of XIa – an example of the amplifying cascade.

PRODUCTION OF THE 'INTRINSIC FACTOR X ACTIVATING PRINCIPLE' – IXAP
This is a macromolecular complex based on PF3, to which is bound factor VIII, and also factor IXa the binding of which requires calcium ions. The complex has enzymic activity towards factor X. This comes from the IXa component, although IXa in isolation has virtually no enzymic activity; the change in molecular configuration resulting from the binding to the PF3–VIII complex reveals the active site (see Fig 58).

Although factor VIII is not activated from a precursor and thus is not involved in an amplifying cascade, the activity of the whole complex is enhanced if the VIII is first gently treated with thrombin. Further thrombin treatment, however, inactivates the VIII, disabling it from forming the proper macromolecular complex:

$$\text{VIII} \xrightarrow{\text{Thrombin}} \text{VIIIt} \xrightarrow{\text{Thrombin}} \text{VIIIi}$$

VIII moderate activity → VIIIt enhanced activity → VIIIi inactive

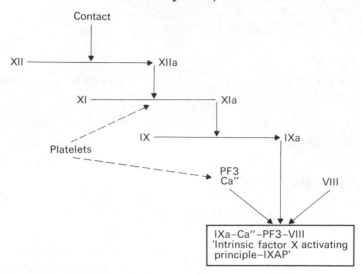

Fig. 58. The formation of intrinsic factor X activating principle.

Extrinsic system

Adding an '*ex*trinsic' tissue extract (T.E.) to freshly drawn whole blood greatly accelerates the clotting time. The active principle is a lipoprotein which, in the presence of calcium ions, interacts with factor VII to produce *extrinsic factor X activating principle*, another macromolecule—EXAP. (See Fig 59.)

GENERATION OF PROTHROMBINASE

Prothrombinase – or the prothrombin activating principle – is the modern term for factor III, formerly known as 'thromboplastin' or 'thrombokinase'. Because of potential confusion with tissue factor, these terms are best discarded.

Like the factor X activating principle, prothrom-

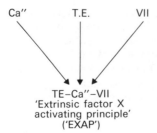

TE–Ca''–VII
'Extrinsic factor X
activating principle'
('EXAP')

Fig. 59. Formation of extrinsic factor X activating principle.

binase is a macromolecule based on phospholipid (P.L.). This may come either from PF3 or tissues. Xa is bound, via calcium ions, to the phospholipid and factor V. The analogy is clear.

IXa–Ca''–PF3–VIII = 'IXAP'.

Xa–Ca''–P.L.–V = 'Prothrombinase'.

Like factor VIII, factor V does not exist in precursor forms, but its activity is enhanced and then destroyed by thrombin.

GENERATION OF THROMBIN

Prothrombin becomes adsorbed to the surface of the lipid micelle of prothrombinase via a unique peptide portion (see below) and is acted on by the active site of the complex, provided by the Xa, releasing free thrombin.

The chemistry of prothrombin and thrombin
The structure of prothrombin is known in detail. It is synthesized in the liver; the final steps require a vitamin K-dependent enzyme system which converts 10 glutamic acid residues among the 42 amino terminal residues into the unique form 'γ-carboxylated glutamic acid'.

The section of the molecule binds to the phospholipid micelle of prothrombinase, calcium ions bridging the negative ionic charges. Similar regions are found on the molecules of VII, IX and X, which

$$-N-C-C- \qquad -N-C-C-$$

$$C \qquad \qquad C$$

$$+ \text{ Vit. K} \longrightarrow$$

$$C \qquad \qquad C$$

$$\text{COOH} \qquad \text{HOOC} \qquad \text{COOH}$$

Glutamic	*γ-carboxyglutamic*
acid	*acid*

also require vitamin K for their final synthesis. In vitamin K deficiency, the precursor molecules of II, VII, IX and X are found in the plasma without γ-carboxyglutamic acid residues. Because they cannot partake in the micellar reactions, blood clotting is delayed. This situation occurs in severe malabsorption, obstructive jaundice and in babies, particularly if premature – *haemorrhagic disease of the newborn*.

Prothrombinase breaks two peptide bonds on the prothrombin, producing two chains – the 'propiece' (which contains all the γ-carboxylated residues) and thrombin. Thrombin has two peptide chains, joined by —S-S— bonds, and the active site is on the longer (B) chain.

Interaction of extrinsic and intrinsic systems
In life, tissue injury and vascular damage usually occur together. The extrinsic system generates thrombin which aggregates platelets causing them to initiate the intrinsic system. Recent experiments have also shown interactions between factors VII, IX and X, which also share physiological inhibiting mechanisms.

FIBRIN FORMATION AND CONSOLIDATION

This is complex but over-simplification leads to loss of understanding.

Chemistry of fibrinogen and fibrin
Fibrinogen (factor I) is a glycoprotein, MW 344 000. There are three pairs of peptide chains, A α (MW 67 000), Bβ (MW 58 000) and γ (MW 47 000). There are many intramolecular disulphide bonds, the unravelling of which is still providing problems for the protein chemist. The abbreviated formula is $(A\alpha\,B\beta\gamma)_2$.

Thrombin acts at the amino-terminal end of the Aα and Bβ chains, breaking off small residues – fibrinopeptides A and B, which have 16 and 14 amino acids respectively.

The result is fibrin monomer – $(\alpha\beta\gamma)_2$, or I_m. In the presence of calcium ions, the denuded portions of the molecule attract other fibrin monomers to form a relatively weak fibrin polymer $(\alpha\beta\psi)_{2p}$, or I_p.

The final step in forming a consolidated fibrin mesh requires peptide-bond cross-links between adjacent fibrin polymers, the formation of which requires the enzymic action of activated factor XIII. Activation of XIII requires thrombin. XIIIa then links a glutamine residue of one fibrin monomer to a lysine residue of another, releasing ammonia.

These bonds produce a stable fibrin mesh relatively resistant to digestion by plasmin. It is not possible to give a sensible abbreviated formula for 'cross-linked fibrin' other than 'I_x'.

The mechanisms are shown diagrammatically in Figs. 60 and 61.

CLOTTING FACTOR LEVELS

Pooling a large number of fresh plasma samples from normal people gives a preparation which can be regarded as having 100 per cent of each clotting factor, and which can be used as a reference standard. However, the activities of the various factors in each contributing sample may differ quite widely from the pool. The 'normal ranges' of each factor among normal persons is usually 60–150 per cent. Factor VIII has a wider range (50–200 per cent) although most persons fall between 85 and 115 per cent. Factors XI and XII have even wider normal ranges.

Samples with '100 per cent' of a given clotting factor have also been described as having '1 unit per ml' or even '100 units per 100 ml'. This is a useful concept, as it gives an indication of how much factor activity one may expect in a given patient's circulation after calculating their expected plasma volume, thus helping treatment with clotting factor preparations. On this basis the National Institute of

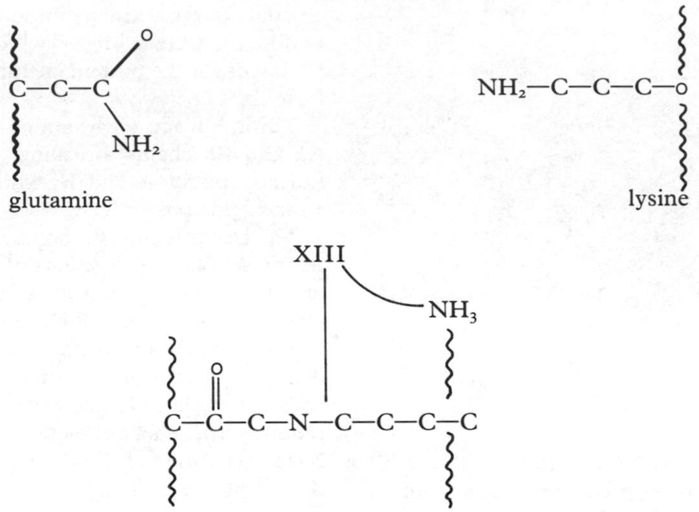

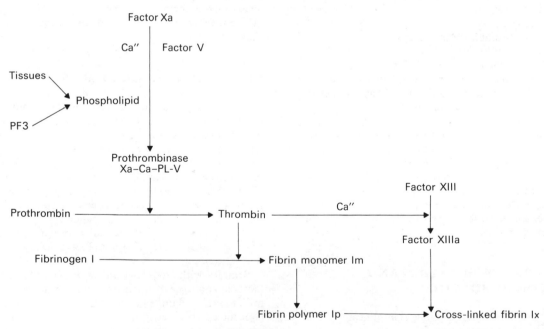

Fig. 60. The action of factor XIII in this cross-linking of fibrin.

Fig. 61. The generation of thrombin and formation of fibrin.

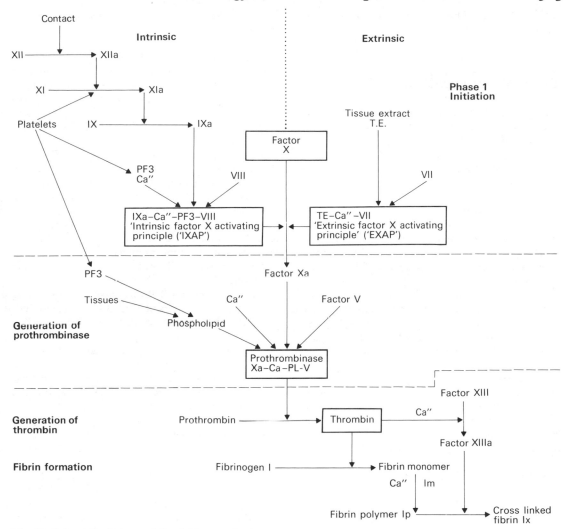

Fig. 62. Schematic diagram of the clotting mechanism.

Biological Standards and Controls is preparing dried plasma reference standards, the activities of which have been pre-determined.

ANTITHROMBINS

Most thrombin generated during clot formation is rapidly neutralized by absorption on to the fibrin. This capacity of fibrin has been called 'antithrombin I'. Any remaining thrombin is further neutralized by an α_2 globulin in the plasma – 'antithrom-

bin III' (AT III). This is the physiological neutralizer of thrombin. Neutralization is slow, but is considerably accelerated by heparin, which binds in a one-to-one molecular relationship to AT III. This heparin–AT III complex is also important for inhibiting prothrombinase and activated factor IX, and probably for neutralizing the active forms of factors VII, IX and XI. 'Antithrombin VI' is the name which has been given to the products of fibrin or fibrinogen when degraded by plasmin. These inhibit thrombin by competing with fibrinogen for the active site, or by blocking the formation of long fibrin polymers. They are discussed again in the section on fibrinolysis (see p. 531).

Tests of coagulation

All should be carried out at 37°C and within 2 hours of collection. Normal controls are usually run in parallel. For most tests, platelet-poor plasma from centrifuged blood, anticoagulated with 1 volume of 3·2 per cent citrate to 9 volumes of venous blood, is used.

Fibrinogen assays

1 Clot from 2 ml of plasma plus thrombin dried and weighed. Normally 2–4 g/l plasma.
2 Fibrinogen titre. Thrombin added to dilutions of plasma and clot formation observed. Normal end point 1:32 to 1:64.
3 Chemical analysis, precipitations, etc. May not measure clottable fibrinogen, especially in the presence of fibrinolysis.
4 Immunological analysis. May cross-react with products of fibrin or fibrinogen degradation.

Thrombin time

Standard amount of bovine thrombin and calcium added to citrated plasma. Clotting time normally adjusted to 10–15 s (depends on amount of thrombin). Prolonged by 'antithrombin', especially heparin and degraded fibrinogen (see p. 531).

Reptilase time – Arvin time

A snake venom, *reptilase*, also 'clots' fibrinogen. It is not affected by heparin, but is altered by products of degraded fibrinogen. Commercial preparations available produce a normal clotting time of 15–20 s. Another venom product, *Arvin*, has very similar properties.

Prothrombin time

Initially thought only to reflect the plasma prothrombin content, but it is actually sensitive to the extrinsic system and final common path, i.e. factors V, VII, X, as well as II. Standardized tissue extract (usually mammalian brain) and calcium are added to citrated plasma. Clotting time is normally 12–15 s. Prolonged clotting times are best expressed as a ratio of test time to control – *prothrombin time ratio*, or 'P.T.R.'. The formerly used 'prothrombin index' or 'P.T.I.' – which is the reciprocal of the 'P.T.R.' expressed as a percentage – is now outmoded.

Whole blood clotting time – W.B.C.T.

Depends on intrinsic factors, final common path and platelet function. Whole, non-anticoagulated blood is taken into standardized glass tubes – clotting time normally 4–12 min. The wide range reduces sensitivity and clinical application.

Kaolin–cephalin clotting time – K.C.C.T.

Formerly called *partial thromboplastin time* – P.T.T. Also sensitive to intrinsic factors and final common path; but as it uses citrated plasma deprived of platelets, cephalin is added as substitute for PF3. Contact activation is standardized by exposure to kaolin prior to adding cephalin and calcium. Clotting time is normally 30–60 s, depending on precise conditions. At any time it is quite reproducible.

Platelet function may be assessed by substituting platelets, i.e. slowly centrifuged blood to produce platelet-rich plasma, instead of cephalin.

Thromboplastin generation test – T.G.T.

This is now becoming outmoded, although still used in specialist centres for assessing intrinsic factors. Preliminary preparation of serum and treated plasma are required.

Russell's viper venom test – R.V.V.

An extract from the venom of Russell's viper activates factor X directly. With phospholipid – as in the K.C.C.T. – R.V.V. considerably accelerates clotting, depending on the activities of the factors subsequent to X. The R.V.V. can also assess platelet function – PF3 release – if done on platelet-rich plasma, or if platelets are added to the platelet-poor plasma instead of phospholipids.

Clot lysis times

The clotting process of normal blood also activates fibrinolysis (see p. 531) which eventually causes clots in glass tubes to redissolve. However, physiological inhibitors in the blood delay the normal 'whole blood clot lysis time' for at least 24 hours even at 37°C. Removal of these inhibitors, and thus accelerated clot lysis times, is carried out in:
(a) *The dilute blood clot lysis time*. Simple dilution of blood reduces the effect of the inhibitors.
(b) *Modification of the fibrinogen titre* (see above). If the row of tubes is incubated at 37°C, inspec-

tion normally shows disappearance of the clot in the last tube by 2 hours.

(c) *The euglobulin clot lysis time. Euglobulin* is the name given to the precipitate which normal plasma yields when diluted and gently acidified in the cold. It contains fibrinogen, plasminogen and plasminogen activator (and also factor VIII), but the fibrinolytic inhibitors remain in the supernatant. If the precipitate is redissolved and clotted with thrombin, the clot normally dissolves 2–4 hours later.

Interpretation

Low fibrinogen levels may rarely be due to inherited afibrinogenaemia. More usually, defibrination is a consequence of fibrinolytic states. A sample with prolongation of both thrombin and reptilase times indicates active fibrinolysis; but if only the thrombin time is prolonged (and reptilase time normal) heparin must be present in the sample. Active fibrinolysis may also be shown by shortened clot lysis times.

Prolongation of the P.T.R. and K.C.C.T. may rarely result from congenital deficiencies of factors X, V, or II, but usually indicates a general decrease of clotting factors, as in liver failure or in anticoagulant therapy; or the presence of inhibitors such as heparin. Inhibitors can be distinguished from deficiency states by adding some normal plasma to the sample. Correction of clotting times implies deficiencies, and failure of correction inhibitors. A normal P.T.R. with a prolonged K.C.C.T. indicates a specific deficiency of the intrinsic system, and is characteristic of haemophilia. A normal K.C.C.T. with a prolonged P.T.R. specifically indicates a factor VII deficiency.

Factor assays

The effect of the patient's plasma on plasma known to be deficient in a specific factor is a useful preliminary screen; lack of correction by the patient's plasma indicating the same deficiency. By measuring the effect of different dilutions of patient's plasma, the degree of deficiency can be assayed.

The clotting system used may be the T.G.T., or the K.C.C.T., for intrinsic factors; and the prothrombin time for factor VII. Special systems have been devised for the final common path.

Chapter 88
Haematology – Congenital Clotting Deficiencies: Fibrinolysis: Anticoagulant Therapy

Congenital deficiencies of clotting factors

A severe haemorrhagic diathesis affecting boys has been known since antiquity. The blood of such boys was shown to lack an *anti-haemophilic factor* in the 1930s when the prolonged clotting of such blood was found to be shortened after adding some normal blood. In the 1950s two separate factors were identified: in most cases it was factor VIII, but in about one case in five it was a new factor, factor IX – *Christmas factor*, after the surname of the first case.

HAEMOPHILIA A – CLASSICAL HAEMOPHILIA

Definition
X-linked recessive deficiency of factor VIII.

Incidence
Affects about 12 males per 100 000 in the U.K., about a third severely.

Clinical
Severe cases suffer spontaneous bleeds particularly into weight-bearing joints and muscles with resul-

tant crippling. Internal organs may be involved, although cerebral haemorrhages are less common. Mild trauma can produce prolonged bleeding. Capillary wounds, e.g. when performing bleeding time procedures, usually stop bleeding within a few minutes, but oozing may start again after 30 min due to defective clot formation. Venepunctures are usually safe if firm pressure is applied over the wound. Severe cases have no detectable factor VIII activity but there are many less severely affected males. Such boys may have only 4 or 5 per cent of normal factor VIII activity, but even this low activity considerably reduces the severity of the disease; the severity can be divided conveniently into four grades: severe (with less than 1 per cent factor VIII activity), moderate (1–10 per cent), mild (10–30 per cent) and minimal (30–50 per cent).

Diagnosis

HISTORY
Is likely to be life-long and often indicated by excessive bleeding, e.g. after circumcision, while teething and after mild trauma, particularly after about 6 months of age when children start to become more venturesome.

FAMILY HISTORY
Positive in about four cases out of five, involving brothers, maternal uncles, etc. The other fifth probably represent *new mutations*. Although female carriers are not usually affected clinically, some do exhibit a mild bleeding tendency. According to the rules of X-linked recessive inheritance, all sons of haemophilic fathers and normal mothers will be normal and will not transmit the disease to further generations, whereas *all* daughters will be carriers. Homozygous female haemophilics are very rare, and usually result from consanguineous marriage.

LABORATORY FINDINGS
Bleeding time and prothrombin time are normal. Tests of the intrinsic clotting system will be prolonged, e.g. the whole blood clotting time, the T.G.T. and particularly the K.C.C.T. The long K.C.C.T. of uncomplicated haemophilia is shortened when normal plasma is added, and also by the addition of plasma deficient in any clotting factor other than factor VIII. The final diagnosis relies on a definitive clotting factor assay.

An increasing number of haemophilics are receiving therapy with factor VIII (see below) and about 1 in 10 of these develop inhibitors to factor VIII. Treatment of bleeding episodes then becomes very difficult as large quantities of factor VIII are required. Furthermore, the prolonged K.C.C.T. of the plasma of such haemophilics cannot be corrected by adding normal plasma *in vitro*.

Management

BLEEDING EPISODES
Bleeding will stop after intravenous administrations of enough factor VIII. Several preparations are available, all derived from blood, the factor VIII activity of which depends on the donor. Factor VIII is an unstable protein, losing activity at room temperature in a few hours.

PREPARATIONS OF FACTOR VIII
1 *Fresh blood.* Factor VIII activity depends on storage time but most activity is lost after 24 hours.
2 *Fresh frozen plasma – FFP.* Prepared within 2 hours of donation; frozen rapidly and stored at $-30°C$.

Unacceptably large volumes of both 1 and 2 may be required to stop haemorrhages.

3 *Cryoprecipitate.* Until recently this has been the mainstay in the routine management of bleeding in haemophilics and von Willebrand's disease. It was discovered by Pool in 1964, when she observed that the gel-like material retained in the filters of intravenous giving sets after infusion of thawed FFP often contained high concentrations of factor VIII, thus accounting for the frequently observed disappointing recovery rate of factor VIII in patients on FFP. Thorough mixing will, however, dissolve the gel.

In the U.K. cryoprecipitate is usually prepared from FFP at blood transfusion centres.

The content of factor VIII is variable, usually being between 30 and 40 per cent of that in the original plasma. However, the removal of about 90 per cent of supernatant plasma produces approximately five-fold concentration.

Besides factor VIII, cryoprecipitate also contains an apparently inert *cold precipitable globulin*; up to half of the original fibrinogen; *von Willebrand factor* (see p. 529); and small amounts of all the other plasma proteins.

4 *Lyophilized concentrate of human factor VIII.* This is now the most important factor VIII concentrate in use. Some preparations are of intermediate

purity and still contain some fibrinogen but even purer preparations are commercially available. There is growing anxiety that the hepatitis which so commonly follows the use of large pool freeze-dried concentrates may eventually lead to the development of chronic liver disease in haemophilic patients.

5 *Animal A.H.G.* A new generation of animal concentrates is now becoming available. Because of their greater purity they are likely to be less antigenic and may find a role in the management of patients with inhibitors to factor VIII.

STABILITY OF FACTOR VIII

As factor VIII loses activity rapidly *in vivo*, two or three injections a day may be required if replacement therapy needs to be prolonged. It also quickly loses activity *in vitro* and therefore needs to be given as soon after reconstitution as possible.

HOME TREATMENT

Home therapy programmes are now well established so that certain boys and men can treat bleeding episodes at home. Lyophilized preparations are better for these purposes as they are easier to store. Patients on home treatment miss less time from school and work and can lead nearly normal lives. A wider range of the less competitive physical activities, e.g. cycling, swimming and even ski-ing should be encouraged. Genetic advice should be offered to prospective parents in affected families and to the boys themselves when considering parenthood.

Detection of carriers

The factor VIII activity of female carriers of haemophilia will, on average, be half that of the normal population, but because the range of factor VIII activity in the normal population is so wide, the activity of many female carriers will be within the normal range. It is not possible to tell a female relative of a haemophilic if she is, or is not, a carrier, although if her factor VIII activity is below 50 per cent *she probably is.* N.B. Such persons should *not* be pregnant or receiving oral contraceptives at the time of testing as these may induce increased production of factor VIII.

The ability to tell whether possible carriers with factor VIII activity above 50 per cent are affected has been improved by immunological studies. Although it was formerly thought that haemophilia was induced by the *absence* of a clotting protein, it is now established that all haemophilic men carry an inactive analogue – 'dud', i.e. a protein which resembles active factor VIII structurally but which has no clotting activity. When animals such as rabbits are immunized to normal human factor VIII, they produce an antibody which precipitates not only normal factor VIII but also the inactive protein of haemophilics which has been called the *factor VIII related antigen* – VIIIR:AG. Carriers of haemophilia will, on average, have only half of their factor VIII molecules in the *active clotting form* – VIII:C. Hence a female with 70 per cent VIII:C and 140 per cent VIIIR:AG activity can be predicted to be a carrier.

Females have two X chromosomes and males only one. It might be expected therefore that females would have twice as much factor VIII, and other X chromosome products, as males. However, at an early stage of female embryogenesis, one X chromosome of each cell is deactivated (although it persists throughout all subsequent mitoses and of course becomes reactivated in subsequent oocytes). This deactivation (also called Lyonization, after Dr Lyon) is random so that, although the chances are that in each embryo equal numbers of paternal and maternal X chromosomes are inactivated, sometimes inactivation may be unequal. Hence carriers of haemophilia could have almost as much VIII:C as VIIIR:AG (say 120 and 140 per cent respectively). The World Health Organization has made specific recommendations on the techniques to be adopted in the performance and analysis of tests for carrier status.

Antenatal diagnosis

In the last 2 years antenatal diagnosis of haemophilia has become available at a very few centres and these techniques can help to prevent the birth of some severely affected haemophilic boys.

CHRISTMAS DISEASE

Definition

X-linked recessive deficiency of factor IX.

Incidence

About one-fifth as common as haemophilia A.

Clinical and diagnosis

Indistinguishable from haemophilia. Severity also ranges from mild to severe.

Laboratory findings

Like factor VIII deficiency, only the intrinsic clotting tests reveal any abnormality. The final diagnosis is made by noting the lack of correction of the patient's K.C.C.T. after adding plasma known to be deficient in factor IX. Christmas disease was actually discovered as a result of the then puzzling finding of a mutually corrective clotting effect of a mixture of plasma from two apparently classical haemophilics, one only being factor XIII deficient, the other lacking factor IX.

Management

Similar to haemophilia A, but as cryoprecipitate does *not* contain factor IX, other preparations are required. A powdered concentrate of factor IX is now available and also contains factors II and X. FFP can help in milder cases. As factor IX is more stable than factor VIII *in vivo*, prolonged treatment does not require the injections to be so frequent, once every day or two usually being sufficient. As with classical haemophilia, home treatment programmes are assuming greater importance. Hepatitis may also follow the administration of factor IX concentrate.

Detection of carriers

Unfortunately, the majority of men with Christmas disease do not have any analogue of factor IX detectable by antibodies. Their affected female relatives, therefore, will not show a 2:1 ratio of *IX antigen* to *IX procoagulant*. Such carriers can only be detected if their factor IX levels are below normal, but there are several authenticated cases of carriers with normal levels of factor IX, presumably as a result of chance inactivation of most of the faulty X chromosomes during Lyonization (see p. 528). Antenatal diagnosis of Christmas Disease is also now available.

OTHER FACTOR DEFICIENCIES

Rare and all are autosomal. Abnormal fibrinogens have been discovered, e.g. fibrinogen Detroit. This fails to clot and even interferes with the clotting of normal fibrinogen, so that heterozygotes show some tendency to bleed. Other inherited 'afibrinogenaemics' have markedly reduced levels of fibrinogen, even when tested immunologically. The tendency is usually surprisingly mild.

Occasional cases of congenital deficiencies of II,

V, VII, X, XI and XIII have been described. Symptoms are very like haemophilia though factor XII deficiency is usually symptomless.

VON WILLEBRAND'S DISEASE – VWD

Definition

Autosomal dominant deficiency of factor VIII whch has *partial expression*, i.e. heterozygotes are moderately affected, homozygotes severely. Actually it is a group of closely related disorders which together are labelled as *von Willebrand's syndrome*.

Heterozygotes usually have moderate-to-mild deficiency of factor VIII (5–40 per cent clotting activity) but there are some severer cases; homozygotes have very little or no factor VIII.

There is also a defect of platelet function exacerbating the bleeding tendency in both heterozygotes and homozygotes and this is responsible for a prolonged bleeding time.

Pathogenesis

Not completely elucidated but the deficiency of factor VIII is linked to a deficiency of a factor in the plasma of vWd patients which is essential for platelets to partake in normal haemostasis. This factor – *Willebrand factor* – can be demonstrated by:

(a) *The effect of adhesion of platelets to glass.* Platelets in vWd blood adhere much less strongly to glass than do platelets of normal blood.

(b) *Effect of aggregation of platelets by ristocetin.* Ristocetin – an antibiotic now withdrawn, aggregates platelets in normal blood, but not in vWd blood.

(c) *Effect on the bleeding time.* The prolonged bleeding time of vWd patients is caused by lack of Willebrand factor.

All these defects are corrected by the Willebrand factor in normal blood. Attempts to purify this factor have shown that it is part of the same molecule bearing VIIIC and VIIIR:AG activity (see p. 528). It has therefore been called VIIIR:WF – *factor VIII-related Willebrand factor*.

The genetic origin of VIIIC and VIIIR:AG must differ, because haemophilia is an X-linked disease while vWd is autosomally linked. It should also be noted that haemophilics have no lack of

VlIIR:WF and that some atypical cases of vWd have no lack of VIIIC. The two conditions are thus quite separate.

It is postulated that a gene on the X chromosome makes the VIIIC component of the normal factor VIII complex and that an autosomal gene makes the VIIIWF so that the final steps of VIII-complex synthesis involve a combination of these two components.

Response to plasma fractions

Administration of FFP or cryoprecipitate to persons with vWd supplies the missing VIIIR:WF as the bleeding time is rapidly, but only temporarily corrected. A 'new synthesis' of VIII:C not accompanied by a parallel rise in VIIIR:AG or VIIIR:WF follows for the next 12–24 hours. The cellular mechanisms for these events are not known and even more extraordinary is the observation that haemophilic plasmas induce the same response.

Management

Bleeding episodes are well controlled with cryoprecipitate. Elective surgery should be preceded by 6–12 hours with cryoprecipitate to induce the *new synthesis*, and again with the anaesthetic to reduce the bleeding time at operation. Cryoprecipitate will often be required at regular intervals until healing is well advanced.

Antifibrinolytic therapy

Drugs such as tramexamic acid may be valuable in the management of abnormal bleeding in haemophilia or von Willebrand's disease and their use may reduce factor requirements. They are most suitable in the management of 'open bleeds', e.g. dental extraction and tonsillectomy. If antifibrinolytic therapy is used for 'closed' bleeds there is a theoretical risk of the formation of blood clot which will be slow to disperse.

Comparison with haemophilia

Figure 63 shows a comparison of the characteristics of classical von Willebrand's disease with those of haemophilia.

	Haemophilia	*vWd (heterozygous)*
Type of bleeding	Characteristically, joints and muscles	Characteristically, skin, mucous membrane nose-bleeds, menorrhagia
Sex	Males	Either
Inheritance	X-linked recessive	Autosomal dominant
Bleeding time	Normal	Prolonged
Aggregation of platelets by ADP	Normal	Normal
Aggregation of platelets by ristocetin	Normal	Low
Adhesion of platelets to glass	Normal	Low
W.B.C.T.	Prolonged	Normal or slightly long
P.T.R	Normal	Normal
K.C.C.T.	Very long	Moderately long
VIIIC levels	Low or Zero	Moderately low
VIIIR:AG levels	Normal	Moderately low
VIIIR:WF levels	Normal	Moderately low
Other clotting factors	Normal	Normal
Response to cryoprecipitate *in vivo*	Transient rise in VIIIC·	(a) Correction of bleeding time (b) Prolonged rise of VIIIC

Fig. 63. Characteristics of von Willebrand's disease and haemophilia compared.

Fibrinolysis

Mechanism

The effective agent is *plasmin*. This destroys fibrin, releasing *fibrin degradation products* – FDP, which are powerful inhibitors of thrombin and have been called 'Antithrombin VI'. Plasmin also acts on fibrinogen, factors V and VIII and other proteins, and therefore must exist in blood as an inactive precursor – *plasminogen*. Normally plasminogen is laid down with fibrin, and plasmin is slowly released to produce the characteristic autodigestion of the clot. Plasmin release follows the diffusion of activators into the clot. There are two main types of physiological activators: *intrinsic* and *extrinsic* – derived from tissues, e.g. lungs, prostate and vascular endothelium, particularly venous. All tubular organs are kept patent by fibrinolysis; the activator in the urinary system is *urokinase* derived from the kidneys. Non-physiological activators include drugs such as phenformin, and bacterial toxins such as streptokinase. (See Fig 64.)

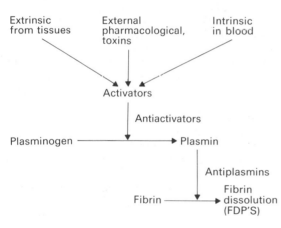

Extrinsic from tissues   External pharmacological, toxins   Intrinsic in blood

→ Activators

Antiactivators

Plasminogen ——→ Plasmin

Antiplasmins

Fibrin ——→ Fibrin dissolution (FDP'S)

Fig. 64. Diagram of fibrinolytic mechanisms.

Hageman factor – XII, is also one of the intrinsic plasminogen activators and hence may contribute another self-limiting mechanism to overall coagulation.

Natural inhibitors of fibrinolysis

ANTIACTIVATORS
Ill-defined at present.

ANTIPLASMINS
These are globulins and are of two subtypes:
1 A fast acting, reversible, 'α_2 globulin'.
2 A slow acting, irreversible, 'α_1 globulin'.
Plasmin bound to the reversible antiplasmin may also be adsorbed on to fibrin clots. Subsequent release may contribute further to the autodigestion.

Pathological fibrinolysis

The physiological balance may be disturbed by:
(*a*) Excessive clot deposition.
(*b*) Excessive activation of plasminogen.

EXCESSIVE CLOT DEPOSITION

Disseminated intravascular coagulation –D.I.C.
Generalized laying down of fibrin due to release of thromboplastic substances into blood stream, e.g. severe tissue trauma, intra-uterine death, amniotic fluid embolism (see p. 127).

Localized intravascular coagulation – L.I.C.
Due to endothelial damage of vessels of certain organs, e.g. kidneys in malignant hypertension or glomerulonephritis, liver in cirrhosis.

In all cases fibrinogen and platelets are 'consumed' leading to hypofibrinogenaemia and thrombocytopenia. Red cells are damaged as they are forced through the fibrin mesh, leading to fragmentation and lysis of circulating red cells – *schistocytes, helmet cells* or *burr cells*, etc. This is also described as *microangiopathic haemolytic anaemia – M.A.H.A.* (see p. 507).

In both D.I.C. and L.I.C., plasminogen activation follows the deposition of fibrin and produces F.D.P. A severe haemorrhagic state therefore develops for three reasons: (*a*) thrombocytopenia; (*b*) diminution of clotting factors, especially fibrinogen; (*c*) antithrombin effect of F.D.P.

EXCESSIVE ACTIVATION OF PLASMINOGEN IN THE BLOOD

Release of tissue plasminogen activators
Into the blood stream, e.g. during surgery to lungs or prostate. Possibly endothelial in origin.

Septicaemia
In bacterial toxaemia, etc., by release of external activators, e.g. streptokinase. These produce free plasmin in plasma, and therefore afibrinogenaemia, low factor V and VIII activity, and F.D.P. But

platelets are not consumed and red cells are not damaged. The free plasmin leads to accelerated clot lysis.

N.B. The F.D.P.'s are technically slightly different from those found in D.I.C., being *fibrinogen* degradation products, but effectively are identical in their antithrombin effect.

Tests for diagnosis of fibrinolysis
1 Blood film, cell and platelet morphology.
2 Platelet count.
3 Thrombin time and reptilase time. These are very useful for the detection of F.D.P. in *plasma*. Both are prolonged.

N.B. Normal reptilase and long thrombin times are indicative of the presence of heparin in the plasma.
4 Timing the lysis of blood clots by various techniques – shorter times indicating the presence of plasmin.
5 Plasmin and plasminogen assays.
6 Fibrin(ogen) degradation products in serum:
(*a*) Immunological – tanned red cells or latex particles, detecting the *fibrin–fibrinogen related antigens*.
(*b*) Staphylococcal clumping.

N.B. Procedures 1–4 may be routine, 5 and 6 are highly specialized.

Treatment of fibrinolytic states

EXCESSIVE CLOT DEPOSITION–D.I.C.
Heparin to stop clot deposition, thereby sparing platelets and halting secondary fibrinolysis. It is better to have platelets, fibrinogen and no F.D.P.'s even with heparin in the blood, than to allow defibrination, thrombocytopenia and the production of F.D.P.'s.

Plasma, fibrinogen and platelet preparations may also be given, though it has been suggested that heparin should be given at the same time if possible.

Acute D.I.C. is the most amenable to this therapy, although if the acute episode, e.g. amniotic fluid embolus, has finished, only 'fresh' blood or clotting factors should be given. Indeed heparin therapy at this stage may actually be harmful. Chronic D.I.C. is more difficult to treat, but if there is progressive renal failure, a course of heparin may be beneficial for a few days or weeks.

There is a growing interest in the use of plasma exchange.

EXCESSIVE ACTIVATION OF PLASMINOGEN
Therapeutic inhibitors of fibrinolysis, e.g. epsilon-amino caproic acid – E.A.C.A., trasylol, or tranexamic acid. These inhibit plasminogen activation and also plasmin. Contra-indicated in D.I.C. as, in these cases, fibrin removal is essential.

N.B. Excessive fibrin deposition and plasminogen activation may occur together in the same patient to varying extents at different stages of the disease. Heparin is the safer therapy but if there is free plasmin in the plasma E.A.C.A. may be added.

THERAPEUTIC FIBRINOLYSIS
Streptokinase and urokinase have been administered in order to 'dissolve' thrombi. There is potentially a dangerous haemorrhagic tendency when these drugs are used (see p. 534).

Anticoagulant therapy

Introduction
In general, venous thrombi are easier to remove than arterial. This probably derives from their contrasting origins, venous thrombi being rather more closely related to the clotting proteins, and arterial thrombi to disease of the arterial wall, e.g. atheroma and possibly to the platelets. Differences in flow dynamics on the two sides of the circulation must also be significant.

Anticoagulation may be given:
(*a*) To reduce thrombotic tendencies during periods of risk, e.g. after surgery, myocardial infarction, heart valve replacement, etc.
(*b*) To prevent extension of already established thrombi.
(*c*) To hasten the removal of already established thrombi.

In the first two situations, conventional therapy with heparin and oral anticoagulants may be useful. Dissolution of thrombi, as in (*c*), is difficult and not always successful. Drugs which interfere with platelet function may help reduce arterial thrombi but even these are probably more effective on the venous side.

On the whole, haematologists are not so concerned with the therapeutic indications for anticoagulation as with their effective control, so that patients do not suffer unduly from any bleeding side effects.

Heparin

Must be given parenterally – 100 units = 1 mg.

Inhibits coagulation at several stages, in particular against IIa, Xa, IXa and XIa, and probably VII (see p. 524).

DOSE AND ROUTE

(a) i.v. continuous infusions 1000–2000 units per hour for adults.

(b) i.v. discontinuous, hourly or 2-hourly, at the same overall dose as (a).

(c) i.v. discontinuous 6000–10 000 units 6-hourly for adults. These are usually given to prevent established thrombi from spreading. However, continuous heparinization, as in (a), is essential during open heart surgery. Six-hourly injections, as in (c), are not as good because immediately after one injection the patient is overanticoagulated; and for about 2 hours before the next injections, he is under-anticoagulated.

(d) s.c. or i.m. 5000–10 000 units b.d. for adults. Usually given prophylactically during and after surgical procedures on patients at risk.

ROUTINE MONITORING

This is only possible for continuous i.v. therapy and is best done by K.C.C.T. which should be kept about 1.5–2.0 times the control time.

Also used are the thrombin time (2–3 × control) and whole blood clotting time (about 2 × control), but neither is as reliable. At therapeutic levels, the prothrombin time is also prolonged to about 1.3–1.5 × normal.

REVERSAL OF OVERDOSE

Heparin disappears rapidly from the circulation, therefore a bleeding state through heparin overdose is likely to stop within a few hours. However, if more immediate reversal is needed, heparin can be neutralized by i.v. protamine sulphate. Ideally, this should not be given in excess as it has mild anticoagulant properties of its own. A required dose can be estimated by assaying the heparin levels.

HEPARIN ASSAY

Heparin is neutralized *in vitro* by protamine sulphate or toluidine blue. The thrombin times of heparinized plasma are progressively shortened by graded additions of protamine sulphate and will enable calculation of the plasma heparin level (1 mg protamine = 1 mg heparin). If the heparin level of the plasma is less than 1 iu/ml, more sensitive techniques are required.

Vitamin K antagonists

Vitamin K is required by the liver to synthesize normal factors II, VII, IX and X. The amounts of such factors are therefore reduced by vitamin K antagonists of which the most widely used is warfarin. This prolongs P.T.R. and K.C.C.T. but leaves the thrombin time normal.

ROUTE

Oral – i.v. preparations of warfarin were available but are now withdrawn through lack of use.

DOSE

Warfarin 1–10 mg/day.

Dosage is highly variable and depends on individual response. This requires frequent checking, e.g. weekly at first, monthly later. Using the *British comparative thromboplastin* and the *prothrombin time ratio* – PTR of patients on these drugs should be 2.0–4.0. Although the K.C.C.T. may theoretically be used to assess blood coagulability, in practice it is found to be less reliable and convenient.

A careful check on other medication is required, e.g. aspirin, antibiotics, as these may render patients more sensitive to vitamin K antagonists. Mild hepatic impairment, e.g. alcohol excess or impending cardiac failure, also increases sensitivity. Conversely, barbiturates lead to increased anticoagulant requirements.

REVERSAL OF OVERDOSE

Vitamin K antagonists may be overcome by the parenteral administration of vitamin K or its analogues, e.g. vitamin K_1, but they may take several hours to become effective. More immediate restoration of the missing factors may be effected by transfusions of blood, plasma, or clotting factor concentrates. Concentrates used for Christmas disease contain factors II, IX and X and sometimes VII, and are indicated if bleeding through overdose occurs in patients with incipient fluid overload, e.g. in congestive cardiac failure.

Persons requiring continuous anticoagulation, who become over-treated, are best managed by stopping the drug for a few days, administering plasma preparations if necessary and recommencing the drug at a lower dose. Vitamin K need not be given. Frequent monitoring of the P.T.R. is required.

Combined heparin and warfarin regimes

This is the conventional approach to instituting anticoagulant therapy for recently established venous thrombosis. A suggested regime is given below. The heparin should be given either continuously or at frequent intervals (1- or 2-hourly). A loading dose of 40–50 u/kg body weight is followed by continuous infusions at the rate of 15–20 u/kg/hour. A K.C.C.T., taken 2–3 hours after starting, should be checked. Warfarin, 0.15 mg/kg should be given shortly after commencing heparin, but note that the sample for K.C.C.T. will be affected by the Warfarin after 2 to 3 hours. Warfarin, 0.07 mg/kg should then be given daily for 3 days. After 72 hours of heparinization, heparin may be stopped and 6 hours later (but no earlier) the first unheparinized sample for the P.T.R. measured. Further warfarin doses can be adjusted from this. There is little point in taking other samples for anticoagulant monitoring during this first 3-day period. The K.C.C.T and P.T.R. will be difficult to interpret as both drugs influence both tests. If necessary, the thrombin time could be measured to check the degree of heparinization.

At the end of warfarin therapy, an immediate cessation of the drug is quite safe. It is not now generally throught necessary to reduce the dose to zero gradually.

Other anticoagulant regimes

THERAPEUTIC FIBRINOLYSIS

Streptokinase – SK

Pharmacological preparations of this substance – initially derived from streptococcal toxins – have been given intravenously for many years in attempts to increase the rate of lysis of established thrombi. Difficulties of dosage arise from its antigenicity and only 7–10 days effective treatment is usually possible. It is extremely potent unless neutralized by antibodies, and when it is administered to patients there is a potentially dangerous bleeding tendency.

Urokinase – UK

This is prepared from human urine or renal cells in tissue culture and is the physiological activator of fibrinolysis in the urinary tract. Like SK it is extremely potent, but, by contrast, is not antigenic. It is expensive because of preparative difficulties. The effect on the blood is similar to that of SK, but the lack of neutralizing antibodies allows longer periods of treatment. Like SK, however, it must be given intravenously.

Therapeutic assessments of SK and UK

Trials have generally been disappointing, their value being doubtful except probably in acute massive pulmonary embolism and in clotted artificially created arteriovenous shunts, e.g. for haemodialysis.

Other means of increasing fibrinolysis

Vascular, especially venous, endothelium is rich in a physiological activator of fibrinolysis. This is released during stress, e.g. anoxia, adrenaline, etc. A more sustained increase in endothelial activator release may result from the administration of various drugs.

A combination of phenformin and ethyloestranol has been used to treat people with a chronic hypercoagulable state associated with decreased levels of endothelial activator. Other drugs include vasopressin analogue and some androgenic steroids.

Defibrinating agents

Snake venom derivatives such as reptilase or arvin can lower circulating fibrinogen to safe levels (*c.* 500 mg/l plasma), thus effecting anticoagulation. As they are derived from non-human sources, their antigenicity may lead to loss of effect after a few days, particularly if given by i.m. or s.c. routes. Therapeutic trials have failed to show any convincing advantage over heparin or warfarin.

Anti-platelet drugs

ASPIRIN

Inhibits prostaglandin synthesis in platelets necessary for their aggregation: 600 mg is sufficient to affect permanently all the platelets circulating at one time in an average-sized adult. This should be borne in mind whenever surgery is contemplated for painful conditions, e.g. peptic ulcer or toothache, for which the patient may have taken aspirin.

PHENYLBUTAZONE AND OTHER ANTI-INFLAMMATORY DRUGS

These may also inhibit platelet prostaglandin synthesis, but usually only transiently. Unfortunately, other side effects, e.g. neutropenia with phenylbutazone (see p. 454), render such drugs unsuitable for prolonged anticoagulant purposes.

DIPYRIDAMOLE – PERSANTIN
Originally developed as a vasodilator. Found to inhibit A.D.P. release from platelets and hence reduce platelet aggregation. May be useful in treating chronic thrombotic disorders particularly in combination with aspirin.

Chapter 89
Haematology – Blood Groups: Transfusion

Blood groups

Introduction

If blood from two normal persons selected at random is mixed, in rather more than half the instances the red cells will agglutinate and sometimes lyse. This results from the interaction of specific factors, *antigens*, on the surface of one of the partner's red cells with correspondingly specific proteins, *antibodies*, in the plasma of the other partner. These antigenic surface factors have specific chemical structures and are integral parts of the red cell membrane. Their structure is determined genetically.

Allelic genes – i.e. genes in exactly corresponding positions on the chromosomes – may code for fac-

tors which differ slightly in structure from person to person. The inheritance of these differences will therefore also be determined genetically.

A group of antigenic factors produced by a set of allelic genes constitutes a 'blood group system'. The different factors in each system may be very similar chemically, i.e. blood group A substance is an oligosaccharide ending with N-acetylgalactosamine whereas B substance is the same oligosaccharide which ends with galactose instead. However, these subtle differences are easily detected by the specific antibodies.

The 'ABO' blood group system is rather exceptional as the antibodies are found naturally in persons without the corresponding antigen. Nevertheless, this makes the system particularly important in blood transfusion.

ANTIGENS AND ANTIBODIES IN THE ABO SYSTEM

Blood group phenotype	Antigens on red cell	Antibodies in serum
A	A	Anti-B
B	B	Anti-A
O	Neither A or B	Anti-A and anti-B
AB	A and B	Neither anti-A nor anti-B

Blood group systems which are genetically distinct may interact on the final structure of the antigens. For example, the ABO and Lewis systems are inherited quite separately, but their antigens are different facets of the same oligosaccharide chain. Other blood group systems are based on substances produced by several closely linked genes. For example, the *rhesus system* has the genetic loci denoted '*D*', '*C*' and '*E*', arranged adjacent to each other on the chromosome in that order. The pattern of inheritance of alternative alleles from each locus nearly always runs true, i.e. persons with the heterozygous arrangement 'DCE/dce' rarely produce any crossing over at meiosis (see p. 000).

Blood group antigens are components of the red cell membrane detectable by specific antibodies. Some, e.g. *rhesus*, may be more fully revealed by gentle enzymic digestion of the membrane, thereby reacting more strongly. Others, e.g. '*M*' and '*N*', are destroyed by such manoeuvres.

BLOOD GROUP ANTIBODIES

Nature
Immunoglobulins, usually IgG or IgM.

IMMUNE
That is, only develop after an individual has been in contact with antigens, e.g. after pregnancy, transfusion, 'blood-brother ceremonies', etc.

NATURAL
That is, develop with other immunoglobulins during first few neonatal months. No specific immunizing stimuli have been detected although they may well abound in natural environment, dust, bacilli, etc.

Physico-chemical properties
Very different for each type.

Natural antibodies
Complete – i.e. agglutinate cells suspended in saline.
Optimum temperature 4°C.
Develop in neonatal period.
IgM in nature (occasionally IgG).
Do not cross placenta.
Example: anti-A.

Immune antibodies
Incomplete – only 'coat' red cells.
Optimum temperature 37°C.
Only develop after immunization.
IgG (occasionally IgM).
Cross placenta (IgG only).
Example: anti-rhesus.

Incomplete immune antibodies are more difficult to detect. They can, however, be just as dangerous as complete antibodies in incompatibility reactions. They may be detected:
(*a*) By adding a macromolecular substance, e.g. albumin, to a mixture of red cell suspension and antibody – agglutination may then be detected.
(*b*) By observing a *blocking* effect on a complete antibody of similar specificity.
(*c*) By the indirect Coombs' test (see p. 540).

BLOOD GROUP SYSTEMS

The following are the more important blood group systems:
ABO
MNSs
P
Rh (Rhesus)
Lewis (Le)
Lutheran (Lu)
Kell
Duffy (Fy)
Kidd (Jk)
Ii

Unfortunately, the naming of antigens and corresponding antibodies has been haphazard.

Sometimes, alleles of newly discovered systems have been given alternative letters, e.g. A and B: on other occasions different cases of the same letter, e.g. C and c. The MNSs system combines both, M and N being one set of alleles, and S and s another set closely linked genetically.

The ABO system

The first to be discovered and the most important. Incompatible transfusions often produce fatal reactions.

ANTIGENS

Oligosaccharides attached to phospholipids. The A and B substances have seven sugar residues, and differ only in the terminal one. Removal of this terminal residue leaves a six-sugared 'precursor' called 'H substance'. The red cell surfaces of group O persons are rich in H substance as these people lack any enzyme capable of adding to it. H substance is also present in small amounts on the cell surface of persons of groups A and B, so it is not specific to O cells.

GENETICS

O is not recessive; A and B are co-dominant. Persons of group O must therefore be homozygous for O.

The A and B genes actually code for a saccharide-transferase enzyme system. The A gene produces 'galactosamine transferase', and the B gene 'galactose transferase'. The structure of these enzymes at present remains unknown, but it may be speculated that any differences are structurally minor.

The 'O' gene is an 'amorph', i.e. produces no enzyme: it may be totally absent.

The pattern of inheritance is summarized in the family tree (Fig. 58) where the parents are heterozygous AO and BO respectively.

FREQUENCY

NB. The phenotypes A or B are either homozygous, AA or BB, or heterozygous, AO or BO (Fig. 59).

Genotype	Phenotype	(%)
AA ⎫ AO ⎬	A	42
BB ⎫ BO ⎬	B	9
AB	AB	3
OO	O	46

Fig. 66. Frequency in the United Kingdom.

UNIVERSAL DONORS AND UNIVERSAL RECIPIENTS

This concept is old fashioned and dangerous. It used to be thought that persons of group AB, because they had no antibodies, could receive any sort of blood – *universal recipients*. Conversely persons of group O, because their cells have no antigens, could give blood to anybody – *universal donors*. However, the antibodies in O blood will react with A, B and AB blood. If a person of unknown group requires transfusion as a life-saving emergency, it is permissible to give blood of group O but such blood should be selected as having only low titre levels of antibody activity.

SUBGROUPS IN ABO SYSTEM

About 20% of persons of groups A and AB have cells which react only weakly with anti-A. Such persons are known as A_2 or A_2B. If the reaction is missed, they will be erroneously grouped as O, or B. It is therefore essential to use well-approved strongly reacting antisera for testing. There are further rarer weaker subgroups of A and B, the detection of which may require special techniques.

SECRETOR STATUS

About 80 per cent of Europeans secrete substances in their saliva and other body fluids which neutralize any ABO antibodies reacting with their blood. These substances have the same oligosaccharides of the ABO factors found on the red cells, but instead of being linked to lipids, they are bound to proteins as glycoproteins. The bond between the oligosaccharide and proteins is effected by an enzyme under the control of a *secretor gene*. The 20 per cent of individuals who are non-secretory lack this

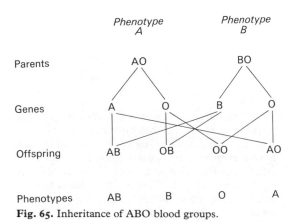

Fig. 65. Inheritance of ABO blood groups.

enzyme, although they still have the ABO factors on their red cells.

ABO GROUPING TECHNIQUES

(a) *Tile.* Blood diluted in saline to about 20 per cent suspension of cells: one drop plus one drop of anti-serum are mixed on a tile and rotated gently. Observe for agglutination after 6 min.

(b) *Tube.* Blood diluted in saline to 5 per cent cell suspension. Two drops plus two drops of anti-serum are incubated for 1 hour at room temperature in a 5×0.3 cm tube. Observe macroscopically for agglutinins.

Rhesus blood group system

Originally thought to be due to factors cross-reacting with antibodies raised in rabbit blood against red cells from the rhesus monkey. About 85 per cent of Europeans were thereby denoted rhesus positive: 15 per cent of blood samples did not react and were called rhesus negative. Now known, however, to be much more complex.

RHESUS D ANTIGEN

The main antigen of rhesus system is *D*. All persons possessing the *D* antigen on their red cells are *rhesus D positive*. Persons whose red cells contain no *D* antigen are *rhesus D negative*. All rhesus antigens are important proteins of the red cell membrane. The *D* antigen is probably slightly below the surface, as gentle digestion of the membrane with enzymes such as trypsin or papain seem to enhance its accessibility to anti-D, although prolonged digestion destroys the *D* antigen.

RHESUS D ANTIBODY

Only found in healthy *rhesus D negative* persons after immunization with the *D* antigen, most commonly as a result of pregnancy with a *rhesus D positive* child, or after receiving *rhesus D positive* blood transfusions.

Antibodies are of the immune type and are best dected using albumin to enhance their agglutinability or by the Coombs' test (see p. 541).

GENETICS

The D antigen, being a protein, develops on the membrane according to normal cell-protein synthetic mechanisms. It was once thought that rhesus D negative persons possess a *d* antigen, and that persons heterozygous Dd are rhesus D positive because *D* is dominant to *d*. However, the *d* antigen has never been identified (see page 540) and is now thought not to exist.

Genotype	Phenotype	Antigen
DD	D – or Rh (D) Pos.	D
Dd	D – or Rh (D) Pos.	D
dd	d – or Rh (D) Neg.	nil

TRANSFUSION REACTIONS TO D

Natural antibodies to *D* are very rare. Therefore blood, whatever its *D* type, may be given to anyone who has not been previously immunized without deleterious effect. If no attempt is made, however, to determine the *D* type of donor or recipient, serious or fatal results may accompany further transfusions. Furthermore, the immunization of women of child-bearing age to rhesus factors is to be deplored except under the most extreme, life-saving circumstances.

Occasionally, several *incompatible transfusions* may be given before detecting antibodies in the recipient. Some persons seem incapable of mounting an immune antibody response even after several immunizing episodes.

OTHER RHESUS FACTORS

Shortly after the rhesus system was discovered, it became apparent that there was a multiplicity of factors. Some persons previously thought to be rhesus positive were found to develop rhesus-type antibodies even though they had apparently been given rhesus compatible blood – i.e. rhesus positive. Even to this day, no truly satisfactory system of nomenclature has been developed, although that developed by Fisher in 1945 still provides a good working hypothesis.

FISHER THEORY OF THE RHESUS SYSTEM

Synthesis directed by three closely linked autosomal gene sites – alleles. Each allelic site is given a generic letter, thus C, D and E. The main alternatives at each allelic site are represented by capital and small type – C and c, D and d, E and e. Other rare alternatives exist, e.g. C^w. Each gene directs the

Genes	Antigens	React with
C	C	anti-C
c	c	anti-c
D	D	anti-D
d	nil	nothing
E	E	anti-E
e	e	anti-e

synthesis of a blood group antigen which has the letter of its gene. Each antigen reacts with a corresponding antibody.

However, antibodies to the *d* antigen – *anti-d* have yet to be found. It is therefore assumed that there cannot be a rhesus factor governed by the *d* gene. *D* is therefore dominant over *d* in the same way that *A* and *B* are dominant over *O*. There is nothing produced by the *d* gene to 'compete' with the product of the *D* gene.

Yet, anti-C, anti-c, anti-E and anti-e are known to exist and the corresponding antigens are therefore real entities. It is important to realize that *c* is co-dominant with *C*, as is *e* with *E*. In these specific instances the use of small type does not imply recessiveness. Cells homozygous *cc* when injected into a person homozygous *CC* can and do result in the production of a strong immune *anti-c*. The genes at the C, D and E loci are closely linked, and are actually in the order D, C, E. In Europeans, about 40 per cent of people carry the gene-complex *dce* either in a heterozygous or homozygous state. Similarly the complex *DCe* is also carried by about 40 per cent. The complex *Dce* is rare among Europeans but common in Africans. Detailed anthropological studies of many populations have been carried out by such means.

Other blood group systems

Many systems are now known but only rarely cause complications, and then usually in persons who have received many transfusions. Although not usually associated with transfusion difficulties, these systems are useful for forensic and anthropological studies. When transfusion problems arise, prompt identification of the offending system is necessary in order to screen for compatible donors.

II BLOOD GROUP SYSTEM

This is a curious system as everyone is born with an *i* antigen, which is replaced during the first year of life by an *I* antigen in most people. Each antigen can be detected by specific antibodies – *anti-i* and *anti-I*. In a few persons, the *I* antigen never appears; this is genetically determined.

Antibodies to both *i* and *I* are well known. They resemble natural antibodies, reacting best at 4°C and being IgM in type. They are rarely found in health, but are particularly found in mycoplasma pneumonia, glandular fever and the lymphomas, and are common antibody types in the cold auto-immune haemolytic anaemias (see p. 506).

GROUPING AND CROSS-MATCHING TECHNIQUES

Whenever possible, transfused blood should be *fully compatible* with that of the recipient. As the genetic characteristics of all blood is highly individual, the ideally perfect compatibility is hardly ever, perhaps never, achieved except with monozygous twins. However, transfusion reactions will be minimized if the major groups are compatible and if the propensity of recipient serum to react with donor cells is checked beforehand by a *cross-match* procedure.

GROUPING

Cell suspensions are exposed to blood group typing sera which contain specific antibodies. Conditions, i.e. tile or tube and temperature, may be adjusted for optimum sensitivity, e.g. room temperature for ABO, 37°C for rhesus typing, etc.

Reverse grouping may be possible with the natural antibodies, e.g. the presence of anti-B in sera of group A persons.

N.B. In some pathological conditions, e.g. myeloma, the level of antibodies in the patient's serum may fall below detectable levels.

CROSS-MATCHING

Donor cells are exposed to patient's (recipient's) serum in order to check on possible reactions. Reactions are detected by:
(*a*) Inspecting for complete agglutination.
(*b*) Albumin technique for incomplete antibodies.
(*c*) Coombs' test for incomplete antibodies.

INDIRECT COOMBS' TEST – INDIRECT ANTI-GLOBULIN TEST
(*a*) Wash donor red cells three times in isotonic saline.
(*b*) Add patient's serum.
(*c*) Incubate 37°. 1 hour.
(*d*) Repeated washing of red cells three times.
(*e*) One drop of 30 per cent saline suspension of red cells plus one drop of Coombs' reagent on tile. Inspected for agglutination.

Interpretation. Agglutination on tile is *positive* and blood is incompatible. *Coombs' reagent* is an antibody raised by injecting animals, e.g. rabbits and goats, with human serum. It is, in effect, an antibody to *human antibody*. It will, therefore, react with cells coated with human antibody and will agglutinate them. Group-compatible blood which passes the cross-match test is fit for transfusion. Occasionally, particularly if blood from previously transfused donors is used, a reversed cross-match using patient's (recipient's) cells and donor plasma is required.

DIRECT COOMBS' TEST – DIRECT ANTI-GLOBULIN TEST
Not a blood transfusion procedure, but used for detecting antibodies that are coating patient's own red cells, e.g. in the diagnosis of autoimmune haemolytic anaemia, haemolytic disease of newborn, etc. (see below).

(*a*) Patient's cells washed three times in saline.

(*b*) One drop of 30 per cent saline suspension of cells added to one drop of Coombs' reagent on tile.

Interpretation. Agglutination is POSITIVE, indicating patient's circulating red cells are coated with antibody.

Transfusion reactions

Blood is potentially very dangerous. It should never be given unless there are good medical indications. Single-unit top-ups for adults, e.g. after surgery, are to be deplored. If anaemias can be treated satisfactorily by other means, e.g. iron or B_{12} therapy, blood transfusion to speed recovery is not indicated. Iron and/or folate deficiency of pregnancy may, however, be treated with transfusion particularly nearing term, as labour is rendered much less risky. However careful the preparations, complications may follow the transfusion of blood.

Immediate complications
(*a*) *Febrile*
   1 Due to pyrogens in drip tubing, container walls, anticoagulant, etc.
   2 Due to pyrogens in donor plasma.
   3 Due to allergic reactions to donor plasma or blood cells.
(*b*) *Infectious organisms in donor blood* – particularly cryophilic bacilli. Can cause fatal shock.
(*c*) *Circulatory overload.* Causing cardiac failure with pulmonary oedema. Treatment is venesection.
(*d*) *Haemolytic reaction.* Due to red cell incompatibility. Stages: (1) anaphylaxis, fever, rash, etc.; (2) shock; (3) oliguria with haemoglobinuria; (4) renal failure (see p. 365); (5) diuresis; (6) recovery.

Except in the last stage, death can occur at any time. The shock phase is characterized by vasodilatation and intravascular coagulation following release of red cell contents into the blood. Renal failure is due to shock and to vascular obstruction by immune complexes. Haemoglobin is present in the small amount of urine excreted because red cell destruction in the blood causes massive haemoglobinaemia.

Long-term complications
(*a*) *Development of immune antibodies*. To plasma proteins, platelets, white cells or red cells.
(*b*) *Iron overload*. Particularly with repeated transfusions (see p. 477). N.B. 1 ml of red cells contains about 1 mg of iron, the usual amount absorbed each day.
(*c*) *Chronic viral infections*. B hepatitis, cytomegalic disease, etc.

Haemolytic disease of the newborn – HDN

Nature
Caused by maternal antibodies crossing the placenta and destroying the foetal blood cells. Antibodies must be IgG, i.e. immune. Natural (IgM) anti-'A' or anti-'B' will not cross placenta. The immunizing episode can arise from previous transfusions or pregnancies. HDN rarely complicates the first pregnancy of a previously non-immunized mother.

The most important time during the previous pregnancy for the mother to become immunized is at labour, especially during placental separation. Several millilitres of foetal blood can become 'transfused' into the maternal circulation.

HDN caused by rhesus incompatibility
Ninety-three per cent of cases are rhesus (D) negative mothers with anti-D. Of the remainder most are due to anti-C.

If mother has not had previous transfusions, the first baby is usually unaffected but immunizes the mother at placental separation. Subsequent babies become increasingly affected.

N.B. If father is homozygous DD, all offspring will be rhesus D positive (genotype Dd) and potentially affected. If father is Dd, only half offspring may be affected.

GENOTYPING OF FATHER

The *d* antigen is impossible to demonstrate directly (see p. 539). Therefore, the father can only be genotyped by family study, i.e. his parents; or by statistical genotyping with anti-C, anti-c, anti-E and anti-e. Thus, if father's cells react as follows:

anti-C	anti-c	anti-D	Anti-E	anti-e
+	+	+	−	+

he has antigens C, c, D and e.

The two alternative genotypes are:
1 CDe/cde.
2 CDe/cDe.

1 is much commoner in the population than 2. He is therefore more likely, but not proven, to be heterozygous, D/d.

MONITORING OF HDN IN PREGNANCY

If there is a history of a previously affected baby, subsequent pregnancies can be monitored by serial estimations of the level of antibody activity in maternal serum – *anti-D titre*. Rising titres indicate an affected baby. Serial amniocentesis, obtaining samples of amniotic fluid by abdominal puncture, may reveal increasing bilirubin staining of the liquor. If the titre is steady and the liquor not significantly stained, pregnancy may be allowed to term. Otherwise, early induction of labour may be indicated.

DETECTION OF AFFECTED BABY AFTER BIRTH
At birth using cord blood:
Blood group.
Blood haemoglobin.
Direct Coombs' test.
Plasma bilirubin.

If blood group shows full rhesus compatibility no further measures need be taken.

If direct Coombs' test is positive, subsequent measurements of haemoglobin and bilirubin should be made. If haemoglobin falls and bilirubin rises, action may be necessary. Bilirubin levels above 350 μmol/l plasma are dangerous as indirect-reacting bilirubin, being fat soluble, is dissolved by cerebral tissue where its toxic effects bring about *kernicterus* which may produce serious neurological disability or death.

TREATMENT
Exchange transfusion – gradual replacement of neonatal blood with fresh donor blood:

(a) *Group*. Although the baby is rhesus D positive, the maternal anti-D makes it vital that rhesus D negative blood be given.
(b) *Cross-matching*. Maternal antibody may be too weak in neonatal blood for easy identification. Therefore, also cross-match donor blood with maternal serum.

PROPHYLAXIS
Only about 10 per cent of rhesus negative mothers have HDN-affected babies. For most of the others, incompatibility, especially for the ABO groups, immediately destroys foetal cells before rhesus immunization occurs, e.g. baby A, Rh D positive; mother O, Rh D negative: foetal cells in mother destroyed by natural maternal anti-A.

Potent preparations of anti-D serum are now available which when given intra-muscularly to any rhesus D negative mother who has just given birth to a rhesus D positive baby or foetus, will destroy the foetal cells before immunization of the mother has occurred. Every potentially sensitized mother is given 100 μg i.m. of IgG anti-D within 72 h of delivery.

Kleihauer test. This detects the presence of foetal red cells in maternal blood at the time of delivery by demonstrating HbF (see p. 502). Positive results indicate need for giving anti-D.

HDN caused by ABO incompatibility

MECHANISM
Usually occurs in mothers who are group O. Sometimes some natural anti-A and anti-B in group O persons is an IgG, but more usually an immune anti-A or anti-B is found which resulted from a previous immunizing episode.

Rarely, the mother is group A (genotype AO) and the baby is group B (genotype BO) – or vice versa.

As with rhesus HDN, the first-born is least affected and the mechanism of immunization by foeto-maternal bleeds is most important at the time of labour.

In absolute numbers, HDN from ABO incompatibility is about as common as with rhesus factors, but it is much milder. Kernicterus is rare in ABO – HDN, though it can be just as serious. Exchange transfusion with blood which is ABO-compatible with maternal serum is required.

PROPHYLAXIS
Can be achieved by use of very strong AB antisera

but it is much more difficult than for rhesus, and is much less often required.

Other blood group systems associated with HDN

Of these, the most important is *Kell* (K) but even this is rarely involved. Sporadic cases involving other systems such as Fy, Lu, etc., have been reported.

Long-term complications of HDN

Without any treatment. It has been found that surviving babies have an increased incidence of spasticity and intellectual impairment.

After adequate treatment by exchange transfusion:

1 *Anaemia in neonatal period.* Due to persisting maternal antibodies suppressing neonatal erythropoiesis. This may require transfusion.

2 *Intellectual impairment.* Difficult to analyse but many mothers claim that affected children are slower than non-affected siblings.

Blood donation, storage and fractionation

Donation

About 450 ml of blood, obtained by clean puncture of the antecubital vein, is drained into a plastic bag containing 75 ml of sterile, pyrogen-free anticoagulant solution.

Two types of anticoagulant:

1 *ACD – Acid–citrate–dextrose.* A somewhat hypertonic solution of citrate at pH about 5.0, fortified by glucose which provides a metabolic source essential for keeping the red cells viable during storage. The final pH immediately after collection is about 7.2.

2 *CPD – Citrate–phosphate–dextrose.* This solution is slightly more alkaline and preserves red cells better. However, the platelets may not be so well protected.

The blood is left at room temperature for 1–2 hours, then cooled to 4°C. If it is not used by 3 weeks, it has to be discarded.

Screening of donors

All donors are asked details of their health, particularly with regard to history of infections, and especially of jaundice. The possibility of previous viral hepatitis is reason for rejection. Inquiry is also made about regular medication, even drugs like aspirin: they are usually rejected if the answer is positive. Donors are also checked for absence of anaemia and for general health. It may not be in the prospective donor's interests to give blood if there is any obvious natural disease, particularly in older persons. Pregnancy is a contra-indication but not oral contraceptive therapy.

The sample is laboratory tested for HB_sAg (see p. 551) and syphilis (see p. 54).

Effects of storage on blood cells

Granulocytes die within hours of transfusion, although lymphocytes are probably more robust.

Platelets deteriorate quite rapidly, although for at least 12 hours they remain viable enough to help haemostasis in thrombocytopenic recipients and they have some effect for up to 48 hours.

Red cells deteriorate slowly, but after 3 weeks of storage about 25 per cent are non-viable and are rapidly destroyed in the recipient's circulation. Asymptomatic hyperbilirubinaemia is quite common after receiving blood.

In the *ACD* solution (see above) red cells become more avid for oxygen after some days but in *CPD* anticoagulant their oxygen affinity remains more normal for up to 2 weeks. Blood near expiry will always be more avid for oxygen, but this rarely seems deleterious. Its potassium content also rises, perhaps to as much as 20 mmol/l, by 3 weeks.

Blood fractionation

The only clinical requirement for *whole blood* is for frank haemorrhage, often operative or traumatic. For the treatment of anaemia, a concentrated red cell preparation is preferable. This can release the supernatant plasma of freshly donated blood for separate use.

The following are the fractions of blood theoretically obtainable:

1 *Packed red cells.* Packed cell volume seldom above 0.60.

2 *Platelets.*

3 *Granulocytes.* Obtained by cell separator from healthy donors.

4 *Plasma:*

(a) Whole; fresh frozen at minus 30°C or lyophilized.

(b) Cryoprecipitate–for factor VIII and fibrinogen (see p. 527). Factor VIII also available as a stable purified dried concentrate.

(c) Cryosupernatant:

   (i) Prothrombin complex (see p. 521).

   (ii) Gamma globulins.

(iii) Plasma protein fraction containing 52 g/l of protein of which 95 per cent is albumin but with no fibrinogen.

Many donor bags are supplied with one or two satellite bags. Soon after donation and gentle centrifugation, about 150–200 nl of platelet-rich plasma is led into the first satellite. This can then be spun, leaving a platelet concentrate. The supernatant plasma can then be separated into the next satellite and either frozen freshly, or further fractionated.

Such schemes obviously allow for the much more economical use of donated blood. Requesting clinicians are therefore urged to ask for packed cells wherever possible.

Chapter 90
Diseases of the Liver – Congenital: Circulatory: Degenerations: Viral Hepatitis

NORMAL LIVER

Weight
1200–1600 g.

Structure
The liver is made up of lobules (see Fig. 67), each of similar structure and comprising a central vein – hepatic vein, draining sinusoids lined by vascular endothelium and Kupffer cells which are part of the lymphoreticular system.

Between the sinusoids are columns of liver cells arranged in a regular and radiate manner and extending to the periphery of the lobule. At the periphery are several portal tracts, each of which contains branches of the hepatic artery, portal vein and intrahepatic bile ducts, together with fibrous connective tissue and lymphatics. The bile ducts drain the numerous intralobular bile canaliculi which lie between the liver cells.

Congenital

ACCESSORY LIVER TISSUE

Separate islands of liver tissue may very rarely be found in the gall bladder wall or serosal coat.

ACCESSORY LOBES

Capsular depressions due to uneven development of the lobes may occur. Occasionally, marked downward enlargement of the right lobe may give rise to a clinical mass – *Riedel's lobe.*

CONGENITAL CYSTIC LIVER – POLYCYSTIC DISEASE

Aetiology
The cysts are presumed to arise due to secretion into malformed bile ducts which result from segmentation or sequestration of the ducts during development.

Macroscopical
Multiple cysts in the hepatic substance may attain a very large size but they do not interfere with function. The cysts are smooth-walled and contain clear fluid. They are demarcated from the hepatic substance by a fibrous capsule, are non-communicating, variable in size and commonly sub-capsular in situation. Sometimes, these multiple cysts are

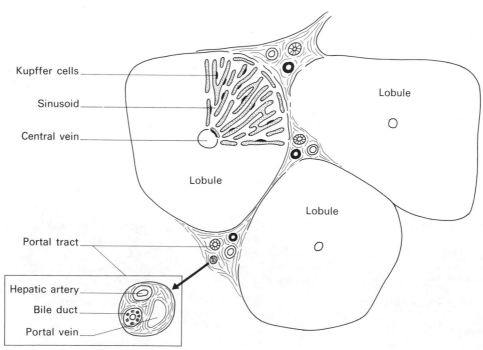

Fig. 67. Liver – lobular structure.

associated with similar lesions in the kidneys and pancreas (see p. 351).

Microscopical
Fibrous-walled cysts with a lining of columnar or cuboidal epithelium similar to that lining the bile ducts.

Effects
The disease causes hepatomegaly but there is no significant interference with liver function.

CONGENITAL HEPATIC FIBROSIS

An autosomally recessive inherited trait presenting predominantly in childhood or adolescence, usually with abdominal distension, respiratory distress and hypertension. Cholangitis, portal hypertension and renal failure are variable accompaniments.

The enlarged liver is firm with diffuse periportal/perilobular fibrosis containing numerous bile ducts and surrounding irregular islands of liver cells.

Mechanical

TRAUMATIC

In spite of protection from the lower ribs, injury to the liver can occur:
1 *Penetrating wounds*, e.g. knife wounds.
2 *Crush injuries*. Laceration, with or without fractured ribs, causing intraperitoneal haemorrhage.
3 *Indirect injury*. Laceration of the liver capsule due to hyperextension or flexion of the trunk following a fall from a height.
4 *External cardiac massage*. Over-vigorous pressure on the lower chest during external cardiac massage.

FURROWS

1 *Transverse*. Rib markings associated with a narrow chest or with tight lacing.
2 *Vertical*. 'Cough furrows' often occur in asthmatics, chronic bronchitics and others with a chronic cough. They are due to the development of abnormal muscular bands in the diaphragm and are visible as deep grooves on the diaphragmatic surface of the liver.

BILE STASIS

Obstruction to the outflow of bile from any cause will lead to green-staining of the liver, dilatation of the bile ducts if the obstruction is extrahepatic and plugs of inspissated bile in the canaliculi – *bile thrombi*. Subsequent degenerative changes which may develop are discussed on p. 564.

Circulatory disorders

CHRONIC PASSIVE VENOUS CONGESTION

Mechanism
This occurs in predominantly right-sided heart failure, commonly due to mitral stenosis, pulmonary hypertension (cor pulmonale) or tricuspid incompetence.

Appearances
A 'nutmeg' liver is produced (see p. 120) which, if severe and prolonged, may result in cardiac fibrosis (see p. 565).

INFARCTION

This is rare, due to the presence of the dual hepatic and portal blood supply. Infarcts are most usually seen associated with tumours in the liver substance.

BUDD–CHIARI SYNDROME

Hepatic venous occlusion is usually due to luminal obstruction, in about 50 per cent thrombus at the site of invasion by a tumour. In other cases the thrombus is associated with oral contraceptive therapy, but in many others the reason is obscure. Initially, there is distension of central veins and sinusoids with formation of '*blood lakes*', parenchymal atrophy and patchy regeneration, sometimes with a true cirrhotic picture. The hepatic vein abnormalities are usually evident, though often patchy.

VENO-OCCLUSIVE DISEASE

This is characterized by occlusion of smaller hepatic vein radicles by loose connective tissue which extends into the lumen to partially or completely occlude them.

Parenchymal cells atrophy, fibrous tissue increases and a cirrhotic picture is later established. The disease usually affects children and is geographically distributed in the Caribbean, South America, South Africa, Egypt and India. It is probably caused by ingestion of a pyrrolizidine alkaloid used in the preparation of medicinal teas.

Degenerations

CLOUDY SWELLING (see p. 103).

FATTY CHANGE – STEATOSIS

This is an indication of 'sickness' of the liver cells. The process and its probable mechanisms are discussed on p. 105.

Causes
1 *'Toxic' conditions and infections.* Including toxaemia of pregnancy.
2 *Poisons.* Inorganic, e.g. phosphorus, or organic, e.g. chloroform and alcohol.
3 *Drugs.* With hepatotoxic effects either direct or indirect (see p. 549).
4 *Anaemia.* e.g. pernicious anaemia and iron-deficiency anaemia.
5 *Nutritional*
(a) Excessive fat intake – this is an extremely rare cause.
(b) Pancreatic insufficiency, e.g. chronic pancreatitis.
(c) Metabolic disorders, e.g. diabetes mellitus.
(d) Inadequate diet, particularly in respect of essential amino acids and other lipotropic factors. This occurs particularly in the following circumstances: Aged persons – self neglect; Famine and war; Chronic alcoholics; 'Cranks' with regard to food; Poverty; Dietetic inhibitions and customs in many geographical areas.
Kwashiorkor. A severe disease occurring in infancy due to an extremely low protein diet. It is characterized by a failure to grow, skin rashes, oedema, anaemia and signs of multiple vitamin deficiencies. There is gross hepatomegaly due to very severe fatty change.

Macroscopical
The liver is enlarged and pale, with a smooth greasy cut surface. The liver parenchyma bulges out from the incised capsule.

Microscopical
The cells are distended by globules of fat, either as multiple fine droplets or single large droplets. The change is most marked in the middle and central zones of the lobule.

Results
If the cause is corrected at a relatively early stage, the changes are completely reversible. Long continued fatty change may however eventually progress to hepatic necrosis and subsequently to cirrhosis (see p. 561).

GLYCOGEN DISORDERS

DIABETES MELLITUS

Glycogen is present not only in the cytoplasm of liver cells in diabetics, but the swollen nuclei also contain glycogen droplets, resulting in a vacuolated appearance.

GLYCOGEN STORAGE DISEASE – VON GIERKE'S DISEASE

A rare disease which is characterized by massive accumulations of glycogen in the liver and kidney and occasionally in the heart and voluntary muscles (see p. 112).

AMYLOID DISEASE

The liver may be the site of severe affection by secondary amyloidosis. In the primary disease, the organ may be only minimally involved with deposits confined to blood vessel walls (see p. 108).

Results
Although some disorder of function may result, deposits are usually present in the kidneys or heart which lead to death before liver failure occurs (see p. 109).

LIPID STORAGE DISEASES

CHOLESTEROL

In abnormal cholesterol metabolism, the liver is rarely involved to a significant degree. In the normocholesterolaemic group, e.g. Hand–Schüller–Christian disease, nests of foamy histiocytes may be present in the liver but these do not cause any interference with function.

GAUCHER'S DISEASE

Nature. A familial disease, occurring mainly, but not exclusively, in Jews, and due to abnormal storage of the cerebroside kerasin in cells of the lymphoreticular system.

Appearances. The spleen is enormously enlarged, the liver only moderately. Bones, particularly those with active marrow, are also infiltrated. The characteristic Gaucher cell with its foamy cytoplasm is seen in the liver substance (see p. 113).

NIEMANN–PICK DISEASE

Also a familial and rare, fatal disease, occurring predominantly in Jews and associated with storage of sphingomyelin in the lymphoreticular system. The liver is invariably enlarged (see p. 113).

Drug and toxin-induced liver injury

Nature and incidence

In the last 20 or so years the importance of liver-cell injury by chemical agents has greatly magnified, more particularly with drugs. At the same time toxic effects of occupational or domestic origin, e.g. chloroform, phosphorus, carbon tetrachloride, have greatly diminished in relative importance.

It is not proposed to identify lists of hepatotoxic drugs but more to deal with the main types of injury, illustrated by common examples.

Classification

1 Intrinsic hepatotoxins:
(a) Direct.
(b) Indirect.
2 Idiosyncratic hepatotoxins:

(a) Hypersensitivity-related
(b) Toxic metabolite-dependent.

INTRINSIC HEPATOTOXINS

The effects are dose-dependent, experimentally reproducible and create a high incidence of hepatic injury in exposed individuals.

1 *Direct hepatotoxins* – The hepatocytes are damaged by a direct physico-chemical effect, e.g. chloroform and carbon tetrachloride.

2 *Indirect hepatotoxins* – The injury is secondary to a metabolic defect produced by the agent interfering with a specific metabolic process or pathway.

This damage can be expressed in two ways:

(a) Cytotoxic – The injury interferes with basic metabolic pathways and leads to steatosis or necrosis, e.g. alcohol, tetracylines, paracetamol.

(b) Cholestatic—Jaundice or impaired function are produced by selective interference with excretory hepatic mechanisms or blood uptake, e.g. anabolic and contraceptive steroids, rifampicin.

IDIOSYNCRATIC HEPATOTOXINS

1 *Hypersensitivity-related* – This is presumed to be allergic in type and certainly often has accompanying fever, skin rash and eosinophilia. Re-exposure to the agent causes prompt reappearance of symptoms.

2 *Toxic metabolite-dependent* – The pattern is uneven without features of hypersensitivity and recurrence with further challenge is variable, e.g. isoniazid, iproniazid.

Types of acute injury

There are two main types:

1 Cytotoxic.
2 Cholestatic.

CYTOTOXIC INJURY

1 *Necrosis* – This may be zonal (usually intrinsic) diffuse or massive (usually idiosyncratic). In *zonal necrosis* three parts of the primary lobule are identified.

(a) Centrizonal – Characteristic of intrinsic toxins including: CCl_4, $CHCl_3$, copper salts, pyrrolizidine alkaloids, aflatoxins, paracetamol. Some idiosyncratic injuries may cause central necrosis including halothane.

(b) Mid-zonal – This is rare in man except for yellow fever virus infection (see p. 555).

(*c*) Peripheral – Phosphorus, allyl alcohol and esters, ferrous sulphate overdose.

2 *Degeneration* – A wide range of appearances may be seen in non-necrotic cells including hydropic degeneration, eosinophilic degeneration and acidophilic bodies. Mallory bodies (MB) are most consistently seen in toxic hepatocyte injury by alcohol.

3 *Steatosis* – Fatty change of either microvesicular or macrovesicular types is a common feature of liver cell injury (see p. 548).

4 *Inflammatory response* – The inflammatory response to most cases of drug-induced necrosis is very slight.

CHOLESTATIC INJURY
Although mixed cytotoxic and cholestatic patterns of injury are common, some agents appear to more or less spare the hepatocytes and cause only interference with bile flow.

The appearances are of canalicular bilirubin casts with a variable, often marked, portal tract inflammatory cell reaction, e.g. with chlorpromazine.

Chronic hepatic injury

1 *Fibrosis* – e.g. alcohol, arsenic, vinyl chloride, chlorpromazine.

2 *Cirrhosis* – Though a rare sequel to drug or chemical injury, it may rarely complicate some inorganic arsenical toxic substances, methotrexate therapy, iproniazid and isoniazid.

3 *Chronic active hepatitis* – Some drugs have been implicated in producing a CAH-like lesion (see p. 552), e.g. α-methyldopa, nitrofurantoin, isoniazid, halothane.

4 Chronic hepatic cholestasis – Clinically, this resembles primary biliary cirrhosis and has been reported with chlorpromazine and other phenothiazines, methyl testosterone, organic arsenicals and tolbutamide.

Alcoholic liver disease

Incidence

Excess alcohol consumption is a serious health problem in many countries and appears to be rapidly increasing. A number of organs show significant lesions due to alcohol abuse including the central nervous system (Wernicke's encephalopathy) (see p. 610) and polyneuritis (see p. 619), pancreas (acute pancreatitis) (see p. 630) and myocardium (fatty change and cardiomyopathy) (see p. 239) but the effects on the liver are probably the most important in relationship to life-threatening situations.

Types of lesion

FATTY LIVER – STEATOSIS
This is the most common abnormality and appears to be a direct effect of the ethanol. It is related in severity to the quantity of alcohol.

The condition is rapidly reversible following withdrawal of the toxin.

In addition to fat accumulation in hepatocytes, which is often maximal in the central part of the lobule, foci of cell necrosis, acidophilic bodies and lipogranulomas (see p. 556) may be seen. Cholestasis is unusual but some fibrosis may be present, particularly related to lipogranulomas.

ALCOHOLIC HEPATITIS
This is defined as a liver lesion with Mallory bodies (MB) or with Mallory bodies together with liver-cell necrosis, fibrosis and focal neutrophil infiltration. The neutrophils are distributed around the hepatocytes containing MB's – *satellitosis*.

The fibrosis is fine and characteristically around centrilobular cells. Extension of this centrilobular fibrosis to the portal tracts results in the formation of nodules. Fatty change is almost always present.

Alcoholics with MB's and thus with alcoholic hepatitis are likely to progress to cirrhosis but it is also reversible if consumption of alcohol ceases.

CIRRHOSIS
A major cause of hepatic cirrhosis is excessive alcohol consumption (see p. 560). Most cases probably progress from alcoholic hepatitis to a micronodular cirrhotic pattern usually with severe fatty change. MB's are also usually seen.

Complications

1 *Hepatocellular carcinoma* – This is an increasing problem seen now in about 10 per cent of known alcoholic cirrhotics.

2 *Infection* – Proneness to infection is common and episodes of gram-negative septicaemia occur quite frequently.

3 *Siderosis* – Alcoholics usually have a degree of iron overload which may be severe and significant in increasing the amount of fibrosis (see p. 563).

4 *Acute alcohol poisoning* – In addition to the

'anaesthetic' effects of alcohol on the brain, acute liver failure can occur with heavy drinking bouts superimposed on previous liver damage.

Viral hepatitis

Nature
Although a wide range of viruses can cause hepatitis, the term acute viral hepatitis is here used in respect of a diffuse inflammatory lesion of the liver, mostly caused by hepatitis A and B viruses, and less commonly by a third agent – non-A, non-B (type C).

Chemicals and drugs can also cause liver lesions closely resembling viral hepatitis (see p. 549).

Aetiology

HEPATITIS A
A naturally acquired infection, sporadic or epidemic with a short incubation period of 15/40 days. Evidence of past infection is very common throughout the population of many countries, even in the absence of a suggestive clinical history.

Carrier states or chronic liver disease do not occur with this organism.

HEPATITIS B
Infection is usually acquired parenterally, e.g. blood and blood products, but may occur as a result of close, usually sexual, personal contact, The incubation period is long – 50–180 days.

Two main antigen/antibody systems are found in blood and liver cells.
1   Surface antigen – HB_sAg/anti HB_s.
2   Core antigen – HB_cAg/anti HB_c.

Microscopical types
The appearances are not separable according to different viral agents though usually the more severe types of change are only seen with B virus infection.

ACUTE HEPATITIS WITH SPOTTY NECROSIS
1   *Fully developed stage* – This shows the following histological features:
(a) Patchy liver cell necrosis, degeneration and regeneration.
  (i) Ballooned cells – leading to lytic necrosis.
  (ii) Acidophilic-body cells – Councilman

bodies. Shrunken eosinophilic cells with pyknotic nuclei.
  (iii) Regeneration – as evidenced by mitotic activity in hepatocytes.
(b) Lobular disarray – Distortion of normal lobular structure by swelling and cell pleomorphism associated with degeneration and regeneration.
(c) Inflammatory cell infiltrate – Consistently present is a centrilobular histiocytic and lymphocytic infiltrate with prominence of Kupffer cells. Plasma cells are uncommon but some eosinophils are common.
(d) Confluent necrosis – Uncommon and usually very patchy.
(e) Cholestasis – Canalicular and intralobular bile pigment is often seen but not, in this type, ductular.
(f) Portal tracts – Oedema and variable inflammatory cell infiltrate of lymphocytes with some histiocytes and polymorphs including eosinophils. The limiting plate of the portal tract remains intact.
(g) Bile ducts – These remain intact.
2   *Late stage* – The parenchymal changes subside but the mesenchymal ones persist. Cell morphology becomes rapidly normal but inflammatory cells around the central part of the lobule persist longer. However, in this type regeneration and restoration of anatomical lobular normality are the rule with elimination of virus particles in dead cells which are phagocytosed.

ACUTE HEPATITIS WITH BRIDGING NECROSIS
1   *Fully developed acute stage.* The key feature is confluent necrosis of variable degree but, in some lobules at least, extending from the central perivenular area to the periphery. Thus bridging between different vascular structures occurs, but reticulin collapse is not inevitable and piecemeal necrosis is not usually seen. Substantial cholestasis is usual.

Changes in the portal tracts are of swelling due to oedema and marked bile duct proliferation, often distended with bile. Appearances need careful distinction from large duct obstruction, particularly as the inflammatory cell infiltrate is often neutrophilic.

The limiting plate of the portal tract may be blurred but piecemeal necrosis of adjacent hepatocytes is not seen.
2   *Late stage.* Regeneration of liver cells is obvious and multinucleate cells are common. Some septa in

the peripheral zones occur from reticulin collapse in some cases. The cholestasis and portal tract changes subside only slowly.

3 *Results*

(a) *Healing* – With substantially normal or slightly scarred liver.

(b) *Liver failure* – The lesion progresses in a small proportion and the confluent necrosis leads to liver-cell failure.

(c) *Chronic active hepatitis* – A proportion of cases persist in this form (see below).

ACUTE HEPATITIS WITH PIECEMEAL NECROSIS

Some cases of B virus or non-A, non-B virus infection show disproportionately severe portal tract inflammation mostly lymphocytic, but commonly also with plasma cells, and piecemeal necrosis of adjacent hepatocytes occurs.

Fibrous spurs develop in the periportal zone and sometimes portal-to-portal bridging is seen. The intralobular changes are otherwise similar to those of the classical acute hepatitis (see p. 551).

Some of these cases inevitably proceed to chronic active hepatitis, most particularly when the infection occurs as a complication of drug addition.

ACUTE MASSIVE NECROSIS – ACUTE YELLOW ATROPHY – FULMINANT VIRAL HEPATITIS

In some cases of viral hepatitis (virtually always B virus) confluent necrosis is so extensive that it becomes panlobular and is associated with some reticulin collapse and usually slight bile duct proliferation.

Death occurs in 70 per cent or more in the first 10 days, but if the patient survives beyond this time then recovery by regeneration can occur.

In those who recover the liver may appear remarkably normal with little or no scarring.

In fatal cases the liver is small with wrinkled capsule and bright green-yellow in colour with loss of pattern and often haemorrhagic foci on the cut surface.

Not all cases of massive necrosis can be shown to be due to hepatitis virus infection, nor indeed to other viral infections.

NEONATAL HEPATITIS

Although originally intended to mean presumed viral infection of the liver in neonates, identical changes have been demonstrated in metabolic disorders such as cystic fibrosis, galactosaemia and fructose intolerance. Viruses implicated include rubella, cytomegalovirus, hepatitis B, herpes simplex, varicella and the coxsackie and echo groups.

The characteristic feature is the presence of multinucleated hepatocytes – *giant cell transformation*, mostly centrally in lobules and associated cholestasis and portal and lobular inflammatory cell infiltrate.

In most cases the prognosis is good but a proportion develop cirrhosis.

Chronic hepatitis

Nature

1 A primary disease of the liver.

2 Inflammation of liver continuing for at least 6 months.

3 Sequel to viral or drug-induced hepatitis or of unknown cause.

Types

1 Chronic active hepatitis – CAH:

(a) Without bridging necrosis.

(b) With bridging necrosis – BHN.

2 Chronic persistent hepatitis – CPH.

3 Chronic lobular hepatitis – CLH.

CHRONIC ACTIVE HEPATITIS – CAH

Nature

A progressive liver disorder characterized by extensive inflammation, liver cell destruction and fibrosis.

Aetiology

Several known causes:

1 Hepatitis B virus.

2 Other types of viral hepatitis.

3 Wilson's disease (see p. 611).

4 Drugs and toxins (see p. 549).

5 Alcoholism.

6 'Lupoid hepatitis' – Usually in young or menopausal women with high serum antibody levels (including ANA, RA and SM) and involvement of several organs. This should not, however, be confused with the usually mild involvement of the liver in SLE (see p. 280).

Without bridging necrosis

MICROSCOPICAL

In this type lobular architecture is preserved, there

is a lymphocyte-rich infiltrate in portal tracts with extension into adjacent parenchyma and with piecemeal necrosis of cells or small groups of hepatocytes in this zone. Regeneration is seen as liver cell rosettes (gland-like formations) or as liver cell plates several cells thick.

PROGNOSIS
Cirrhosis may develop when liver cell destruction is sufficiently advanced and nodular regeneration is also present.

With bridging necrosis – CAH with BHN

MICROSCOPICAL
In addition to the features described previously there is bridging necrosis with broad or narrow septa traversing the lobules and caused by collapse from BHN.

Inflammatory infiltrate is seen in any part of the lobules in addition to portal tracts. Plasma cells are often numerous. In cases due to hepatitis B virus, *'ground glass'* hepatocytes are commonly found in which orcein-positive virus particles can be demonstrated.

PROGNOSIS
This type is more rapidly progressive to cirrhosis.

CHRONIC PERSISTENT HEPATITIS – CPH

Nature
The presence of a cellular infiltrate and enlargement of portal tracts after exclusion of obvious intrahepatic or extrahepatic causes.

Amongst the lesions which need exclusion are those due to:
1 Non-specific reactive hepatitis.
2 Lymphomas involving liver.
3 Acute viral hepatitis.
4 Primary biliary cirrhosis.

The clinical history is usually helpful as 'persistent' is defined as 'more than 6 months'.

Microscopical
Lobular architecture is intact but portal tracts are enlarged and may show short radiating septa. Inflammatory cell infiltrate of mononuclear cells including plasma cells, lymphocytes and a few polymorphs, occasionally together with lymph follicles is variably intense but is normally confined by the limiting plate. Bile duct proliferation is unusual and lobules appear normal, or with at most mild liver-cell damage.

Cholestasis is nearly always absent.

Results
The course is almost always benign and progression to cirrhosis hardly ever occurs.

CHRONIC LOBULAR HEPATITIS – CLH

Nature
If lobular changes of continuing spotty necrosis and inflammatory cell infiltrate which are characteristic of acute viral hepatitis proceed with only mild or absent portal tract changes, then this probably represents a failure of resolution of acute hepatitis.

For this condition the term CLH is preferred to alternatives of protracted acute hepatitis or unresolved hepatitis.

Microscopical
Minimal portal tract changes with usually mild spotty parenchymal necrosis and variably diffuse liver-cell swelling and acidophilic bodies.

Cholestasis may be present.

Results
Progression of the disease to more serious types is uncommon and, although it may persist for many years, spontaneous resolution usually occurs eventually.

Chapter 91
Diseases of the Liver – Other Inflammations

Non-specific inflammations

BLOOD-BORNE – PYAEMIA

ARTERIAL

Pyaemic abscesses may occur in the liver in septi-caemia or in infective endocarditis. The liver contains multiple abscess cavities, mostly small, from which the causative organism may be recovered on culture.

PORTAL

Abscesses also occur in the liver associated with portal pyaemia. This is usually associated with suppuration in the area drained by the portal vein, most commonly an appendix abscess. Multiple abscesses are formed and septic thrombus can usually be found in the intrahepatic portions of the portal vein – *portal pylephlebitis*.

BILIARY – CHOLANGITIS

Ascending cholangitis, with the production of purulent inflammation of the intrahepatic bile ducts, may lead to abscess formation in the portal tracts. It is only rarely seen in the absence of extra- or intrahepatic duct obstruction and is most frequently associated with impaction of a stone in the bile duct (see p. 570).

EXTENSION FROM NEIGHBOURING ORGANS

SUBPHRENIC ABSCESS

Occasionally a subphrenic abscess may penetrate the liver substance.

RETROPERITONEAL

Retroperitoneal abscesses may extend to and penetrate the liver, e.g. perinephric abscess.

GALL BLADDER

Acute cholecystitis and empyema of the gall bladder may cause inflammation in the adjacent liver tissue.

Specific inflammations

VIRAL HEPATITIS

This is described on pp 551–553.

YELLOW FEVER

Aetiology
A virus disease, transmitted to man by the mosquito, *Aedes aegypti*.

Geographical distribution
Tropical Central and S. America and W. Africa.

Macroscopical
Liver. Normal size, pale yellow and greasy with multiple areas of haemorrhage.

Kidneys. Pale, swollen and bile-stained.
Spleen. Congested, slightly enlarged and friable.
Heart. Pale and flabby.
Skin and mucosae. There is generalized capillary damage, resulting in haemorrhages in the skin, gastric mucosa, lungs and other organs.

Microscopical
Liver. There is extensive midzonal necrosis with areas of extravasated blood and fatty change of adjacent liver cells but there is no inflammatory cell reaction. The necrotic cells show hyaline acidophilic areas in their cytoplasm – *Councilman bodies*. The nuclei often contain inclusion bodies but these are not, however, specific as they may also be seen in burns.
Other organs. Haemorrhages, renal tubular degeneration and myocardial degeneration are usually found in fatal cases.

Results
The mortality varies between 20–70 per cent in different epidemics. The remainder recover completely. Cirrhosis does not follow this disease.

WEIL'S DISEASE

Aetiology
Caused by *Leptospira icterohaemorrhagica*, a spirochaete which has its natural reservoir in rats. Transmission to man is usually by contact with rat excreta but sometimes by direct inoculation by rat bites. The organisms may penetrate unbroken skin or mucous membrane, hence infection may also occur by drinking polluted water.

Geographical distribution
World-wide.

Incubation
Two to twenty-one days.

Clinical
Haemorrhages into mucous membranes associated with jaundice in 60 per cent of cases. There is commonly suppression of urine and enlargement of the liver and spleen.

Liver
Macroscopical. Enlarged, firm and deep yellow; almost always there are small haemorrhages.

Microscopical. There is slight to marked centrilobular necrosis, with perisinusoidal oedema, bile stasis and haemorrhages. The portal tracts show an infiltration by lymphocytes and polymorphs. Organisms are demonstrable by silver impregnation techniques.

Kidneys
Macroscopical. Swollen, firm and oedematous with petechial haemorrhages.

Microscopical. Tubular necrosis with glomerular and interstitial haemorrhages.

Diagnosis
1 *Culture.* On special media. Blood – first week. Urine 6–12 days.
2 *Agglutinations.* The patient's serum agglutinates the organism; a rising titre is diagnostic.
3 *Guinea-pig inoculation.* 'Butterfly' lesions are produced in the lungs.
4 *Dark ground examination.* Of infected tissue or occasionally of blood or urine, when the organism may be demonstrable.

Results
The disease usually has a mortality of about 10 per cent, death occurring from renal and/or hepatic failure.

CANICOLA FEVER

This disease, caused by *Leptospira canicola,* is of worldwide distribution and is carried by dogs who infect man by bites or by food or water contamination. The appearances are similar to mild forms of Weil's disease and it is only rarely fatal.

SYPHILIS

Congenital
A diffuse, fine, pericellular fibrosis surrounding each cell and accompanied by a lymphocytic and plasma cell infiltration.

Acquired – gummas
These may be single or multiple and occur in the tertiary stages. There are the characteristic appearances of necrotic masses with thick fibrous capsules. Healing produces deep scars dividing the liver into coarse nodules – *hepar lobatum.* The liver architecture is preserved except in these localized gummatous areas, so the condition is not a true cirrhosis.

HEPATIC GRANULOMAS

These are of two types:
1 Lipogranulomas.
2 Epithelioid.

Lipogranulomas
These are seen in fatty livers particularly in alcoholics and consist of loose collections of macrophages and lymphocytes sometimes with foreign body giant cells. The histiocytic cells usually contain readily demonstrable fat.

Epithelioid granulomas
These are a frequent cause of diagnostic difficulty in percutaneous hepatic needle biopsies.

At one time tuberculosis was by far the most important cause of such lesions but this is now superseded in frequency by many other disorders.

A very large number of conditions have been described as producing hepatic epithelioid granulomas including the following groups of disorders:

Causes
1 Infective diseases:
(*a*) Bacterial – e.g. tuberculosis, brucellosis.
(*b*) Fungal – e.g. blastomycosis, histoplasmosis, actinomycosis, cryptococcosis.
(*c*) Parasitic – e.g. schistosomiasis, amoebae, worms, toxocara.
(*d*) Viral – e.g. cytomegalovirus.
(*e*) Rickettsial – e.g. Q fever.
(*f*) Spirochaetal – e.g. syphilis.
2 Hypersensitivity and other immunologically mediated disorders – e.g. berylliosis, a wide range of drugs (including phenylbutazone and sulphonamides) vascular diseases (polyarteritis nodosa, giant cell arteritis).
3 Tumours – e.g. Hodgkin's and non-Hodgkin's lymphomas.
4 Miscellaneous – including sarcoidosis (which is common) and primary biliary cirrhosis.

ACTINOMYCOSIS

The liver is involved by blood spread from the primary focus in the ileo-caecal region, or rarely in the disseminated type (see p. 57).

Macroscopical

Honeycomb abscesses with '*sulphur granules*' in the pus and dense surrounding fibrosis.

Microscopical

The characteristic '*ray fungus*' is present in smears of the pus. Fibrosis is very marked and polymorphs are abundant.

AMOEBIASIS

In cases of intestinal amoebiasis, spread of the *Entamoeba histolytica* to the liver occurs following penetration of the submucosal portal vein tributaries.

AMOEBIC HEPATITIS

In mild cases, the amoebae multiply and block small intrahepatic portal vein radicles with consequent focal infarction.

Macroscopical

The liver is of 'moth-eaten' appearance with scattered necrotic areas surrounded by zones of congestion.

Microscopical

These areas show necrotic liver cells, scanty mononuclear cells and debris which contains amoebae.

AMOEBIC 'ABSCESS'

In severe infestation of the liver, the amoebic cytolytic enzyme destroys the liver tissue – 'solitary or tropical abscess'.

Appearances

The lesion may be multiple but is usually solitary and in the right lobe on the diaphragmatic aspect. There is a large necrotic area filled with brown-red material – '*anchovy sauce*', and a very shaggy lining. The amoebae are present in the lining of the wall, but pus cells are absent unless there is secondary infection.

Results

1   *Secondary infection.*
2   *Rupture.*
(*a*) Through the diaphragm into the pleural cavity.
(*b*) Into the peritoneum.
(*c*) Into the mediastinum.
(*d*) Into the gastro-intestinal tract.
3   *Healing.* Energetic and early therapy may result in the elimination of the amoebae and healing of the cavity by granulation tissue.

Diagnosis

Demonstration of amoebae:
(*a*) In the colon or faeces.
(*b*) In scrapings from the wall of the 'abscess'.
(*c*) Indirect haemagglutination test on serum.

HYDATID DISEASE

Nature

An infestation by the cysticercus stage of *Echinococcus granulosus* (*Taenia echinococcus*).

Geographical distribution

Cases of hydatid disease are found wherever dogs abound, since dog is the definitive host, but particularly in Australasia and Africa. The disease occurs in Great Britain, especially in Wales, but the total numbers are small.

Life cycle

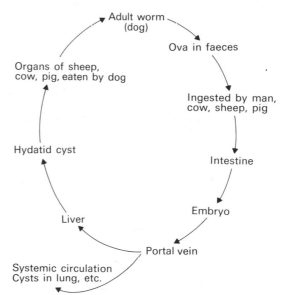

Fig. 68. Life cycle—*Taenia echinococcus*.

Man, cow, sheep and pig are, therefore, intermediate hosts.

Sites
Liver – 70 per cent; lungs – 20 per cent; systemic – 10 per cent (kidney, bones, etc.)

Appearances
The ectocyst is formed by fibrous tissue and may calcify after the parasite dies. The cyst is usually solitary, especially in the right lobe. The lesion increases in size whilst alive with budding off of numerous daughter cysts and some may attain an enormous size – 15 cm in diameter or more – causing hepatomegaly.

Results
1 *Aseptic degeneration*. Death of the parasite, commonly followed by calcification.
2 *Secondary infection*. The parasite dies but an abscess cavity is formed.
3 *Rupture into*:
(a) *Peritoneum*. Peritoneal cysts.
(b) *Biliary tree*. Obstructive jaundice and infection.
(c) *Intestine*. Elimination of the parasite in the faeces.
(d) *Chest*. To produce pleural and pulmonary cysts.
(e) *Blood*. Secondary metastatic cysts.
(f) *External*. Fistula formation through the skin.

Diagnosis
1 *Complement fixation test*. Positive in 70–80 per cent of cases with living cysts, but only becomes positive when some leakage of cyst fluid has occurred.
2 *Casoni test*. Intradermal injection of sterile hydatid cyst fluid produces a positive reaction in 90 per cent of active cases.
3 *Eosinophilia*. Not specific but is usually present.
4 *Cyst contents*. Cysts should not be aspirated but fluid removed at operation may contain hooklets or scolices.
5 *Haemagglutination test*. This is the test of choice.

SCHISTOSOMIASIS – BILHARZIASIS

Nature
An infestation with the trematodes *Schistosoma mansoni* or *S. japonicum*. *S. haematobium* causes disease of the urinary tract, but only very rarely affects the liver (see p. 388).

Geographical distribution and life cycle
These are described on p. 72.

Pathogenesis
The disease is acquired in humans by contact of the skin with water infected with the cercariae which will penetrate intact skin. The disseminated parasites, after reaching the abdominal viscera, pass through the capillaries into the portal venous radicles and thence to the liver where they mature and produce ova.

Liver
Ova produced by the mature parasite in the liver migrate throughout the portal vascular tree and cause a marked inflammatory reaction.
Early. There is a granulomatous reaction around the ova with foreign body giant cells, epithelioid cells and a zone of eosinophils, lymphocytes and plasma cells. The presence of ova distinguishes the granuloma from a tubercle.
Later. Fibrosis around the ova leads to periportal fibrosis and sometimes to cirrhosis in which nodular regeneration is not prominent (see p. 565). The larger portal veins are surrounded by a dense fibrous cuff giving rise to the characteristic '*pipe-stem*' appearance.

Effects
1 *Portal hypertension*. This is progressive and is usually marked with considerable splenomegaly.
2 *Liver-cell failure*. Rarely prominent.

Results
Slowly progressive over 10 years or more with death usually resulting from portal venous hypertension.

Diagnosis
1 *Identification of ova in the faeces*. These are very scanty in the late stages of the disease.
2 *Liver biopsy*.
3 *Serological tests*. Complement fixation and intradermal tests are usually positive.
4 *Haemagglutination tests*. This indirect test on serum has largely superceded (3) above.

KALA-AZAR – VISCERAL LEISHMANIASIS

In this infestation with *Leishmania donovani*, the liver is involved in respect of its cells of the phagocytic system.

Liver
Enlarged and fatty with narrowed congested sinusoids due to swelling of the Kupffer cells which contain the parasite – Leishman–Donovan bodies (see p. 62).

Chapter 92
Diseases of the Liver – Cirrhosis : Tumours

Cirrhosis of the liver

Definition

The result of failure of the liver to return to normal after injury. A simple definition is 'diffuse fibrosis associated with parenchymal nodules'. There is also the inference that such structural alterations will have major effects:

1 Portal hypertension.
2 Shunting of blood from portal to systemic circulations.
3 Disordered liver-cell function.

Appearances of liver

In all types of hepatic cirrhosis the liver is firmer than normal with a thickened opaque capsule and a nodular surface of yellow-brown or green colour, greatly variable in size. On section the organ is diffusely replaced by round or oval brown-yellow or green nodules separated by bands of grey fibrous tissue. Histologically, there is great variability in nodule size and loss of normal lobular pattern, with marked absence of central veins and hepatic cell plates several cells thick. The surrounding fibrous tissue contains variable numbers of mononuclear cells and portal tracts in which there are often prominent bile ducts.

There are two main varieties which are merely descriptive terms without any aetiological significance.

1 Macronodular – most nodules more than 0.3 cm.
2 Micronodular – most nodules 0.3 cm or less.

MACRONODULAR TYPE – SYN. TOXIC CIRRHOSIS, POST-NECROTIC CIRRHOSIS.

There is a very wide range of nodular size up to 3 cm or more. Mostly there is no identifiable vascular pattern of hepatic vein radicles though some may have normal vascular relationships. Hepatocytes show hyperplastic effects and most portal tracts have evidence of collapse and approximation suggesting previous necrosis.

MICRONODULAR TYPE – SYN. LAËNNEC'S CIRRHOSIS, PORTAL CIRRHOSIS, SEPTAL CIRRHOSIS.

The fibrous tissue is rather finer and the nodules smaller and more even in size – 0.1–0.5 cm. Histologically, hepatic venous radicles (central veins) are hardly ever seen and the nodules consist of multi-layered hepatic cell plates.

Pathogenesis

The common event associated with liver injury is liver-cell necrosis, the result of a wide range of insults from viral hepatitis and alcohol to metabolic disorders with less severe but continuous cell damage. Although theoretically, regeneration following necrosis of cells and collapse of supporting connective tissue and reticulin framework would explain the origin of the features identified, in practice, in man, cell increase is not commonly detected in cases in which cirrhosis subsequently develops. Chronic active hepatitis (see p. 552), with or without bridging hepatic necrosis, appears to be a mechanism in cirrhosis arising after viral hepatitis (see p. 551). However, some types of cirrhosis are predominantly fibrous with little or no liver-cell damage in the early stages, but presumably true cirrhosis only develops if cell necrosis later appears. Accumulation of toxic bile constituents or direct chemical injury to liver cells are additional features to be considered.

Once cirrhosis is established its speed of progression is determined by the rate of continuing liver-cell loss as opposed to hepatocyte regeneration. With more rapid cell loss cirrhosis is designated 'active' as evidenced by 'spotty (focal)' or 'piece-meal' necrosis. When more static, the cirrhosis is referred to as 'inactive'.

Though many patients with cirrhosis have evidence of immunological abnormalities (see p. 562), it is not clear that this reflects a primary pathogenetic mechanism and is probably an important associated effect of the agent responsible for the original injury, e.g. in chronic active hepatitis.

AETIOLOGICAL CATEGORIES

ESTABLISHED ASSOCIATIONS

1 *Viral hepatitis* – B hepatitis virus but hardly ever a sequel of A virus infection. This is the most common factor in developing countries where high levels of population have HB_sAg or other associated markers in their serum for a long time after a clinically acute attack or after a more insidious subacute infection (see p. 551). This may be of either micronodular or macronodular type, more commonly the latter: fat and Mallory bodies are not present in hepatocytes but cholestasis and increased copper levels may be present.

2 *Alcoholism* – This is the most common cause in

Western countries. The liver is of micronodular type, usually with fat and Mallory bodies and also often with cholestasis (see p. 576).

3 *Metabolic diseases*

(a) *Haemochromatosis* – The cirrhosis is usually macronodular with abundant iron in hepatocytes and portal tracts and is of a very regular lobular pattern. Fat is seldom obvious and cholestasis is not usually present (see p. 562).

(b) *Wilson's disease* – Usually macronodular with excess copper as a dominant feature, sometimes with fat and cholestasis (see p. 563).

(c) *α-1-antitrypsin-deficiency* – This deficiency is associated with panlobular pulmonary emphysema (see p. 653) and also with cirrhosis, mostly macronodular but sometimes micronodular or mixed. Bile duct proliferation is usually striking and liver cells contain acidophilic cytoplasm inclusions which stain intensely with PAS. These are variable in size and usually numerous in individual cells. There is also a marked increase in hepatic copper content.

The pathogenesis of this condition is not known.

(d) *Other metabolic causes of cirrhosis*
(i) Glycogen storage disease (see p. 112).
(ii) Cystic fibrosis (see p. 632).
(iii) Galactosaemia.
(iv) Hereditary fructose intolerance.
(v) Amino acid disorders.
(vi) Abetalipoproteinaemia

4 *Biliary disease – biliary cirrhosis*

(a) Primary biliary cirrhosis (see p. 564).

(b) Major bile duct obstruction (see p. 576).

5 *Venous outflow obstruction*

(a) Budd–Chiari syndrome (see p. 547).

(b) Veno-occlusive disease (see p. 548).

6 *Drugs and toxins* (see p. 549).

7 *Intestinal by-pass for obesity* – Operations designed to reduce intestinal absorption of fatty substances and thus correct obesity have been complicated by cirrhosis, particularly when the anastomosis is jejuno-colic. This appears to be a toxic injury and is associated with severe fatty change.

8 *Others* – Occasional causes include sarcoidosis and hereditary haemorrhagic telangiectasia (see p. 516).

DEBATABLE FACTORS

1 *Auto-immunity* – Some immunological parameters are associated with cirrhosis of the liver but it seems likely that these are secondary rather than primary events. They are, however, of value as markers, e.g. smooth muscle antibodies in cryptogenic and other forms of cirrhosis and mitochondrial antibodies in primary biliary cirrhosis.

2 *Toxins* – Whereas some toxins and chemical poisons are known to cause cirrhosis and are included above there are some, e.g. aflatoxins, where evidence that they cause cirrhosis in humans is inconclusive.

3 *Parasitic* – Most parasitic infections if they involve the liver cause only slight fibrosis but severe portal fibrosis is seen in schistosomiasis and can lead to true cirrhosis (see p. 558).

4 *Malnutrition* – There is no evidence that malnutrition on its own can cause cirrhosis but, as a complication of other agents, e.g. viral hepatitis, alcohol, it may predispose to a significant degree. Kwashiorkor does not lead directly to cirrhosis.

UNKNOWN AETIOLOGY

1 *Cryptogenic cirrhosis* – No definite clinical or morphological pattern. This is the case in at least 15 per cent of patients with hepatic cirrhosis.

2 *Indian childhood cirrhosis* – This condition affecting children from 6 months to 5 years old has a female predilection and also has a high morbidity and mortality. Almost all cases are from India and the features are of fatty change, progressing to cell degeneration and necrosis with abundant fibrosis but little parenchymal regeneration. The cirrhosis is micronodular.

The aetiology is obscure but believed to be due to action of an exogenous agent. Viral hepatitis, malnutrition and other identified agents of cirrhosis elsewhere do not appear to play a role.

CLINICAL MANIFESTATIONS

The previously identified basic effects of cirrhosis (see p. 560) determine most of the clinical features.

1 *Ascites* – Mostly from combination of portal hypertension and low plasma osmotic pressure due to decreased albumin synthesis. Later renal function and electrolytic disturbances also play a part.

2 *Jaundice* – This is usually due to liver-cell failure, even though there is also an increased risk of gall stones in cirrhotics.

3 *Splenomegaly* and oesophageal varices – the result of portal venous hypertension.

4 *Haemorrhagic tendency* – deficiency of blood coagulation factors due to liver-cell dysfunction (see p. 533).

5 *Encephalopathy* – Mental deterioration and hepatic coma are largely the result of liver-cell failure and porto-systemic shunting.

6 *Infections* – Predisposition to infection is common and is multifactorial.

7 *Toxaemia* – Failure of the detoxification mechanisms of the liver leads to accumulation of drugs, metabolic and infective products which can cause endotoxaemia, e.g. 'liver palms', gynaecomastia and oestrogen retention in both sexes.

8 *Asymptomatic* – It is clear that many patients remain in a compensated asymptomatic state for years. This can quite frequently be demonstrated by needle biopsy or by an unexpected autopsy finding.

DIAGNOSIS

1 *Jaundice.* If present this is of hepatocellular pattern (see p. 577).

2 *Enzymes.* Serum alkaline phosphatase is raised, as is 5-nucleotidase, but not to the levels anticipated in obstructive jaundice.

SGPT and γ-glutamyl transpeptidase levels are usually high.

3 *Prothrombin time.* Normal in compensated cases, but usually prolonged when liver failure supervenes.

4 *Serum proteins.* Albumin is low and γ-globulins are often relatively or absolutely high, particularly in IgG and IgA components.

5 *Autoantibodies*
(a) *Mitochondrial* – High titre in 90 per cent of cases of primary biliary cirrhosis and in some patients with cryptogenic cirrhosis, and others with chronic active hepatitis. Present in less than 1 per cent of normal persons and virtually never in 'pure' extrahepatic duct obstruction.

(b) *Smooth muscle* – Levels above 1 in 40 are hardly ever seen except in cases of chronic active hepatitis and cryptogenic cirrhosis.

(c) *Others* – Antinuclear factor is found in 50 per cent of patients with chronic active hepatitis and in some patients with rather aggressive cryptogenic cirrhosis. Occasional cases have high titre rheumatoid factor blood levels.

6 *Biopsy.* Currently percutaneous needle biopsy is the most satisfactory diagnostic agent. The risk from complications is small and diagnostic accuracy is high. By definition, cirrhosis is a diffuse disease and thus random biopsy should be representative, but fibrosis can be readily misinterpreted and exaggerated and in macronodular examples particularly the large size of the nodules may create confusion.

RESULTS

1 *Liver-cell failure.* Death in hepatic coma with 'liver palms', foetor hepaticus, spider naevi and a haemorrhagic diathesis.

2 *Portal hypertension.* Haemorrhage from oesophageal varices is clinically most relevant. Mortality of the first bleed has been reduced by endoscopic and gastric surgical procedures. Anastomoses between portal and systemic venous systems, e.g. porto-caval shunt, are effective in reducing pressure in the portal venous system and in prolonging life.

3 *Hepatocellular carcinoma.* Development of liver cell carcinoma in cirrhosis is frequent, particularly in cases due to hepatitis B virus, alcohol and haemochromatosis (see p. 566).

HAEMOCHROMATOSIS – BRONZE DIABETES – IRON OVERLOAD

Nature

Whereas the terms siderosis and haemosiderosis denote increase of haemosiderin in tissues without reference to its location or the presence of tissue damage, in haemochromatosis iron deposition in parenchymal cells is associated with tissue damage and, in the liver, with development of cirrhosis (see p. 560). The mechanisms in relationship to iron metabolism are explained in Chapter 80 on p. 477.

Aetiology

1 *Primary – Idiopathic – Haemochromatosis* – Due to an inherited defect of iron metabolism, with increased absorption from a normal diet. There is a familial autosomal recessive inheritance.

2 *Haemochromatosis with anaemia* – Anaemia treated with blood transfusion usually overloads the phagocytic cell system but in certain anaemias, particularly those with accelerated erythropoiesis or defects of cell maturation, parenchymal cell deposition can occur (see p. 478), e.g. thalassaemia, sideroblastic anaemia.

In some cases changes identical to haemochromatosis occur.

3   *Dietary excess* – In Bantus and less commonly in others, excess ingestion of iron in a soluble form may cause excess tissue deposition of iron.

4   *Cirrhosis* – In many cases of hepatic cirrhosis, heavy parenchymal iron deposition is secondary and is particularly common in alcoholic cirrhotics.

Incidence
Male to female 10:1; peak age incidence 45–55 years.

Organ changes
Liver: *Macroscopical*. Enlarged, red-brown in colour, wrinkled, firm and nodular, indicative of cirrhosis.

Microscopical. There is iron pigmentation of liver cells and fibrosis varying from portal tract fibrous tissue to wide fibrous bands. Bile duct proliferation is marked but fatty change is not seen. The Prussian blue stain reveals the presence of iron in the liver cells and in the fibrous tissue.

Pancreas: *Macroscopical*. Deep brown and firm.

Microscopical. Interacinar and interlobular fibrosis with parenchymal degeneration. The islets of Langerhans are pigmented and atrophic, thus causing diabetes (see p. 635).

Spleen: *Macroscopical*. About twice the normal size, brown and firm.

Microscopical. Pigmentation and fibrosis.

Heart. Pigmented, with atrophy of myocardial fibres. Severe coronary atheroma is commonly found.

Skin pigmentation. There is increased melanin in the basal layer of the epidermis and iron-containing pigment in the dermis, especially around the skin appendages.

Testes. Atrophic and pigmented.

Other organs. The pituitary gland, adrenals and thyroid may also be affected by pigmentation and become atrophic with resulting functional deficits.

Pigment
The pigments in this condition are haemosiderin which is iron-containing, and haemofuscin which is not iron-containing.

Results
In uncomplicated cases the disease is slowly progressive with about 20 years' duration of life from the time of clinical recognition. Death is, however, inevitably due to:

1   Myocardial involvement or coronary occlusion.
2   Diabetes mellitus and its complications.
3   Liver-cell failure.
4   Portal venous hypertension.
5   Hepatocellular carcinoma, which is a common complication.

HEPATOLENTICULAR DEGENERATION — KINNIER WILSON'S DISEASE

Nature
An autosomal recessively inherited disease, characterized by the deficiency of a copper-binding plasma protein, ceruloplasmin, and deposition of copper in the liver, brain and kidneys as a result of increased intestinal absorption.

Organ changes
Liver. The liver contains an excess of copper and shows changes resembling a chronic active hepatitis, later proceeding to a macronodular cirrhosis (see p. 552).

Brain. Symmetrical degeneration of the basal ganglia with excess copper in astrocytes (see p. 611).

Cornea. Kayser–Fleischer ring on the cornea due to deposition of a brownish-green pigment in Descemet's membrane.

Kidney. Deposition of copper in the glomeruli and renal tubules associated with amino-aciduria.

Results
Progressive, with death usually before the age of 30 years from intercurrent infection associated with the neurological disturbance which is the dominant clinical feature. Occasionally, death may be due to liver failure.

SECONDARY BILIARY CIRRHOSIS

Nature
Prolonged obstructive jaundice – extrahepatic cholestasis, leads to liver damage and biliary cirrhosis.

Pathogenesis
From studies of congenital bile duct atresia it is clear that true cirrhosis can occur in 5–6 months but

there is dispute about the role of superimposed cholangitis on obstruction in relationship to development of true cirrhosis as opposed to hepatic fibrosis (see p. 576).

Causes

EXTRAHEPATIC OBSTRUCTION OF THE BILE DUCTS
1 Calculus
2 Stricture.
3 Tumour.
4 Congenital atresia.
5 Cystic fibrosis.

INTRAHEPATIC OBSTRUCTION OF THE BILE DUCTS
1 Primary intrahepatic bile duct carcinoma.
2 Metastatic tumour.

Macroscopical

The liver is enlarged and dark green in colour with a finely nodular or granular surface. The distended bile ducts may be visible on the cut surface and the cause of the biliary obstruction may also be apparent, e.g. stone.

Microscopical

The appearances vary from a portal tract fibrosis – perilobular fibrosis, to dense coalescing bands of fibrous tissue in the portal tracts associated with nodular regeneration to produce a true cirrhosis. Bile thrombi and distended dilated bile ducts are conspicuous, as is bile duct proliferation, but the regenerated nodules have a clear margin and there is no fatty change. An inflammatory cell infiltration is often present around the distended bile ducts.

Effects

In addition to the effects of the causative obstructive jaundice, portal hypertension and liver-cell failure occur but develop relatively late and progress slowly. Relief of the obstructive cause will lead to some improvement of function, even when severe damage to the liver has already occurred. Complicating ascending cholangitis is common.

PRIMARY BILIARY CIRRHOSIS – PBC

Nature

An uncommon disorder of middle-aged women in which there is chronic non-suppurative obstruction of small intrahepatic bile radicles, followed by true cirrhosis.

Aetiology

This is not known although there is some evidence to implicate an immune complex disorder.

Clinical features

Male to female ratio – 10–15 : 1; age range 30–70 but most are 50–70 years.

Pruritis usually precedes jaundice, skin pigmentation and hepatomegaly. Portal hypertension develops in 50 per cent and may present before cirrhosis has become established.

Biochemical

1 Bilirubin – mildly raised to 34–68 mmol/l.
2 Alkaline phosphatase – raised 3–5 times normal.
3 Amino-transferase – moderate rise.
4 Immunoglobulins – IgM increased consistently to about 150 per cent.

Immunology

1 Other diseases – Sjögren's syndrome is common (50 per cent). Other immune disorders are less commonly associated.
2 Mitochondrial antibody – present in 90 per cent or more of patients, usually in titres greater than 1 in 128.

Stages

1 *Florid duct lesion* – Focal changes with inflammatory cell infiltrate around and in the wall of swollen intrahepatic bile ducts, with disruption of duct basement membrane and development of small granulomas.
2 *Ductular proliferation* – Inflammatory reaction extends beyond the portal tracts with periportal hepatocyte piecemeal necrosis and intense ductular proliferation.
3 *Scarring* – Progressive fibrosis in portal tracts and adjacent parenchyma.
4 *Cirrhosis* – Regenerative nodules appear and the fibrosis progresses.

Results

Many patients die within a few years from progressive liver-cell failure. Portal hypertension with bleeding oesophageal varices is a cause of death in about one third of the patients.

Some survive for 10 years or more.

CARDIAC FIBROSIS

Severe chronic passive venous congestion may lead to centrilolobular necrosis involving the reticulin framework with collapse of liver structure in these areas. Subsequently, there is fibrosis which extends outwards and may coalesce with fibrous areas of other lobules. Nodular regeneration is never conspicuous and the condition causes little clinical effects. Liver-cell failure and portal hypertension do not occur, but the serum bilirubin level may be raised. Only very occasionally does a true cirrhosis occur in these circumstances.

SCHISTOSOMIASIS

The 'pipe-stem' fibrosis, sometimes with true cirrhosis, is described on page 558.

Tumours of the liver

BENIGN

These are rare and only very seldom give rise to symptoms.

HAEMANGIOMA

Incidence
This is the commonest primary 'tumour' of the liver.

Macroscopical
Although usually solitary, these tumorous malformations may be multiple and attain a size of 5–8 cm in diameter. They are often subcapsular in position, wedge-shaped and on section are dark red with a honeycomb appearance.

Microscopical
Cavernous endothelial-lined spaces filled with blood and with a fibrous framework.

ANGIOSARCOMA

A relatively recently recognized highly malignant vasoformative primary liver tumour of which many examples have been shown to be associated with exposure to vinyl chloride and associated chemicals.

PELIOSIS HEPATIS

Multiple blood-filled cysts in the liver usually without endothelial lining and often associated with therapy by anabolic/androgenic steroids.

BENIGN EPITHELIAL LIVER TUMOURS AND TUMOUR-LIKE LESIONS

Nature
These lesions are uncommon but appear to be increasing and uniform nomenclature as established by the W.H.O. classification is important.

Types
1 *Liver-cell adenoma* – Mostly in women 30–40 years of age and quite commonly on oral contraceptive therapy. Rupture and intraperitoneal haemorrhage are clinically important complications.

There is a solitary nodule, 2–15 cm in size, in an otherwise normal liver and composed of large but uniform hepatocytes in a regular arrangement without bile ducts and portal tracts but with a more or less normal reticulin pattern.

2 *Focal nodular hyperplasia* – Female to male 2 : 1: any age but often 30–50 years. Symptoms are rare from this solitary mass, usually less than 5 cm in diameter projecting from the liver surface and with a histological pattern reminiscent of cirrhosis and containing proliferating bile ducts in the fibrous septa.

3 *Partial nodular transformation* – Nodular formation throughout much of the liver and sometimes producing portal hypertension.

4 *Nodular regenerative hyperplasia* – Nodular hyperplasia without fibrous bands. This sometimes complicates therapy by anabolic steroids.

5 *Mesenchymal hamartoma* – This lesion of childhood is often very large, well demarcated and solitary. It is predominantly composed of loose oedematous connective tissue with cyst-like spaces, bile ducts and irregular islands of hepatocytes.

MALIGNANT – PRIMARY

There is a very wide geographical difference in incidence of primary malignant liver tumours, rare in Europeans but in some countries the most frequent cause of death from malignant disease.

There are four main types:

1 Hepatocellular carcinoma – 80 per cent.
2 Cholangiocarcinoma – 20 per cent.
3 Hepatoblastoma – rare.
4 Others – rare, including angiosarcoma (see p. 567).

HEPATOCELLULAR CARCINOMA – LIVER-CELL CARCINOMA

Nature
A primary carcinoma of liver cells.

Epidemiology
Very high incidence rates – up to 50 per cent, are found in East and South Africa and in South-East Asia (particularly China, Singapore, Malaysia, Indonesia). Although relatively uncommon in Western countries there is clear evidence that the incidence is rising.

Aetiological factors
1 *Hepatitis B virus infection* – There is no doubt that the presence of HB_sAg is carcinogenic and this is probably a dominant force in many countries (see p. 551).
2 *Mycotoxins* – Of these the most studied and probably the most relevant are aflatoxins, produced by *Aspergillus flavus* and *A. parasiticus*. These fungi are widely distributed in soil and produce the toxins which get into foodstuffs, particularly in tropical countries where fungal growth is climatically encouraged. In such areas a strong body of circumstantial association with hepatocellular carcinoma exists and there are some supportive experimental studies.
3 *Alcohol* – The incidence of hepatocellular carcinoma is rising in alcoholic cirrhosis.
4 *Genetic* – There is a particular association with some HLA types.
5 *Haemochromatosis* – Iron overload in general is a clear predisposing factor in some patients.

Macroscopical
Liver-cell carcinomas are usually large, soft haemorrhagic and sometimes bile-stained. Massive solitary tumours are usually found in non-cirrhotic livers, but in cirrhotics multiple neoplastic nodules are common. A rare variant is a diffuse infiltrative type. Gross evidence of intrahepatic vascular spread is frequently seen but it is also likely that multifocal primary tumours occur.

Microscopical
The tumour cells are identifiable as hepatocytes but are variably pleomorphic and arranged in trabecular or pseudoglandular pattern. Bile production is present in only a small proportion but glycogen is commonly present and fat not unusually so.

Effects
1 Rapid clinical deterioration of a known cirrhotic.
2 Blood-stained ascites.
3 Rapid increase in liver size.
4 Increasing levels of α-fetoprotein in serum in about 85 per cent of patients with these carcinomas.

Results
Nearly all cases are rapidly fatal – a few months from diagnosis. Less frequently the course is longer and occasionally long-term survivals following surgery for well-differentiated tumours have been recorded.

Intrahepatic blood spread is common but distant metastases are infrequent.

CHOLANGIOCARCINOMA – BILE DUCT CARCINOMA

Nature
A primary adenocarcinoma of intra-hepatic bile duct origin and which is not associated with cirrhosis.

Aetiology
The high (and increasing) incidence in parts of South-East Asia is closely related to the distribution of infestation with *Clonorchis sinensis* (see p. 72) and less often by other liver flukes.

Macroscopical
These tumours are either hilar or central in position presenting with intra-hepatic bile duct obstruction, or are more like the more peripheral liver-cell carcinomas. A dense fibrous reaction is usually present and often infiltration alongside biliary channels is obvious.

Microscopical

Variably tubule-forming, mucus-producing adenocarcinomas, nearly always with a marked scirrhous fibrous reaction.

Results

Intrahepatic vascular spread and lymphatic spread to para-aortic abdominal nodes are common as is peritoneal involvement and coelomic spread.

The course may be relatively prolonged to many months or years but the ultimate prognosis is very poor.

HEPATOBLASTOMA

Nature

This 'embryonal' highly malignant tumour presents in the first 2 years of life and is much less common than the nephroblastoma (see p. 378).

Appearances

Usually bulky, haemorrhagic and necrotic, the histological appearances are variable and usually dominated by an epithelial 'foetal' element with variable amounts of mesenchymal tissues, e.g. fibroblastic tissue, cartilage, osteoid.

Course

The tumour is rapidly progressive and, except in cases treated by early surgical excision, death occurs within a few months.

OTHERS

This group includes:

1   Combined liver-cell and bile duct carcinoma.
2   Bile duct cystadenoma and cystadenocarcinoma.

3   Adenosquamous and squamous cell carcinoma.
4   Sarcomas including angiosarcoma (see p. 155).

SECONDARY TUMOURS

Incidence

Metastatic tumour in the liver is extremely common, occurring in about 30 per cent of all fatal cases of cancer.

Origin

1   *Via the portal vein.* From any malignant intestinal tumour, e.g. stomach, large intestine.
2   *Via the systemic circulation*, e.g. carcinoma of the breast and bronchus.

Occasionally, direct invasion of the liver occurs from adjacent organs, e.g. stomach, pancreas, gall bladder.

Macroscopical

The appearances vary with the number and size of the deposits, but these can be extremely extensive so that the liver occupies two-thirds or more of the abdomen. The deposits are often variable in size with haemorrhagic or necrotic centres which, when near the surface, may lead to 'umbilication'.

Effects

1   Hepatomegaly.
2   Ascites.
3   Intrahepatic biliary obstruction with jaundice.
4   Portal vein obstruction or thrombosis.
5   Infarcts of the liver.
6   Haemorrhage. From oesophageal varices or from the liver.
7   Obstruction of the inferior vena cava.
8   Liver-cell failure.

Chapter 93
Diseases of the Gall Bladder and Biliary Tract

Functions of the gall bladder
1 Concentration of bile – ten times.
2 Acts as a reservoir of bile – holds 60–90 ml. The liver secretes 600–900 ml/day.
3 Regulates pressure in the biliary tract.
4 Controls the discharge of bile into the duodenum.

Composition of bile
1 Bile pigments – mainly bilirubin – 50 mg/dl.
2 Bile acids and salts – 1 g/dl.
3 Cholesterol – 60 mg/dl.
4 Mucin – variable amounts.

Functions of bile

1. Bile salts:
(*a*) Emulsify fat.
(*b*) Assist in the absorption of calcium and the fat soluble vitamins.
(*c*) Their presence in the intestine encourages the liver to produce more bile.
2 Excretion of bile pigments, cholesterol and alkaline phosphatase.
3 Excretion of some drugs and poisons – e.g. heavy metals, quinine, salicylates, strychnine.

Congenital

Numerous congenital abnormalities may occur which are commonly detected by radiological examinations. Most produce little effect or no clinical effect but are important anatomical variations to the surgeon.

Absence of the gall bladder
Rare and often associated with other anomalies of the biliary tract.

Double gall bladder
Vary rare; the cystic duct is single.

Accessory bile ducts
Rare but of surgical importance.

Left-sided gall bladder
Very low in position under the left lobe of the liver.

Folded (kinked) gall bladder
Occurs in approximately 20 per cent of normal persons.
(*a*) Kinking between the body and the fundus.
(*b*) Kinking between the body and the infundibulum.

Hour-glass gall bladder
An exaggerated form of folding.

True diverticula
Rare, but false diverticula are common, occurring in chronic cholecystitis as Rokitansky–Aschoff sinuses (see p. 570).

Intrahepatic gall bladder
The organ may be almost completely buried in the liver substance and in such circumstances is often diseased.

Floating gall bladder
There is a mesentery formed by two serosal layers in 4–5 per cent of persons, which may be as much as 2–3 cm long. This may predispose to torsion leading to infarction.

Anomalies of the cystic duct and artery
Variations in the site and anatomical relations of these structures are of surgical importance.

Choledochal cyst
Cystic dilation of the bile duct.

Congenital obliteration (atresia) of the bile ducts

ORIGIN
1 Failure of development of the bile ducts leading to complete absence. This is exceedingly rare.
2 Failure of canalization of the biliary bud with variable lengths of solid ducts.

EFFECTS
Obstructive jaundice apparent soon after birth and leading to biliary cirrhosis, liver–cell failure or haemorrhage due to hypoprothrombinaemia or varices.

RESULTS

Usually fatal by 24 months of age; a few cases may be amenable to surgery when only a localized segment is involved.

Inflammations

ACUTE CHOLECYSTITIS

Organisms
Streptococci, coliforms, *Salmonella typhi*, clostridia, etc. In the early stages, 90 per cent are sterile, but in the first 24 hours 35 per cent become infected and after the third day, 80 per cent are infected.

Aetiological factors
The exact mechanism is unknown, but factors and theories suggested include:
1 Obstruction of the cystic duct by calculus. This is the most important factor and is found in 96 per cent of cases. Stasis of bile, associated probably with chemical injury, results in mucosal damage and subsequent secondary bacterial infection.

2   The condition can be experimentally produced by increasing the concentration of the bile salts in the gall bladder.

3   Enzyme action from reflux of pancreatic secretions.

4   Infarction of the wall with subsequent infection.

Routes of infection
Organisms may reach the gall bladder:
1   In the blood.
2   From the liver via lymphatics.
3   From the intestine via peribiliary lymphatics.
4   In the bile via the biliary tree.
5   By direct extension from neighbouring organs.

Macroscopical
The organ is intensely congested and often haemorrhagic. There is marked oedema of the wall and the organ is distended unless preceded by chronic cholecystitis. The bile is turbid or even frankly purulent – *empyema of the gall bladder*, in which case blockage of the cystic duct is invariably found. Fibrinous mucosal and serosal exudates are common, as is ulceration of the mucosa, particularly when stones are present in the lumen.

Microscopical
Congestion, infiltration of the mucosa and later other layers of the wall by polymorphs, with mucosal ulceration and, in severe cases, gangrene.

Results
1   Complete resolution – rare.
2   Suppuration – empyema.
3   Gangrene leading to perforation and peritonitis.
4   Chronic cholecystitis.

CHRONIC CHOLECYSTITIS

Nature
Although this may follow acute inflammation, chronic cholecystitis is much more commonly a separate entity of insidious onset and slow progression.

Aetiology
Associated with gall stones in at least 90 per cent of cases.

Macroscopical
The contracted organ shows marked fibrous thickening of the wall and the mucosal surface is scarred and atrophic. Cystic spaces may be seen deep within the wall. The bile, in addition to stones, may contain a sediment of debris – biliary mud.

Microscopical
There is usually considerable fibrosis of the wall. The mucosa initially becomes hypertrophied or sometimes papillary, but later atrophies. Protrusion of epithelium into the muscular coat leads to sinuses which may reach the serosal coat or produce cysts – the *Rokitansky-Aschoff sinuses*, and these may simulate carcinoma. There is an accompanying chronic inflammatory cell infiltration of all coats. Sometimes stones or abscesses are seen within the wall.

CHOLECYSTITIS GLANDULARIS PROLIFERANS

In this condition there is a 'stricture' dividing the organ into two loculi. At the site of the stricture of the lumen, the wall is thickened due to epithelial sinus formation and marked muscular hypertrophy and there is a fundal 'adenoma' comprising a localized area of similar appearance. This fundal lesion may simulate a tumour on palpation and shows as a filling defect on cholecystography.

Initially there is no inflammation but this commonly develops later due to stasis in the upper loculus and results in fibrous thickening of the wall. The wall of the lower loculus may remain histologically normal.

The aetiology is unknown. Stones are not commonly associated with the condition except by secondary formation when chronic inflammation supervenes. Muscular inco-ordination seems a possible aetiological factor.

Gall stones – cholelithiasis

Incidence
Found in about 10 per cent of the adult population.

Age
Rare in the young, common from about 40 years onwards.

Sex

M:F 1:4

Aetiology

Factors:

1 Abnormal bile composition.

2 Infection.

3 Stasis.

   The actual deposition of stones is due to precipitation from an already supersaturated solution. The most important factor is alteration of the cholesterol:bile salt ratio by changes in hepatic bile secretion or by infection which leads to absorption of bile salts.

Types of stones

PURE STONES (10 per cent.)

These are usually due to primary changes in the composition of the bile excreted by the liver and are thus metabolic or hepatogenous stones.

Cholesterol

The stone is often solitary and large – 1–5 cm in diameter, round or oval and yellow; they may be translucent. On section there is a typical glistening and radiate appearance – 'solitaire'. They may be associated with cholesterosis of the gall bladder (see p. 572) and are radiolucent.

Calcium bilirubinate – Pigment Stones

Due to increased haemolysis of red cells and liver excretion of the excess breakdown products. They are multiple, jet black, small, ovoid or spherical and are often faceted. The cut surface is homogeneous and they can be readily crushed.

Calcium carbonate

The aetiology is unknown and these stones are very rarely due to abnormalities of calcium metabolism. Small, ovoid, smooth, chalky in appearance, they are purely inorganic.

MIXED STONES (90 per cent)

Composed of cholesterol, bile pigment, calcium salts and a protein matrix derived from the gall bladder. They are virtually always associated with cholecystitis, are multiple, variable in size from minute to 5 cm or more in diameter and are brownish-grey in colour. The surface is often faceted and the cut surface usually shows a cholesterol centre with surrounding concentric laminations of pigment. As most contain calcium, they are usually radio-opaque.

Sites

Most arise in the gall bladder but stones may rarely form in other parts of the biliary tract.

Effects

1 *Nil.* The gall stones remain *in situ* with no clinical symptoms.

2 *Potentiate chronic cholecystitis.* With frequent acute exacerbations.

3 *Cause acute cholecystitis.*

4 *Obstruct cystic duct*

(a) *Completely.* Leading to mucocoele or empyema of the gall bladder.

(b) *Incompletely or intermittently.*

5 *Migrate.* To the common bile duct where they may:

(a) *Obstruct completely.* Progressive obstructive jaundice.

(b) *Obstruct incompletely.* Fluctuating level of obstructive jaundice.

(c) *Pass to the duodenum.*

(d) *Precipitate acute pancreatitis.*

6 *Gall stone ileus.* Acute cholecystitis due to stones may lead to perforation and formation of a fistula with a loop of adherent intestine. Stones may pass into the lumen of the intestine with resulting intestinal obstruction.

Mucocoele of the gall bladder

Aetiology

Total obstruction of the cystic duct in the absence of infection usually caused by a stone and especially when impacted in Hartmann's pouch.

Macroscopical

The organ is grossly distended and contains clear watery mucoid fluid, the mucus having been secreted by the mucosa. The wall is thin with a smooth lining. Evidence of previous cholecystitis may or may not be present together with the cause of the obstruction. Occasionally, a mucocoele may become infected – *empyema of the gall bladder.*

Cholesterosis – 'strawberry' gall bladder

Incidence
Found in 10 per cent of autopsies.

Aetiology
Not definitely known. The condition is not associated with generalized abnormalities of cholesterol metabolism and so local factors must be present. Suggested causes include:
1   Excessive absorption of cholesterol from bile.
2   Failure of the mucosa to secrete cholesterol into the bile.

Macroscopical
The mucosa is studded with small, yellow or pale flecks with an intervening background of red-coloured mucosa, thus mimicking the surface of a strawberry.

Microscopical
Enlargement and distension of mucosal folds due to aggregates of foam cells in the subepithelial layer. Later, cholesterol crystals may be present, together with an inflammatory reaction.

Effects
This does not predispose to cholecystitis although the two conditions may occur coincidentally.

Normally symptomless, although the lipid collections may be the starting point for the formation of cholesterol stones.

Benign stricture of the bile ducts

Aetiology
Eighty per cent follow surgery, i.e. ligature or surgical trauma.

They may occur spontaneously; following perforation or penetration of a duodenal ulcer, associated with chronic pancreatitis, due to benign bile duct tumours or scarring at the site of stone impaction.

Appearances
The stricture is usually an area of fibrous scarring of the wall with narrowing or occlusion of the lumen. The bile duct above the obstruction is dilated and the liver shows bile stasis or, in longstanding cases, biliary cirrhosis.

Effects
1   Obstructive jaundice.
2   Cholangitis.

Results
If obstruction is complete and unrelieved, death occurs from biliary cirrhosis. If the condition is surgically relieved liver damage already caused by the obstruction may improve considerably.

Tumours of the biliary tract

BENIGN

These are very rare. Papillomas and adenomas are small and composed of regular overgrowth of the columnar epithelial cells; when the tumour is pedunculated – papilloma, or when sessile – adenoma.

Most so-called 'adenomas' of the gall bladder are in fact localized areas of marked epithelial sinus formation as part of cholecystitis glandularis proliferans, particularly in the region of the fundus (see p. 570).

MALIGNANT

CARCINOMA OF THE GALL BLADDER

Incidence
About 1 per cent of cancers.

Age
Sixty to seventy years.

Sex
M:F 1:4

Aetiology
1   Stones.
2   Cholecystitis

Gall stones are found in about 90 per cent of cases and cholecystitis is also very commonly associated. It has therefore been postulated that chronic irritation is a potent aetiological factor, particularly in the formation of squamous cell carcinoma.

Cholic acid derivatives, which are present in bile, are amongst the most powerful experimental carcinogenic agents known.

Macroscopical

1 *Infiltrating*. Poorly defined areas of diffuse thickening of the wall, which is very hard. Ulceration of the mucosal surface and invasion of the serosal surface or the liver bed are common. On section, the wall is replaced by hard white gritty tumour.

2 *Papillary*. The tumour grows largely into the lumen, as irregular papillary cauliflower masses but, by the time the disease is clinically apparent, the wall and neighbouring organs are usually invaded.

Microscopical

1 *Adenocarcinoma*. Ninety per cent – columnar cell type with mucus secretion. They are mostly well differentiated.

2 *Squamous cell carcinoma*. Ten per cent.

Spread

1 *Local*. Invasion of liver, bile ducts, etc., commonly causing jaundice.

2 *Lymphatic*. Metastases to nodes in the porta hepatis which may lead to external pressure on the bile ducts and jaundice.

3 *Blood*. Metastases in the liver, lungs, etc.

Results

Five-year survivors are very few; the average duration of life from the time of diagnosis is 1 year.

CARCINOMA OF THE EXTRAHEPATIC BILE DUCTS

Incidence

This tumour is only slightly less frequent than gall bladder carcinoma.

Age

Sixty to seventy years.

Sex

M:F 2:1.

Aetiology

Stones are found in about 30 per cent of cases but inflammation does not appear to be a significant factor.

Sites

In order of frequency:

1 Common bile duct.
2 Hepatic bile ducts.
3 Cystic duct.
4 Region of the ampulla of Vater.

Macroscopical

These tumours are very small and readily missed surgically but seldom metastasize. There is scirrhous thickening of the duct wall and narrowing or occlusion of the lumen.

Microscopical

Adenocarcinomas which are usually solid, but rarely papillary.

Effects

1 Obstructive jaundice is an early manifestation and is usually progressive.

2 Enlarged gall bladder (Courvoisier's Law) with a dilated duct above the site of the obstruction.

Results

The average survival time from diagnosis is 6 months.

Chapter 94
Diseases of the Liver and Biliary Tract: Jaundice

Definition
The normal blood bilirubin level is 5–17 μmol/l. Clinical jaundice usually appears when the blood bilirubin exceeds 35 μmol/l.

Normal bile formation and circulation
This is diagrammatically illustrated in Fig. 69 on p. 575.

Types of jaundice

Haemolytic
The rate of bilirubin formation is greater than the rate at which it can be excreted by the liver cells. Jaundice of this type, therefore, represents increased breakdown of haemoglobin and is due to retention. The bilirubin is mainly of the 'pre-hepatic' type; it is thus not conjugated with glycuronic acid and does not pass through the kidneys into the urine, e.g. acholuric jaundice and other inherited and acquired haemolytic anaemias (see pp. 486–507).

Parenchymatous – hepatocellular
Bilirubin production is normal, but the liver cells are functionally incapable of excreting all the pigment – retention jaundice. Some of the pigment excreted is reabsorbed into the blood due to intralobular obstruction and disorganization – regurgitation jaundice. The bilirubin is thus a mixture of conjugated and non-conjugated types.

Obstructive – cholestasis
Bilirubin production is normal but the pigment excreted by the liver cells is prevented from reaching the intestine by obstruction of the biliary tract at some level. The excess bilirubin is thus mainly of the conjugated type, giving a direct van den Bergh reaction and also, having a smaller molecule, it can pass into the urine via the kidney.

There are two types:
1 Extrahepatic.
2 Intrahepatic.

HAEMOLYTIC JAUNDICE

Introduction
The normal daily bile pigment production is 300 mg from 6.25 g. of haemoglobin broken down. The normal life span of erythrocytes is 120 days but in haemolytic states this may be reduced to as little as 15–20 days. In such conditions, bile pigment production may increase to as much as 1500 mg/day. The depth of haemolytic jaundice depends

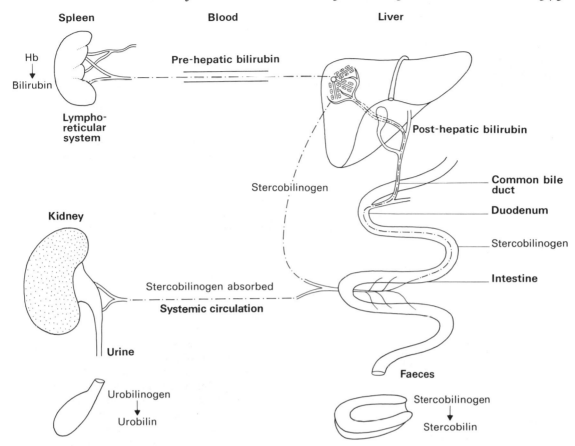

Fig. 69. Normal bile formation and circulation.

upon the rate of red cell destruction, but the degree of anaemia is related to the hyperplastic ability of the bone marrow to compensate for the red cell destruction.

Causes

The haematological conditions which give rise to excessive haemolysis and haemolytic jaundice are described on pp. 486–494 and on pp. 504–507.

Effects

Jaundice. Usually mild and a lemon yellow colour.

Changes in blood, urine and faeces are indicated in the table on p. 577.

Gall stones. Pigment stones may form in the gall bladder.

Spleen. Splenomegaly with siderosis – increased

iron in the organ, is often, but not invariably, present.

Liver. Normal size with a reddish-brown colour due to excess iron present as haemosiderin in granular form in the Kupffer cells and macrophages in the portal tracts. This haemosiderosis should not be confused with haemochromatosis (p. 562).

HEPATOCELLULAR JAUNDICE

The changes in blood, urine and faeces are listed on p. 577. The jaundice is often a mixture of conjugated and non-conjugated bilirubin.

Causes

1 Liver-cell damage by infection, e.g. viral hepa-

titis (see p. 577), cytotoxic effect of drugs (see p. 549).

2 Chronic active hepatitis (see p. 552).

3 Cirrhosis (see p. 560).

Jaundice is not always present at all stages of the process or in all cases, particularly if the cirrhosis is well compensated.

Obstructive jaundice

Types

EXTRAHEPATIC – LARGE DUCT OBSTRUCTION
This may occur at any site in the main biliary tree with resulting resorption of conjugated bilirubin into the blood. Obstruction may be:
(*a*) Total – e.g. tumour.
(*b*) Incomplete – e.g. early stages of tumour or with a stricture or calculus.
(*c*) Intermittent – e.g. stone in the common bile duct.

Causes
1 *Lumen.* Calculi in the common bile duct, hepatic ducts, or at the ampulla of Vater; cystic fibrosis (see p. 632).
2 *Wall:*
(*a*) Stricture.
(*b*) Atresia.
(*c*) Tumour of the bile duct or the hepatic duct.
(*d*) Primary biliary cirrhosis.
3 *External:*
(*a*) Carcinoma of the pancreas.
(*b*) Carcinoma of the duodenum and ampulla.
(*c*) Metastatic tumour in the liver or lymph nodes.
(*d*) Chronic pancreatitis.
(*e*) Ligature.

INTRAHEPATIC – CHOLESTASIS
(*a*) Intralobular – Pure intrahepatic intralobular bile duct obstruction may be found in the cholestatic type of drug jaundice (see p. 550), viral hepatitis, metabolic disorders, pregnancy, etc.
(*b*) Extralobular – e.g. primary biliary cirrhosis (see p. 564)

Appearances

JAUNDICE
This may be intense and of dark green colour.

Xanthelasmas of the skin and conjunctiva may be present.

LIVER

Macroscopical
Enlarged and dark green. Initially smooth, but a fine nodularity may appear as biliary cirrhosis develops. The bile ducts are usually dilated above the site of obstruction and may be varicose. At first, the bile is dark, but later the rise in pressure causes suppression of hepatic bile secretion and it becomes colourless – *white bile*, containing mucus secreted by glands in the duct wall. Cholangitis and abscess formation in the liver may occur as complications.

Microscopical
1 *Large duct obstruction:*
(*a*) Early – lobular cholestasis with portal oedema and inflammation and a little later duct dilatation and proliferation.
(*b*) Later – there is increase in intracellular bile thrombi, feathery degeneration of hepatocytes may be apparent, and liver-cell necrosis develops. Inflammatory cell infiltrate increases with polymorphs and mononuclear cells. Eosinophils may be numerous.
(*c*) Infection – stasis encourages infection and this is a common concomitant to large duct obstruction – *ascending cholangitis* (see p. 570).
(*d*) Later changes – in long continued obstruction there is increasing fibrosis in portal tracts leading to secondary biliary cirrhosis – though this is only in the very advanced stages a true cirrhosis.
2 *Intrahepatic cholestasis.* There is mild centrilobular bile accumulation and bile thrombi in bile canaliculi but little change in portal tracts and normal interlobular bile ducts. Variable, usually modest evidence of liver-cell damage is seen.

Effects
1 *Acholia.* Steatorrhoea leading to multiple deficiencies of absorption, manifest particularly as: osteomalacia, hypoprothrombinaemia with haemorrhages, malnutrition, etc. (see p. 209).
2 *Liver.* If unrelieved and complete, obstruction leads to: liver-cell dysfunction, biliary cirrhosis, liver-cell failure, portal hypertension and death.

Laboratory tests in jaundice

	Haemolytic	Obstructive			Hepatocellular	
		Carcinoma of the pancreas	Stones in C.B.D.	Intrahepatic cholestasis	Hepatitis	Cirrhosis
Urine						
Bilirubin	Absent	+ +	+ or + + or intermittent	+ +	+	Usually − or sl. +
Urobilinogen	+ +	NOT +	NOT +	NOT +	+ +	± to + +
Faeces						
Colour	Dark	Silver	Pale or normal	Pale or normal	Pale or normal	Normal (or with blood)
Occult blood	NEG.	POS.	Usually	NEG.	NEG.	Often POS.
Blood						
Bilirubin	Unconjugated + +	Conjugated + + +	Conjugated + to + +	Conjugated + to + +	Conjugated + to + + +	(most Conjugated) + to + + +
Alkaline phosphatase	N	+ + + +	+ + to + + +	+ + to + + +	+	±
5′-Nucleotidase	N	+ to + +	+ to + +	+ +	+ + + +	+ to + +
Aspartate transaminase (SGOT)	N	N	N	N to + +	+ + + +	+ to + +
Alanine transaminase Aminotransferase) (SGPT)	N	+	+ to + +	+ to + +	+ + + +	+ to + + +
γ-Glutamyl transpeptidase	N	+ + +	+ + +	+ +	+ + +	+ to + + +
Proteins	N	N	N	N	γ Globulin ↑	Albumin ↓ γ Globulin ↑
Prothrombin time	N	Prolonged corrects with vitamin K$_1$	Prolonged corrects with vitamin K$_1$	Prolonged usually corrects with vitamin K$_1$	Prolonged does NOT correct with vitamin K$_1$	Prolonged NOT corrected by vitamin K$_1$

Chapter 95
Diseases of Lymph Nodes

Normal

Sites
Lymphoid tissue is widespread throughout the body, but is particularly aggregated in the lymph nodes, spleen and gastro-intestinal tract (Waldeyer's ring and Peyer's patches).

Structure
This is diagrammatically illustrated in Fig. 70. The lymph nodes vary in size from a few millimetres up to 2 cm in diameter and are surrounded by a fibrous

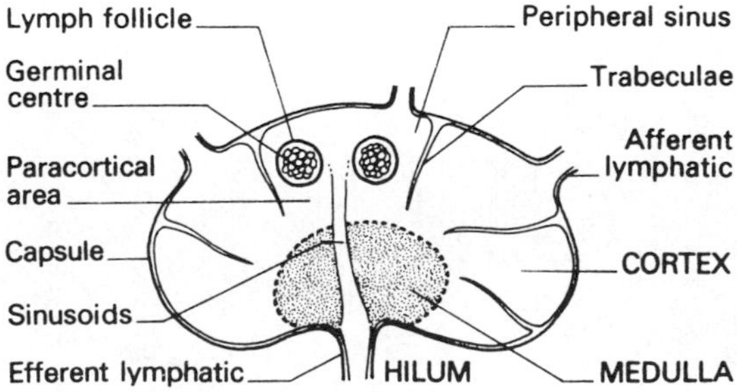

Fig. 70. Normal lymph node structure.

Lymph follicle — Peripheral sinus
Germinal centre — Trabeculae
Paracortical area — Afferent lymphatic
Capsule — CORTEX
Sinusoids —
Efferent lymphatic — HILUM — MEDULLA

capsule through which afferent lymphatics lead into the peripheral sinus. The lymph node is divided into a cortex and medulla.

The cortex contains the lymphoid follicles which are composed of an outer zone of darkly staining small lymphocytes and a central paler germinal centre. The latter contains a variety of lymphoid cells, dendritic cells and macrophages. The follicles are the main site of B-lymphocyte activity in the lymph node. The interfollicular and deep part of the cortex is designated the paracortical area. It contains numerous small lymphocytes, and the postcapillary venules which are an important site for the traffic of lymphocytes between the vascular and lymphatic compartments. In contrast to the follicles and the medullary cords the paracortical area is thymus dependent and is populated by T lymphocytes.

The medulla comprises the sinusoids which connect the peripheral sinus with the hilum of the node and which are lined by fixed macrophages, and the medullary cords which contain small lymphocytes, free macrophages and plasma cells.

Functions
1   To receive, via the macrophage system, and process antigenic material from the drainage area.
2   In response to the presence of antigenic material, to mount an immunological response, either humoral antibody production (B-cell activity) or cell mediated (T-cell activity).

Inflammatory and reactive

NON-SPECIFIC

Lymph nodes, in their protective role, react to infection in local or more distant sites, but in the majority of infections the changes produced are microscopically and macroscopically identical. There is a variable reactivity of the follicles, paracortical areas and sinusoids – *non-specific reactive hyperplasia*. In the case of acute infections the node may be very swollen and tender – *acute lymphadenitis* (e.g. cervical lymph nodes in acute tonsillitis). The node usually returns to normal after the infection subsides, but chronic infection may lead to fibrosis in the node – *chronic lymphadenitis*. Reactive hyperplasia can also be recognized in lymph nodes draining malignant tumours, in

particular proliferation of free macrophages in the sinusoids – *sinus histiocytosis*.

SPECIFIC

Many inflammations result in characteristic and often diagnostic histological changes in the lymph nodes. Most of these conditions have already been described in the appropriate section but the following are reminders of the type of disease which may often be diagnosed from lymph-node biopsy:

1   *Bacterial*, e.g. tuberculosis, brucellosis, granuloma inguinale.
2   *Viral*, e.g. infectious mononucleosis, measles.
3   *Chlamydial*, e.g. lymphogranuloma venereum, cat-scratch disease.
4   *Fungal*, e.g. histoplasmosis, blastomycosis.
5   *Parasitic*, e.g. toxoplasmosis, filariasis, trypanosomiasis, leishmaniasis.
6   *Others*, e.g. sarcoidosis, dermatopathic lymphadenopathy, rheumatoid disease, angio-immunoblastic lymphadenopathy.

CAT-SCRATCH DISEASE

Aetiology
The chlamydia (see p. 43) are organisms classified between bacteria and viruses and cause psittacosis, trachoma and lymphogranuloma venereum. A similar agent almost certainly causes cat-scratch disease, although positive identification has not yet been achieved. Transmission is by the scratch of a cat or sometimes other animals. A small local lesion appears at the site of the scratch which resolves, followed by enlarged regional lymph nodes 2–3 weeks later.

Microscopical
The lymph nodes show reactive hyperplasia with foci of epithelioid cells and some giant cells. At a later stage, the centres of these foci undergo necrosis and produce oval, flattened or stellate abscesses containing nuclear debris and polymorphs. There is a surrounding zone of epithelioid cells in a palisaded arrangement. The appearances are thus very similar to lymphogranuloma venereum (see p. 406).

Results
The disease pursues a chronic course, but the

lymphadenopathy usually regresses with scarring. Sometimes the lymph node suppurates and extends to involve the overlying skin with sinus formation and secondary infection.

TOXOPLASMOSIS

Aetiology
A worldwide zoonosis caused by the protozoan parasite *Toxoplasma gondii*. This may exist extra-cellularly, but usually multiplies in the cytoplasm of cells. The organisms may be highly virulent, but adult human infection is usually of low virulence. Clinical presentation varies from isolated lympha-denopathy to generalized lymphadenopathy with pyrexia resembling glandular fever.

Microscopical
There is usually follicular hyperplasia with enlarged germinal centres. Numerous small granu-lomas composed of epithelioid macrophages are present in the follicles and paracortical areas, where post-capillary venules are prominent. The sinu-soids are closely packed with macrophages.

Results
The diagnosis should be confirmed by toxoplasma fluorescent antibody studies on serum. Symptoms may persist for several weeks or months, but the lymphadenopathy eventually resolves without scarring.

DERMATOPATHIC LYMPHADENOPATHY

Nature
A characteristic change occurring in the lymph nodes draining areas of chronic skin disorders in which there is breakdown of epithelial cells, i.e. may occur with any chronic dermatitis.

Microscopical
There is often follicular hyperplasia, with an ac-cumulation of large macrophages in cortex and medulla. The macrophages contain varying amounts of phagocytosed lipid, melanin pigment and haemosiderin derived from the breakdown of skin structures.

Results
There are no important sequelae but the condition requires differentiation from other and more sinis-ter causes of lymphadenopathy, e.g. malignant lymphoma.

ANGIOIMMUNOBLASTIC LYMPHADENOPATHY

Nature
A recently recognized disease complex of unknown aetiology which has features of hyperimmunity and immune deficiency, but can behave like a malignant lymphoma. Patients have constitutional symptoms, generalized lymphadenopathy, hepatosplenomeg-aly and skin eruptions. There is hypergammaglo-bulinaemia, anaemia which may be Coombs' positive haemolytic, and auto-antibodies are frequently detected.

Microscopical
The lymph node architecture is effaced, with prominent vascular 'arborization' (possibly post-capillary venules), and a polymorphic cellular in-filtrate including prominent immunoblasts, plasma cells, lymphocytes, eosinophils and macrophages. They may be deposition of PAS-positive intercell-ular material. Care must be taken not to mistake the appearances for Hodgkin's disease; Reed–Stern-berg cells are not found.

Results
The natural history is not yet clearly defined. There is a high mortality and although a 40 per cent remission rate can be achieved with corticosteroids, some combination of steroids and cytotoxic drugs is the preferred treatment. Some cases appear to evolve into immunoblastic sarcoma (see p. 583).

Tumours

MALIGNANT LYMPHOMA

Nature
Primary tumours of the lymphoreticular system, arising mainly in lymph nodes.

Incidence
This group of tumours, excluding the leukaemias, accounts for over 2500 deaths annually, approxima-tely 2 per cent of all deaths from malignant disease.

Types

Many of the difficulties in classification have now been resolved and there is general agreement on a basic subdivision into Hodgkin's disease and non-Hodgkin's lymphoma. The finer classification of the non-Hodgkin's lymphomas is, however, still to be agreed. The two main groups will be discussed separately.

Much of the difficulty in the correct diagnosis of the lymphomas stems from poor technical quality. It is essential to ensure proper fixation of material, careful processing and embedding, and preparation of thin sections sensitively stained.

HODGKIN'S DISEASE

Aetiology

The cause of Hodgkin's disease is unknown. The current theory is that there is a virus-induced neoplastic transformation of T lymphocytes, but conclusive evidence is lacking.

Incidence

This is the commonest of the lymphomas, accounting for about 40 per cent of cases.

Age and sex

There is a bimodal age incidence, with the larger peak at 15–34 years and the smaller after 55 years. Males are affected about twice as frequently as females, except in the nodular sclerosing type (see below) which has a predilection for young females.

Clinical manifestations

The clinical presentation varies; the commonest presentation is painless, firm, mobile, lymph node enlargement. The cervical nodes are most frequently involved, followed by the axillary and inguinal nodes. Mediastinal nodes are initially involved in only a small proportion of cases, but this increases in later stages. Hepatosplenomegaly may be present and other viscera may be affected. Constitutional symptoms such as pyrexia and weight loss are occasionally encountered (see Staging below).

Macroscopical

The lymph nodes are enlarged, firm, sometimes lobulated and usually discrete. On section they appear rubbery, homogeneous, pale and often show fibrous strands.

Microscopical

The lymph node architecture is destroyed and the node replaced by a polymorphic infiltrate composed of Reed-Sternberg cells, atypical mononuclear cells, lymphocytes, plasma cells, macrophages and eosinophils. The Reed-Sternberg cell is the pathognomonic feature. These are very large cells with binucleate or multilobed indented nuclei having prominent inclusion-like nucleoli, and abundant pink-staining cytoplasm.

There have been a number of attempts to subdivide the histological appearances of Hodgkin's disease, but there is now worldwide acceptance of the Rye classification which employs four subgroups.

1 *Lymphocyte predominance.* There is an intense infiltrate of small lymphocytes and only scanty eosinophils, atypical cells and Reed–Sternberg cells. A careful search of multiple sections may be required to identify the latter. Approximately 15 per cent of cases.

2 *Nodular sclerosing.* In this form broad bands of collagen divide the node into nodules. Within the nodules the characteristic polymorphic infiltrate is present, together with a variant of the Reed–Sternberg cell, the 'lacunar' cell which is artefactually shrunken from the adjacent tissue and appears to occupy a space or lacuna. Approximately 40 per cent of cases.

3 *Mixed cellularity.* This is 'classical' Hodgkin's disease, in which the typical polymorphic infiltrate described above is seen. Reed–Sternberg cells are easily identified. Approximately 30 per cent of cases.

4 *Lymphocyte depletion.* In this group numerous atypical mononuclear cells are present, with numerous Reed–Sternberg cells, and there is a corresponding lack of small lymphocytes. There are often areas of necrosis, and there is little fibrosis. Approximately 15 per cent of cases.

Staging

In recent years it has become apparent that the prognosis of Hodgkin's disease is related in part to the extent of disease at the time of presentation. In order to assess this more accurately lymphangiography is undertaken together with bone biopsy and, in some centres, laparotomy with splenectomy, para-aortic lymph node biopsy and liver biopsy. The Ann Arbor Staging Classification arises from a consideration of this approach:

Stage I. Involvement of a single lymph node region.

Stage II. Involvement of two or more lymph node regions on the same side of the diaphragm.

Stage III. Involvement of lymph node regions on both sides of the diaphragm and/or involvement of the spleen (IIIS).

Stage IV. Involvement of one or more extra lymphatic organs, e.g. liver, marrow, lung.

Systemic symptoms absent – A.

Systemic symptoms present – B.

Prognosis

With the advent of combination chemotherapy and more accurate staging, survival has improved dramatically. Both prognosis and stage are related to histological type:

Lymphocyte predominance

   70 per cent Stage I,

   70 per cent 10-year survival;

Nodular sclerosing

   35 per cent Stage I,

   45 per cent 10-year survival;

Mixed cellularity

   35 per cent Stage I,

   20 per cent 10-year survival;

Lymphocyte depletion

   10 per cent Stage I,

   0 per cent 5-year survival.

NON-HODGKIN'S LYMPHOMA

Aetiology

Unknown. Burkitt's lymphoma has been shown to have an association with the Epstein–Barr virus, but the implications of this are not fully understood.

Age and sex

Occurs at any age, but the peak is between 50 and 70 years. Slight male predominance.

Clinical manifestations

Painless lymph-node enlargement is the commonest form of presentation, but disease is often more widespread than in Hodgkin's disease. Similarly, extranodal disease is more common and hepatosplenomegaly frequently occurs. Staging procedures may be carried out as for Hodgkin's disease, but are not so useful.

Macroscopical

The nodes are enlarged and fleshy, often stuck together to form a large mass. There may be foci of haemorrhage and necrosis. In follicular lymphoma (see below) the cut surface may have a prominent nodular appearance.

Microscopical

In recent years a number of new classifications have been devised, based on light microscopy, ultrastructure and immunological techniques. Most have some merit, but universal agreement has yet to be reached. To be practically useful a classification must be simple, and have prognostic value. For the present, the following classification is recommended.

GOOD PROGNOSIS GROUP

Follicular lymphoma

The lymph node is replaced by a nodular lymphomatous infiltrate. The nodules are neoplastic follicles composed of varying proportions of small and large follicle centre cells, recognized by their cloven (cleaved) nuclei. They are therefore of B-cell origin. Even if the node shows a partly diffuse pattern it is still classified as follicular lymphoma.

Great care is needed to distinguish this neoplastic follicular pattern from reactive and, therefore, benign, follicles seen in non-specific reactive hyperplasia. Extension of follicles throughout the whole node, condensation of reticulin fibres in inter-follicular areas, and spread of lymphoid cells outside the capsule are all points in favour of follicular lymphoma.

Diffuse lymphoma

Two of the non-Hodgkin's lymphomas with a diffuse pattern have a relatively 'good' prognosis:

Small follicle centre cell. The nodal architecture is replaced by a monotonous infiltrate of small lymphoid cells which have cloven nuclei. This is the diffuse counterpart of the follicular lymphoma. Good quality sections and imprint preparations are of value in distinguishing the cloven nuclei in this type.

Small lymphocyte. The node is diffusely infiltrated by small lymphocytes with darkly staining nuclei and scanty cytoplasm. Their histological appearance is similar to normal small lymphocytes. The great majority of these lymphomas are of B-cell origin, and this is the tissue counterpart of chronic lymphatic leukaemia.

POOR PROGNOSIS GROUP
The rest of the diffuse lymphomas fall into the poor prognosis group.

Large lymphocytic. In this type, although small lymphocytes may be present, the majority of cells are large lymphocytes with more vesicular nuclei in which nucleoli can be seen. The cytoplasm is pyroninophilic. Neoplastic cells frequently extend through the capsule of the node. The majority of these tumours are thought to be of B-cell origin, although in some cases specific markers cannot be identified.

Undifferentiated. Without benefit of specialized techniques this is inevitably a mixed group and includes tumours which are almost certainly of lymphoid origin and some which may be histiocytic. The tumour cells are large and irregular, variable in size and shape, often multinuclear and usually with abundant cytoplasm and a high mitotic count.

Burkitt's lymphoma. This lymphoma, originally described as having a specific geographical distribution in tropical Africa, has also been reported sporadically in New Guinea, Europe and the United States. It usually occurs in children between 5 and 10 years. Classically the lesion presents as single or multiple tumours in the jaw and there may be spread to testes, ovaries and other organs; lymph nodes are relatively spared. Microscopically the tumour is composed of very large lymphoid cells with finely stippled nuclei and abundant basophilic cytoplasm. There are numerous benign macrophages in the tumour tissue, giving the characteristic 'starry sky' appearance. The Epstein-Barr herpes virus, which has been isolated from cultured tumour cells, is thought to play a part in the pathogenesis.

Histiocytic. True histiocytic lymphomas are very rare, and most cases previously included in this category are probably of lymphoid origin.

Other Non-Hodgkin's Lymphomas
A number of other and rare types of non-Hodgkin's lymphoma are recognized including:

(i) Sézary syndrome. This is characterized by erythrodermia and generalized lymph node enlargement. The malignant cells, which may be present in peripheral blood, are convoluted lymphocytes of T-cell origin.

(ii) Immunoblastic sarcoma. Some cases of angio-immunoblastic lymphadenopathy (see p. 580), develop a progressive proliferation of cells resembling transformed lymphocytes – *immunoblasts*. This usually proves to be rapidly fatal. N.B. In some classifications the term immunoblastic lymphoma is used to denote non-Hodgkin's lymphoma with plasmacytoid differentiation.

(iii) Malignant histiocytosis – histiocytic medullary reticulosis. A rapidly fatal condition characterized by fever, splenomegaly, anaemia and lymphadenopathy. There is widespread infiltration by abnormal histiocytes which exhibit *erythrophagocytosis*.

Prognosis
Because of the terminological difficulties referred to previously and continuing improvements in chemotherapy, precise survival figures for each histological type are difficult to obtain.

The lymphomas in the 'good' prognosis group tend ultimately to prove fatal, but progression of the disease is slow, with remissions. Survival ranges from 5 to more than 10 years, with a substantial proportion living for many years.

In the 'poor' prognosis group the mortality is high, the average survival being 1–2 years. In the minority of cases, particularly if disease is localized, long-term remission and even cure may be achieved. This is particularly true of Burkitt's lymphoma.

Secondary tumours

Metastases in lymph nodes from a carcinoma arising in any organ of the body are extremely common, much more so than primary tumours of lymphoid tissue. Secondary sarcomatous deposits in lymph nodes are considerably less common.

Chapter 96
Diseases of the Mediastinum

Acute mediastinitis

Nature
A spreading infection in the tissue planes of the mediastinum which carries a high mortality. The infection is nearly always secondary to a pathological process affecting structures and organs within the mediastinum, neck or rarely from the abdomen. Mediastinitis may also be associated with penetrating wounds or follow thoracic surgical procedures, e.g. pneumonectomy.

Aetiology
The more common causes are:
1 *Oesophageal perforation*. By foreign body, e.g. bone, bougies and other instruments, oesophageal carcinoma, 'spontaneous' perforation (see p. 185) and oesophageal peptic ulcer.
2 *Pharyngeal perforation*. Following operations or due to carcinoma.
3 *From the neck*. As a result of spreading cellulitis.
4 *From bone*. Spread of infection from osteomyelitis of the spine.

5 *From the abdomen*. Spread of infection through the diaphragm.
6 *Carcinoma*. Infection of necrotic tumour in lymph nodes in the mediastinum, most commonly secondary deposits from a carcinoma of the bronchus.

Macroscopical
There is a cellulitis of the loose connective tissues of the mediastinum. Abscess formation is rare.

Results
Localization of the infection rarely occurs and thus there is a very high mortality.

Mediastinal masses

Most other lesions of the mediastinum are abnormalities which present as masses and are frequently found on routine radiology of the chest. It is thus important to know the types of lesion which may occur.

THYMIC ENLARGEMENT

LYMPHOID HYPERPLASIA

Moderate enlargement, which is due to marked overgrowth of the thymic lymphoid tissue with pronounced lymphoid follicle formation. This may be associated with myasthenia gravis or be unassociated with any clinical abnormality. In the young age group thymic enlargement has in the past been blamed as a cause of sudden death – status thymolymphaticus. There is, however, no justification for the retention of this term as there is no evidence that this condition predisposes to death.

THYMIC CYST

A simple unilocular cyst with fluid contents containing cholesterol crystals, lined by fibrous tissue, and with thymic tissue in the wall.

THYMIC LIPOMA

A large benign fatty tumour may arise within the thymus.

THYMIC TUMOURS

These tumours are rare but are one of the commonest causes of a mass in the anterior mediastinum. Their pathology is complex due to the fact that the thymus consists of two main elements:
1 *Epithelium.* Forming the Hassall's corpuscles.
2 *Lymphoid tissue.* Thymic tumours may be composed of pure epithelium, pure lymphoid tissue or variable mixtures of both. Macroscopically, they are usually round or oval and appear encapsulated. On cross-section they have a fibrous lobulation and may contain cysts. The macroscopic appearance gives little guide to their histological features.

They can be classified as follows:

EPITHELIAL THYMOMA
Composed of well-differentiated epithelial cells reproducing recognizable Hassall's corpuscles or are composed of oval- or spindle-shaped cells. These epithelial thymomas are slowly growing and rarely metastasize. They are, however, sometimes associated with myasthenia gravis (see p. 590) or with a pure red cell aplastic anaemia, both of which may improve dramatically after thymectomy. There is a variable lymphocytic infiltrate.

GRANULOMATOUS THYMOMA
Composed of a mixture of lymphoid and epithelial cells. In addition there are mononuclear cells, giant cells and a fibrous stroma. This is the thymic tumour which histologically and clinically closely mimics Hodgkin's disease. Metastases are commonly seen in the cervical and internal mammary lymph nodes, and later in more distant sites.

LYMPHOID TUMOURS
Rarely, a lymphoid lymphoma may arise from the thymic lymphoid tissue and although apparently localized, initially, will eventually result in generalized malignant lymphoma.

LYMPHOEPITHELIOMA
A tumour of similar appearance to the undifferentiated nasopharyngeal and tonsillar carcinomas (see p. 172), consisting of sheets of undifferentiated malignant epithelial cells with a diffuse and usually marked lymphocytic infiltration. In spite of the histological appearances the tumour is usually encapsulated and carries a good prognosis.

THYMIC TERATOMA
A rare tumour of neonates and infants which may be fully differentiated and organoid or variably dedifferentiated.

GERM CELL TUMOUR
Rare and usually highly malignant tumours mostly in young adult males. Areas may closely resemble seminoma (p. 401) or yolk-sac tumours (p. 403 and p. 439). Immunoperoxidase studies may show α-fetoprotein and/or HCG in the tumour cells which may be reflected in these substances being found in serum.

RETROSTERNAL GOITRE

An intrathoracic goitre may be part of a generalized nodular colloid goitre palpable in the neck or may arise from the lower pole of the thyroid and be the only manifestation of thyroid enlargement. Rarely, ectopic thyroid tissue may be present in the mediastinum from birth and may be the site of enlargement in later life. The intrathoracic goitres shows the appearances of nodular colloid goitre (see p. 309). Results include pressure on the trachea, occlusion of the great veins with superior vena caval obstruction, pressure on the recurrent laryngeal nerves with laryngeal paralysis and on the oesophagus causing dysphagia.

MALIGNANT LYMPHOMA

Hodgkin's and non-Hodgkin's lymphomas may arise in the lymphoid tissue of the mediastinum and thus produce a mass of enlarged lymph nodes which may attain very considerable size and produce marked pressure effects (see p. 587).

TRACHEAL AND BRONCHIAL CYSTS

These arise as a result of a developmental abnormality of the trachea or main bronchi and may thus be found in the mediastinum or in the lung (see p. 645). They are simple cystic structures lined by ciliated respiratory epithelium.

ENTEROGENOUS CYSTS — GASTRIC AND OESOPHAGEAL

Cysts may occur in the posterior mediastinum related to and communicating with the oesophagus. They are simple cysts with a muscular wall lined by squamous or gastric epithelium. They are probably congenital in origin.

NERVE TUMOURS

TUMOURS OF SYMPATHETIC NERVES

Tumours may arise from the sympathetic nerve tissues in the posterior mediastinum.

The most common is *ganglioneuroma* (see p. 621) which is composed of interlacing nerve bundles in which there are sympathetic ganglion cells. These tumours are encapsulated, often mucoid or cystic and frequently show areas of calcification. They are benign and removal is curative.

The least well differentiated is the *neuroblastoma*; these highly malignant tumours are described on p.

295. It should be reiterated that they are formed by sheets of darkly staining undifferentiated neuroblasts often showing a rosette configuration. They are not encapsulated and the prognosis is extremely poor.

Intermediate between these two tumours is the *ganglioneuroblastoma* which contains both neuroblasts and ganglion cells. These tumours are only partially encapsulated and the prognosis is unpredictable but is generally poor.

PERIPHERAL NERVE TUMOURS

Neurofibromas, neurinomas and neurofibrosarcomas may arise from peripheral nerves anywhere in the chest. They are most commonly seen related to intercostal nerves and may extend from the intervertebral foramina of the spine to produce 'hour-glass' tumours in the posterior mediastinum.

PERICARDIAL CYST

Rare cysts which arise as developmental abnormalities of the pericardium. They are unilocular simple cysts containing clear fluid – '*spring water*' *cysts*, are lined by pericardial cells and have a fibrous wall. The most common situation is in the cardiophrenic angle where they may attain a very large size.

PARATHYROID ADENOMA

Although the lower parathyroid glands may be the site of adenoma formation in the mediastinum, these seldom attain a size where they can be visualized radiologically. However, they may be functionally active, producing hyperparathyroidism (see p. 316) and the possibility of a mediastinal position of such a tumour is therefore of importance in the surgical correction of this condition.

OTHER MEDIASTINAL MASSES

SECONDARY TUMOURS

Enlargement of mediastinal lymph nodes due to metastatic tumour is very common. Small primary carcinomas of the bronchus may present clinically due to the effects of massive mediastinal metastases.

BONE TUMOURS

Chondromas, chondrosarcomas, osteosarcomas, etc., are very rare in this region but may arise from the spine, sternum or costal cartilages.

VASCULAR

Aneurysm of the aortic arch and the giant left atrium in mitral stenosis may produce pressure effects on adjacent structures, e.g. dysphagia, vertebral erosion, in addition to characteristic radiological appearances.

CONNECTIVE TISSUE TUMOURS

Lipomas, fibromas, etc., are very rare.

TRAUMA

A haematoma may result from injuries to the chest. This may localize in the anterior superior mediastinum and so produce a mass.

EFFECTS OF MEDIASTINAL MASSES

1 *Pressure on trachea.* Causing cough, respiratory distress, stridor and predisposing to pulmonary infection.
2 *Pressure on vessels.* Pressure on the large veins results in a 'full face' with prominence of veins and oedema of the head, neck and arms.
3 *Recurrent laryngeal nerve palsy.* Changes in the voice.
4 *Sympathetic nerve palsy. Horner's syndrome.*
5 *Infection.* The cystic lesions frequently produce no symptoms until they become infected, when rapid increase in size may occur with dramatic and serious pressure effects.
6 *Haemorrhage.* Haemorrhage into the lesions may similarly produce rapid and commonly dangerous increase in size. This is particularly liable to occur in retrosternal goitres and in cystic masses.

Chapter 97
Diseases of Muscle

Normal muscle

Skeletal muscle is composed of many muscle bundles – *fasciculi*, which are bound together by the *perimysium*; individual muscle fibres are surrounded by an *endomysium*. The muscle cells – myocytes, have closely applied sarcolemmal cells, each with a peripheral nucleus. The myocytes also have nuclei and their cytoplasm is formed by *myofibrils* which extend the whole length of the cell and show cross-striations approximately 3 μm apart. Skeletal muscle fibres are approximately 40–50 μm in diameter, thus, in adults, a diameter less than this implies atrophy and greater than this indicates hypertrophy.

Muscle biopsy

Muscle biopsies taken for diagnosis should be placed on, or preferably slightly stretched over, a thin card or glass slide to prevent distortion before being immersed in fixative and both longitudinal and transverse sections examined. Alternatively, allowing the biopsied muscle tissue to die (20–30 min) before placing into fixative, will also prevent distortion due to violent contraction of the fibres. Enough material should be taken in the biopsy to include both blood vessels and nerves supplying the muscle. A segment should also be taken for histochemical tests, rapidly frozen from the fresh state.

ATROPHY

Nature
Progressive loss of bulk of muscle fibres, which is later followed by fibrous replacement.

Aetiology
1 *Disuse*, e.g. following prolonged immobilization.
2 *Senility*.
3 *Ischaemia*. Due to any arterial disease – e.g. atheroma.

4 *Neuromuscular disorders*, e.g. peripheral neuritis, traumatic severance of motor nerves, progressive muscular atrophy, amyotrophic lateral sclerosis, poliomyelitis, peroneal muscular atrophy.

5 *Nutritional and metabolic*, e.g. wasting diseases, malignant cachexia, malnutrition, malabsorption syndromes, thyrotoxicosis.

Macroscopical

The muscle is smaller than normal and loses its normal red colour, becoming yellow or brown and later firm and grey due to fibrous replacement.

Microscopical

Shrinkage of muscle fibres from the normal 40–50 μm to 20 μm in diameter, or less. There is diminution of the myofibrils but the cross striations are initially preserved. With the decrease in cytoplasm, the sarcolemmal nuclei become more prominent and, in severe cases, the atrophic muscle appears as nucleated sarcolemmal tubes with no muscle substance. Sometimes, an excess of lipochrome is apparent in the muscle cells which imparts a yellow or brown coloration. There is virtually no inflammatory cell infiltration, but in the later stages there is fibrous replacement.

The distribution of atrophy may be of diagnostic importance. The atrophy of senility and vascular occlusion usually affects all fibres of a muscle group equally, whereas, in denervation, the atrophy is patchy with groups of atrophic fibres alternating with normal muscle bundles. In these latter examples, degenerate nerve fibres may also be visible in the section.

MUSCULAR DYSTROPHIES — MYOPATHIES

Nature

A group of primary degenerative diseases of muscle.

Aetiology

There are a number of clinical syndromes, most of which are hereditary (p. 17) and are of similar pathological appearances, but which vary in their distribution. The aetiology remains unknown, but inborn errors of creatine and creatinine metabolism have been postulated, since the patients have an increased serum creatine phosphokinase and excretion of creatine and a decreased excretion of creatinine.

Clinical types

The clinical types include:

1 *Pseudo-hypertrophic muscular dystrophy*. A severe generalized familial muscular dystrophy.

2 *Facio-scapulo-humeral dystrophy*. A mild muscular dystrophy restricted to certain areas.

3 *Dystrophia myotonica*. Atrophy associated with prolonged contraction and slow relaxation of muscles – *myotonia*.

Macroscopical

The affected muscles are smaller than normal and usually pale and soft. In the pseudo-hypertrophic form, the muscles may be of normal size or more bulky than normal.

Microscopical

A mixture of degenerate and necrotic muscle cells with some normal fibres and others which appear larger than normal. This variability in the size and the appearances of the fibres is characteristic of the group and, in addition, there is increased fat between the muscle fibres. The degeneration seen may take several forms, from cloudy swelling to coagulative necrosis – Zenker's degeneration. There is always loss of striations and an increase in the number of subsarcolemmal nuclei. The presence of necrotic fibres induces a mild inflammatory cell reaction but the nerve fibres and blood vessels in the muscle are normal.

MYOSITIS AND POLYMYOSITIS

Nature

Inflammation in muscle.

Aetiology

Many agents may be responsible:

1 *Pyogenic*. Spread of pyogenic infection from neighbouring organs into muscle with acute suppurative inflammation.

2 *Septicaemia*. Scattered pyaemic abscesses in muscles in many parts of the body.

3 *Gas gangrene*. Clostridial infection, producing saccharolytic and proteolytic toxins, gas formation and rapidly spreading necrosis of infected muscles (see p. 131).

4 *Parasites*. Especially trichiniasis and cysticer-cosis (see pp. 68 and 71).

5 *Viruses*. Coxsackie virus – Bornholm disease, influenza

6 *'Toxic'*. Zenker's degeneration, especially in typhoid, pneumonia and diphtheria.

7 *Connective tissue diseases*. Dermatomyositis (see p. 284), rheumatoid arthritis (see p. 285), rheumatic fever (see p. 241), polyarteritis nodosa (see p. 282).

Appearances

These vary with the aetiological agent and thus may show suppurative inflammation, reaction to para-sites, interstitial inflammation or Zenker's degene-ration.

In the connective tissue diseases, the 'poly-myositis' is interstitial and consists of a variable interstitial inflammatory cell infiltration, associated with changes in the collagen, blood vessels and muscular degeneration. These changes vary slightly amongst the various members of the group and have been described in the section on connec-tive tissue diseases (pp. 280–287).

TRAUMATIC – MYOSITIS OSSIFICANS

A localized form of myositis ossificans may follow trauma to muscle when haemorrhage into the muscle is followed by organization into fibrous tissue and later replacement by cartilage upon which enchondral ossification occurs. The osteo-blasts are probably derived from the periosteum, but when the localized area of myositis ossificans occurs entirely within soft tissues, it is probable that they are derived by metaplasia from fibro-blasts. This is not the same disease as *myositis ossificans progressiva*, a rare disease of young sub-jects which is described on p. 115.

ISCHAEMIA

Ischaemia produces simple atrophy of the muscle (see p. 135). When restricted to certain areas the localized changes produce clinical syndromes which merit mention. Ischaemia, possibly asso-ciated with faulty venous drainage, may be respon-sible for the *'sternomastoid tumour'* of infants which results in torticollis. Fractures around the elbow joint may be complicated by *Volkmann's contrac-ture* of the forearm due to interference with venous drainage. In both these conditions, the muscle is progressively replaced by fibrous tissue. A recently described condition is the *anterior tibial syndrome* where oedema, usually due to muscular activity in young persons, raises the pressure in the compara-tively rigid anterior tibial compartment of the lower leg and causes avascular necrosis of the anterior tibial muscles with subsequent fibrous replacement and contractures.

Disorders of function

Nature

There are certain diseases in which the muscle is functionally abnormal and yet no consistent histo-logical abnormality can be demonstrated. *Myotonia congenita* and *periodic familial muscular paralysis*, the latter being associated with low levels of serum potassium, fall into this category but the most important disease of this group is myasthenia gravis.

MYASTHENIA GRAVIS

Nature

A disease characterized by weakness of muscles and exacerbated by fatigue.

Aetiology

Essentially there is a functional acetyl choline deficiency. There is a neuromuscular block due to a humoral agent interfering with neuromuscular transmission. An anti-striated muscle antibody is present in the serum in 30 per cent of all cases but in 90 per cent of patients with associated thymoma. There is a high incidence of other immune dis-orders, e.g. thyroid and S.L.E.

Thymus gland

In about 25 per cent of cases there is a thymoma, usually of the epithelial type (see p. 585). In about 50 per cent of cases there is enlargement of the thymus due to lymphoid hyperplasia. In the remainder, the thymus is either atrophic or histolo-gically normal. Removal of the thymus in myas-thenics may be followed by dramatic improvement of the disease, but a significant proportion are only ameliorated and some are even made worse.

Muscles

These are macroscopically normal until a later stage when there is disuse atrophy. Microscopically, the muscles are frequently completely within normal limits or show simple disuse atrophy. In a small proportion, foci of lymphocytes – *lymphorrhages*, may be present.

Tumours

RHABDOMYOMA

These are not true tumours but are developmental abnormalities of striped muscle which form tumour-like lesions in the heart and occur in other organs associated with tuberose sclerosis (see p. 593).

RHABDOMYOSARCOMA

Excessively rare tumours, mostly occurring in young patients. They present as large, often lobulated or polypoid tumours, which are composed of pleomorphic sarcoma cells in a mesenchymal stroma containing 'strap' cells with visible cross-striations. The prognosis is extremely poor. It should be stressed that atypical muscle cells occur in areas of degeneration and similar changes may also be seen at the site of muscular invasion by any tumour. Hence the diagnosis has to be made with special care and the cross-striations must be present within malignant cells.

DESMOID TUMOUR — MUSCULO-APONEUROTIC FIBROMATOSIS

Nature

A connective tissue mass occurring within muscle, often in the rectus abdominis of middle-aged parous women but even more frequently elsewhere in diverse muscle groups.

Appearances

A firm, locally infiltrative, grey, gritty mass in the anterior abdominal wall. Microscopically it shows the appearances of a cellular fibroma growing between the muscle fibres which become separated by the tumour cells. There is no capsule but the cells are regular in size, shape and staining, and mitotic figures are infrequent.

Results

These infiltrating tumours require wide excision to avoid local recurrence. Desmoids are sometimes named 'recurring fibromas of Paget' and it is probably wise to regard them as low-grade fibrosarcomas which are locally invasive and destructive; a very small proportion may metastasize if untreated.

'MYOBLASTOMA' — GRANULAR CELL MYOBLASTOMA

Origin

Probably of nerve/nerve ending origin.

Sites

The commonest site is the tongue or gum (see p. 173) but they also occur dermally in many areas.

Macroscopical

They are small, firm, yellow or grey nodules, usually associated with thickening of the overlying skin.

Microscopical

The lesion consists of sheets of pink-staining strongly PAS-positive granular cells which infiltrate the subcutaneous tissues. The overlying skin shows acanthosis and hyperkeratosis.

Results

These are almost certainly not true tumours and local excision is curative.

Introduction
Many disease processes which affect other organs
or tissues of the body also produce pathological
changes in the C.N.S., but the appearances are
modified by differences in structure. Although H.
and E. staining may at times be adequate for

histological examination, recourse has frequently to be made to special stains demonstrating myelin sheaths, e.g. Weigert–Pal, Loyez, or neuroglia, e.g. silver impregnation techniques, phosphotungstic acid haemotoxylin (P.T.A.H.).

Structure

Brain tissue is composed of:

1 *Neurones*. These consist of a nerve cell body, with small cytoplasmic processes – dendrites, and a long process – the axis cylinder or axon, which is surrounded by a myelin sheath (see Fig. 80 on p. 619).

2 *Neuroglia*. There is no fibrous tissue within the brain parenchyma, the supporting tissue being formed by three main types of neuroglia:

(a) *Astrocytes*. Of neuroectodermal origin; these are star-shaped cells with long cytoplasmic processes.

(b) *Oligodendroglia*. Also neuroectodermal in origin; they are fewer in number, smaller, rounded and more darkly staining cells with fewer and shorter processes.

(c) *Microglia*. Of mesodermal origin and part of the lymphoreticular system; these cells are the equivalent of histiocytes being actively phagocytic.

3 *Blood vessels*.

4 *Meninges*. In three layers, pia, arachnoid and dura.

Congenital abnormalities of the brain

ANENCEPHALY

Failure of development of a large portion of the brain and cranial bones, usually maximal in the frontal region and incompatible with life.

MICROCEPHALY

Congenital smallness of the brain which is otherwise anatomically and proportionately normal. This results in varying grades of mental deficiency.

SPASTIC DIPLEGIA – LITTLE'S DISEASE

A disease present at birth and associated with signs of pyramidal tract degeneration. It may possibly be due to birth trauma, but more probably is a developmental abnormality of the brain tissue. There is nerve cell degeneration and replacement gliosis which results in a small brain with areas of shrunken gyri.

TUBEROSE SCLEROSIS – EPILOIA

A disease in which sclerotic glial masses in the brain are associated with mental deficiency, adenoma sebaceum on the face and multiple hamartomatous tumours in various viscera. The brain contains multiple nodules of varying size, composed of glial fibres and deformed nerve cells.

MICROGYRIA

A localized or generalized cerebral deformity with shrunken convolutions and absence of the secondary fissures.

PORENCEPHALY

Multiple cystic spaces in the brain substance. These may communicate with the ventricles and are filled with fluid.

MONGOLISM

A condition of idiocy associated with characteristic body build and mongoloid facial features. The brain is grossly abnormal with diminished numbers of gyri and cortical neurones (see p. 13).

Congenital abnormalities of spinal or cranial fusion

This group of conditions is characterized by varying degrees of failure of fusion of the neural tube and the spinal canal. Surgical correction with closure of the more severe forms of failure of fusion allows preservation of life but with a severe penalty on occasions of neurological disability. It is now possible to identify many cases at early stages of intrauterine life by estimation of α-fetoprotein assays of blood and, more accurately, amniotic fluid. It is then possible, in the case of definite positive tests, to recommend to terminate the pregnancy.

SPINA BIFIDA OCCULTA

This is a common but minor defect of one or more spinal neural arches in the lumbo-sacral region. The cord is normally formed in a normal position and the condition is usually a chance radiological finding (see Fig. 71). Minor neurological abnormalities may occasionally result, e.g. enuresis.

SPINA BIFIDA VERA – RACHISCHISIS

COMPLETE RACHISCHISIS – MYELOCOELE

This extreme error of fusion is incompatible with life. The cord is poorly formed and lies exposed in the base of a complete defect of the neural arches (see Fig. 71).

SYRINGOMYELOCOELE

The spinal cord is complete, but there is dilatation of the central canal associated with a severe defect of the vertebral arches (see Fig. 71). There is a considerable neurological deficit and early death occurs.

MENINGOMYELOCOELE

There is herniation of meninges and spinal cord through defects in neural arches into a skin-covered sac in the thoraco-lumbar region. The nerve roots are abnormally situated so that paralysis below the level of the deformity is usual (see Fig. 71).

MENINGOCOELE

This is fairly common and is a simple herniation of meninges through a defect of neural arches, usually in the thoraco-lumbar region (see Fig. 71). The cord is normal but the condition is frequently associated with other deformities, especially the Arnold–Chiari malformation. In addition to some

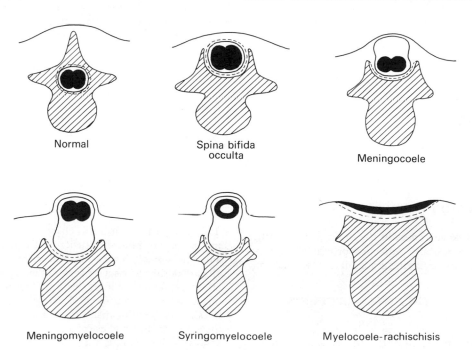

Normal   Spina bifida occulta   Meningocoele

Meningomyelocoele   Syringomyelocoele   Myelocoele-rachischisis

Fig. 71. Abnormalities of fusion of the spinal canal.

neurological disability there is a grave risk of infection and subsequently of meningitis of this thin-walled, skin-covered sac.

ENCEPHALOCOELE

Protrusion of the brain and its coverings through a mid-line defect in the occiput. The bony defect is usually narrow.

ARNOLD – CHIARI MALFORMATION

There is protrusion of the ventro-medial portion of the cerebellum, fourth ventricle and medulla into the cervical spinal canal. This deformity is commonly associated with other abnormalities, particularly with varying grades of rachischisis, but may not produce neurological symptoms until adulthood.

SPONDYLOLISTHESIS

Defective union between vertebral bodies, usually L.5 and S.1. As a result, the vertebral column may dislocate forwards on the sacrum and produce symptoms due to pressure on nerve roots.

PLATYBASIA

Indentation of the base of the skull by the cervical vertebrae with narrowing of the foramen magnum. Although commonly congenital in origin, the condition may be acquired due to softening of the cranial bones by Paget's disease.

KLIPPEL – FEIL DEFORMITY

Fusion of the cervical vertebrae, producing shortness of the neck. This condition may be associated with platybasia.

Hydrocephalus

Nature
An excessive amount of cerebrospinal fluid.

Normal C.S.F. pathways

The C.S.F. is secreted by the choroid plexus into the lateral ventricles, passes through the foramen of Monro to the third ventricle, through the aqueduct of Sylvius to the fourth ventricle and out into the subarachnoid space via the median foramen of Magendie and the lateral foramina of Luschka. It then passes downwards into the spinal theca and also upwards over the brain surface, where it is absorbed by the arachnoid granulations into the large dural venous sinuses. This circulation is illustrated in Fig. 72.

Composition of C.S.F.

Protein	Glucose	Lange gold curve	Cells	Other features
0.150–0.450 g/l	2.75–4.4 mmol/l	000000	Up to 5 lymphocytes c.mm	Crystal clear

Types

Hydrocephalus is probably always due to obstruction and the site of this obstruction will determine whether the hydrocephalus is communicating or non-communicating.

1 *Communicating.* This implies that the C.S.F. has access to the spinal theca and that dye injected into the ventricular system can be recovered from the spinal C.S.F. on lumbar puncture. The obstruction must therefore be around the base of the brain, preventing access of fluid to the supratentorial sites of resorption.

2 *Non-communicating.* This implies obstruction at a point within the ventricular system. The sites where this is especially common are at the foramen of Monro, in the aqueduct, or in the roof of the fourth ventricle.

CLINICAL VARIETIES

CONGENITAL HYDROCEPHALUS

Nature
Hydrocephalus present at birth or developing soon afterwards in infancy.

Aetiology
1 *Anatomical defects.* With stenosis of the C.S.F.

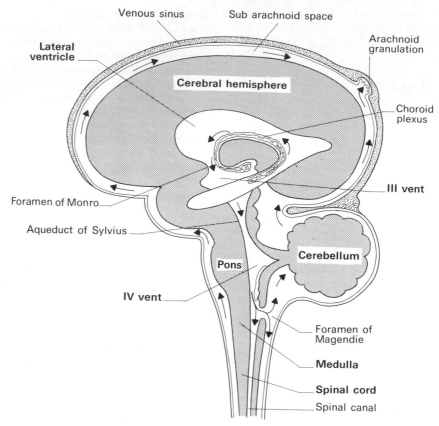

Venous sinus Sub arachnoid space

Arachnoid granulation

Lateral ventricle

Cerebral hemisphere

Choroid plexus

III vent

Foramen of Monro

Aqueduct of Sylvius

Cerebellum

Pons

IV vent

Foramen of Magendie

Medulla

Spinal cord

Spinal canal

Fig. 72. Circulation of cerebrospinal fluid.

pathways within the brain, especially by stenosis of the aqueduct.

2 *Arnold–Chiari malformation* (see p. 595).

3 *Intra-uterine infections*. Especially tuberculosis, pyogenic meningitis, toxoplasmosis.

4 *Space-occupying lesions*, e.g. tumour or abscess.

Appearances

Distension of the cranium occurs with wide separation of the suture lines of the skull, stretching of the scalp and prominence of the superficial veins. The brain is distended by C.S.F., with only a thin rim of residual compressed and largely degenerate cerebral tissue.

Results

There are varying grades of severity depending on the degree of completeness of the obstruction. In some cases the process becomes arrested without

any substantial neurological impairment. This may occur spontaneously, or be due to surgical techniques which shunt the excess C.S.F. from the ventricles into veins or into the right atrium of the heart.

ACQUIRED HYDROCEPHALUS

Nature

Hydrocephalus occurring in older persons in a previously normal brain.

Aetiology

1 *Infections*. As in the congenital form, especially from the various types of basal meningitis.

2 *Space-occupying lesions*. Especially tumours of the brain stem.

3 *Arnold–Chiari malformation*. With late clinical presentation.

Appearances

The suture lines are closed so the skull is incapable of gross enlargement but, as a result, the brain tissue rapidly becomes compressed and destroyed. The ventricular system is distended by C.S.F. proximal to the site of obstruction. Sustained rise of intracranial pressure may produce areas of thinning of the cranial bones.

Vascular disorders – Haemorrhage

Intracranial haemorrhage may be either meningeal or intracerebral.

MENINGEAL HAEMORRHAGE

EXTRADURAL HAEMORRHAGE

Nature

Haemorrhage into the extradural space, i.e. between the skull and the dura.

Aetiology

Trauma to the temporal region with laceration of the middle meningeal artery.

Macroscopical

Blood clot strips the dura away from the skull, which usually shows a fracture. The artery or one of its branches is severed and a haematoma forms which indents the brain substance.

Results

There is a progressive rise of intracranial pressure, unconsciousness and death, unless the bleeding is rapidly controlled by surgical intervention.

SUBDURAL HAEMORRHAGE

Nature

A collection of blood in the subdural space, i.e. between the dura and the arachnoid.

Aetiology

Trauma, which produces two types of lesion:
1 *Acute.* With severe head injuries lacerations of the brain and arachnoid are common which thus allows accumulation of blood derived from severed cortical veins in the subdural space. The already damaged and oedematous brain is compressed and distorted by the haematoma.
2 *Chronic.* Particularly in the very young following birth trauma and in the elderly following relatively minor degrees of trauma, there is rupture of one of more cerebral veins as they cross the subdural space to enter the dural venous sinuses. Blood escapes slowly with a gradual increase in the size of the clot and organization at the margins by a fibroblastic and vascular membrane to produce an encapsulated mass. This slowly increases in size as a result of osmotic attraction of fluid into the haematoma and it is only at this stage, weeks or months after the injury, that symptoms and signs due to pressure on adjacent brain tissue, may become apparent.

Macroscopical

There is a collection of blood clot most commonly in the parietal region of the subdural space. The clot will be of varying age and may show, in the chronic type, considerable variation in the amounts of organization, with haemosiderin staining of adjacent tissues. The brain is commonly indented.

Results

1 *Acute.* The subdural blood is a complicating factor in severe brain injury and the prognosis is usually very poor.
2 *Chronic.* If the condition is recognized in time, surgical evacuation of the haematoma is life-saving and curative. Without treatment, most patients die from increasing cerebral compression; rarely spontaneous limitation occurs followed subsequently by resorption of the blood.

SUBARACHNOID HAEMORRHAGE

Nature

Blood in the subarachnoid space, i.e. between the arachnoid and pia.

Incidence

Spontaneous subarachnoid haemorrhage accounts for about 3000 deaths each year in England and Wales.

Aetiology

1 *Traumatic.* Leakage of blood into the space may occur after any closed or penetrating head injury.

2 *Spontaneous*

(a) *Aneurysms*. Leakage of a congenital 'berry' aneurysm, most of which arise from one of the vessels of the circle of Willis, is the most common cause of subarachnoid haemorrhage (see p. 272). Occasionally, mycotic or atheromatous aneurysms may produce similar effects.

(b) *Extension from intracerebral haemorrhage*. Which ruptures into the space through the cortex or via the ventricles.

Macroscopical

Much of the blood is centred around the lesion of origin and may clot, but commonly there is intermingling with the C.S.F. throughout the system.

Results

These vary according to the cause of the haemorrhage and the amount of blood leaking into the space. Small amounts may cause only irritative meningitic signs, but with substantial quantities, the rise of pressure may interfere with vital centres and death ensues.

In cases of subarachnoid haemorrhage due to aneurysms treated conservatively, 60 per cent die at the first bleed; 20 per cent are crippled and 20 per cent recover. With surgical treatment, the prognosis in accessible situations is much improved, thus 75 per cent of those surviving the operation are alive 5 years later (see p. 271).

INTRACEREBRAL HAEMORRHAGE

Introduction

Cerebral vascular lesions cause some 75 000 deaths each year in England and Wales, which is approximately 15 per cent of deaths from all causes and nearly 90 per cent of the deaths due to diseases of the C.N.S. The term 'cerebral vascular accident' is often used to include both haemorrhage and vascular insufficiency, as the clinical differentiation may be difficult, particularly in the early stages.

MASSIVE CEREBRAL HAEMORRHAGE

Nature

A large area of haemorrhage within the cerebral substance.

Aetiology

1 *Hypertension and arterial diseases*. Especially atheroma.

2 *Trauma*. Penetrating or closed injuries.

3 *Rupture of an intracranial aneurysm*, e.g. congenital or mycotic.

4 *Anticoagulant therapy*.

5 *Haemorrhage into tumours*.

6 *Cerebral angiomatous malformations*.

7 *Haemorrhagic diatheses*, e.g. thrombocytopenic purpura.

Appearances

An extensive area of haemorrhage with destruction of adjacent brain tissue, frequently arising from the lenticulo-striate artery in the internal capsule, or from arteries in the pons. The blood may rupture into the ventricular system to gain access to the C.S.F. in the subarachnoid space.

Results

The bleeding is usually progressive with a rapidly fatal outcome. A haematoma, limited to a relatively small area within the parenchyma, may occasionally occur and rarely may be beneficially evacuated by surgical means. Spontaneous recovery may occur when the haemorrhage is small, but this is most unusual.

PUNCTATE CEREBRAL HAEMORRHAGES

Nature

Multiple small haemorrhages into the brain substance.

Aetiology

1 *Traumatic*. Contusion of the brain following trauma. Repeated injuries may affect the basal ganglia, e.g. 'punch drunk' boxers. An area of punctate haemorrhages is commonly seen in closed head injuries at the opposite pole to the site of the primary point of impact – '*contre coup*' injury.

2 *Infections*. Petechial haemorrhages associated with toxic capillary damage in septicaemia and other bacterial diseases. In addition viral and rickettsial infections of the brain may also show punctate haemorrhages.

3 *Asphyxia*. Extreme venous congestion and anoxia due to a respiratory obstruction may cause haemorrhages.

4 *Haemorrhagic diathesis.* Any bleeding disorder, e.g. acute leukaemia.

5 *Vitamin B deficiency.* Wernicke's encephalopathy (see p. 610).

6 *Embolism.* Petechial haemorrhages in the brain due to emboli of thrombus, fat or air (see p. 126).

Appearances

Multiple small haemorrhages in the grey and white matter, in most cases of a generalized distribution.

Vascular insufficiency

ARTERIAL

Nature

Partial or complete obstruction of the carotid, vertebral or cerebral arteries. This may occur in any part of their course in the neck or intracranially and produces anoxia in the area of the brain supplied by the affected vessel.

Aetiology

1 *Arterial disease.* Especially atheroma and hypertension. Rarely endarteritis obliterans due to syphilis or a necrotizing arteritis, e.g. polyarteritis nodosa, may be causative.

2 *Thrombosis.* Usually superimposed on arterial disease.

3 *Embolism.* Particularly from left atrial thrombus in mitral stenosis and from a mural thrombus over an area of myocardial infarction.

Macroscopical

An area of cerebral softening results due to ischaemic colliquative necrosis. If the patient survives, an '*apoplectic*' cyst with surrounding gliosis results.

Microscopical

Softening of brain tissue with phagocytosis of the degenerate myelin by microglia which become '*compound granular corpuscles*'. Astrocytic proliferation walls off the area with glial tissue. The destroyed brain substance and all dead nerve elements are removed by phagocytes leaving fluid contents.

Results

This disease process is the commonest cause of 'strokes' but the results depend on the site and the size of the area of brain tissue permanently destroyed. Occasionally, especially in hypertensive encephalopathy, the ischaemia is transient and is not followed by permanent brain damage; vascular spasm has been postulated to explain this clinical syndrome.

VENOUS

Nature

Thrombosis of cortical veins or venous sinuses.

Aetiology

1 *Cortical veins.* This is rare and the cause remains unknown. There may be transient paralyses associated with headache.

2 *Venous sinuses*

(*a*) *Infection of adjacent structures.* With a spreading thrombophlebitis of communicating or emissary veins, e.g. ear to lateral sinus, scalp to longitudinal sinus, nose and lip to carotid sinus.

(*b*) *Dehydration.* Especially in children, predisposes to thrombosis of the superior longitudinal sinus.

Results

Obstruction of the venous sinus circulation results in vascular congestion, oedema of brain tissue and sometimes hydrocephalus. Extension of infection may occur to produce meningitis or cerebral abscess.

Chapter 99
Nervous System – Infections:
Suppurative, Tuberculosis, Syphilis

Suppurative infections

SUPPURATIVE MENINGITIS

Nature
Any pyogenic infection of the meninges.

Organisms
The most common organisms found are meningococci, pneumococci and *Haemophilus influenzae*, but occasionally other pyogenic organisms may produce a suppurative meningitis, e.g. coliforms, staphylococci.

Incidence
Although not as common as in pre-antibiotic days, there were still over 300 deaths in England and Wales from meningitis in 1977.

Routes of infection
1 *Blood-borne.* As part of a bacteraemia or septicaemia from a distant focus, e.g. from the lungs.
2 *Direct spread.* From suppurative infection in adjacent tissues, e.g. middle ear, mastoid, nasal sinuses, dural venous sinuses, osteomyelitis of vertebrae or the skull.
3 *Penetrating wounds.* Including compound fractures of the skull.

Macroscopical
Hyperaemia of the meninges which rapidly become covered by purulent exudate in the subarachnoid space. Usually abundant fibrin fills the sulci and the

600

exudate is commonly particularly profuse in the basal region.

Microscopical

An intense acute inflammatory reaction in the meninges with polymorphs and fibrin-rich exudate, particularly around blood vessels, and which extends into the depths of the sulci and into the Virchow–Robin spaces. Numerous organisms may be demonstrable by Gram's stain and the causative organism identified by cultural methods.

C.S.F.

Protein	Glucose	Lange gold curve	Cells	Other features
Increased 1–10	Decreased 0–2.5	Meningitic	Polymorphs 200–3000	Purulent. Organisms present on Gram's stain and culture

Results

When treated early, resolution occurs. In the untreated or neglected cases, there is a substantial mortality. Rarely, organization of the exudate may occur, with subsequent adhesion formation, blockage of C.S.F. pathways and hydrocephalus (see p. 595).

MENINGOCOCCAL INFECTIONS

Organism

Gram-negative diplococci which are commonly observed intracellularly in polymorphs.

Incidence

Now a rare condition.

Pathogenesis

The organisms gain access to the pharynx by inhalation from infected individuals or carriers. Sporadic cases of meningococcal infection occur in addition to rather explosive epidemics, in which a high percentage of the population become carriers of the infection.

Phases of infection

1 *Initial stage.* A localized nasopharyngitis.
2 *Bacteraemia.* This may result in:

(*a*) Acute fulminating meningococcal septicaemia with a rapidly fatal outcome.
(*b*) Chronic meningococcal septicaemia lasting months or even years.
(*c*) Clinically not apparent.

In this bacteraemic phase, haemorrhages from small vessels are common and may produce skin rashes – 'spotted fever', or occasionally massive adrenal haemorrhages – Waterhouse–Friderichsen syndrome (see p. 290).

3 *Meningitis*

The clinical prominence and duration of these phases are extremely variable and meningitis does not invariably occur.

Macroscopical

In addition to the purulent exudate on the meninges, which in children is maximal around the base of the brain – 'posterior basic meningitis', there may be a complicating endocarditis, suppurative arthritis, haemorrhagic skin rashes, adrenal haemorrhages producing adrenal insufficiency and marked constitutional disturbances.

CEREBRAL ABSCESS

Nature

Suppurative inflammation of the brain substance.

Incidence

This is now uncommon, but caused 100 deaths in England and Wales in 1977.

Aetiology

1 *Spread from an adjacent focus of pyogenic infection*, e.g. venous sinus, nasal sinus, middle ear, mastoid, in association with a cholesteatoma, or osteomyelitis of the skull bones.
2 *Implantation of organisms.* From a penetrating wound.
3 *Blood-borne infection.* Especially from suppurative disease in the lung, e.g. lung abscess, empyema, bronchiectasis.
4 *Septic infarction*, e.g. in acute endocarditis.

Sites

The site varies with the aetiology:
Temporal lobe or cerebellum from the ear.
Frontal lobe from frontal air sinuses.
Frequently frontal lobe from suppurative pulmonary disease.

These are the most common sites, but any area of the brain may be involved. The lesion is commonly solitary but when the infection is blood-borne, abscesses may be multiple and occasionally numerous.

Macroscopical
A localized area of pus formation surrounded by oedematous brain tissue and resulting in distortion of the brain substance.

Microscopical
A central area of purulent material with an inflammatory cell infiltration of the adjacent oedematous brain. A capsule of glial tissue develops later.

C.S.F.

Protein	Glucose	Lange gold curve	Cells	Other features
Slight Increase 0.45–1.0	Normal 2.75–4.4	Normal	Lymphocytes and a few polymorphs 10–100	Dramatic changes do not occur unless there is rupture of the abscess

Results
Produces a space-occupying lesion which enlarges progressively unless treated. Rupture into a ventricle or into the subarachnoid space produces a meningitis and this complication is almost invariably fatal. Increased intracranial tension may result in distortion or herniation of the brain substance – *coning*, and a fatal outcome due to interference with vital cerebral functions. A late manifestation in survivors is the onset of epilepsy due to the subsequent glial scarring; this occurs in approximately 50 per cent of cases.

Non-suppurative infections

Nature
Infections of the brain or meninges by non-pyogenic organisms.

TUBERCULOUS MENINGITIS

Incidence
This is now a rare condition in most countries. In the U.K. it may occasionally be seen in immigrant children. About 90 new cases annually in England and Wales.

Features
Blood borne spread from lung as part of miliary disease (see p. 666). Tubercles are seen on the membranes particularly basally where they may cause obstruction to C.S.F. flow and non-communicating hydrocephalus. The tubercles are usually, histologically, not well formed and caseation is unusual.

Occasionally, a solitary *tuberculoma* is present in the brain substance.

C.S.F.

Protein	Glucose	Lange gold curve	Cells	Other features
Increased 0.6–4.0	Decreased 0.55–2.75	Meningitic	Lymphocytes and some polymorphs 50–500	Clear or slightly turbid. 'Spider' clot. Organisms present on Z.N. staining

Results
In spite of antituberculous chemotherapy there is still a significant mortality usually due to obstruction by adhesions.

NEUROSYPHILIS

Syphilis affects the C.N.S. in two main forms:
1 Meningovascular.
2 Parenchymatous.

MENINGOVASCULAR

Nature
This is an early manifestation of acquired tertiary syphilis affecting predominantly the meninges and blood vessels and usually occurs about 3 years following the primary infection. This type of disease may also occur in congenital syphilis.

C.S.F.

Protein	Glucose	Lange gold curve	Cells	Other features
Increased 0.6–1.0	Usually normal 2.75–4.4	Paretic or Luetic	Lymphocytes 10–500	Positive W.R.

Effects

Endarteritis obliterans of small blood vessels with subsequent ischaemic effects. The vessels show a plasma cell and lymphocyte cuff. The meninges, are thickened and opaque. Cranial nerve palsies and a transverse myelitis of the cord are relatively frequent sequelae.

PARENCHYMATOUS NEUROSYPHILIS

Nature

A later tertiary manifestation of acquired syphilis or occurring in adolescence in the congenital type. There is destruction of C.N.S. parenchymal tissue which is of two main types:

GENERAL PARALYSIS OF THE INSANE – G.P.I.

Macroscopical

The meninges are opaque, thickened and adherent; the brain is atrophic with wide sulci and shrunken convolutions. Internally, the ventricles are dilated and show a granular ependymal lining. On section, there is loss of the normal clear line of demarcation between the narrowed cortex and the white matter.

Microscopical

There is loss of cortical nerve cells which are replaced by neuroglia. Perivascular cuffing by plasma cells and lymphocytes is seen.

C.S.F.

Protein	Glucose	Lange gold curve	Cells	Other features
Normal or increased 0.3–1.0	Usually normal 2.75–4.4	Paretic	Lymphocytes 40–100	Positive W.R.

Results

The loss of neurones produces deterioration of intellect and other mental disturbances. The changes of G.P.I. may be associated with tabes dorsalis – *taboparesis*. Typical Argyll Robertson pupils are usually present.

TABES DORSALIS

Macroscopical

Decrease in size of the dorsal columns, maximal in the lumbar region with atrophy of the posterior roots and thickening of the meninges, especially posteriorly.

Microscopical

The meninges are thickened by fibrous tissue and there is degeneration of the fibres in the posterior columns with replacement gliosis (Fig. 65).

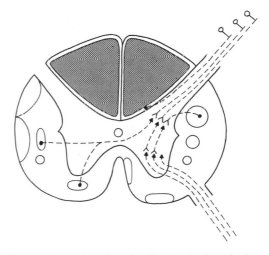

Fig. 73. Tabes dorsalis – site of lesions in the spinal cord.

C.S.F.

Protein	Glucose	Lange gold curve	Cells	Other features
Normal or increased 0.3–0.8	Normal 2.75–4.4	Weak paretic or luetic	Lymphocytes 10–50	Positive W.R.

Results

Sensory loss due to involvement of the posterior columns results in trophic disturbances, e.g. Charcot's joints and trophic ulcers, and in loss of postural sensation which causes the staggering gait.

OTHER NON-SUPPURATIVE INFECTIONS OF THE C.N.S.

FUNGAL INFECTIONS

The brain or meninges may be involved in the disseminated type of actinomycosis (p. 57); in European blastomycosis (cryptococcosis) (p. 57); in coccidioidomycosis (p. 60). Such infections are particularly likely to complicate long-term corticosteroid and immunosuppressive therapy (see p. 375).

PROTOZOAL INFECTIONS

The brain is commonly involved in toxoplasmosis, particularly in the congenital type (see p. 63). In cerebral malaria, areas of cerebral softening or 'malarial granulomas' may be seen (see p. 64).

WORMS

Infestation by the cystic stage of *Taenia solium* – cysticercosis, or *Taenia echinoccus* – hydatid disease, may result in parasitic cysts in the brain substance (see pp. 70 and 71). The brain may likewise be infested in trichiniasis (see p. 68).

Chapter 100
Nervous System – Virus Infections

INTRODUCTION

The C.N.S. can be attacked by many different viruses which have some features in common:
1 There is a generalized viraemia which, in a proportion of cases, is followed by localization in the C.N.S.
2 The virus may attack:
  Predominantly the meninges – viral meningitis, e.g. lymphocytic choriomeningitis, *or*
  Predominantly the brain – encephalitis, e.g. encephalitis lethargica, *or*
  Predominantly the spinal cord – myelitis, e.g. poliomyelitis.
3 The virus multiplies within the nerve cell which, as a result, shows changes varying from reversible degeneration to irreversible necrosis.
4 There is a mononuclear cell inflammatory response with a tendency to perivascular lymphocytic cuffing.

Acute anterior poliomyelitis

Nature
Infection by the poliovirus, one of the enterovirus group, was formerly responsible for worldwide epidemics usually in summer months. There was a high mortality, often in younger persons, as a result of destruction of anterior horn cells of the spinal cord and neurones in the brain stem causing paralysis. In particular, this affected respiratory muscle innervation and cranial nerves – *bulbar poliomyelitis*.

Stages
1 *Preparalytic.* A viraemia with general systemic symptoms. A proportion of cases proceeded to:
2 *Paralytic.* Lower motor neurone lesions of variable distribution.

C.S.F.

	Protein	Glucose	Lange gold curve	Cells	Other features
Pre-paralytic	Normal 0.15–0.45	Normal 2.75–4.4	Normal	Polymorphs 50% Lymphocytes 50% 100–200	Clear or hazy
Paralytic	Increased 0.45–1.0	Normal 2.75–4.4	Weak paretic or luetic	Lymphocytes 100–150	Slightly hazy

Prevention

Vaccination of susceptibles by attenuated virus has virtually eliminated the disease.

Viral encephalitis

Introduction

A group of virus diseases which appear sporadically, but in past years have been responsible for many epidemics due to different viruses which presented slight variations of clinical pattern. All show similar basic changes due to viral invasion of nerve cells of the brain and are, therefore, true encephalitides.

Organisms

Most of the causal agents belong to the Coxsackie group or other groups of enteroviruses including poliovirus. Similar manifestations may, however, be produced by very numerous viral species which more usually produce clinical diseases without neurological involvement and of a different distribution and character, e.g. mumps, herpes.

Macroscopical

Congestion of the meninges and brain with petechial haemorrhages in the brain substance, particularly in the basal ganglia, at the base of the brain and in the floor of the fourth ventricle.

Microscopical

All show petechial haemorrhages and congestion of the brain with perivascular cuffing by mononuclear cells and a patchy or diffuse infiltration of the brain parenchyma with similar cells. There is nerve cell degeneration of variable distribution which may lead to loss of nerve fibres and glial replacement.

The sites particularly affected are the basal ganglia, substantia nigra, pons, medulla and oculomotor nuclei. The cerebral cortex may be involved but the spinal cord only rarely – encephalomyelitis.

Results

In the acute stage, there is pyrexia, changes often in the level of consciousness and extremely variable neurological signs with paralyses, tremors and rigidity.

The mortality rate is high, particularly in the epidemic types of the past. Of the cases which recover, many have residual neurological deficiencies with post-encephalitic Parkinsonism a common sequel.

C.S.F.

Protein	Glucose	Lange gold curve	Cells	Other features
Normal or increased 0.40–1.0	Normal 2.75–4.4	Usually normal	Lymphocytes 50–200	In the early stages there may be lymphocytes and polymorphs

Epidemic encephalitis

In the first half of the 20th century a series of epidemics of viral encephalitis occurred in humans and horses. Some of these were responsible for large numbers of deaths and those who recovered often had serious neurological sequelae.

This group included:

1 Encephalitis lethargica.
2 St Louis encephalitis.
3 Japanese B and Australian 'X' disease.
4 Eastern and western equine encephalitides.

Other viral diseases causing encephalitis

In many virus diseases the nervous system is usually spared but, in certain infectious diseases, C.N.S. involvement may be a complicating factor of variable severity.

Mumps. A usually transient and uncommon

complication with a very low mortality and no sequelae.

Herpes simplex. This infection of the skin may occasionally cause a severe cortical form of encephalitis with a high mortality, particularly in children and infants.

Infectious mononucleosis. A mild encephalitis may occasionally be clinically prominent in cases of this virus infection (see p. 449).

Others. Encephalitis may occur rarely in many other viral diseases and occasionally minor epidemics of pyrexia associated with rather obscure neurological disorders occur, which are almost certainly viral in origin.

Rabies – Hydrophobia

Incidence
Quarantine regulations have eliminated the disease from this country, but it is still widespread amongst domestic and wild animals in many parts of the world, from whom man may be infected.

Pathogenesis
A virus infection transmitted to man by the bite of a rabid animal, usually a dog. From the bite wound the virus travels up nerves to the C.N.S., the incubation period being dependent upon the distance of the bite from the brain or spinal cord.

Macroscopical
Congestion and oedema of the meninges and brain.

Microscopical
Perivascular cuffing by lymphocytes with widespread nerve cell degeneration, particularly marked in the basal nuclei, medulla and mid-brain and especially in the segment of the cord related to the site of the bite. Negri bodies, which are probably aggregates of the virus, are diagnostic. They are circular acidophilic bodies, found in the paranuclear regions of all nerve cells, but are most readily observed in the hippocampus.

Results
There is intense irritability of the nervous system, the slightest touch causing pain, muscular contractions and convulsions. Unless rapidly treated by antiserum – '*virus fixé*', the disease is invariably fatal.

Benign aseptic lymphocytic choriomeningitis

Aetiology
A virus infection of humans contracted from mice who are the natural reservoir of the organisms.

Macroscopical
Intense congestion of the meninges and choroid plexuses.

Microscopical
An intense lymphocytic infiltration of the meninges, choroid plexuses and ependyma of the brain.

C.S.F.

Protein	Glucose	Lange gold curve	Cells	Other features
Increased 0.45–1.0	Normal 2.75–4.4	Normal	Lymphocytes 50–1500	Fluid clear or slightly turbid

Results
Produces signs of meningitis for a period of about 7–10 days with subsequent full recovery in all but very rare cases.

Herpes zoster

This disease is caused by the chickenpox virus which, for reasons unknown, sometimes localizes in dorsal root or cranial nerve ganglia to produce degenerative changes in the ganglion cells, a vesicular eruption with pain and sensory disturbances over the distribution of the affected nerves (see p. 42).

Slow virus infections

Nature
A group of viral neurological diseases with a very long incubation period affecting both animals and man and characterized also by lack of antibodies and of inflammatory cell reaction. The diseases are, however, transmissible.

Types
1 *Kuru.* A subacute human disease with incuba-

tion period of 4–20 years affecting cannibal tribes of Papua, New Guinea, and now less frequent as the particular indulgence of eating poorly cooked brain becomes less frequent.

2   *Creutzfeld–Jakob disease*. There are a number of variants of this fatal disease which has occasionally become accidentally transmitted from man to man with an incubation period of about 10 weeks.

3   *Scrapie and other veterinary diseases*. The scrapie agent is filterable and causes disease in inoculated sheep in about $2\frac{1}{2}$ years. *Visna* and *maedi* are similar slow virus diseases of sheep.

4   *Other possible slow virus infections of C.N.S.* Amongst other well-recognized neurological diseases considered to be possibly caused by slow virus infections are: Multiple sclerosis; Alzheimer's disease; Motor neurone disease, etc.

Appearances

Although affecting many organs, it is usual for brain and spinal cord lesions to dominate the clinical picture. The common findings, histologically, are of variable distribution and severity but are:

1   Spongiform degeneration.
2   Neuronal loss and degeneration.
3   Astrocytic proliferation with variable gliosis.

Chapter 101
Nervous System – Demyelination: Degenerative Disorders: C.S.F. Changes in Nervous Diseases

Demyelinating diseases

Nature
This is a group of diseases in which, at some stage, there is demyelination of nerve fibres, although there is preservation of the axis cylinders, at least initially.

POST-INFECTIVE ENCEPHALOMYELITIS

Aetiology
A disease first described in 1921 when it followed primary vaccination for smallpox. A clinically iden- tical disease may also follow measles, German measles, chickenpox, smallpox and influenza. The disease is not directly due to the virus but results from an auto-immune response in the C.N.S.

Macroscopical
Hyperaemia of the brain and cord both of which are softer than normal.

Microscopical
Perivascular cuffing by lymphocytes and plasma cells and later by histiocytes, with focal areas of demyelination in the white matter.

Results
Presents as a neurological disorder following the

exanthemata, with coma, paraplegia or other cerebral or spinal manifestations. It is usually followed by complete recovery and is only very rarely fatal.

METACHROMATIC LEUCODYSTROPHY – ENCEPHALITIS PERIAXIALIS DIFFUSA

Nature
A disease of unknown aetiology, formerly called *Schilder's disease*, which affects children and is occasionally familial as an autosomal recessive.

Macroscopical
There is progressive involvement of the occipital, temporal, parietal and frontal lobes in that order, with demyelination of the white matter but sparing of the cortical tissue.

Microscopical
Demyelination of the white matter with eventual destruction of axis cylinders which is followed by gliosis. There is cellular infiltration by histiocytes together with perivascular cuffing by lymphocytes and an accumulation of sulphatide in the white matter.

Results
A progressive course with blindness and eventual decortication, terminating fatally. Diagnosis can be made from examination of the urine which shows excess excretion of sulphatide and a metachromatic spot with toluidine blue.

MULTIPLE SCLEROSIS – DISSEMINATED SCLEROSIS

Nature
A relapsing and remitting demyelinating disease of unknown aetiology which is most common in young adults.

Aetiology
This remains unknown but many factors have been incriminated, including virus and slow virus infections (see p. 608), hypoxia, chemical poisons and allergy. None of these agents, however, have been substantiated as causative.

Incidence
A fairly common disorder responsible for about 1000 deaths in England and Wales annually.

Macroscopical
The disease is primarily one of patchy plaques of demyelination of the white matter of the brain and spinal cord. Recent lesions are soft and pink; the older lesions are grey, firmer and semi-translucent. These plaques show a predilection for the white matter of the brain and spinal cord, especially in the paraventricular regions, the optic nerves, cerebellar peduncles, dorsal tracts of the spinal cord and the brain stem.

Microscopical
The early lesions show demyelination with intact axis cylinders and some oedema. Later, axis cylinder degeneration occurs and there is replacement by gliosis.

C.S.F.

Protein	Glucose	Lange gold curve	Cells
Normal or increased 0.2–1.0	Normal 2.75–4.4	Normal or paretic	Lymphocytes 10–50

Results
The clinical picture is remarkable for its variation in neurological signs due to the scattered and patchy distribution of the plaques, and for its remissions, which become less complete as a progressive amount of C.N.S tissue is involved. The speed of progression varies from a few weeks or months to a more gradual deterioration extending over many years. Ocular disturbances, cerebellar ataxia, posterior column sensory loss, limb spasticity and mental changes are among the more common clinical manifestations. Death usually occurs from intercurrent infection associated with these grave disabilities.

Other disorders of the C.N.S.

WERNICKE'S ENCEPHALOPATHY

Aetiology
Due to thiamine deficiency associated with chronic

alcoholism, hyperemesis gravidarum and other types of prolonged vomiting and with other causes of malnutrition.

Macroscopical
Congestion with a brown discoloration or haemorrhages in the mammillary bodies, the wall of the third ventricle, around the aqueduct of Sylvius and in the floor of the fourth ventricle where the nuclei of the ocular muscles are involved.

Microscopical
The changes are primarily vascular, with proliferation of endothelium resulting in luminal narrowing and with the escape of red blood cells into the surrounding brain tissue. Later, there is gliosis in the untreated cases.

Results
There are general changes of mental confusion together with focal signs, e.g. nystagmus and palsies of ocular muscles.

AMAUROTIC FAMILIAL IDIOCY – TAY–SACHS DISEASE

Nature
A lipid storage disease with accumulation of a ganglioside in nerve cells. A familial disease of recessive inheritance: 1 in 30 carriers are Jews.

Macroscopical
The brain appears firm and smaller than normal.

Microscopical
The cytoplasm of all nerve cells is distended by foamy vacuolated material which can be shown by histochemical methods to be a ganglioside.

Results
Progressive mental deterioration and blindness. The latter is due to retinal involvement which shows the characteristic 'cherry-red' spot at the macula.

HEPATOLENTICULAR DEGENERATION – KINNIER WILSON'S DISEASE

Aetiology
This is a recessively inherited error of metabolism whereby copper is absorbed from the intestine in excessive amounts, and is deposited in the liver cells, in the cornea – Kayser–Fleischer ring, in renal tubular epithelium and in cerebral astrocytes.

Macroscopical
The brain shows a brown discolouration or cavitation of the lenticular nucleus, with similar changes in the tips of the frontal lobes and sometimes in the dentate nucleus.

Microscopical
The histological changes are more widespread than the naked-eye appearances would indicate. The changes are maximal in the lenticular nucleus, especially in the putamen, but they are also present in the thalamus, red nucleus and dentate nucleus. The astrocytes, containing copper pigment, are increased in number and in size and many are multinucleated. Degeneration of the adjacent nerve cells occurs, together with cavitation in the advanced cases.

Results
The neurological disturbances of tremor and rigidity are clinically dominant and are progressive with death, usually from intercurrent infection, before the age of 30. Occasionally, the hepatic lesions may cause death from liver-cell failure (see p. 563).

HUNTINGTON'S CHOREA

Nature
A rare disease, inherited as a Mendelian dominant, of entirely unknown aetiology and which produces symptoms in middle life.

Macroscopical
There is atrophy of the brain, maximal in the cortex and basal ganglia. The caudate nucleus is chiefly involved and, instead of producing the normal convex contour of the lateral ventricular wall, is atrophied to a thin ribbon of tissue. The cerebral cortex, especially of the frontal lobe, is also atrophic.

Microscopical
There is extensive loss of the nerve cells with replacement gliosis in the affected areas.

Results

The disease presents clinically with choreiform movements, but progresses to complete mental and physical incapacity with premature death.

PARKINSON'S DISEASE – PARALYSIS AGITANS

Nature

This common condition, recorded as responsible for nearly 2000 deaths in England and Wales in 1975, may follow encephalitis – post-encephalitic Parkinsonism, but much more commonly presents in the 50–70 age group with tremor and rigidity. The aetiology in this latter group is completely unknown and most cases are unassociated with vascular disease.

Macroscopical

The changes are minimal, but there may be some shrinkage of components of the basal ganglia.

Microscopical

There is loss of nerve cells in the substantia nigra, globus pallidus and sometimes of the putamen and caudate nucleus, but the significance of these changes is poorly understood.

Results

Progressive rigidity (spasticity) and tremor produce great disability. Recently, stereotactic operative procedures with destruction of nerve tracts in the region of the globus pallidus, have been successful in abolishing the tremor and rigidity with astonishingly little neurological deficit.

ALZHEIMER'S DISEASE

Nature

A common cause of dementia due to progressive cortical atrophy from nerve-cell loss and additional features.

Incidence and age

Originally considered to be confined to the elderly, it is now clear that many cases occur in the fourth and fifth decade. Recognition of the condition as a cause of pre-senile as well as senile dementia has recently increased.

Aetiology

Unknown. Though small amounts of amyloid material are present, this is believed to be a secondary effect and not the result of systemic amyloidosis.

Macroscopical

The brain shows diffuse atrophy, particularly of the cerebral cortex with compensating hydrocephalus of non-obstructive communicating type.

Microscopical

1 *Senile plaques* – Eosinophilic fibrillar spheres up to 100 μm in diameter with central hyaline eosinophilic core of amyloid material and radial or haphazard peripheral fibrils.
2 *Neurofibrillary tangles* – These can only be recognized by silver stains or electron microscopy. They are intra-cytoplasmic condensates of neuro-tubules forming a tangled mass of fibrils. They occur mostly in the large cortical cells.
3 *Granulovascular changes* – The cells of the hippocampus in particular contain haematoxyphilic and argyrophilic cytoplasmic granules with non-staining vacuoles.

Results

Progressive nerve-cell loss with increasing atrophy and dementia usually without any localizing neurological signs. Clinical differentiation from other causes of dementia, particularly multi-infarct and other arteriosclerotic changes is often difficult, though pathologically the lesions of Alzheimer's disease are readily identifiable.

C.S.F. Changes in nervous diseases

Examination of the C.S.F. may yield diagnostic information in the investigation of nervous system diseases. The important features of the changes found in certain diseases are given in the table on p. 613.

Disease	Protein	Glucose	Lange gold curve	Cells	Other features
Normal	0.15–0.45 g/l	2.75–4.4 mmol/l	0–0	Up to 5 lymphocytes c.mm	Crystal clear
Suppurative meningitis	Increased 1–10	Decreased 0–2.5	Meningitic	Polymorphs 200–3000	Purulent. Organisms present on Gram's stain and in cultures
Cerebral abscess	Slight increase 0.45–1.0	Normal 2.75–4.4	Normal	Lymphocytes and a few polymorphs 10–100	Marked changes do not occur unless there is rupture of the abscess
Tuberculous meningitis	Increased 0.6–4.0	Decreased 0.5–2.7	Meningitic	Lymphocytes and some polymorphs 50–500	Clear or slightly turbid. 'Spider' clot. Organisms present on ZN-staining
Meningovascular syphilis	Increased 0.6–1.0	Usually normal 2.75–4.4	Paretic or luetic	Lymphocytes 10–500	Positive WR
G.P.I.	Normal or increased 0.3–1.0	Usually normal 2.75–4.4	Paretic	Lymphocytes 40–100	Positive WR
Tabes dorsalis	Normal or increased 0.3–0.8	Normal 2.75–4.4	Weak paretic or luetic	Lymphocytes 10–50	Positive WR
Poliomyelitis Pre-paralytic	Normal 0.15–0.45	Normal 2.75–4.4	Normal	Polymorphs 50% Lymphocytes 50% 100–200	Clear or hazy
Paralytic	Increased 0.45–1.0	Normal 2.75–4.4	Weak paretic or luetic	Lymphocytes 100–150	Slightly hazy
Viral encephalitis	Normal or increased 0.4–1.0	Normal 2.75–4.4	Usually normal	Lymphocytes 50–200	In the early stages there may be polymorphs and lymphocytes
Lymphocytic choriomeningitis	Increased 0.4–1.0	Normal 2.75–4.4	Normal	Lymphocytes 50–1500	Fluid clear or slightly turbid
Multiple sclerosis	Normal or increased 0.2–1.0	Normal 2.75–4.4	Normal or paretic	Lymphocytes 10–50	Clear
Froin's syndrome	Increased 1.0–20	Normal 2.75–4.4	Meningitic	Normal 0–5	Xanthochromia, large clot, Queckenstedt test positive
Cerebral tumour	Usually increased 0.4–1.0	Normal 2.75–4.4	Normal	Normal 0–5	The protein level is variable and occasionally may attain high levels, e.g. acoustic neuroma

Chapter 102
Nervous System – Spinal Cord and Peripheral Nerves

Spinal cord

SPINAL CORD COMPRESSION – CAUSES

Bone disorders	*Extra-medullary*		*Intra-medullary*
Fracture-dislocation	Neurofibroma	Secondary carcinoma,	Gliomas,
Crush fracture	Schwannoma	e.g. breast, bronchus and	especially
Prolapsed intervertebral disc	Meningioma	prostate	ependymoma
	Tuberculosis	Paget's disease	
	Osteoporosis	Tumour deposits	
	Myeloma	Extradural abscess	
	Primary bone tumours	Gumma	

Pathogenesis

The spinal cord may be compressed by direct pressure; venous obstruction may cause oedema and impairment of function; or arterial occlusion, with ensuing ischaemia, may produce necrosis and transection of the cord.

Macroscopical

The affected area of the cord is swollen and softened or distorted by compression. In prolonged compression with blockage of the spinal C.S.F., there is xanthochromia below the site of the block – *Froin's syndrome.*

C.S.F.

Protein	Glucose	Lange gold curve	Cells	Other features
Increased 1–20	Normal 2.75–4.4	Meningitic	Normal 0–5	Xanthochromia, large clot, Queckenstedt test positive

Effects

1 *At the site of compression.* The affected segment shows colliquative necrosis as a sequel of ischaemia. The local lesion produces motor or sensory disturbances of root distribution in the areas supplied by the necrotic segment.

2 *Below the site of compression.* There is a descending degeneration of the motor tracts to give upper motor neurone signs below the level of the compression (see Fig. 74).

3 *Above the site of compression.* There is an ascending degeneration of the sensory pathways, causing sensory loss below the level of the lesion (see Fig. 74).

Staining reactions

In the early stages of ascending or descending tract degeneration, the myelin sheath breaks up into multiple fatty globules stainable by Marchi's method. The myelin is not completely oxidized by the bichromate solution and is thus able to reduce perosmic acid. These degenerated areas, therefore, stain black and this reaction will remain positive for several months until all the myelin has been absorbed.

In the late stages, Weigert–Pal or Loyez staining techniques are employed. These methods stain normal myelin black so that the degenerated tracts appear as pale areas in the sections.

SYRINGOMYELIA

Nature

A rare disease, mainly of young adults and probably of developmental origin, in which there is gliosis and cavity formation in the cord, usually presenting clinically as 'dissociated' anaesthesia.

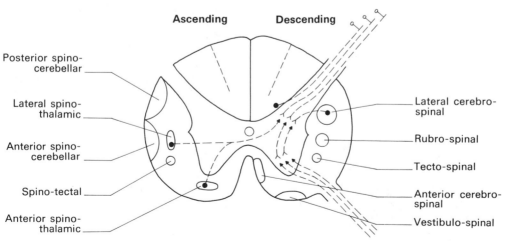

Fig. 74. Spinal cord showing the normal sites of nerve tracts, motor on the right and sensory on the left. The diagram also indicates the tracts affected by ascending and descending degeneration in spinal cord compression.

Macroscopical

The changes in the cord are usually confined to the cervical region, but may extend into the medulla – *syringobulbia*, or also occasionally involve the lumbar region. The cord at the site of involvement is tense and swollen with thickening of the meninges. On section, there is a cyst occupying several segments of the cord which, in early cases, is anterior to the central canal. As it enlarges, the cord becomes grossly deformed with compression of many of the spinal cord tracts.

Microscopical

The cyst has no connection with the central canal and no ependymal lining. The cavity is of variable size and has a glial wall. It appears that the gliosis precedes the cavitation.

Effects

1 The fibres of pain and temperature which cross the cord to pass up the spinothalamic tracts are interrupted, hence there is loss of pain and temperature sensation in the hands (see Fig. 75).

2 The fibres of touch and vibration sense pass up the posterior columns of the same side and remain normal; thus the sensory loss is 'dissociated' (see Fig. 75 (*a*)).

3 As the cyst enlarges, pressure on long tracts, especially the pyramidal tract, produces signs of an upper motor neurone lesion in the legs (see Fig. 75 (*b*)).

4 The anterior horn cells also become involved in the affected segments producing a lower motor neurone lesion in the arms (see Fig. 75 (*b*)).

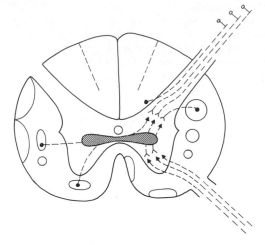

Fig. 75b. Syringomyelia – effects in the later stages.

Results

Progressive neurological loss and great disability over a course of many years. The anaesthesia predisposes to severe 'trophic' ulceration of the hands and neuropathic arthropathy – Charcot's joints, e.g. the shoulder (see p. 710).

MOTOR NEURONE DISEASE

Nature

A disease of unknown aetiology, usually presenting insidiously between 35–50 years of age, and characterized by degeneration of the anterior horn cells of the spinal cord, cells of the cranial motor nuclei and the fibres of the pyramidal tracts.

Types

Depending on the predominant site of involvement and on whether upper or lower motor neurones are maximally involved, there are four main clinical types:

Spinal Cord

Progressive muscular atrophy – lower motor neurone lesion predominates.

Amyotrophic lateral sclerosis – upper motor neurone lesion predominates.

Brain Stem.

Progressive bulbar palsy – lower motor neurone lesion predominates.

Pseudo-bulbar palsy – upper motor neurone lesion predominates.

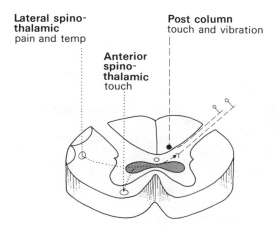

Lateral spino-thalamic
pain and temp

Post column
touch and vibration

Anterior spino-thalamic
touch

Fig. 75a. Syringomyelia – effects in the early stages.

PROGRESSIVE MUSCULAR ATROPHY

Appearances
There is a diminution in the size of the anterior horns and the peripheral nerves, resulting in wasting of muscles. The disease usually starts in the cervical region of the cord with muscle atrophy maximal in the hands. The anterior horn motor cells disappear and are replaced by glial tissue. The motor nerves and muscles are atrophied (see Fig. 76).

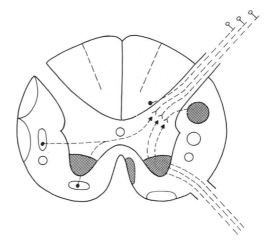

Fig. 77. Amyotrophic lateral sclerosis – site of spinal cord lesions.

frequently the tenth, seventh and the motor nucleus of the fifth. This is associated with degenerative changes of the pyramidal tracts. Clinically, therefore, the tongue, lips, larynx and pharynx are maximally involved.

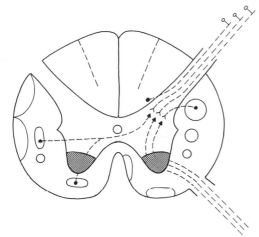

Fig. 76. Progressive muscular atrophy – site of spinal cord lesions. In poliomyelitis similar areas are affected (see p. 605).

AMYOTROPHIC LATERAL SCLEROSIS

Appearances
There are degenerative changes of both the anterior horn cells producing a lower motor neurone lesion, and of the long motor tracts causing an upper motor neurone lesion. The pyramidal tracts are maximally involved, but the anterior and lateral white columns are also degenerate; however, the posterior columns are spared (see Fig. 77).

BULBAR PALSY

Appearances
In the bulbar forms, there is degeneration of the cranial nerve nuclei in the pons and medulla affecting especially the eleventh and twelfth and

RESULTS OF MOTOR NEURONE DISEASE

In all types, the disease is progressive with death resulting in 2–5 years from the time of diagnosis.

FRIEDREICH'S ATAXIA

Nature
An hereditary autosomal recessive disease which presents at about the time of puberty and is progressive.

Macroscopical
The cord is smaller than normal, especially in the lower segments.

Microscopical
There is degeneration of the posterior and lateral white columns with a replacement gliosis of a characteristic whorled pattern. In addition, there is involvement of the spinocerebellar tracts and atrophic posterior roots (see Fig. 78).

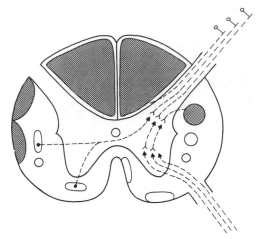

Fig. 78. Friedreich's ataxia – sites of spinal cord lesions.

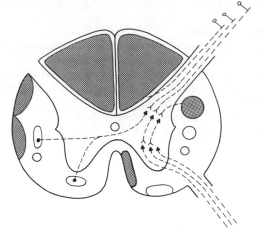

Fig. 79. Subacute combined degeneration of the cord – sites of spinal cord lesions.

Results

These patients develop scoliosis and pes cavus with progressive pyramidal and posterior column signs. They are completely disabled within a few years of the onset. Death is frequently due to an associated myocarditis in which there is necrosis of the myocardial cells and increased fibrosis (see p. 239).

SUBACUTE COMBINED DEGENERATION OF THE CORD

Aetiology

A peripheral neuritis and cord degeneration found only in cases of pernicious anaemia and curable in the relatively early stages by the administration of vitamin B_{12} (see p. 482).

Appearances

There is a patchy degeneration involving the long tract fibres of the posterior columns and later the pyramidal tracts, particularly in the thoracic segments. Histologically, there is phagocytosis of degenerate myelin sheaths and later degeneration of axis cylinders but no gliosis. Similar changes occur in the peripheral nerves.

Results

The peripheral neuritis produces paraesthesiae of the hands and feet with evidence of diminished vibration sensation or sensory ataxia due to posterior column involvement (see Fig. 79). At a later stage, the pyramidal tract signs become evident.

Administration of adequate doses of vitamin B_{12} is curative unless the disease has long been neglected. Folic acid cures the megaloblastic anaemia, but may unmask the neurological condition or make it worse (see p. 483).

Peripheral nerves

Structure

Peripheral nerves are composed of axons of motor or sensory fibres with sheath (neurilemmal) cells and interstitial connective tissue. The cell bodies are in the spinal cord ganglia (see Fig. 80). Blood supply by the vasa nervosum is within the outer fibrous sheath.

TRAUMA

The commonest cause of peripheral nerve disease is injury produced by direct severance, pressure or traction. When a peripheral nerve is injured the following changes occur:

1 *Proximal end*. There is proximal degeneration of the myelin sheaths for one or two segments above the line of section. The sheath (Schwann or neurilemmal) cells subsequently proliferate, accompanied by growth of the axis cylinders towards the distal portion of the cut nerve. If there is a gap – '*union gap*', between the severed ends of the nerve, a nodule of proliferating fibrous tissue will

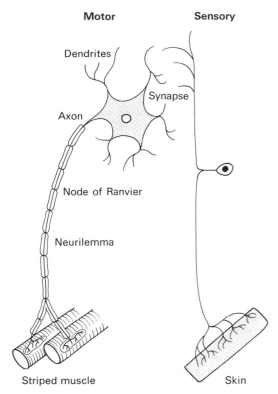

Motor   Sensory

Dendrites

Synapse

Axon

Node of Ranvier

Neurilemma

Striped muscle   Skin

Fig. 80. Motor and sensory neurones.

form containing axis cylinders and sheath cells – 'traumatic neuroma'. This delays functional regeneration of the nerve.

2 *Distal end.* The distal portion of the nerve undergoes Wallerian degeneration. The axis cylinders swell and disintegrate, whilst the myelin breaks up to be phagocytosed by histiocytes and sheath cells; the myelin at this stage can be demonstrated by the Marchi method. The sheath cells proliferate and the degenerate material is absorbed. At a later stage, the sheath cells become rearranged in linear fashion and are then in a position to receive the regenerated axons growing from the proximal end.

Results

If the severed portions are closely apposed and correctly orientated, the regenerating nerve axons, derived from the proximal end, will successfully grow down the columns of sheath cells at the rate of between 1–2 mm/day and a satisfactory functional end-result ensue. If the 'union gap' is large or as a

result of an 'amputation neuroma' or interposition of other tissues, the regenerating axons will fail to pass down the nerve sheaths. Thus, the motor and sensory end-plates will not become re-innervated and the functional result will be poor.

POLYNEURITIS – PERIPHERAL NEURITIS

Nature
Impairment of the motor and/or sensory function of peripheral nerves commonly presenting clinically with pain, paraesthesiae and muscular weakness.

Aetiology
There are many causes including:
1 *Poisons*
(a) Organic, e.g. carbon bisulphide, sulphonal, chloral, chloretone, aniline and sulphonamides.
(b) Metals – arsenic, copper, mercury, antimony, phophorus, bismuth and lead.
(c) Drugs e.g. nitrofurantoin, isoniazid.
2 *Metabolic diseases*, e.g. diabetes mellitus, porphyria, pernicious anaemia, myxoedema, amyloid disease.
3 *Nutritional diseases*, e.g. starvation, beriberi and other vitamin-deficiency disorders, alcoholism, malabsorption syndromes, pregnancy.
4 *Infective.* Leprosy, diphtheria, tetanus, toxic effects of many acute or chronic infections.
5 *Guillain–Barré Syndrome–Landry's Paralysis.* Acute, rapidly progressive, predominantly motor paralysis, with very high protein levels in C.S.F. (0.4–2.0 g/l) without cells. Comparison with allergic experimental neuritis suggests an immunological basis.
6 *Connective tissue diseases*, e.g. rheumatoid arthritis, polyarteritis nodosa.
7 *Malignant disease.* Malignant neuropathy, which is most commonly associated with carcinoma of the bronchus.

Appearances
In the early stages the nerves may show no histological abnormality but later there is Wallerian degeneration with breakdown of myelin which is phagocytosed by hyperplastic Schwann cells and histiocytes. The changes are non-specific and do not indicate the aetiological agent.

Results

Although the distribution of affected nerves varies from case to case and from cause to cause, the symptoms and signs are usually symmetrical and most marked in the extremities. If the cause of the disease is corrected, regeneration of the axons usually occurs with restoration of function, although in severe cases there may be some residual functional deficit.

TUMOURS OF PERIPHERAL NERVES

Tumours of peripheral nerves include neurofibroma and neurofibromatosis, schwannoma and ganglioneuroma as well as their malignant counterparts.

'Traumatic neuroma' is often included as a tumour but this is a nodule on a nerve following section or injury and is formed by proliferating sheath cells, fibroblastic tissue and regenerating axons and is thus a reparative and not a neoplastic condition (see p. 618).

NEUROFIBROMA

Nature

A tumour of peripheral nerves probably arising from the peri- or endo-neural fibrous tissue; however, some authorities regard it as derived from Schwann cells.

Sites

These may be single but are frequently multiple and may be numerous in neurofibromatosis – von Recklinghausen's disease. They most commonly occur on the cranial and spinal nerve roots, the large nerves of the neck and trunk and also on the smaller nerves of the dermis, viscera and limbs. Nerves of the autonomic system may also be the site of formation of neurofibromas.

Macroscopical

A diffuse, irregular, cylindrical swelling of the nerve which is soft and elastic. On section it is pale and has poorly defined borders which frequently merge with adjacent tissues.

Microscopical

The tumour is comparatively acellular and is composed of wavy bundles of fibroblastic cells with long thin nuclei, separated by a loose connective tissue in which groups of nerve fibres are readily visible. Large vascular channels, areas of cystic and myxomatous degeneration and foam cells are seldom seen.

Results

The nodules slowly increase in size and may cause pressure effects, e.g. on the spinal cord. Malignant transformation to neurofibrosarcoma may occur in a very small proportion of cases of solitary neurofibromas.

NEUROFIBROMATOSIS – VON RECKLINGHAUSEN'S DISEASE

Nature

A familial condition transmitted as an autosomal dominant of incomplete penetrance, in which there are numerous neurofibromas of variable size on many of the cranial or peripheral nerves.

Appearances

The nodules usually show the appearance of neurofibromas but some are Schwannomas and the condition is frequently associated with one or more of the following abnormalities:
1 Intracranial Schwannomas.
2 Intraspinal Schwannomas.
3 Skin pigmentation – '*café au lait*'.
4 Elephantiasis, due to hamartomatous connective tissue overgrowth.
5 Gliomas of brain and spinal cord.
6 Meningiomas.
7 Bone rarefaction.
8 Kyphoscoliosis.
9 Neurofibrosarcoma.

Results

The distribution of the lesions and clinical features are extremely variable but most cases are diagnosable in young adult life. The tumours grow slowly over many years and one or more may ultimately become sarcomatous in about 5–10 per cent of cases.

SCHWANNOMA – NEURILEMMOMA

Nature

A tumour derived from the Schwann cells of the nerve sheath. Usually solitary occasionally multiple it with von Recklinghausen's disease.

Sites
1 *Intracranial.* Most occur on the auditory nerve in middle-aged females, less commonly on the trigeminal nerve. The acoustic Schwannomas, which form about 8 per cent of all primary intracranial tumours, arise at the internal auditory meatus, expanding the bony foramen and, as they increase in size, produce a mass in the cerebellopontine angle deforming and indenting the cerebellum and brain stem.

2 *Spinal.* These arise mainly from the posterior nerve roots in the thoracic region and slowly enlarge to indent the spinal cord. Occasionally, the tumour grows through the intervertebral foramen to produce a tumour mass inside and outside the spine in continuity through the enlarged foramen – 'dumb-bell' or 'hour-glass' tumour.

3 *Peripheral nerves.* Schwannnomas occur less frequently than neurofibromas on peripheral nerves. The main nerve trunks in the neck and the smaller nerves on the flexor aspects of the limbs are the sites of election, whilst the posterior mediastinum is a common site for a tumour arising from the intercostal nerves.

Macroscopical
The tumours are firm, encapsulated and discrete. The nerve bundles are usually stretched over the capsular surface of the tumour and do not extend into the tumour substance to the same extent as in neurofibroma. On section the tumour is pale, myxomatous, and is frequently vascular with yellow or cystic areas.

Microscopical
Two types of tissue patterns are seen usually mixed in the same tumour:

1 *Antoni type A.*—Compact interwoven fascicles of spindle cells often with a palisaded appearance.

2 *Antoni type B*—A looser texture often with degeneration, pleomorphism and plumper cells. Foam cells, haemosiderin pigment and proliferated abnormal blood vessels are often noted.

Results
The intracranial and spinal tumours slowly increase in size and indent the adjacent C.N.S. tissue with increasing symptoms of compression, but only rarely does malignancy supervene. In the peripheral nerves, the growth is usually extremely slow, although rarely more rapid growth, with atypical cellular proliferation and giant cell forms in the tumour, indicates malignant transformation.

GANGLIONEUROMA

Nature
Benign tumours of the autonomic nervous system.

Origin
They arise from sympathetic nerve tissue and contain ganglion cells.

Incidence
Rare; they mostly occur in young adults below the age of 30.

Sites
Most are found in the posterior mediastinum, less commonly in the abdomen where they may arise from any sympathetic nerve, or from the adrenal medulla.

Macroscopical
Large, firm, encapsulated, spherical tumours which sometimes show mucoid areas.

Microscopical
Composed of a myxomatous fibrous stroma incorporating both nerve fibres and large, mature, ganglion cells.

Results
These are slowly growing benign lesions and only produce symptoms when they have attained a large size in the chest or abdomen. They are often chance radiological findings within the chest, whilst others may extend intrathecally through an intervertebral foramen as an 'hour-glass' tumour and then produce cord compression.

GANGLIONEUROBLASTOMA

This is a rare tumour intermediate in differentiation between the benign ganglioneuroma and the highly malignant neuroblastoma. Although it usually appears encapsulated and may appear macroscopically similar to a ganglioneuroma, neuroblasts are present in addition to ganglion cells, nerve fibres and connective tissue stroma. The behaviour of such tumours is unpredictable but many are frankly malignant.

NEUROBLASTOMA

These rare and highly malignant tumours of neuro-blasts arise most commonly in the adrenal medulla, although they may also be found in the posterior mediastinum and at other sites where there is sympathetic nerve tissue. They are described on p. 295.

Chapter 103
Nervous System – Tumours

INTRODUCTION

The histogenesis of the tumours arising from the nervous system has been the subject of very considerable study and many complex concepts have been suggested. From these, elaborate classifications of tumours based on the many stages in the normal development of C.N.S. tissues have been propounded, resulting in a profusion of names, particularly in respect of tumours of glial cells.

It is generally agreed that most of the C.N.S. tissues arise from primitive neural epithelium – neuroectoderm, which subsequently differentiates in different directions and through numerous stages to produce, in mature form, two main types of cell:

1 Nerve cells.
2 Glial cells.

Tumours of nerve cells within the C.N.S. are exceedingly rare and more than 45 per cent of intracranial tumours are gliomas, i.e. tumours of glial origin.

Primary brain tumours are responsible for about 2 per cent of all deaths from malignant disease.

Gliomas

Classification

This is schematically represented in Fig. 81.

ASTROCYTOMA

Incidence

Approximately 75 per cent of gliomas fall within this group, in which there is marked variability in both their appearance and in their degree of malignancy.

Age

They occur mostly in adults but occasionally in children.

Sites

Usually in the cerebral hemispheres in adults and in the cerebellum in children.

Macroscopical

Indistinctly demarcated or grossly infiltrative tumours which are grey in colour, firmer than the surrounding brain tissue and vary in size from a few centimetres in diameter, to those which occupy a whole lobe. They are commonly haemorrhagic with areas of necrosis and extensive oedema in and around the tumour mass. Cystic changes occur, particularly in the less malignant types, and in the tumours of children there may be only a small tumour nodule in the wall of a relatively large cystic cavity.

Microscopical

They can be subdivided on their histological appearances into Grades I–IV in ascending degrees of malignancy.

Grade I astrocytoma – Fibrillary or protoplasmic astrocytoma. The tumour shows an increased cellularity due to an excess of astrocyte cell bodies and fibres which form a felted mass of processes somewhat thicker than those of normal adult astrocytes. Individually, however, the cells closely resemble mature astrocytes and are regular with no pleomorphism or giant cells.

Grade II astrocytoma – Astroblastoma. The cells are still recognizable as astrocytes, but are more abundant than in the Grade I tumours and there is some variation in cell size, although mitoses are, at the most, scanty.

Grades III and IV astrocytoma. These are by far the commonest types, forming 50–60 per cent of gliomas. The Grade III tumours still show recognizable astrocytes but pleomorphism is marked, mitoses are present and occasional giant cell forms are seen. Proliferation of the endothelial cells of blood vessels is present.

Grade IV tumours are extremely cellular and

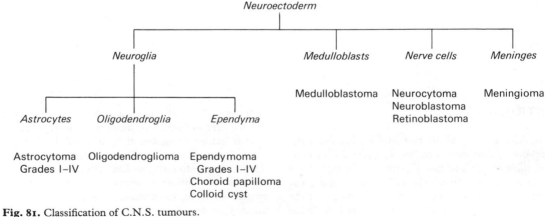

Fig. 81. Classification of C.N.S. tumours.

only very occasional cells are recognizable as astrocytes. Pleomorphism, mitoses, giant cell forms and endothelial cell proliferation are all prominent.

Behaviour
All astrocytomas are malignant but the prognosis varies according to the grade:

Grade I – may survive for many years.

Grade IV – usually survive only weeks or a few months.

Glioblastoma Multiforme
Though often used synonymously with Grade IV astrocytoma, these rapidly growing pleomorphic gliomas may sometimes be derived from glia other than astrocytes.

EPENDYMOMA

Origin
Tumours arising from the lining cells of the ventricles, central canal of the spinal cord or from the choroid plexus, the cells of which have an ependymal origin.

Incidence
About 10 per cent of gliomas.

Age
Average 25–30 years of age but they can occur in children, where they usually arise in the cerebellum.

Sites
Fourth ventricle, thoracic portion of spinal cord and also in relation to other ventricles.

Macroscopical
The appearances are variable and they may be cystic, papillary or solid. The commonest is the solid type which is seen as an infiltrating, grey, homogeneous, softish mass adjacent to a ventricle. Fifteen per cent contain areas of calcification.

Microscopical
This is also very variable and the tumours may be divided into Grades I-IV of malignancy as with the astrocytomas according to their cytological features of pleomorphism, mitoses, etc. Fifty per cent are in Grades I or II. The commonest histological appearance is that of a cellular solid mass of uniform oval-shaped cells with indistinct cell membranes and pseudo-rosette formation – solid or cellular ependymoma. Grades III and IV are composed of similar ependymal cells but with increased anaplasia.

Occasionally, the cells are columnar and epithelial in appearance, resembling those of the normal ependyma – *epithelial type*. In these, tubules or acinus formation may be prominent. A rare type is that with a papillary structure around cores of mucoid material – *myxo-papillary type*. Tumours of the choroid plexus in infants are often of large size within the ventricle of origin and resemble the normal choroid – *choroid papilloma*.

Variants
Ependymoblastoma. Grade IV ependymomas are sometimes known by this name.

Colloid cysts. Thin-walled cysts, usually in the third ventricle, filled with mucoid material. The lining tissue resembles the normal choroid.

Behaviour
Colloid cysts. Benign, slowly growing lesions, but they obstruct the C.S.F. circulation and are surgically inaccessible.

Choroid papilloma. Slowly growing and of low-grade invasiveness but they frequently give rise to seedling deposits in the spinal theca via the C.S.F.

Others. The behaviour varies according to the grade. The group are more slowly growing than astrocytomas with an 80 per cent 3-year survival but all are malignant and the eventual prognosis is extremely poor.

OLIGODENDROGLIOMA

Incidence
Approximately 5 per cent of gliomas.

Age
Occur almost exclusively in adults

Sites
Usually situated in the cerebrum, commonly in the white matter of the frontal lobe.

Macroscopical
Grey tumours of soft consistency which may be very large; 20 per cent are cystic but necrosis and haemorrhages are rare. They often appear well

demarcated and frequently contain substantial amounts of calcium.

Microscopical
A cellular tumour with little or no stroma. The cells are small with regular nuclei and the cytoplasm stains poorly giving a halo or 'boxed-in' appearance.

Variant
Oligodendroblastoma. Moderately pleomorphic with a less orderly cellular arrangement and a greater degree of malignancy.

Behaviour
Slowly growing tumours which are locally infiltrative. The natural history is an approximate 50 per cent 5-year survival with tumour present, but the ultimate prognosis is poor.

MEDULLOBLASTOMA

Origin
It is probable that these tumours arise from residual foetal cells of the cerebellar external granular layer which normally migrate inwards to augment the neurones of the cerebellum. These are thus really tumours of potential nerve cells rather than gliomas, but are usually classified with the latter.

Incidence
Five to seven per cent of gliomas.

Age
Children.

Site
Mid-line of the cerebellum, from the roof of the fourth venticle.

Macroscopical
A soft grey mass connected to the cerebellum and extending into the fourth ventricle, resulting in blockage of the C.S.F. pathway and hydrocephalus. They are non-haemorrhagic, rarely necrotic and often appear encapsulated.

Microscopical
Densely cellular tumours with small, oval, 'carrot-shaped' cells, often clustered around blood vessels to form 'pseudo-rosettes'.

Behaviour
They expand within the cerebellum and commonly seed through the C.S.F. to produce numerous deposits on the surface of the spinal cord. Initially, they are very radiosensitive tumours but the ultimate prognosis is very poor; 15 per cent are alive at 3 years but only 1–2 per cent at 10 years.

Microglioma and lymphomas

The lymphomas seldom involve brain parenchyma but meningeal lesions are more frequently seen in leukaemias, Hodgkin's and non-Hodgkin's lymphomas. A 'primary' lymphoma of the brain – *microglioma or Hortega cell tumour*, is rare and resembles histiocytic lymphoma in other sites (see p. 583).

Pineal tumours

These are very rare but the following types occur:
1 *Pinealoma.* Mostly occur in males between 15–25 years of age. They have a characteristic histological appearance with groups of large 'epithelioid' cells in a background of small dark cells of lymphocytic appearance. This is the commonest type of pineal tumour.
2 *Glioma.* Astrocytoma or ependymoma.
3 *Atypical teratoma – Germinoma.* Although typical teratomas and teratoid tumours occur, the most frequent pineal tumour is a seminoma-like germ-cell tumour.

Nerve cell tumours

Tumours of nerve cells are exceedingly rare within the central nervous system but are more commonly found arising from the autonomic nervous system – ganglioneuroma (see p. 621) and neuroblastoma (see p. 295), and in the retina – retinoblastoma (see p. 342).

NEUROCYTOMA

Nerve-cell tumours are very rare in the brain and consist of neurocytes in a gliomatous stroma.

NEUROBLASTOMA

These are very rare in the central nervous system. They are highly malignant tumours of similar appearance and close histogenetic relationship to the medulloblastomas but contain neuroblasts – primitive nerve cells, which form neurofibrils and have a rosette arrangement. The adrenal neuroblastoma is described on p. 295.

RETINOBLASTOMA

This intra-ocular malignant tumour forms 0.5 per cent of all C.N.S. tumours and is described in the eye section on p. 342.

Blood vessel tumours

'ANGIOMA'

These are not true tumours but are congenital abnormalities, consisting of masses of malformed tortuous vessels of variable size.

Incidence
They form about 2 per cent of intracranial tumours.

Sites
The cerebral hemispheres, often superficially, are the commonest sites but they may also occur in the pons and the midbrain.

Age
Although probably present from birth they frequently do not become clinically manifest until 30–40 years of age.

Macroscopical
May be multiple and associated with similar lesions in the retina – von Hippel–Lindau syndrome (p. 341), the face – Sturge–Weber syndrome, or viscera – Osler's hereditary haemorrhagic telangiectasia (see p. 516). They commonly consist of a mass of tangled blood vessels.

Microscopical
Poorly developed blood vessels with irregular walls which are deficient of muscle.

Effects
1 Space-occupying lesion.
2 Leakage or rupture producing cerebral haemorrhage.
3 Interference with the blood supply to the surrounding brain resulting in areas of cerebral ischaemia.

HAEMANGIOMA

A true benign vasoformative tumour is exceedingly rare in the nervous system and is only slightly more common in the meninges. The tumours may be of the capillary or cavernous type and are described on p. 155.

HAEMANGIOBLASTOMA

A rare but highly cellular neoplasm occurring most frequently in the cerebellum of children. Macroscopically, they are hemispherical cysts with a solid mural nodule and histologically show neoplastic vascular endothelium – together with foam cells containing lipid material. They are slowly growing and clearly demarcated, thus excision may be technically possible and lead to cure, but 10 per cent are multiple.

Meningeal tumours

MENINGIOMA

Incidence
Fifteen per cent of all primary intracranial neoplasms.

Origin
From the arachnoid which is of neuroectodermal origin.

Age
Adults, typically between 45–55 years of age, but can occur at any age.

Sites
They can occur anywhere where there is arachnoid but the common sites are:
1 Parasagittal.
2 Spinal cord.

3 Sphenoidal ridge.
4 Olfactory groove.

Macroscopical

Usually seen as spherical, well-demarcated, homogeneous masses – 'golf ball' tumours, of firm, tough, granular or gritty, grey-coloured tissue. They are attached to the meninges and indent the brain. Occasionally, they arise from the meninges deep within a sulcus and many then appear to be buried within the cerebral substance.

Microscopical

The basic cell is the arachnoid fibroblast which may appear as a spindle cell or as a cell having a more epithelial appearance. Most characteristically, there is a whorled pattern of these cells enclosing a central calcified spherule – *psammoma body*. Others show a more solid epithelial appearance with little fibroblastic tissue – *meningo-epithelial type*, but occasionally a tumour is predominantly fibrous – *fibroblastic type*, or extremely vascular – *haemangiomatous type*.

Behaviour

Ninety per cent are slowly growing, non-invasive masses, dangerous because of their progressive increase in size which produces local pressure effects and indentation of the brain.

Ten per cent are more cellular and show invasion of adjacent brain tissue or the overlying skull.

Variant

A pigmented melanotic variety which behaves like a malignant melanoma is occasionally seen – *melanotic meningioma*.

Secondary tumours

It is probable that at least 20 per cent of intracranial neoplasms are secondary, mostly carcinomas. Any tumour can metastasize to the brain but the common sites of origin are the lung, breast, kidney and malignant melanoma.

Pituitary tumours

These tumours, mostly benign, and accounting for about 15 per cent of all primary intracranial neoplasms, are described on p. 301.

Notochord tumour

Chordoma

Chordomas may arise from the basi-sphenoid and then invade the brain from this site. The features of this tumour are described on p. 719.

Chapter 104
Diseases of the Pancreas

Development

Formed by dorsal and ventral buds which grow from the duodenum and subsequently fuse. The dorsal bud forms from the body and tail and its main duct persists. The ventral bud forms the head of the pancreas and its main duct usually disappears but occasionally persists as the accessory duct of Santorini.

Structure

There are two components:

1 *Exocrine*. A lobular arrangement of groups of acini connected by interlobular ducts which drain into the main pancreatic duct and thence into the duodenum. The cells secrete three groups of enzymes which digest:

(*a*) Protein – trypsin and chymotrypsin.

(*b*) Fat – lipase.

(*c*) Carbohydrate – (amylase) diastase.

The duct epithelium is tall, columnar and mucus-secreting.

2 *Endocrine*. Islets of Langerhans.

(*a*) A cells – formerly α cells – secrete glucagon – 20 per cent.

(*b*) B cells – formerly β cells – secrete insulin – 75 per cent.

(*c*) D cells – formerly δ cells – secrete somatostatin – 5 per cent.

These and other cells in the islets may normally also elaborate gastrin, vasoactive intestinal peptide (VIP) and pancreatic polypeptide (PP).

Congenital

ECTOPIC PANCREAS

Found in 2 per cent of post-mortem subjects as nodules of histologically normal pancreatic tissue in the wall or serosa of the intestine.

Sites

In order of frequency: stomach and duodenum; jejunum; Meckel's diverticulum; ileum.

Size

Usually a few millimeters in diameter but may rarely be up to 4 cm.

Effects

Nearly always asymptomatic but they may rarely cause symptoms from involvement in inflammation or intestinal obstruction. A focus of ectopic pancreas in the gastric wall may be seen in the floor of a gastric ulcer for the origin of which it is conceivably responsible.

ANNULAR PANCREAS

The head of the pancreas encircles the duodenum as a collar and may cause obstructive symptoms. This is due to persistence of the ventral bud of the pancreas.

DUCT ANOMALIES

These are common and may have important surgical implications.

1 Accessory duct of Santorini persists.

2 Main duct drains into the common bile duct.

3 Main duct enters the duodenum above the ampulla of Vater.

4 Main duct is in the situation expected for the accessory duct.

MISCELLANEOUS CONGENITAL ABNORMALITIES

1 Agenesis.

2 Hypoplasia.

3 Persistence of separate dorsal and ventral portions.

Inflammations

ACUTE PANCREATITIS – ACUTE HAEMORRHAGIC PANCREATITIS

Nature

Sudden diffuse enzymatic destruction of the pancreatic substance due to the escape of active, lytic, pancreatic ferments.

Clinical

Presents as an 'acute abdomen' with severe pain, shock and circulatory collapse.

Age

Usually over the age of 40.

Sex

Females more commonly than males, especially when they are obese.

Incidence

Uncommon, but accounts for 400 deaths annually in England and Wales.

Aetiology

The disease is due to the digestive action of liberated enzymes. What triggers off the release of these enzymes is not known with certainty, but factors include:

1 *Reflux of duodenal contents*. There is evidence to suggest that pancreatic enzymes can only be activated by duodenal secretions. Malfunction of the sphincter of Oddi to allow reflux is more common in biliary tract disease, particularly when associated with calculi. Certainly 60 per cent of cases have concomitant biliary system stones.

2 *Alcoholism*. Ethyl alcohol stimulates secretion of pancreatic juice and raises pressure within pancreatic ducts. It also increases protein concentration in pancreatic juice. There is a marked increase in incidence in chronic alcoholics.

3 *Vascular*. Embolism, thrombosis, accelerated hypertension and polyarteritis are all occasionally associated conditions which may initiate pancreatitis through infarction.

4 *Others*. Conditions occasionally complicated by acute pancreatitis are infections (septicaemia), corticosteroid therapy, renal dialysis and hypothermia.

Macroscopical

Peritoneum. Blood-stained peritoneal fluid and areas of omental and mesenteric fat necrosis. These are chalky white or yellow, hard nodules due to lipolytic actions of free lipase on adipose tissue with the liberation of fatty acids and glycerol.

Pancreas. The gland is swollen and firm throughout, with areas of haemorrhage, loss of lobular pattern by necrosis and foci of chalky fat necrosis.

Microscopical

1 Proteolytic destruction of the pancreatic substance causing coagulative necrosis.

2 Necrosis of blood vessels resulting in extensive interstitial haemorrhage.

3 Fat necrosis with granular foamy histiocytes and later foreign body giant cells. Calcium granules are commonly found deposited in these areas.

4 An accompanying inflammatory reaction of polymorphs of variable degree, but usually not marked.

Diagnosis

Serum and urinary amylase levels are raised and are often diagnostic (greater than 800 i units) in the acute phase, but may fall to normal within 12 hours. However an elevated urinary level of amylase may persist for up to 48 hours. Later, there is a fall in the serum calcium level due to its deposition in areas of fat necrosis.

Results

1 *Death*. The mortality rate in severe cases is approximately 50 per cent. Death during the first week is from shock with peripheral circulatory failure. The mortality is reduced by antibiotics, presumably due to reduction of secondary infection.

2 *Resolution*. May occur in mild cases, but it is usually incomplete and associated with areas of residual fat necrosis, fibrosis or cyst formation.

3 *Chronic pancreatitis*.

4 *Suppuration*. Rare.

5 *Gangrene*. A fulminating and fatal type of acute pancreatitis.

ACUTE INTERSTITIAL PANCREATITIS

Mild acute interstitial inflammation may occur in cases of mumps, typhoid, scarlet fever and in infections with Coxsackie viruses. The symptoms are mild and resolution usually occurs.

CHRONIC PANCREATITIS

Aetiology

1 Following acute pancreatitis.

2 Haemochromatosis.

3 Vascular – arteriosclerosis of abdominal arteries.

4 Duct obstruction – calculi or strictures.

5 Idiopathic – the commonest form.

Macroscopical

The gland is firm, fibrous and shrunken, with areas of calcification and duct dilatation or cysts.

Microscopical

Loss of acinar tissue with fibrous replacement and

calcification, often associated with a focal and interstitial lymphocytic infiltration. The islet cells are usually preserved and appear normal.

Results

1 *Steatorrhoea.* In 25–50 per cent of cases.
2 *Mild symptoms.* Recurrent episodes of vague abdominal discomfort – chronic relapsing pancreatitis.
3 *Asymptomatic.*
4 *Diabetes mellitus.* Only rarely follows but when it does, it is characteristically difficult to control.
5 *Obstructive jaundice.* An area of chronic pancreatitis, especially in the head of the organ, may result in a hard fibrotic lesion which compresses the common bile duct. The condition then produces an obstructive jaundice and has to be differentiated from a carcinoma at this site.

Cysts

TRUE CYSTS

1 *Congenital cysts.* Anomalies of development of the pancreatic ducts.
(*a*) *Solitary.* These simple unilocular cysts are lined by a single layer of cuboidal epithelium and are rare.
(*b*) *Multiple.* They are often part of polycystic disease and are then associated with cysts in the liver and kidneys (see p. 351). They are of variable size with walls of fibrous tissue lined by a single layer of flattened or cuboidal epithelium. They are filled with clear mucoid or serous fluid and do not communicate with the duct system.
2 *Retention cysts.* Small, multiple, thin-walled cysts communicating with the duct system and associated with duct obstruction and chronic pancreatitis.
3 *Neoplastic cysts*
(*a*) Cystadenoma – see p. 636.
(*b*) Cystadenocarcinoma – see p. 637.

FALSE CYSTS – PSEUDO-CYSTS

Nature
A collection of fluid in a fibrous-walled space which has no epithelial lining and is usually outside the substance of the pancreas.

Aetiology
1 The majority are associated with a previous acute pancreatitis.
2 Trauma, resulting in an area of pancreatic necrosis followed by cyst formation, causes a few of these lesions.
3 Idiopathic.

Appearances
Solitary and may be large. The contents vary from clear serous fluid to fluid which is bloodstained or purulent. Although it is frequently stated that these cysts do not communicate with the duct system, injection studies have demonstrated that there is a communication from the ducts through the pancreatic tissue into the lumen of the cyst.

Sites
1 Lesser sac of the peritoneum.
2 Peripancreatic tissues.
3 Within the pancreatic substance – rarely.

Cystic fibrosis – mucoviscidosis

Nature
A generalized disease due to the accumulation of thick, viscid mucus in the mucous glands of many organs.

Incidence
Uncommon, but accounts for 3–4 per cent of deaths in children's hospitals and 5 per cent in the white population are carriers. High prevalence in Caucasians of about 1 in 2000 live births but rare in Africans and almost unknown in Asians.

Sex
M:F equal

Aetiology
The cause is unknown but the disease is hereditarily transmitted by a single autosomal recessive gene. Families affected have a 1 in 4 chance of producing affected siblings.

Pathogenesis
The underlying nature is obscure but may result from a single biochemical anomaly – the inhibition of movement of water and electrolytes through secretory cells of affected glands. Patients and

heterozygous carriers of cystic fibrosis show an abnormal metachromasia in cultured fibroblasts.

Clinical

1 *Birth – Meconium ileus.* A plug of viscid mucus and meconium in the intestinal lumen causing intestinal obstruction.
2 *Neonatal*
(a) Failure to thrive.
(b) Respiratory symptoms and infections.
3 *Adolescence.* In mild cases, the patients may survive to adolescence and then present with:
(a) Failure to mature normally.
(b) Chest infections.

Organ changes

GENERAL

Marked emaciation by the time of death with depletion of depot fat and wasting of muscles. Skeletal and body underdevelopment is frequently marked, with skin lesions due to multiple vitamin deficiencies.

PANCREAS

Macroscopical. Progressive shrinkage with replacement by fibrous tissue and dilatation of the ducts which may become cystic. The ducts are blocked by plugs of tenacious mucus.

Microscopical. Duct distension with mucus plugs in the lumen and fibrous replacement of the atrophic acinar tissue. There is a variable lymphocytic infiltration but the islet cells usually remain intact.

LUNGS

Affected in 80–90 per cent of cases.

Macroscopical.
Alternating patches of collapse and emphysema with bronchiolar mucus plugs and secondary infection. Bronchiectasis, bronchopneumonia and lung abscesses may also occur.

Microscopical. The mucous glands of the bronchial and bronchiolar walls are prominent and distended by mucus.

LIVER

Bile in the gall bladder is more viscid than normal and this may lead to chronic obstruction of the bile ducts and biliary cirrhosis.

SALIVARY GLANDS

These are also affected, with atrophy and fibrosis.

Effects

1 Pancreatic insufficiency – steatorrhoea and malabsorption syndromes.
2 Respiratory infections.
3 Biliary cirrhosis.

Diagnosis

1 *Duodenal intubation.* Lack of lipase, trypsin and diastase in the duodenal juice.
2 *Sweat test.* The patients always have excessive sweating, the sweat containing increased concentrations of sodium and chloride.

Prognosis

Poor; most cases are diagnosed a few months after birth, but in spite of the administration of pancreatic enzymes and antibiotics and the maintenance of the child in nutritional balance, few survive beyond 10–15 years of age.

Calculi

Pancreatic stones are relatively common in the older age groups. They consist of calcium carbonate with small amounts of phosphate. Their causation is unknown and many remain asymptomatic although in some cases they cause duct obstruction or chronic pancreatitis.

Pancreatic duct obstruction

Causes

1 *Lumen.* Mucus (cystic fibrosis), calculi, gall stones.
2 *Wall.* Fibrous strictures, tumours, e.g. carcinoma of pancreatic duct.
3 *External.* Acute and chronic pancreatitis, primary carcinoma of the ampulla of Vater, ligature, carcinoma of acinar tissue.

Results

Fibrosis follows the atrophy of the acinar tissue and steatorrhoea may result. The islet cells usually remain normal and thus diabetes is an extremely uncommon sequel.

Diabetes mellitus

Nature

A disease of disordered metabolism due to a relative or absolute deficiency of insulin.

Incidence

This is a common disease affecting about 1 per cent of the population. Diabetes is the certified cause of death in 4000 patients annually in this country but is almost certainly a major contributory factor in the causation of many other deaths certified as due to its cardiovascular or renal complications.

Aetiology

The precise causation of this multifactorial disturbance of carbohydrate metabolism remains obscure, but certain factors are known.

The blood glucose level is controlled by a balance between the amount of circulating insulin and other hormones, including the pituitary growth hormone, adrenal glucocorticoids, glucagon and adrenaline, all of which antagonize insulin action. Insulin secretion from the cells of the islets is stimulated by a rise of blood sugar and inhibited by a fall.

The changes of diabetes are essentially due to a deficiency of available insulin in the tissues. This deficiency can be caused by destruction or removal of pancreatic tissue so resulting in an absolute reduction of insulin production. Alternatively, the insulin deficiency may only be relative when the insulin antagonists are being formed in excess. Thus, diabetes may be symptomatic of the following diseases:

1 *Pancreatic destruction*, e.g. chronic pancreatitis, pancreatectomy, haemochromatosis – causing an absolute reduction.
2 *Adrenal causes*. Due to an excess of glucocorticoids – Cushing's syndrome.
3 *Pituitary causes*. Due to an excess of growth hormone (in respect of its diabetogenic action) produced by the anterior pituitary, e.g. in acromegaly.

The adrenal and pituitary causes result in diabetes from a relative deficiency of insulin but together the above three groups only account for 3 per cent of clinical diabetics. In the remaining 97 per cent the cause of the apparent insulin insufficiency is not due to any known or detectable abnormality. In this, the most common form of diabetes, it appears possible that one or more of the following factors may be operative:

1 There is a decreased secretion of insulin from the cells of the islets.
2 Insulin activity is decreased by an antagonist, possibly associated with some degree of pituitary or adrenal dysfunction.

3 There is a relative deficiency of insulin due to excessive bulk of the tissues, e.g. in obesity.
4 Glucagon, secreted by the A cells of the islets increases gluconeogenesis in experimental circumstances and may be a factor in the production of the raised blood sugar.
5 Some individuals develop immunological reactions to insulin with the development of anti-insulin antibodies.

Other factors

1 *Racial*. The disease is common in Jews and rare in the Chinese.
2 *Heredity*. A familial history is found in 35 per cent of diabetic children (see p. 18).

Age

Classically a disease of middle and late life, but a considerable number of patients are in a younger age group and diabetes may even present soon after birth.

Sex

M:F 1:3.

Clinical

Two groups:
1 *Requiring insulin – Growth-onset type*. Often younger persons who, without insulin, lose weight and develop ketosis.
2 *No insulin required – Maturity-onset type*. Mostly obese and older individuals who only develop ketosis when their disease is complicated by infection. Reduction of the obesity and a controlled diet often leads to correction of the diabetes. The insulin lack is only relative and often sufficient is produced for ordinary requirements, but the reserve is inadequate should obesity, dietary excess or infections occur.

Effects of insulin

1 Lowers the blood sugar.
(a) More rapid transport into cells by alteration of the permeability of the cell membrane.
(b) Facilitates intracellular utilization.
(c) Promotes glycogen storage in liver and muscle.
2 Inhibition of the gluconeogenesis from protein and fat.

These effects are antagonized by adrenal corticosteroids and pituitary growth hormone which stimulate glucose formation from non-carbohydrate sources. The opposite effects are therefore seen in insulin lack with, in severe cases, ketosis, dehydration, acidosis, coma and death.

Appearances

Pancreas. Only very rarely is the diabetes caused by islet cell destruction but this occasionally occurs in haemochromatosis, chronic pancreatitis, carcinoma of pancreas and following surgical extirpation.

In 'idiopathic' diabetes, the pancreas is macroscopically normal and microscopically the islet cells show variable changes:

1 All cases show decrease in total amount of islet tissue mostly loss of B cells.
2 Hyalinization.
3 Hydropic degeneration of B cells.
4 Fibrosis.
5 Degranulation of B cells.

Kidneys. Twenty-five to thirty per cent die of renal failure. The lesions are usually of mixed appearance (see p. 358).

(*a*) Pyelonephritis and papillitis necroticans – due to the general predisposition to infections.
(*b*) Diabetic nephropathy – diffuse or nodular – Kimmelstiel–Wilson lesion.
(*c*) Glycogen infiltration of tubular epithelium.
(*d*) Benign nephrosclerosis.

Cardiovascular. Atherosclerosis develops at an earlier age and progresses more rapidly in diabetics. This may possibly be related to the hypercholesterolaemia (see p. 21).

(*a*) *Heart.* Coronary atheroma; myocardial infarction; hypertension with left ventricular hypertrophy.
(*b*) *Kidneys.* Benign nephrosclerosis.
(*c*) *Brain.* Cerebral atheroma; thrombosis or haemorrhage.
(*d*) *Limbs.* Peripheral arterial narrowing usually due to atheroma and leading to gangrene.

Liver. Fatty change and glycogen infiltration (see p. 548).

Eyes. Cataract, diabetic retinitis, microaneurysms, haemorrhages and microangiopathy (see p. 337).

Skin.

(*a*) Trophic changes in areas of poor blood supply which become infected so that gangrene may supervene, e.g in the feet.
(*b*) Boils, carbuncles, etc., as manifestations of poor resistance to infection.
(*c*) Xanthelasmas – particularly on the eyelids (see p. 326).

Lungs. Infections are common, both non-specific, e.g. bronchopneumonia, and specific, e.g. tuberculosis.

Nerves. Peripheral neuritis (see p. 619).

Causes of death

In approximate order of frequency these are:
1 Myocardial infarction.
2 Cerebral vascular accident.
3 Renal failure.
4 Congestive heart failure.
5 Bronchopneumonia and other infections.
6 Gangrene.
7 Diabetic coma – now very uncommon.
8 Hypoglycaemic coma – overdose of insulin.

Diagnosis

1 *Blood.* A fasting true glucose level of greater than 5.5 mmol/l.
2 *Glucose tolerance test.* Peak values of 8.8 mmol/l or above, with maintenance of a high level and a slow fall.
3 *Urine.* Sugar is present and ketones and acetone may also be found.

Prognosis

1 *Children.* Poor.
2 *Young adults.* Death from atheromatous or renal complications 15–25 years after the onset of the disease.
3 *Adults.* In the older age groups there is only a slight or moderate depreciation of life expectancy.

Haemochromatosis

Nature

A primary disorder of iron metabolism mostly occurring in males and characterized by:
1 Pigmentation of the skin, mostly due to increased melanin in the basal layer but associated with some haemosiderin in the upper dermis.
2 Cirrhosis of the liver.
3 Diabetes mellitus – diabetes is due to haemochromatosis in about 1 in 600 cases.

Pancreas

Brown and firm with haemosiderin deposition in the acinar cells, duct epithelium and islets. There is increased fibrosis and hyalinization of the islets (see p. 562).

Tumours

FIBROMA, LIPOMA, HAEMANGIOMA

All very rare.

ADENOMA AND CYSTADENOMA

Very uncommon. They are composed of regular columnar epithelium with villous processes and cyst-like spaces. They arise from duct epithelium, are solitary and may attain a large size.

ISLET CELL TUMOURS

Adenoma and carcinoma.

Incidence
Uncommon, but important due to their secretory activity.

Age
Most occur between 30–50 years.

Sex
Slightly more common in males.

Macroscopical
Solitary or multiple, small, firm, circumscribed, yellow-brown or red nodules anywhere in the pancreas, but most frequently in the tail. They are multiple in 20 per cent of cases and are commonly very small and difficult to find.

Microscopical
There is reproduction of the cell types of the islet cells. Histologically, it is extremely difficult to distinguish between the benign and malignant types, except in the rare anaplastic tumours. The only real criterion is the development of metastases in lymph nodes, liver, lung or bones.

Endocrine effects
In about 60 per cent of cases of islet-cell tumour there is clinical evidence of excessive hormone (insulin, gastrin, glucagon) secretion. However, there is immunohistochemical evidence that at least some of the remainder may be endocrinologically active, although the clinical effects may be unrecognized.

1 *Insulin-secreting–Insulinoma*. Manifest by attacks of hypoglycaemia. The attacks typically remain undiagnosed for several years.
2 *Gastrin-secreting – Zollinger-Ellison syndrome*. Intractable progressive peptic ulceration in the duodenum or jejunum associated with gastric hypersecretion of up to 100 mEq of hydrochloric acid in a 12-hour overnight sample (see p. 188). The tumours are multiple in 40 per cent and many are malignant. They may be composed of A cells or the tumour cells may contain no granules.
3 *Glucagon-secreting – glucagonoma*. Rare tumours of A cells which result in a syndrome of diabetes mellitus with an unusual serpiginous skin rash.
4 *Vasoactive-intestinal-peptide secreting – VIPoma – Werner Morrison syndrome*. Intractable watery diarrhoea follows excessive secretion of VIP, with profound hypokalaemia and alkalosis. In 20–30 per cent of cases, the pancreatic islet-cell tumour is accompanied by adenomas of one or more other endocrine glands including parathyroid and pituitary – multiple endocrine adenoma (MEA 1) syndrome (see p. 317).

Behaviour
1 Eighty per cent – morphologically and clinically benign.
2 Ten per cent – morphologically malignant but clinically benign.
3 Ten per cent – morphologically and clinically malignant.

CARCINOMA OF THE PANCREAS

Incidence
Moderately common. Tumours in this site are stated to cause 3–4 per cent of deaths from malignant disease, but such a figure probably includes tumours of the ampulla of Vater and the bile ducts.

Age
Average 55–65 years.

Sex
M:F 2:1.

Sites
1 Head – 60 per cent.
2 Body – 25 per cent.
3 Tail – 15 per cent.

Macroscopical

Infiltrating, hard, white, irregular masses with early involvement of neighbouring structures. They may be quite small and yet have massive and extensive metastases. Cystic tumours – cystadeno-carcinomas, also occur.

Microscopical

ADENOCARCINOMA
1 Mucus-secreting, of duct origin.
2 Acinar origin without mucus secretion.

Spread

1 *Direct*. Invasion of adjacent organs, particularly the duodenum, common bile duct with obstructive jaundice, and the spine.
2 *Lymphatic*. Usually occurs early and is found in 75 per cent of fatal cases.
3 *Blood*. Common and early with metastases in the liver and lungs, particularly.
4 *Peritoneum*. Invasion of the peritoneum by tumours in the body or tail, may cause carcinomatosis peritonei.

Effects

1 *Biliary obstruction*. Obstructive progressive jaundice which is classicially stated to be painless but, in fact, pain is present in 75 per cent of cases although not usually colicky in nature. Eventually, biliary cirrhosis may develop if the patient lives for a sufficient length of time (see p. 564).
2 *Pancreatic obstruction*. This is seldom clinically relevant.
3 *Portal vein obstruction*. With thrombosis a common sequel.
4 *Diabetes mellitus*. Occurs in about 5 per cent.

Prognosis

Very poor and most patients are dead within 6 months of the time of diagnosis. A few long-term survivors occur following surgery.

SECONDARY TUMOURS

Infrequent, except by direct spread from the stomach. Surrounding lymph nodes are commonly invaded by lymphomas and secondary carcinomas, when the resulting masses may produce any of the obstructive effects of a primary pancreatic tumour.

Chapter 105
Respiratory System – Nose : Nasal Sinuses: Nasopharynx : Larynx

Nose : nasal sinuses : nasopharynx

RHINOPHYMA

Nature
An enlargement and deformity of the nose associated with acne rosacea and occurring in patients with seborrhoea. It is often, but falsely, regarded as alcoholic in causation.

Macroscopical
The nasal skin is irregularly thickened with associated erythema, telangiectases and a mottled dusky discoloration.

Microscopical
Dilatation of the sebaceous ducts which are filled with epithelial debris and inspissated sebaceous material. The sebaceous acini show hypertrophy and the surrounding dermal tissues are fibrotic and infiltrated with lymphocytes.

Results
The overgrowth of sebaceous glands and the associated scarring result in the visible deformity which is surgically remediable.

ACUTE RHINITIS

Aetiology
Inflammation of the nasal mucosa due to viruses, e.g. the common cold, by bacteria, or by allergens – *vasomotor rhinitis*. These all produce the clinical condition of 'catarrh'.

Pathogenesis
The initial inflammatory response is usually caused by viruses or allergens, e.g. pollens, bacterial infection being secondary to breakdown of the local defence barriers.

Macroscopical
In the initial stages the nasal mucosa is red, oedematous and swollen with enlargement of the turbinates. The mucosal surface is bathed by a watery or mucoid fluid which becomes mucopurulent when secondary bacterial infection supervenes.

Microscopical
At an early stage there is marked oedema of the submucosa with vascular dilatation, hyperactivity of the mucous glands and a sparse inflammatory infiltration with eosinophils predominating in the allergic types. The onset of bacterial invasion produces a marked polymorph infiltrate.

Results
If the bacterial infection persists, frank suppuration with mucosal ulceration may ensue. However, more frequently the inflammatory exudate resolves and the nasal mucosa returns to normal. In some individuals the inflammatory process persists in a chronic form to result in fibrous scarring of the nasal submucosal tissues, diminished vascularity, atrophy of the mucous glands and atrophy or squamous metaplasia of the surface epithelium. These changes lead to a dry, shiny appearance of the nasal mucosa with lack of normal secretions – *atrophic rhinitis*.

RHINOSCLEROMA – SCLEROMA

Nature
A chronic infectious disease of the nose and upper respiratory tract associated with the production of hard plaques and nodular masses. The disease is due to *Klebsiella rhinoscleromatis* and responds to antibiotic therapy. It is endemic in Mediterranean countries and also in some areas of Central Europe, e.g. Poland. Histologically, these short gram-negative rods can be demonstrated in the large foamy histiocytic cells which are diagnostic – *Mikulicz's cells*.

RHINOSPORIDIOSIS

Nature
A fungus infection of the nasal mucosa, due to *Rhinosporidium seeberi*, which is endemic in India and Ceylon and occurs sporadically elsewhere. Polypoid masses containing the double-contoured sporocysts in a fibroblastic stroma remain localized to the nose.

SINUSITIS

Aetiology
The aetiological factors are similar to those previously described for acute rhinitis, i.e. viral,

allergic or bacterial. However, the anatomical structure of the air sinuses with a hollow cavity and a narrow draining outlet may produce different end-results. Additionally, the maxillary antrum is frequently infected from tooth sockets or following dental extractions.

Results

1 Blockage of the outlet in the early stages of excess mucus formation may produce a mucocoele or, in the later purulent stages, an empyema.

2 Maxillary sinusitis with suppuration may follow tooth infection directly through the floor of the antrum or the trauma of extraction may perforate the sinus and allow the free access of infected material into the cavity.

3 In any of the nasal sinuses blockage of the drainage outlet may result in increased pressure so that the infection passes through the lining into the surrounding bone and produces an osteomyelitis or periostitis with reactive new bone formation. This may occur in the maxillary area to produce one form of *leontiasis osseum* (see p. 176), but it also occurs in the frontal sinus and results in osteomyelitis of the skull. From this site, infection may spread further via communicating veins to the brain producing cerebral abscess or sometimes a suppurative meningitis (see p. 600).

NASAL AND SINUS POLYPS

Nature
The polyps are not true tumours and probably arise due to longstanding allergic rhinitis.

Macroscopical
Single or multiple gelatinous polyps in the cavities of the nose or sinuses, usually attached to the mucosa by a narrow pedicle.

Microscopical
Benign respiratory type epithelium covering an oedematous connective tissue core infiltrated by eosinophils and commonly showing myxomatous degeneration. Mucous glands are often present.

Results
Polyps commonly produce nasal or sinus obstruction which may lead to secondary pyogenic infection. They are not true tumours and do not predispose to malignancy.

NASOPHARYNGEAL FIBROMA – JUVENILE ANGIOFIBROMA

Nature
Tumour-like masses which develop in the nasopharynx of young boys.

Macroscopical
A polypoid vascular mass filling the nasopharynx or posterior nasal space which bleeds profusely on the slightest manipulation.

Microscopical
Very numerous blood vessels in a loose but sometimes cellular fibrous tissue stroma.

Results
They may extend below the soft palate from their site of origin or into the nasal cavity and rarely into the antrum. They are not malignant and frequently regress when the patient reaches maturity. However, operative procedures are frequently attended by torrential haemorrhage and the space-occupying lesion predisposes to secondary infection of the sinus cavities, bones and soft tissues in the region.

'MALIGNANT GRANULOMA' – MID-LINE GRANULOMA

Nature
A rare, progressive, destructive and ulcerative process affecting the nose, antrum or palate. The lesion is commonly situated in the mid-line.

Types
1 *Arteritic.* The granuloma is associated with a necrotizing arteritis with fibrinoid necrosis. The condition may remain localized to the upper respiratory tract but evidence of polyarteritis nodosa usually develops in other organs, e.g. lungs, kidneys, etc., and the prognosis then becomes that of polyarteritis nodosa (see p. 282).

2 *Wegener's granuloma.* In this type there is also a necrotizing arteritis but in addition there is necrosis of the tissue collagen and the inflammatory reaction contains Langhans' type giant cells. The nasal lesion is, eventually, always associated with cavitating necrotic granulomas of similar appearance in the lungs and other organs. A severe focal and segmental necrotizing, fibrin-rich, proliferative glomerulonephritis with abundant

crescent formation frequently develops with acute renal failure (see p. 363). Untreated the disease is fatal, usually within a year. However, recent experience with cytotoxic drugs and corticosteroids is encouraging for long-term survival.

3 *Lymphoma.* A rather similar ulcerative lesion occurs due to infiltration by non-Hodgkin's lymphoma often of histiocytic type (see p. 583). Even if this appears to be the only clinical manifestation at the time of presentation generalized disease appears to be inevitable.

Tumours of the upper respiratory tract

HAEMANGIOMA

A vascular and frequently polypoid tumour in the nose which may bleed profusely. Secondary infection and ulceration commonly occur.

PAPILLOMA

Nature
A true tumour of the respiratory mucosa.

Macroscopical
A papillary tumour in the nose or sinuses which is often exuberant and multifocal.

Microscopical
The papilloma shows delicate fibrous tissue fronds covered by respiratory or squamous epithelium. The respiratory epithelium readily undergoes metaplasia to the squamous type.

Results
Although initially benign, local recurrences usually occur following excision due to the difficulty of adequate surgical clearance. Frank malignancy as a squamous cell carcinoma, or rarely as an adenocarcinoma, eventually supervenes in a substantial proportion of cases.

CARCINOMA

Types
Carcinomas may arise *de novo* without a preceding papilloma. The majority of these are squamous cell carcinomas arising from metaplasia of the respiratory type mucosa, although rarely there may be a columnar cell adenocarcinoma. Occasionally, 'transitional cell' or 'lymphoepithelioma' types are found, particularly in the nasopharynx (see p. 172).

Results
These tumours usually completely fill the sinus of origin before clinical symptoms become manifest and, in all sites, have usually extended to adjacent structures, e.g. cranial nerves or bone of the base of the skull, by the time of diagnosis. Adequate surgical removal of tumours in these regions is impossible and the 5-year survival is only approximately 10 per cent.

PLASMACYTOMA

Nature
A rare, progressively destructive, plasma cell tumour arising in soft tissues of the upper respiratory and alimentary tracts.

Macroscopical
A polypoid or sessile mass, frequently presenting with nasal obstruction.

Microscopical
Composed of sheets of atypical plasma cells with little supporting stroma.

Results
The tumour slowly destroys and invades the adjacent soft and bony tissues. Many examples remain solitary and are thus not related to multiple myeloma. However, a small proportion do eventually develop terminal manifestations of generalized bone myeloma or rarely involve other soft tissues, e.g. lung, stomach (see p. 470).

NERVE TUMOURS

Rarely, peripheral nerve tumours, e.g. neurofibromas may arise from nerves in the region.

A rare polypoid tumour is composed of gliomatous tissues – *nasal glioma*. This may be due to extension from an intracranial glioma but more frequently arises from ectopic brain tissue in the nose.

MUCOUS GLAND TUMOURS

All types of mucous gland tumours may be found in the nasopharynx, palate and nasal sinuses. In this region the more aggressive adenocystic carcinoma and muco-epidermoid tumour are relatively more common than the pleomorphic adenoma. In view of the anatomical difficulties of adequate surgical excision, the long-term prognosis is often poor (see p. 179).

Larynx

NON-SPECIFIC LARYNGITIS

Aetiology
The larynx is only rarely primarily infected and laryngitis usually follows an upper respiratory infection, e.g. common cold, or streptococcal sore throat, a mouth infection, e.g. thrush, or as part of a generalized laryngotracheobronchitis. A sometimes dangerous and rapidly fatal infection, particularly affecting the epiglottis can occur with *Haemophilus influenzae*.

Appearances
The larynx is smooth, swollen, red and congested due to a non-specific inflammatory reaction.

Results
Laryngeal inflammation usually resolves, but if very severe and accompanied by much swelling, can cause laryngeal stridor which may progress to obstruction. This occurs particularly in young children.

TUBERCULOSIS

This occurs secondarily to active pulmonary tuberculosis and is an example of spread via the natural passages of such an infection (see p. 665). It presents with voice changes and macroscopically shows swelling or ulceration of the cord. Biopsy reveals the tuberculous giant cell systems.

DIPHTHERIA

Nature
Infection of the pharynx and upper respiratory tract by *Corynebacterium diphtheria* is now very rare, following inoculation programmes. The organisms remain superficial, produce a *false membrane* locally and severe toxaemia by a powerful exotoxin which may cause death by myocardial or nerve damage. The local membrane and association oedema may cause respiratory obstruction.

LARYNGEAL NODULE – SINGER'S NODE

Nature
A nodule appearing on the vocal cord alleged to be common in persons who use their voices excessively, hence Singer's node.

Macroscopical
A small, rounded nodule, usually on the anterior part of the vocal cord.

Microscopical
The nodule is covered by benign squamous epithelium with an underlying core of the oedematous and often myxomatous fibrous tissue, but this is variable and may alternatively be extremely vascular or very fibrous. The lesion is thus variously named 'myxoma', 'haemangeioma' or 'fibroma' of the larynx.

Results
The lesion is benign but causes a change of voice; this is remedied by local removal.

Tumours of the larynx

PAPILLOMA

Nature
Papillary lesions of the larynx frequently appear in young persons but the older age groups are not exempt.

Appearances
Squamous cell papillary tumours with an intact basement membrane.

Results
They frequently recur following removal although, histologically, they remain benign for many years. In some cases they progress to invasive carcinoma

after a variable time interval, frequently 10–20 years from the time of first diagnosis.

LEUKOPLAKIA

This condition may affect the vocal cords where it commonly progresses to squamous cell carcinoma after a variable time interval.

'CARCINOMA *IN SITU*'

'Carcinoma *in situ*' rarely occurs in the larynx but has the same significance as in other sites. A proportion of cases, if untreated, will ultimately progress to invasive carcinoma. The lesion produces a change of voice and is cured by local excision.

CARCINOMA OF THE LARYNX

Incidence
About 900 deaths a year in England Wales – 1 per cent of all malignant deaths.

Age
Usually about the age of 60 years.

Sex
M:F 10:1

Sites
The majority (70 per cent) arise from the vocal cords – *intrinsic* carcinomas. The remainder arise from adjacent structures, e.g. epiglottis and aryepiglottic regions – *extrinsic* carcinomas.

Aetiology
A small proportion of cases have evidence of a preceding papilloma, leukoplakia or 'carcinoma *in situ*'. Excessive tobacco smoking has been incriminated.

Appearances
Diffuse, ulcerated or papillary, some show evidence of a pre-existing pre-malignant lesion at the periphery. They are squamous cell carcinomas usually showing some keratin formation.

Spread
Direct. Along the cord and across the anterior commissure to the opposite cord, but the tumour is confined by the laryngeal cartilages for a considerable period of time. It also spreads in a vertical direction to the epiglottis or to the subglottic region.

Lymphatic. Once the tumour extends into the extralaryngeal tissues, metastases to the cervical lymph nodes occur rapidly.

Blood. Blood spread occurs late, usually to the lungs.

Effects
The extrinsic tumours kill by local invasion, by associated secondary infection of the ulcerated tumour or by bronchopneumonia.

Results
The 5-year survival is about 20 per cent, the majority of these being of intrinsic type as they commonly remain confined within the larynx for a longer period and are thus more amenable to treatment.

OTHER TUMOURS

Haemangiomas, chondromas and fibromas occur rarely in this site.

Chapter 106
Respiratory System – Congenital: Inflammations of Trachea and Bronchi: Circulatory

Normal
Bacteriology
Dead space

FUNCTIONS

Ventilation
   Tidal volume
   Vital capacity
   Residual air

Respiratory gas exchange

Congenital

Abnormal fissures

Sequestration segment

Abnormal bronchi

Congenital cystic disease

*Tracheo-oesophageal and
   broncho-oesophageal fistulae*

Congenital alveolar dysplasia

**Inflammations of the
   trachea and the bronchi**

ACUTE TRACHEOBRONCHITIS
Nature
Aetiology
Macroscopical
Microscopical
Results

CHRONIC BRONCHITIS
Nature
Incidence
Aetiology
Clinical
Macroscopical
Microscopical
Effects
Results

BRONCHIAL ASTHMA
Nature
Aetiology
Clinical
Macroscopical
Microscopical
Results

BRONCHIECTASIS
Nature
Incidence
Aetiology
Pathogenesis
Sites
Macroscopical
Microscopical
Results

Circulatory disorders

CHRONIC PASSIVE VENOUS
   CONGESTION
Aetiology
Macroscopical
Microscopical
Results

PULMONARY OEDEMA
Aetiology
Macroscopical
Microscopical

PULMONARY EMBOLISM

PULMONARY INFARCTION
Aetiology
Macroscopical
Microscopical
Results

PULMONARY HYPERTENSION

Secondary

Primary

RESPIRATORY DISTRESS
   SYNDROME
Nature
Pathogenesis
Macroscopical
Microscopical
Results

HYALINE MEMBRANE IN ADULTS
Nature
Causes

Normal

Bacteriology

The lung parenchyma is in direct continuity via the air passages with the external air and yet healthy lung is sterile. This is due to the protective mechanisms of the upper respiratory tract, including nasal hairs, the lymphoid tissue of the oro- and nasopharynx, the cilia of the tracheal and bronchial mucosa, the upwardly directed peristalsis of the large bronchi and trachea and the cough mechanism. All of these promote the expulsion of material from the lungs and maintain cleanliness of the bronchial tree – 'bronchial toilet'.

Dead space

The trachea, bronchi and bronchioles are not static tubes as, with inspiration, their capacity increases due to lengthening and widening. The air contained in the upper respiratory passages and bronchial tree is the dead space air.

FUNCTIONS

Pulmonary functions include:

VENTILATION

This is the function concerned with the movement of air into the alveolar spaces and is produced by action of the respiratory muscles, especially the diaphragm.

Tidal volume. The volume of air inhaled and exhaled during a natural cycle of breath – normally about 500 ml.

Vital capacity. The volume of air expelled by maximal voluntary expiration after a maximal voluntary inspiration – normally about 4000 ml.

Residual air. The volume of air remaining in the lung after forced expiration – normally about 1200 ml.

Diseases can:

1 Reduce the air-containing capacity of the lung by collapse or pathological replacement of lung tissue, or
2 Prevent the flow of air through the respiratory passages by obstruction.

RESPIRATORY GAS EXCHANGE

The diffusion of oxygen and carbon dioxide across the alveolar walls, which is dependent upon the state of the alveoli and their circulation. Thus, oedema fluid, inflammatory exudate or fibrous tissue intervening between the alveolar air and the alveolar capillaries, will diminish respiratory gaseous exchange. Similar effects will be produced by diminution of blood flow.

Congenital

Although these are largely unimportant in this site, minor congenital abnormalities are not uncommon.

ABNORMAL FISSURES

There may be additional fissures, absence of one or more of the normal fissures or extra fissures due to displaced structures, e.g. azygos vein creating the azygos lobe. They are symptomless and unimportant.

SEQUESTRATION SEGMENT

This is a separated segment of lung, associated with an abnormal artery arising from the aorta above or below the diaphragm which supplies an area of the lower part of the lung. The bronchi in this segment are usually dilated or cystic due to their failure to communicate with the main respiratory tract and subsequent retention of secretions.

ABNORMAL BRONCHI

Both supernumerary and abnormally distributed bronchi may occur but are only of significance to the thoracic surgeon.

CONGENITAL CYSTIC DISEASE

Congenital cysts of the lung are bronchial or alveolar in origin. The bronchogenic cysts may be single or multiple, communicating or non-communicating and are lined by bronchial-type mucosa.

Alveolar cysts are also either single or multiple, are frequently multilocular and mostly apical or subpleural in position. Their importance lies in the complications which may occur:

1 *Progressive enlargement*. Resulting in compression of normal lung tissue.

2 *Accumulation of secretions*. Which become infected with resulting lung abscess, empyema or bronchopleural fistula.

3 *Rupture*. With haemoptysis, pneumothorax or haemothorax.

TRACHEO-OESOPHAGEAL AND BRONCHO-OESOPHAGEAL FISTULAE

Rare developmental abnormalities presenting soon after birth with inhalation of food via the fistula into the lung parenchyma (see p. 181).

CONGENITAL ALVEOLAR DYSPLASIA

A rare condition in which there is a failure of alveolar development associated with the presence of excessive interstitial tissue. There is thus a deficiency of functioning lung tissue.

Inflammations of the trachea and the bronchi

ACUTE TRACHEOBRONCHITIS

Nature
An extremely common acute inflammation of the air passages which can be caused by a large number of agents.

Aetiology
1 *Infective*. The more common causative organisms include pneumococci, streptococci, *Haemophilus influenzae*, *H. pertussis*; viruses, e.g. influenza, measles, common cold.

2 *Irritants*. Particulate matter, e.g. dust, atmospheric pollution; chemical irritants, e.g. smoking, industrial fumes.

3 *Allergic*. Protein sensitization may occur in the respiratory tract or may be part of a systemic allergy. In both circumstances there is a predisposition to secondary bacterial infection.

Macroscopical
The mucous membrane is swollen and red producing the appearance of the catarrhal, fibrinous, membranous, haemorrhagic or purulent types of acute inflammation.

Microscopical
Acute inflammation of the tracheal and bronchial mucosa and submucosa together with loss of epithelium and hence of protective cilial action.

Results
1 *Recovery*. With restitution of the mucosa, although the regenerated epithelium may be lacking in cilia.

2 *Chronic bronchitis*. The condition may persist and become chronic.

3 *Bronchopneumonia*. Extension of the infection into the lung parenchyma or interference with the protective mechanisms and subsequent secondary bacterial infection, may result in bronchopneumonia.

CHRONIC BRONCHITIS

Nature
A pathological definition is chronic inflammation of the bronchial tree but, from the clinical point of view, this is frequently enlarged to include most patients with a chronic cough. The restriction of the clinical use of the term to those cases having a productive cough with mucoid sputum for 3 months or more in each year would seem preferable. Because of its close association with emphysema and the lack of correlation between pathological and clinical manifestations, the term *chronic obstructive airways disease* is now widely used.

Incidence
An extremely common and important disease in temperate climates though with some evidence of a recent decline in mortality: in England and Wales from 29 000 in 1965 to 26 000 in 1973. The geographical distribution is closely related to climatic and atmospheric conditions, being most common in the industrial Northern and Midland regions of England and less common in rural areas.

Aetiology
This is predominantly a disease of males which commonly starts in young adults but, although

inflammatory in nature, infection is not constantly present. Many factors are contributory:

1 Tobacco smoking. Cigarette smoking in particular, is probably the most important factor.

2 Repeated attacks of acute bronchitis producing damage to protective mechanisms and thus predisposing to subsequent lung infections.

3 Maintenance of chronic infection in the lower respiratory tract due to chronic infection, often with pus formation, in the upper respiratory tract, e.g. nasal sinuses, nasopharynx.

4 Failure of maintenance of adequate 'bronchial toilet', associated with concomitant disease, e.g. bronchiectasis.

5 Chronic irritation produced by inhalation of particulate matter and chemicals in the polluted atmosphere, and by cold damp climates.

6 Maintenance of low-grade infection due to the inefficiency of protective mechanisms. The organisms most commonly involved are pneumococci and *H. influenzae* and these are usually responsible for the acute clinical exacerbations.

Clinical

A progressive disease with chronic cough and mucoid sputum, usually occurring in the winter months, in which there are acute exacerbations recurring with ever-increasing severity during succeeding years.

Macroscopical

The bronchi may be dilated and the mucous membrane is roughened, thickened, red, granular and bathed in mucous secretions. 'Webbing' of the mucosa is usually seen. The trachea and bronchioles may show a similar appearance. In advanced cases, emphysema is nearly always present (see p. 652).

Microscopical

The major change is an increase in mucous glands in the submucosa with a variable chronic inflammatory cell infiltration and some increased fibrosis. The epithelium invariably shows marked increase in goblet cells and later may show loss of cilia and other metaplastic changes. Hyperplasia of mucous glands with marked increase in their volume is a prominent feature.

Effects

Cough with excessive viscid, mucoid, sputum which becomes mucopurulent during infective exa-

cerbations. Dyspnoea from obstruction of airways due to excess secretions occurs and predisposes to the development of emphysema. There is also associated bronchial spasm, possibly due to an allergic reaction to the presence of organisms.

Results

Unless the multiple aetiological factors are controlled there is gradual progression over many years with episodes of pneumonia and the development of emphysema due to bronchiolar obstruction. As a result, there is right heart strain, cor pulmonale and heart failure in addition to obstruction to the free flow of air and thus impairment of ventilation. There is thus a marked disability and commonly a considerable shortening of the life span.

BRONCHIAL ASTHMA

Nature

An allergic condition, manifest by bronchospasm and producing expiratory wheezing with prolongation of expiration.

Aetiology

1 *Heredity*. A large proportion of asthmatics have a family history of asthma or some other allergic disorder.

2 *Allergic substances*. Any foreign protein substance or derivative may be the allergen. These may be inhaled, or the pulmonary symptoms may be the manifestations of injected or ingested antigens. Common allergens include dust, pollens, protein foods, drugs and bacteria.

3 *Predisposing factors*. There is frequently an abnormal emotional background and acute attacks may be psychogenically precipitated.

Clinical

Occurs as intermittent acute attacks of wheezing which subside, either spontaneously or with appropriate therapy. Severe prolonged attacks – *status asthmaticus*, may be difficult to control and cause severe mental and physical exhaustion.

Macroscopical

The lungs may appear normal or show one or more of the following features: tenacious mucus and mucous plugs in the lumen of the bronchi and bronchioles, thickening of the bronchioles, focal areas of collapse. Emphysema is rarely found.

Microscopical

The bronchiolar walls are thickened due to muscular hypertrophy, overgrowth of the mucous glands with thickening of basement membrane due to deposition of IgA and IgG and an infiltration with eosinophils. There is stringy mucus in the lumen, together with eosinophils, Charcot–Leyden crystals and Curschmann's spirals. In status asthmaticus there is also extensive desquamation of the cilia and epithelium which impedes the removal of mucus.

Results

Death is only rarely a direct result of asthma but it may follow status asthmaticus or massive pulmonary collapse due to bronchial obstruction by mucus. Cor pulmonale and the predisposition to concurrent bronchitis and bronchiolitis are important additional factors.

BRONCHIECTASIS

Nature

Dilatation of the bronchi.

Incidence

At one time a common sequel to measles and whooping cough it is now much less frequently derived from childhood.

Aetiology

The main factors are infection associated with bronchial obstruction. The obstruction may be due to:

1 Intraluminal foreign bodies, mucus, inflammatory exudates (particularly in whooping cough and measles), pus, etc.
2 Tumour or stricture of the wall.
3 Pressure from outside the wall by enlarged lymph nodes, due to tumour invasion, tuberculosis, etc.

Pathogenesis

The usual sequence of events in the production of bronchiectasis is:

1 Partial or complete bronchial obstruction.
2 Resorption of air with an area of pulmonary collapse.
3 Accumulation and stasis of secretions within the obstructed bronchi.

4 Infection occurs with extension into the bronchial wall.
5 Dilatation of the damaged wall by the effect of negative intrapleural pressure transmitted through the collapsed lung tissue and by the distension effect of retained excessive secretions in the blocked bronchi.

Sites

Most commonly occurs in the basal segments of the lower lobes, middle lobe and lingula.

Macroscopical

There are distended, pus-containing fusiform or saccular dilatations of the bronchi with inflamed walls. The adjacent lung tissue and pleura is frequently fibrous due to organized collapse and chronic inflammation.

Microscopical

Variable infiltration of part or all of the bronchial wall by chronic inflammatory tissue with fibrous replacement. The mucosa is usually replaced by inflammatory tissue with foci of respiratory mucosa and areas of squamous metaplasia. The adjacent lung tissue shows fibrosis and organized inflammatory exudate with carnified, collapsed areas.

Results

The production of copious purulent sputum with respiratory dysfunction due to pulmonary fibrosis and the risk of abscess formation in the lung with subsequent metastatic brain abscess. Furthermore, the condition predisposes to repetitive inflammatory episodes due to aspiration of infected material into other areas of the lungs, so that chronic bronchitis may be perpetuated or pneumonia may occur.

Circulatory disorders

CHRONIC PASSIVE VENOUS CONGESTION

Aetiology

Associated with chronic failure of the left side of the heart, e.g. mitral stenosis, chronic hypertensive heart failure.

Macroscopical

Brown induration of the lung with vascular thickening (see p. 120).

Microscopical

Congestion of alveolar vessels with fibrous thickening of the walls, heart failure cells in the alveoli, and atheroma of the larger vessels.

Results

This is a common cause of pulmonary hypertension (see p. 269).

PULMONARY OEDEMA

Aetiology

1 *Cardiac failure.* Especially acute left ventricular failure, e.g. acute hypertensive heart failure, cardiac infarction.

2 *Inflammatory.* In the early stages of all infections, oedema fluid is part of the inflammatory exudate and is especially pronounced in virus infections, e.g. influenza.

3 *Renal disease.* Associated with hypoproteinaemic oedema from any cause (see p. 373) and also with uraemia.

4 *Raised intracranial pressure.* Usually due to a space-occupying lesion of the brain but the precise mechanism of the pulmonary oedema is unknown.

Macroscopical

The lungs are firm, heavy and pit on pressure. On section, fluid wells from the cut surface.

Microscopical

Pale, pink-staining, protein-containing fluid fills the alveolar spaces. There is usually some associated pulmonary congestion, and commonly a variable degree of inflammatory change which may be pre-existing or be due to secondary infection, e.g. hypostatic pneumonia.

PULMONARY EMBOLISM

This common cause of sudden death or of pulmonary infarction usually develops as a complication of femoral or pelvic venous thrombosis. The changes are described on p. 128.

PULMONARY INFARCTION

Aetiology

Usually associated with embolism but may rarely occur due to a primary vascular thrombosis associated with an abnormal circulation, e.g. in pulmonary hypertension.

Macroscopical

The lower lobes are involved in 75 per cent of cases. The infarcts are pyramidal-shaped and haemorrhagic with their base at the pleural surface, over which there is a fibrinous reaction.

Microscopical

The infarcted area shows coagulation necrosis with nuclear death, profuse red cells in the alveoli, and an inflammatory reaction at the margins.

Results

1 Loss of functioning lung tissue, therefore cyanosis may ensue.

2 Large infarcts cause right ventricular strain and may precipitate cardiac failure or induce pulmonary hypertension (see p. 269).

3 Pleural involvement causes pain and may be followed by effusion.

4 Healing results in a fibrous scar.

5 Septic infarction – the infarct may be infected from a septic embolus or become secondarily infected from the lung. The appearances of this infarct are modified by softening and suppuration, eventually producing a lung abscess (see p. 663).

PULMONARY HYPERTENSION

SECONDARY TO A KNOWN DISEASE

This is the more common form and is seen in excessive pulmonary blood flow – shunts, chronic passive venous congestion and obstructive lung disease, organic obstruction of pulmonary vessels, e.g. pulmonary fibrosis, emphysema, etc.

PRIMARY

A rare condition in which there is pulmonary hypertension with no pre-existing or known cause.

The subject is further considered on p. 270.

RESPIRATORY DISTRESS SYNDROME – HYALINE MEMBRANE DISEASE

Nature
A disease affecting infants during the first few days of life. It most commonly occurs in premature infants, those delivered by caesarian section and children of diabetic mothers.

Pathogenesis
The relationship to prematurity and foetal distress *in utero* is clear. Moreover, there is an absence of surfactants at birth, which normally facilitate pulmonary expansion. This would suggest a deficiency of Type 2 pneumocytes which produce surfactants, but this is not consistently found.

Macroscopical
The lungs are solid, dull red like liver and engorged. They are poorly aerated and sink in water.

Microscopical
There is widespread atelectasis with over-distended respiratory bronchioles and alveolar ducts lined by the characteristic eosinophilic hyaline membrane. This is PAS-positive and contains some fat but iron and fibrin are usually absent. Ultrastructurally, this is an amorphous ground substance with a granular or fibrillar matrix, cell remnants, amniotic squamous and osmiophilic lamellar bodies but fibrin is unusual.

Results
Mortality from hypoxia is high.

HYALINE MEMBRANES IN ADULTS

Nature
A similar histological appearance to that described above for premature infants is seen occasionally in adults.

Causes
1 'Shock' lung. Particularly if the 'shock' is toxic in origin.
2 Oxygen excess. Excess oxygen administration by positive-pressure ventilatory techniques—*ventilator lung*.
3 Influenza. Some fatal cases of this pure virus infection.
4 Chemical. Following some inhaled irritant chemicals.

Mechanical disorders

PULMONARY ATELECTASIS

Nature
A failure of aeration of the lung at birth.

Aetiology
1 *Birth trauma.* With brain damage involving the respiratory centre and resulting in inadequate respiratory efforts.
2 *Bronchial obstruction.* By mucus or inhaled liquor amnii.

Macroscopical
Small, non-crepitant, blue or grey-coloured lungs which sink in water and which may show petechial haemorrhages due to asphyxia or show obstructing material in the bronchial lumen.

Microscopical
Non-aerated alveoli with crowding of the alveolar walls which appear thicker than normal. There may be mucus or keratinous debris from the amniotic fluid in the bronchi and alveoli.

Results
This depends upon the amount of atelectatic lung. Death ensues when large areas are involved; smaller areas may subsequently expand or remain airless thus predisposing to infection, bronchiectasis or pulmonary fibrosis.

PULMONARY COLLAPSE

Nature
The term implies an airless condition of lung tissue which has previously contained air.

Aetiology

1 *Compression.* Compression of the lung parenchyma by any space-occupying lesion, e.g. pneumothorax, pleural fluid, tumours, aneurysms, etc.

2 *Obstruction.* Obstruction of the lumen of bronchi or bronchioles with subsequent resorption of air. The more common causes of the obstruction are:

(a) *Lumen.* Foreign bodies, mucus, pus, aspirated material including vomit, inflammatory exudate. This is a common post-operative feature due to a combination of tenacious mucus, poor respiratory movements and depression of the cough reflex.

(b) *Wall.* Tumours and stricture.

(c) *External.* Pressure from enlarged lymph nodes due to tuberculosis or tumour, or due to aneurysms and cysts.

Macroscopical

Collapse may be patchy and peripheral, segmental, lobar, or involve the whole lung. If most of the lung is involved it is called *massive collapse* and this is the type which may occur as a serious acute post-operative complication. Small areas show a grey-blue colour and are depressed below the surface of the surrounding, normal pink, aerated zones. A large collapsed portion is non-crepitant, wrinkled on the pleural surface, feels like wet leather and sinks in water. The compressive or obstructive cause is usually obvious.

Microscopical

The alveoli are airless and crowded together, the bronchi and vessels thus appear more prominent than normal.

Results

If the cause of the collapse is removed at an early stage, the lung will re-expand and return to normal. If the collapse persists, organization may lead to *carnification*, so called because of the firm, fibrous, fleshy appearance. In addition, the collapsed area of lung is frequently the site of bronchiectasis at a later date (see p. 648). Thus it is important to promote the re-expansion of collapsed lung, especially in children, e.g. in whooping cough, measles, etc.

Emphysema

Nature

The most acceptable definition is of 'a condition of the lung characterized by increase, beyond the normal, in the size of air spaces distal to the terminal bronchiole, either from dilatation or from destruction of their walls'. It will be appreciated that the essential feature is distinction between dilatation of small air passages and destruction.

The older classification of emphysematous lungs into atrophic and hypertrophic is no longer acceptable. Studies of lungs by controlled inflation–fixation with the application of the whole lung section and barium impregnation techniques, have shown anatomical abnormalities in emphysema related to the lung lobule and varying in distribution.

Anatomical

The lung lobule is the smallest component bounded by fibrous tissue septa and is 1–2 cm in diameter. Seen poorly in normal lungs, but clearly seen in lungs heavily pigmented by coal dust which outlines the septa. Each is virtually a miniature lung and in emphysema irregular distribution may cause variability in severity between different lobules. The structure is diagrammatically represented in Fig. 82 on p. 653.

The term *acinus* should be utilized for the unit of respiratory tissue distal to the terminal bronchiole.

Classification

1 *Dilatation (mainly) of air passages alone*

(a) Unselective distribution:
  (i) Compensatory emphysema.
  (ii) Emphysema due to main bronchus obstruction.
  (iii) Non-obstructive overdistension emphysema.

(b) Selective distribution:
  (i) Focal emphysema of dust diseases – focal dust emphysema.
  (ii) Focal emphysema non-industrial nature.

2 *Destruction of the walls of air passages and distal air spaces*

(a) Unselective distribution:
  (i) Panacinar emphysema – including paraseptal – syn. panlobular, diffuse, vesicular, diffuse lobular.
  (ii) Senile or ageing lung.

(b) Selective distribution:
  (i) Centrilobular emphysema – non-industrial centrilobular emphysema.

(c) Irregular distribution:
  (i) Emphysematous change related to scars – paratractional.

(ii) Giant bullous emphysema.

(iii) Unilateral translucent lung – MacLeod's syndrome.

(iv) Acute tension cysts of infancy.

Pathogenesis

Although in some cases and varieties of emphysema concomitant factors are clearly identified, e.g. bronchial obstruction or compensation following scarring or surgical excision, it is far from clear in most types what mechanisms operate to produce permanent and often progressive structural changes.

There are four main theories of causation:

1 Emphysema is caused by obliteration and destruction of respiratory bronchioles causing '*air-trapping*'. This causes secondary distension and eventually disruption of alveoli and air passages distal to the obstruction which then form a '*common pool*'.

2 Emphysema results from inflammatory weakening and destruction of the walls of either respiratory bronchioles or more distally situated structures together with the peribronchiolar alveolar walls.

3 Emphysema is primarily the result of vascular obliteration leading to ischaemic atrophy of lung tissue. This theory has gained little favour, though experimentally supportable in part.

4 Emphysema is caused by narrowing of terminal and respiratory bronchioles, preventing normal expiration.

None of these explanations satisfactorily fits all types of emphysema and it will be appreciated that the major difficulty in human lung disease is identifying the sequence of events, i.e. which features are primary and which are secondary.

A number of cases are due to disruption of alveolar walls by congenital α-1-antitrypsin deficiency (see p. 561) and others by injurious chemical fumes, notably cigarette smoke.

Varieties

I DILATATION OF AIR PASSAGES ALONE

(*a*.i) *Compensatory emphysema* – Overdistension in remaining lung tissue is seen after surgical excision of a part or whole lung.

(*a*.ii) *Main and lobar bronchial obstructive emphysema* – Partial or total major bronchial obstruction may cause air trapping and a valve-like effect with over-distension. Infection usually follows and adds destruction.

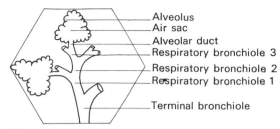

(a) Lobule

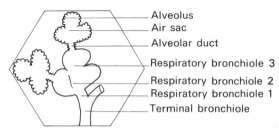

(b) Centrilobular emphysema

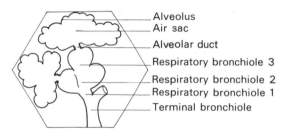

(c) Panacinar emphysema

Fig. 82. (*a*) Normal lung lobule (diagrammatic); (*b*) Diagrammatic representation of centrilobular emphysema; (*c*) Diagrammatic representation of panacinar emphysema.

(*a*.iii) *Non-obstructive overdistension emphysema* – A rare type seen in infancy or childhood and associated with metabolic or structural deficiencies.

(*b*.i) *Focal emphysema of dust diseases* – This mostly relates to coal dust, occasionally to other inert dusts. Dust ingested by macrophages collects in the alveoli and lymphoid tissue with a minimal reticulin reaction and resulting dilatation of second and third orders of respiratory bronchioles giving a *centrilobular* distribution of the emphysema (see above). Upper lobes are mainly affected.

This usually gives rise to relatively little functional disability.

(*b*.ii) *Focal emphysema of non-industrial nature* – This results from the deposition of sooty anthracotic particles, in city dwellers in particular. When severe and possibly due to the presence of adsorbed acids, a type of centrilobular emphysema can develop.

2 DESTRUCTION OF WALLS OF AIR PASSAGES AND SPACE

(*a*.i) *Panacinar emphysema – Panlobular emphysema* – There is disruption, destruction and enlargement of the alveoli and alveolar ducts (see p. 653).

Although some cases are associated with α-1-antitrypsin deficiency, this is not so for the majority, most of whom are heavy cigarette smokers or have repetitive episodes of infection. A variant is restricted to the *paraseptal* part of the lobule.

Lower lobes are usually most severely affected and destruction can be very severe but variable from one lobule to another. Strands of tissue containing vessels bridging across large air spaces which later form bullae, are seen.

Functional disorder is frequently increasingly severe in this common type of emphysema.

(*a*.ii) *Ageing senile lung* – Although some degenerative changes do occur with increasing age and may exacerbate lung damage from other causes, the older descriptions of 'senile emphysema' were inaccurate and exaggerated in importance. However, over 70 years of age, some functional deterioration can often be detected, irrespective of the presence or absence of other conditions.

(*b*.i) *Centrilobular emphysema – Non-industrial* – This is caused by inflammatory destruction of distal respiratory bronchioles and adjacent alveoli. Spaces are traversed by strands of tissue containing vessels. It is more severe in males particularly in the upper lobes and is closely related to chronic bronchitis (see p. 647). The central parts of the lobule show not only destructive dilatation but also some chronic inflammatory changes. This helps to distinguish the histological appearances from the centrilobular, dust-related, focal dust emphysema (see p. 653).

(*c*.i) *Emphysema related to scars* – The distribution of this type has a direct relationship to scars, most frequently apical from old tuberculous disease. Large bullae may form as a result of tractional forces.

(*c*ii) *Giant bullous cysts* – These may reach 19 cm or more and can cause disproportionate symptoms due to compression of adjacent more normal lung tissue. There is also a considerable risk of rupture and resulting pneumothorax. They probably result from post-inflammatory bronchial stenosis and 'air trapping'.

Effects

1 Obstruction to the movement of air leads to inadequate ventilation. Furthermore, there is loss of diffusing capacity at alveolar level due to destruction of the alveolar-capillary membrane and disordered distribution because of distension of some areas and compression of others. The physiological dead space is therefore increased and abnormalities of blood flow, induced by the ventilating and structural changes, result in diminished oxygenation of blood.

2 The ventilatory and structural changes, together with the increased intra-alveolar pressure, which causes compression of capillaries in the alveolar walls, lead to pulmonary hypertension and right ventricular hypertrophy. This may be followed by heart failure – *cor pulmonale*.

3 Rupture of bullae may give rise to pneumothorax.

INTERSTITIAL EMPHYSEMA

Nature
Air in the interstitial tissue framework of the lung.

Aetiology
1 *Spontaneous*. Tearing of alveolar walls may result from violent coughing, especially in patients with asthma, whooping cough, other types of emphysema or chronic bronchitis.

2 *Trauma*. Surgical or traumatic injury to the chest wall with involvement of the lung, oesophagus, or trachea.

Results
Air bubbles gain access to the interstitial tissue of the lung and mediastinum and may then track up into the neck to produce 'surgical emphysema',

characterized by crepitus on palpation. The air usually reabsorbs without significant sequelae.

Asphyxia

Nature
Death from asphyxia is due to a decreased oxygen content of the blood and tissues which falls below the level necessary for the maintenance of life. Thus, the terms anoxia or hypoxia are more accurate than asphyxia: the latter term should probably be restricted to those cases dying from anoxia due to obstruction of the air passages.

Causes
All the causes have lack of oxygen as their common feature.

1 *Lack of oxygen in the blood*
(a) Respiratory obstruction by external pressure, e.g. gags, strangulation, pillows, hanging.
(b) Respiratory obstruction from internal causes, e.g. laryngeal spasm or oedema, impacted foreign bodies.
(c) Drowning (see below).
(d) Prevention of normal gaseous exchange by pulmonary disease, e.g. pulmonary oedema, pulmonary fibrosis.
(e) Acute pulmonary collapse, e.g. penetrating chest wounds with pneumothorax, spontaneous tension pneumothorax, massive collapse due to bronchial obstruction.
(f) Respiratory paralysis, e.g. medullary injury from birth trauma or cerebral haemorrage, or paralysis of the muscles of respiration in poliomyelitis and in poisoning, e.g. strychnine, barbiturates.

2 *Lack of circulating blood*
(a) Peripheral circulatory failure, e.g. shock and severe haemorrhage.
(b) Cardiac failure with stagnant anoxia.

3 *Loss of oxygen carrying power of the blood*
(a) Severe anaemia.
(b) Carbon monoxide poisoning.

4 *Inability of tissue cells to utilize oxygen*
(a) Breakdown of the cellular oxygenation systems utilizing cytochrome by cyanide or, in a lesser degree, by barbiturates.
(b) Insufficient foodstuffs to maintain the cell metabolism, e.g. hypoglycaemia.
(c) The presence of lipid-soluble anaesthetics, e.g. chloroform, ether, trilene.

(d) Retention of metabolites within the cell, e.g. uraemia, carbon dioxide posioning.

Tissue changes of anoxia
These are similar in all types. All parenchymal cells show degenerative changes of varying degrees of severity. The brain tissues are the most affected and show the most advanced findings, with oedema or areas of obvious softening due to necrosis in severe or prolonged cases.

Other appearances
It should be stressed that many examples of anoxia leave little evidence of their causation and the post-mortem appearances are then those of simple anoxia, e.g. anaemia, overdose of anaesthetics, etc. In those examples due to respiratory obstruction – asphyxia, the findings are more dramatic:

External. The skin shows cyanosis, especially of the lips and the nailbeds, whilst the face may show a florid colour with petechial haemorrhages, maximal in the conjunctiva. Froth may be present in the mouth and nose.

Internal. The blood is extremely dark and all the organs show marked venous congestion with distension of the great veins. The cause of the obstruction may be apparent, e.g. impacted foreign body, laryngeal oedema, etc. Owing to the terminal congestion and the increased intrapleural negative pressure associated with strenuous agonal attempts to breathe, multiple petechial haemorrhages are almost invariably present in the pericardium and pleura – *Tardieu's spots.*

Drowning

Fatalities due to immersion in cold water may be:
1 Due to reflex glottic or laryngeal spasm with asphyxia or immediate cardiac arrest, possibly induced by a vagal reflex. This accounts for 10–15 per cent of fatal cases.
2 The remaining 85–90 per cent have water in the lungs.

FRESH-WATER DROWNING

Inhaled fresh water in the alveoli, being hypotonic, is rapidly absorbed into the blood. This produces rapid haemodilution with decreased electrolyte levels and red-cell haemolysis which results in a raised blood potassium level (up to 8 mmol/l). The combination of haemodilution with increased cardiac volume, anoxia due to prevention of respiratory gaseous exchange in the water-filled lungs and the raised serum potassium, result in death 2–5 min after the immersion.

SALT-WATER DROWNING

Aspirated salt water induces withdrawal of fluid from the blood due to the osmotic differential and thus haemoconcentration results. Magnesium ions are absorbed into the blood from the sea water but the blood sodium and potassium ratios are not significantly altered, nor does haemolysis occur. Death in sea-water drowning is delayed for 7–9 min and is due either to cardiac arrest, possibly associated with an increased magnesium blood level, or to respiratory paralysis following the eventual anoxia.

Chapter 108
Respiratory System – Pneumonia

DEFINITION OF PNEUMONIA

Consolidation of lung tissue by the presence of intra-alveolar inflammatory exudate of variable distribution and aetiology.

INTRODUCTION

At one time pneumonia was entirely classified on the basis of anatomical distribution of the consolidation into (1) lobar (2) bronchopneumonia. In more recent times, attempts have been made to classify according to the aetiological agents and these include:
1 Bacteria.
2 Viruses.
3 Rickettsiacae.
4 Fungi.
5 Chemicals.
This is highly desirable but there are difficulties in subclassification of bacterial pneumonias caused

657

by specific organisms, mainly due to the problems, in a significant number of cases, of cultural isolation and identification during life. This is partly related to technical inadequacies of sputum culture as a diagnostic test and also to some extent to the difficulties in laboratory isolation when antibiotic therapy has already been commenced.

It is, therefore, still important that the anatomical distribution of the consolidation and the resulting classification is retained in part, though wherever possible it should be qualified, i.e. pneumococcal lobar pneumonia, staphylococcal bronchopneumonia.

Lobar pneumonia

Nature
A condition seen often in previously healthy young adults in which large areas of uniform consolidation affect a lobe or lobes of the lungs.

Aetiology
The bacterial agents are usually pneumococci: occasionally Klebsiella bacilli, β-haemolytic streptococci or staphylococci may be responsible. Atypical types may be due to Legionella (see p. 660).

Predisposing factors
Sometimes there is a history of a recent mild upper respiratory infection but more commonly the subject was previously healthy.

Mode of infection
The exact mechanism of infection is still controversial but it seems almost certain the organisms reach the alveoli via the bronchial tree. It has been further suggested that a local hypersensitivity reaction to the organism in the lung may be an important factor in the production of the consolidation.

Sites
The process is usually sharply confined to a lobe which is diffusely affected; rarely more than one lobe may be involved.

Appearances
The changes are descriptively subdivided into four phases, but these overlap in different regions of the affected lobe.

STAGE I – CONGESTION
Macroscopical. A deep red, firm lobe which still contains air.

Microscopical. Congestion of the alveolar walls with early inflammatory changes and bacteria in the alveoli.

STAGE II – RED HEPATIZATION
Macroscopical. Firm, red consolidation of the lobe which is, therefore, airless and sinks in water. There is often a fibrinous pleurisy.

Microscopical. Congestion is still present and the airless alveoli contain a profuse, fibrinous and polymorphonuclear inflammatory exudate together with phagocytosed organisms and red blood cells.

STAGE III – GREY HEPATIZATION
Macroscopical. The lobe is firm, grey, dry and airless but of normal or slightly increased size.

Microscopical. The exudate is still present in the alveoli but the red cells have lysed and the alveolar walls are no longer congested. The lung architecture is, however, preserved.

STAGE IV – RESOLUTION
The inflammatory exudate is digested and absorbed with great rapidity so that the lung returns to normal. It will be noted that pus is not formed at any stage of lobar pneumonia. There is concomitant rapid improvement in the clinical state, the fever disappearing over the course of a few hours – resolution by crisis. This is probably the effect of a massive antibody response.

Results
The disease is profoundly modified by chemotherapy. Before antibiotics were available, there was a considerable mortality, but this is now very small. Complete resolution is the usual outcome in most treated cases although complications which may occasionally occur include:

1 *Cardiac.* Mechanical effects due to right heart strain associated with redistribution of blood due to the lobar consolidation. Rarely pericarditis or endocarditis may occur.

2 *Septicaemia.* Blood spread of the organisms with meningitis, suppurative arthritis or pyaemic abscesses in many organs or tissues.

3 *Suppuration.* Gross pleural infection with effusion followed by empyema. Occasionally, the alveo-

lar walls may break down in the consolidated area to produce a lung abscess.

4 *Incomplete resolution*. Resolution may be incomplete with organization of residual exudate resulting in pulmonary and/or pleural fibrosis.

Bronchopneumonia – lobular pneumonia

Nature
Bronchopneumonia is a patchy consolidation centred around inflamed bronchi which is multifocal and usually bilateral.

Aetiology
This may be caused by a large number of different organisms of varying pathogenicity. Of the acute bacterial infections, staphylococci, streptococci, *Haemophilus influenzae* and pneumococci are the organisms most commonly isolated. Viruses, tuberculosis and organisms of low pathogenicity may also cause bronchopneumonia which, however, varies in its appearance according to the aetiological agent.

Predisposing factors
A disease typically of the very young and the old; in both groups the general resistance of the host is low. Any other condition which lowers general or local resistance also predisposes to bronchopneumonia, particularly pre-existing tracheobronchitis, pulmonary oedema, cardiac or renal disease, diabetes mellitus, malignant disease, anaesthesia, chilling, malnutrition and exposure.

Mode of infection
The infection starts in the bronchi and bronchioles and subsequently extends to produce foci of alveolar consolidation around these inflamed bronchi.

Sites
Commonly bilateral, the basal segments of the lower lobes are the most frequently involved areas.

Macroscopical
Externally, the pleura shows a fibrinous or purulent exudate. On palpation there are multiple firm areas of consolidation distributed around bronchi and the bronchial tree is inflamed and filled with mucopurulent material. On section, the lung is congested with pale, consolidated areas of variable size which exude pus from the central bronchus on pressure. Intervening lung tissue appears normal but, with progression of the disease, the consolidated areas may become confluent.

Microscopical
1 *Bronchi*. A suppurative bronchitis and bronchiolitis with an inflammatory exudate and pus in the lumen.

2 *Lung*. The peribronchial alveoli are filled with an acute inflammatory exudate containing polymorphs, fibrin and organisms. In addition to these consolidated areas, patchy collapse, associated with bronchial obstruction due to blockage by the mucopurulent exudate, is frequently seen. The centres of the consolidated areas show destruction of alveolar walls and suppuration, thus distinguishing this type of pneumonia from the lobar variety.

Results
Bronchopneumonia is a suppurative disease producing breakdown of tissue so that complete resolution is most unusual.

1 *Resolution*. This can only occur if treatment is instituted early and before there is any structural damage.

2 *Lung fibrosis*. Usually the exudate is not completely absorbed but becomes organized with repair to the central area of suppuration and residual fibrous scarring.

3 *Bronchial damage*. The bronchial wall may not be restored to normal. Resulting scarring of the bronchi, particularly in children, and imperfect restitution of the protective mucosa, predisposes to further infection and to bronchiectasis.

4 *Suppuration*. Single or multiple pulmonary abscesses may form following confluence and suppuration of the pneumonic areas. Extension of the inflammation to involve the pleura may result in empyema.

5 *Pericarditis*. Direct extension of the infection to involve the pericardium rarely occurs but may produce a suppurative pericarditis.

6 *Death*. Bronchopneumonia is a very common cause of death, occurring frequently as a terminal manifestation of many diseases. Moreover, death is not uncommon when extensive bronchopneumonia occurs in the absence of other serious disease.

Bacterial pneumonias

PNEUMOCOCCAL – STREPTOCOCCUS PNEUMONIAE

Pneumonia due to *S. pneumoniae* is virtually always of classical lobar type. There are several serological subtypes (I–VIII) of which Type I is most common in man and Type III has a rather mucoid appearance in both culture and lung tissue.

STAPHYLOCOCCAL – STAPHYLOCOCCUS PYOGENES

Coagulase-positive staphylococci (*Staph. aureus*) are not infrequently relatively or absolutely antibiotic resistant, and this pneumonia carries therefore a high morbidity and mortality both in childhood and in adults.

It is nearly always bronchopneumonic in distribution, becomes confluent early and suppuration is a common complication with multiple abscess formation frequent.

Staphylococcal pneumonia is a common secondary infection superimposed on respiratory tract virus infections, e.g. an important cause of death in influenza. It is also particularly likely to occur in hospital in-patients who are post-operative or who are debilitated by other illnesses. In these circumstances the strains of staphyloccoci are often antibiotic-resistant.

STREPTOCOCCAL – STREPTOCOCCUS PYOGENES

Pneumonia due to Group A, *β*-haemolytic streptococci (*Strep. pyogenes*) was at one time a very common and highly lethal disease but is now infrequent.

The consolidation is of bronchopneumonic distribution and is often haemorrhagic.

KLEBSIELLAL – KLEBSIELLA PNEUMONIAE

Pneumonia due to Klebsiella pneumoniae (formerly Friedländers bacillus) may be either primary (acute or chronic) or secondary to another bacterial lung infection or complicating non-infective pulmonary disease such as carcinoma of bronchus, asthma and bronchiectasis.

The primary pneumonia is usually a complication of oral sepsis and is of bronchopneumonic type in the distribution seen in inhalational infections. Chronic suppurative disease may follow or occur *de novo*.

INFLUENZAL – HAEMOPHILUS INFLUENZAE

In this bacterial pneumonia the organism is the gram-negative bacterium *H. influenzae* and not the pneumonia due to the influenza virus.

It is a relatively more common infection in the bronchi of children and may then spread to the lung parenchyma to produce a bronchopneumonia. The organism is also a secondary invader which complicates the damage caused by other organisms including viruses and though only a moderate pathogen may cause serious progressive consolidation and death in these circumstances and also in those with some impairment of immunological response.

LEGIONELLAL PNEUMONIA – LEGIONELLA PNEUMOPIIILA

Nature
A commonly severe lobar or lobular type of epidemic pneumonia relatively recently identified and due to *L. pneumophila*.

Organism
L. pneumophila is a gram-negative rod which stains poorly with conventional stains but can best be morphologically identified by silver stains or by electron microscopy. Growth requirements for cultural isolation are exacting and critical. The organism is widespread and epidemics are mostly spread by water often through the cooling towers of air-conditioning systems. Case-to-case contact does not appear to occur.

Lungs
There is a significant mortality, possibly as high as 10 per cent in clinically severe cases, from respiratory failure and response to antibiotic therapy is often disappointing. It is this and failure of usual cultural techniques which alerts to the 'atypical pneumonia' course and awareness of the poss-

ible diagnosis. Immunofluorescent serological tests are diagnostic though several strains of Legionella have now been identified.

OTHER BACTERIA

Organisms which less frequently cause pneumonia, usually of bronchopneumonic distribution include:

1 Coliforms – pseudomonas, proteus, *Escherichia coli*. These are often secondary invaders or are involved in aspiration pneumonia (see below).

2 Plague – *Pasteurella pestis* (see p. 39).

3 Anthrax – *Bacillus anthracis* – wool-sorter's disease (see p. 39).

4 Tularaemia – *Pasteurella tularensis* – Particularly in some parts of the U.S.A., Scandinavia and Japan.

5 Brucella – *Brucella sp.* – occasional reports only of pneumonia due to several different strains of this organism.

6 Meningococci – *Neisseria meningitidis* – rare.

7 Salmonella – *Salmonella typhi* and others – rare.

ASPIRATION PNEUMONIA

This is bronchopneumonia following aspiration of gastric contents or infected material from the oropharynx into the bronchial tree.

If the aspirated material is frankly infected then bronchopneumonia due to the organisms present develops, particularly in persons otherwise debilitated by disease.

When the material is gastric juice there is a violent chemical reaction to the gastric acid with damage to alveolar and bronchiolar walls and progressive oedema with acute inflammatory reaction – *Mendelson's syndrome*.

In occasional cases putrefactive pneumonia will follow inhalation of anaerobic organisms of the clostridial and bacteroides groups.

Aspiration of fatty material leads to a rather special type of *lipid pneumonia* (see p. 663).

When aspiration of gastric contents is involved, portions of vegetable and other foreign matter may be identified in the pneumonic foci.

NEONATAL PNEUMONIA

By definition this is pneumonia occurring in the first month of life.

1 In the first 48 hours. Most or all of these start in intrauterine life and are probably largely due to inhalation of amniotic fluid.

2 After 48 hours. The majority are due to the same range of organisms as previously identified for adults, though lower-grade pathogens are responsible for a higher proportion of fatal cases.

A minority of cases of neonatal pneumonia are from inhalation of milk or gastric contents.

Differentiation from hyaline membrane disease (see p. 650) can be clinically difficult.

CASEOUS BRONCHOPNEUMONIA

The cheesy consolidation of tuberculous bronchopneumonia is described on p. 666.

Virus and mycoplasma pneumonia

Nature
Virus infection of the lungs causes a primary interstitial inflammation with a mononuclear cell response. Similar changes occur in infections due to mycoplasma.

Aetiology
Several viruses may cause respiratory disease which is often confined to the upper respiratory tract, e.g. common cold. True pneumonic disease may occur with the following organisms:

1 Influenza – A & B strains.

2 Measles and giant cell pneumonia.

3 Cytomegalovirus.

4 Adeno-virus infection.

5 Chickenpox, smallpox and vaccinia.

6 Other virus infections of infancy, e.g. Coxsackie, herpes simplex and respiratory syncytial virus infection.

7 Mycoplasma pneumonia – primary atypical pneumonia.

8 Pertussis (whooping cough).

Clinical
The disease varies from extremely mild pulmonary involvement to a fulminating, highly lethal form.

Macroscopical

The lungs show a patchy involvement varying from multiple small foci to consolidation of large areas of lobes. These areas are firm and intensely red, sometimes with haemorrhagic foci and a similar intense and often violaceous congestion of the trachea and bronchi is invariably seen. The lungs are commonly very oedematous but there is no suppuration in the uncomplicated cases.

Microscopical

Trachea and bronchi. Intense congestion with a mononuclear cell infiltration.

Lungs. There is oedema and a mononuclear cell infiltration in the interstitial tissue with congestion and often haemorrhages in the alveolar walls. The lumen of the alveoli contain only moderate amounts of exudate and small numbers of mononuclear cells. There is no pus formation.

In the *giant cell pneumonia* of children, in addition to the above changes, large numbers of extremely large giant cells are present in the mononuclear cell infiltrate. The great majority of these cases are caused by the measles virus.

Results

1 These changes may resolve and the patient may recover. In severe cases, however, particularly with influenza virus, death may occur with great rapidity.

2 Secondary infection may alter the appearances due to the superimposed changes of a pyogenic infection. This occurred in the pandemic following World War I and in some of the epidemics of Asian influenza in recent years.

The dangerous secondary invaders are: staphylococci, β-haemolytic streptococci, pneumococci and *Haemophilus influenzae*, which convert the viral changes to those of a severe suppurative bronchopneumonia.

Rickettsial pneumonia

Nature

Pneumonia occurs in a number of rickettsial and Bedsonial infections, particularly typhus, Q fever and psittacosis. In the last named the pulmonary infection is often dominant and transferred to humans by psittacine birds (parrots) (see p. 43).

Fungal pneumonia

Appearances

Widespread parenchymal pulmonary disease due to fungal infection is very uncommon and mycotic lesions in lungs are usually focal and solitary or multiple and necrotic.

Cavitation may render differentiation from tuberculosis difficult and, indeed, most of the lesions are granulomas in that there is a mass of inflammatory granulation tissue containing the organisms or cavities lined by tissue containing giant cell granulomas.

Some fungal infections of the respiratory tract are restricted to the bronchial mucosa with no 'invasive' tendencies and declare their presence as a result of symptoms due to hypersensitivity or allergy, e.g. aspergillus.

Aetiological agents

The most frequent causes of pulmonary fungal infection are:

1 *Phycomycetes* – mucormycosis and coccidioidomycosis.

2 *Fungi imperfecti* – aspergillus, blastomycosis, histoplasmosis, sporotrichosis, moniliasis.

Effects

These lesions are usually slow growing, solitary or few in number though in the circumstances of immunocompromise may be intensive and serious. Cavitation may be followed by rupture into a bronchus or pleura with fistula formation.

Identification

The responsible organism may not be readily seen on culture of sputum nor easily identified in tissue. Gridley's aldehyde fuchsin and Grocott's silver stain may be particularly helpful.

Immunoperoxidase stains using specific fungal antisera are diagnostic.

Blood serology is particularly helpful if consecutive samples are examined.

Chemical pneumonia

An inflammatory reaction in alveoli may occur due to a number of inhaled or ingested chemicals. These include irritant gases, e.g. chlorine, cadmium or liquids, e.g. paraquat, but most particularly fatty material – lipid pneumonia.

LIPID PNEUMONIA

Nature

Pulmonary inflammatory reaction to lipid materials. It can be:

1 *Endogenous*. Related to bronchial obstruction and infection, particularly in bronchial carcinoma.

2 *Exogenous*. Inhaled fat or oily substances, particularly liquid paraffin taken as an aperient or as a base for nasal sprays, throat medicines etc., or fat in food, e.g. in milk particularly if there is delay in oesophageal emptying, e.g. achalasia of the cardia (see p. 182).

Macroscopical

The area or areas involved are usually in one or both lower lobes. On section there is either a yellowish consolidation or, when more chronic, a firm fibrous wall surrounding a semi-cystic mass which contains droplets of the oily substance. The oily material is also found in the enlarged regional lymph nodes.

Microscopical

There is replacement of the lung tissue by free droplets of the oily substance, foam cells, foreign body giant cells, inflammatory cells and fibrous tissue.

Results

These granulomatous lesions produce a mass or masses which radiologically may be confused with lung tumours and other lesions. When extensive and bilateral, some functional loss may occur.

'Embolic pneumonia'

This term is sometimes applied to pulmonary suppuration due to blood borne infection.

1 *Pyaemia*. As part of a generalized pyaemia with multiple abscesses scattered throughout the lungs.

2 *Septic infarction*. Single or multiple septic infarcts which suppurate to produce areas of pneumonic consolidation and lung abscesses.

Lung abscess

Nature

An area of suppurative destruction of lung tissue usually caused by staphylococci, streptococci or pneumococci.

Aetiology

1 *Aspiration of infected material*. Aspiration of teeth or tonsils during operations, or foreign bodies accidentally. A further common cause is aspiration of pus from the upper respiratory tract, especially from the nasal sinuses. The right main bronchus is anatomically more in line with the trachea than the left and thus abscesses are more frequent in the right lung.

2 *Following pulmonary infection*. Abscesses may follow bronchopneumonia, bronchiectasis, lobar pneumonia, or infection associated with bronchial obstruction, particularly when this is due to carcinoma.

3 *Blood borne*. Pyaemic abscesses and septic infarcts (see p. 649).

Appearances

There is a pus-filled cavity in the lung parenchyma surrounded by a variable thickness of fibrous tissue.

Results

1 Communication with a bronchus and copious purulent sputum.

2 Communication with the pleural cavity leading to empyema and commonly associated with a bronchopleural fistula.

3 Metastatic abscesses, particularly in the brain (see p. 601).

Chapter 109
Respiratory System – Tuberculosis and other Granulomatous Infections

Pulmonary tuberculosis

Incidence

The lungs are by far the commonest and most important site of tuberculosis. Although the death rate from pulmonary tuberculosis has decreased in recent years, in England and Wales from 20 000 in 1945 to 3500 in 1959, 2000 in 1965 and 1000 in 1976. This is still a common and important disease, particularly in the economically less-well-developed countries where, in many areas, the infection is still rife. Notification of new cases of respiratory tuberculosis fell from 12 000 in 1966 to 7700 in 1976 (England and Wales). A high proportion was in the 65–74 age group.

Organism

Mycobacterium tuberculosis

Predisposing factors

1 *Access of organisms*. Close contact with open cases of the disease. The infection is therefore particularly liable to occur in crowded and unhygienic working conditions or in unhygienic and overcrowded living conditions.

2 *Susceptibility*. There is individual and, to some extent, racial variability in susceptibility.

3 *Local factors*. The presence of pre-existing chronic lung disease is an established predisposition.

4 *General factors*. Social and economic factors are important as this is predominantly a disease of the undernourished and underprivileged. Thus there is an increase in the elderly, partly resulting from dietary factors.

5 *Corticosteroid therapy*. Patients with longstanding inactive lesions may develop serious clinical manifestations when on prolonged corticosteroid or immunosuppressive therapy. Additionally, generalized diseases, e.g. diabetes mellitus, confer a further predisposition.

Mode of infection

The organisms are inhaled in the form of droplets or in dust particles.

PRIMARY INFECTION – GHON FOCUS

Macroscopical

The primary focus is in the lung parenchyma, usually subpleural and most commonly in the apex of the lower lobe or the lower portion of the upper lobe. The focus is small and shows central caseation. This is associated with a caseous lymphadenitis of the hilar lymph nodes. The lung lesion is the Ghon focus; the combination of the lung lesion and the hilar lymphadenopathy is the primary complex (see p. 48).

Microscopical

The lung lesion and the hilar lymph nodes show the typical tuberculous giant cell granulomas with acid and alcohol-fast organisms visible on Ziehl–Neelsen staining.

Results

1 *Healing*. This is the result in a very high proportion of cases. The lung and lymph node lesions heal by fibrosis followed by calcification, but viable organisms may remain within the calcified scar and in the lymph nodes.

2 *The disease may progress:*

(*a*) Progressive caseation and destruction of the lung tissue – progressive primary complex (see p. 48).

(*b*) Spread via the bronchial tree to produce:
Caseous bronchopneumonia or foci of infection in other parts of the lung.
Laryngeal tuberculosis.
Tuberculous enteritis due to swallowed infected sputum.

(*c*) Haematogenous spread to produce:
i Generalized miliary tuberculosis.
ii Single organ tuberculosis, e.g. bone, joint, kidney, etc.

At the time of primary infection, the Mantoux test becomes positive indicative of the development of an hypersensitivity. Any subsequent tuberculous infection is of the secondary or adult type (see p. 47).

POST-PRIMARY – SECONDARY TUBERCULOSIS

Nature

This is the phase of reinfection of a person who has recovered from the previous primary type of tuberculosis. The reinfection may be caused by inhalation of further organisms or be due to the reactivation of quiescent but still viable organisms lurking in the primary complex.

Sites

The apex of one or both lungs is the usual site.

Types of pulmonary lesion

Unlike the primary type, secondary disease almost always produces clinical manifestations, mostly by direct spread.

EARLY APICAL LESION – ASSMANN FOCUS

The secondary or Assmann focus is in the apex and is an area of active caseous tuberculosis which spreads directly and usually with concomitant fibrous repair but with no lymph node involvement. The area is thus converted into a mass of fibrous tissue enclosing caseous material which subsequently becomes quiescent – the healed Assmann focus. Alternatively, organisms may remain viable in the area, or the healing processes may be inadequate to prevent further spread of the disease and so produce any of the following commonly seen types.

APICAL CAVITATING FIBROCASEOUS TUBERCULOSIS

As a result of direct extension and continuing caseation, a progressive area of lung destruction ensues and if a bronchiole is eroded, the caseous material is expectorated leaving an apical cavity. There is a thick fibrous wall lined by caseous tuberculous granulation tissue. The blood vessels in the wall appear as thickened cords due to endarteritis which tends to prevent blood dissemination. This area may subsequently:

1 *Heal*. By slowly progressive fibrosis to produce chronic healed fibrotic apical tuberculosis.

2 *Spread*. By:

(*a*) Direct extension.

(*b*) Bronchial tree.

(*c*) Lymphatics.

(*d*) Blood.

PROGRESSIVE CAVITATING PULMONARY TUBERCULOSIS

If the disease spreads by direct extension, a progressive amount of lung becomes replaced by cavitating caseous tuberculosis with little fibrous reaction. The multiple irregular caseous cavities show no endarteritis obliterans and little evidence of fibrous healing. This type of disease may spread throughout the lung by direct, bronchial and lymphatic spread and end fatally due to:

1 Progressive destruction and cavitation of the lung.
2 Tuberculous caseous bronchopneumonia.
3 Laryngeal tuberculosis.
4 Tuberculous enteritis by swallowing infected sputum.
5 Blood dissemination – miliary tuberculosis.

TUBERCULOUS BRONCHOPNEUMONIA
In the previous types it has been stated that the tubercle bacilli may disseminate via the bronchial tree. The infected material from a tuberculous cavity may:

1 Be coughed up and the pulmonary focus subsequently heal.
2 Give rise to laryngeal or intestinal tuberculosis.
3 Spread the disease throughout the lung with the establishment of new foci of the disease, or in highly susceptible and highly sensitized individuals produce tuberculous bronchopneumonia.

This 'galloping consumption' is manifest by extensive areas of firm or cheesy bronchopneumonic consolidation. Histologically, the usual features of tuberculosis may not be obvious as they are modified by an exudate filling the alveoli which is composed of fibrinous material and histiocytes. Frankly caseous necrosis occurs later with, in some areas, abortive tubercle formation, but there is seldom any significant proliferative response in this frequently fatal type of pulmonary tuberculosis.

BLOOD DISSEMINATION – MILIARY
TUBERCULOSIS
Erosion of a blood vessel or lymphatic involvement may disseminate the organisms into the blood-stream and so produce miliary tuberculosis. The lymphatics may drain the organisms into the right heart via the main lymphatic trunks and jugular vein to produce a miliary picture localized to the lungs; if a vein is eroded the tuberculosis will be disseminated systemically. Pulmonary miliary tuberculosis appears as the 'snow-storm' appearance due to multiple tubercles scattered throughout the lung parenchyma.

These various descriptive types of pulmonary tuberculosis are not always present in pure form and the clinical and pathological picture is capable of many variations due to the combination of progression, healing or the influence of treatment.

Pleural involvement
This is common in all varieties of pulmonary tuberculosis, with active, caseous tubercles found on pleural biopsy. A pleural effusion is frequent and this has the characteristics of an exudate with a Relative Density of 1.020 or more, protein present in excess of 3 g per cent, a fibrin clot and a cellular content of lymphocytes. The pleura heals by fibrosis to result in fibrous obliteration of the space or areas of local pleural thickening and adhesion.

Effects
In addition to the results of spread indicated above, the disease is accompanied by fever, malaise, loss of weight and other general manifestations of variable severity and incidence. In severe cases, wasting is very marked. Many complications may occur including:

1 Massive haemoptysis from erosion of a large vessel or sometimes due to aneurysmal dilatation of the vessel associated with loss of support due to infection within its wall – *mycotic aneurysm* (see p. 274).
2 Considerable fibrosis in the healing or chronic fibrotic types results not only in loss of ventilating capacity, but is attended by compensatory emphysema and pulmonary hypertension. Occasionally, 'honeycomb lung' may be a late sequel (see p. 673).
3 Involvement of bronchial walls may cause narrowing, particularly when fibrous scarring supervenes and causes a stricture with resulting functional loss, bronchiectasis or collapse.
4 Severe infection of the pleura may lead to a tuberculous empyema; this is usually associated with rupture of a parenchymal lesion into the pleura and sometimes a bronchopleural fistula develops.
5 Spread to involve neighbouring organs:
(a) Chest wall.
(b) Mediastinum, especially the pericardium.
(c) Spine.

Diagnosis
This is confirmed by isolation of the organism:
1 From sputum.
2 From early morning stomach washings.
3 From material obtained by bronchoscopic aspiration.
4 Occasionally from tissue; histological examination may also be diagnostic.
5 From pleural fluid or pleural biopsy.

Pulmonary sarcoidosis

Aetiology
This remains unknown (see p. 50).

Incidence
The lung is the most frequently affected organ and is involved in approximately 90 per cent of all cases.

Macroscopical
The pulmonary manifestations are variable:
1 *Hilar lymphadenopathy*. Enlargement of the lymph nodes by sarcoid tissue.
2 *Miliary sarcoidosis*. This gives a radiological 'snow-storm' appearance due to multiple miliary sarcoid lesions throughout the lung parenchyma.
3 *Diffuse fibrosis*. The sarcoid tissue may heal by fibrosis.
4 *'Honeycomb lung'*. This occasionally occurs as a late result of fibrosis (see p. 673).

Microscopical
The histology shows sarcoid granulomas with circular foci of epithelioid cells, giant cells, lymphocytes and sometimes inclusion bodies. Later, there may be progression to fibrosis. There is no caseation and no organisms are present on Ziehl–Neelsen staining.

Results
1 The early active stages of pulmonary sarcoidosis may resolve with no residual pulmonary symptoms or sequelae.
2 Pulmonary fibrosis may ensue in a small proportion of cases and this may be associated with the subsequent development of cor pulmonale or occasionally of 'honeycomb lung'. Functional disability may be severe in these cases.
3 Active pulmonary tuberculosis may rarely develop and is then probably a superimposed infection.

Pulmonary actinomycosis

This rare disease due to *Actinomyces israeli* may affect the lung and adjacent tissues. It shows typical honeycombed abscesses, frequently involving adjacent chest structures, and is surrounded by a dense fibrous reaction with the fungus, in the form of 'sulphur granules', in the pus (see p. 59).

Pulmonary syphilis

Pulmonary syphilis is now extremely rare but congenital pneumonia alba or gummata in congenital or acquired forms is still occasionally found.

'Coin lesions'

A common finding on radiological examination of the chest is the presence of a peripherally situated shadow in the lung parenchyma of approximately circular outline which commonly has no specific or distinguishing radiological features. Moreover, diagnosis of the exact nature of the lesion by macroscopical examination of the tissue is often very difficult. The term 'coin lesion' has been applied to such masses and the causes include:
1 *Granulomas*. Tuberculosis, lung abscess (see p. 663), 'paraffinoma' (see p. 663), aspergillosis (see p. 59), actinomycosis (see p. 57), European blastomycosis (cryptococcosis) (see p. 58), North American blastomycosis (see p. 58), histoplasmosis (see p. 58), moniliasis (see p. 60), coccidioidomycosis (see p. 60), eosinophil granuloma (see p. 691), gumma.
2 *Parasitic cyst*. Hydatid disease (see p. 557).
3 *Tumours*. Carcinoma, metastatic carcinoma, hamartoma (see p. 677), carcinoid tumour (see p. 677).

The relative incidence of these lesions shows considerable variation from one geographical region to another.

Chapter 110
Respiratory System – The Pneumoconioses: Pulmonary Fibrosis

The pneumoconioses

Nature
A group of diseases, mostly of occupational or industrial origin, caused by the inhalation of dusts.

SILICOSIS

Aetiology
This is produced by the inhalation of silica-containing dust. It is most commonly found in miners of gold, iron and occasionally of coal, quarry workers, stone masons and sand blasters.

Pathogenesis
The larger particles of silica are arrested by the normal protective mechanisms and are expectorated. The smaller particles, of 3 μm or less, gain access to the alveoli, are ingested by macrophages and are transported along lymphatics which they

block. A fibrous reaction to the presence of the silica then occurs, but its exact mechanism is controversial. Possible mechanisms include:

1 The slow production of silicic acid which acts as a tissue poison inducing fibrosis and sometimes tissue necrosis.

2 Phospholipids released by disintegrating phagocytes may be fibrogenic.

3 Silica may combine with body protein to form an antigen and the resulting antigen–antibody reaction produces the tissue damage.

Macroscopical

The pleura is grossly thickened, the fibrosis extending into the fissures. On section, there are multiple, circular, hard nodules of varying size scattered throughout the lung parenchyma, but usually maximal in the upper zones. In addition, there are almost always areas of focal emphysema and bronchiectasis and the pulmonary arteries show hypertensive thickening, often with atheroma. The majority of cases show areas of active pulmonary tuberculosis by the time of death.

Microscopical

The nodules consist of concentric, laminated layers of hyaline collagen around central collections of particles of silica. There are also hypertensive changes in the pulmonary arteries (see p. 269), bronchiectasis, focal emphysema and frequently active tuberculosis.

Incineration

Normal lung contains up to 0.2 per cent of silica. A markedly fibrotic silicotic lung contains about 1 per cent and 1.6 per cent indicates severe silicosis.

Results

The disease is slowly progressive over very many years producing respiratory cripples and death in all but the mildly affected cases. The usual results are:

1 Fibrosis of pulmonary tissue and emphysema result in gross pulmonary dysfunction which is commonly associated with cor pulmonale due to pulmonary hypertension.

2 In about 60 per cent of cases of silicosis, tuberculosis co-exists and is commonly responsible for the rapid clinical progression of the disease in the later stages and for death.

ANTHRACOSIS

Carbon particles are present in the lungs and hilar lymph nodes of all town dwellers. Dust particles produced by atmospheric pollution are inhaled into the alveoli where they are phagocytosed by histiocytes and subsequently carried in lymphatics. There is, however, no significant direct clinical or pathological effect on the parenchyma from the presence of this amount of carbon. The continued irritant effect of particulate matter in the bronchial tree is, however, an important factor in chronic bronchitis and emphysema (see p. 647).

Coal miners, who inhale large amounts of carbon particles in their dusty surroundings, do get a pneumoconiosis but this is of rather special type and is preferably considered separately from anthracosis.

COAL-WORKER'S PNEUMOCONIOSIS

Nature

A lung disease of common occurrence in coal workers due to the dusty nature of their occupation. It occurs in two distinct types:

SIMPLE PNEUMOCONIOSIS

This is due to the action of the dust alone. The changes are focal and discrete and are related to the respiratory bronchioles where phagocytosed particles are aggregated. There follows a little reticulin formation, but only rarely is any significant amount of collagen produced. These fibres are irregularly and radially arranged causing the X-ray appearances of 'dust reticulation'. There is a concomitant focal emphysema due to dilatation of the surrounding respiratory bronchioles around these heavily pigmented areas.

The disease may remain in this simple form regardless of the amount of contained dust or the length of exposure, in which case there is little or no clinical disability. However, the disease may progress.

NODULAR COAL-WORKER'S LUNG

Nodular reticulation

In these nodules the collagen is arranged radially rather than concentrically and the nodules are poorly circumscribed, small in size and contain coal dust rather than silica, giving them a softer outline, radiographic shadow and, on section, less gritty appearance.

Silicotic and compound silica – coal dust nodules

These are essentially silicotic lesions with coal dust less important. They particularly occur in coal miners exposed to risk of silicosis, e.g. hardheaders and other rock-workers. The appearances, histologically, are of central silicotic nodules of concentric appearance with surrounding zone of more radially-arranged collagen.

Progressive massive fibrosis – P.M.F.

NATURE

In this type there is massive fibrosis in the upper lobes, particularly posteriorly, in addition to the heavily pigmented zones of the simple pneumoconiosis.

The nodules are usually intensely black and more than 3 cm in diameter.

Originally thought to be a complication of silica content and subsequently the result of a complicating tuberculous infection, the evidence for both theories is incomplete and immunological factors are also poorly supported as of prime aetiological importance.

The reason for P.M.F. developing in some coal miners is, therefore, not clearly understood though tuberculous infection is identifiable in a significant number.

MACROSCOPICAL

Upper lobe or lobes replaced by jet black confluent masses with central cavitation and surrounding fibrosis.

MICROSCOPICAL

The periphery is densely collagenous and the centre is acellular with amorphous proteinaceous material replacing the collagen bundles.

RESULTS

1 In the early stages, the focal emphysema results in 'miner's asthma'.
2 Death from respiratory failure.
3 Death from cor pulmonale.
Overt clinical manifestations of tuberculosis

cause death in only a small proportion of cases – 4 per cent.

ASBESTOSIS

Aetiology
Due to inhalation of the fibres of asbestos – a magnesium silicate. The disease is encountered in persons exposed to these fibres.

Macroscopical
There is dense, bilateral, pleural thickening over the lower lobes. On section the lung parenchyma is shrunken by a diffuse fibrosis affecting mainly the basal areas. Pleural plaques are always present.

Microscopical
A diffuse fibrosis of the lung tissue associated with macrophage and foreign body giant cell reactions around the diagnostic 'dumb-bell' *asbestos bodies* which are present in the respiratory bronchioles.

Results
1 Pulmonary fibrosis with cor pulmonale.
2 Increased incidence of pulmonary tuberculosis.
3 Increased incidence of bronchial carcinoma and pleural mcsothelioma (see p. 680).

SILICO-SIDEROSIS – HAEMATITE LUNG

Aetiology
Inhalation of silica-containing iron ore in haematite quarry workers.

Macroscopical
The lungs are grossly and diffusely fibrotic and are a rusty red colour. Pleural thickening is marked and sometimes tuberculosis or a carcinoma of the bronchus complicate the appearances.

Microscopical
Dense, diffuse fibrosis with extensive iron deposition in the tissues. This brown pigment, which contains free iron, may also be present in the lymphoreticular cells elsewhere in the body, e.g. in lymph nodes and in the liver.

Results
1 Pulmonary fibrosis with cor pulmonale.

2 Pulmonary tuberculosis as a complication.

3 Predisposes to bronchial carcinoma.

BERYLLIOSIS

Aetiology

The inhalation of beryllium-containing dust in those processing beryllium ores or employed in the manufacture of fluorescent lighting tubes. Metal welders in the radio and television industries are also exposed to beryllium-containing dust.

Macroscopical

Focal fibrotic areas in the lung parenchyma, without significant pleural involvement. The fibrosis is later more diffuse and there are associated areas of emphysema.

Microscopical

The focal areas are beryllium granulomas which show a picture very similar to that of sarcoid with a centre composed of epithelioid-like cells. Sometimes the centre becomes necrotic and then mimics tuberculosis but organisms are not present. The only certain method of proving the aetiology of the granuloma is by chemical analysis.

Results

The same tissue reaction may occur in other organs, e.g. liver, lymph nodes and spleen, but the lung effects are the most serious and may, in severe cases, lead to death from respiratory or cardiac failure.

OTHER FIBROTIC DUST DISEASES

A number of other inhaled particles may produce significant fibrotic reactions including:

1 *Talc* – This type of hydrated magnesium silicate induces a considerable fibrous reaction when inhaled either for a long period of time or in very high concentrations for quite a short time.

2 *Kaolin* – Heavy exposure to china clay may cause severe and rapidly progressive fibrosis of lungs, particularly if associated with tuberculous infection.

3 *Aluminium* – Pure aluminium powder may cause severe pulmonary fibrosis.

4 *Fuller's earth* – Pneumoconiosis due to inhalation of this aluminium silicate is uncommon.

EXTRINSIC ALLERGIC ALVEOLITIS

Nature

A group of diseases caused by inhalation of vegetable dusts and often occupational in origin. Most cause a hypersensitivity type of immunological reaction in which immune complexes are formed consisting of large molecular aggregates containing antigen, antibody and complement. Some of these conditions may also cause a granulomatous inflammatory reaction in the lung.

Pathogenesis

Most of these diseases occur only in a small number of individuals exposed to the inhaled antigen as a manifestation of personal idiosyncrasy.

The hypersensitivity is quite frequently due to fungal contaminants and not to the vegetable matter itself.

In other disorders dried animal protein dusts initiate the hypersensitivity, e.g. pigeon-handler's lung.

Types of disease

There is an ever-growing list of conditions in this group.

VEGETABLE DUSTS

1 *Farmer's lung* – This follows the handling and close contact with mouldy hay, grain or silage. Inhalation of this fungally contaminated material results in granulomas of sarcoid-like appearance around terminal bronchioles and with a more diffuse interstitial mononuclear cell infiltrate. These changes may be very widespread throughout both lungs and severe bronchiolar damage may ensue with permanent functional disability.

2 *Bagassosis* – The waste material left after sugar has been extracted from cane is now used to manufacture insulating board, explosives and poultry food. When this is handled dry, the dust may cause severe allergic pulmonary manifestations with asthma, desquamative alveolitis and granulomas, later with some fibrosis. Fungi are probably responsible for the hypersensitivity. Severe disability can occur associated with capillary damage and alveolar fibrosis.

3 *Bysinnosis* – Originally described in cotton-workers in England, it has now been identified in other cotton-manufacturing countries and in workers with hemp and flax. There is marked bronchospasm but little damage to lung tissue

except in a minority of patients who develop some alveolar fibrosis and small granulomas around cotton fibres.

4 *Other vegetable dusts* – Rather similar, predominantly asthmatic conditions, sometimes with significant fibrosis and granuloma formation, are increasingly recognized amongst numerous groups of workers with dry vegetable products. These include:

(*a*) Maple-bark-stripper's lung – maple logs.
(*b*) Capsicum lung – paprika preparation.
(*c*) Mushroom-picker's lung – mushroom compost.
(*d*) Malt-worker's lung – preparation of malt from barley.

ANIMAL PROTEIN DUSTS

These are conditions of idiosyncrasy to a variety of inhaled allergens of animal origin, particularly bird droppings, e.g. pigeon-breeder's lung, budgerigar-fancier's lung and furrier's lung.

Although granulomas and interstitial inflammatory cell infiltration of lungs have been reported, the dominant clinical picture is of bronchospasm with fibrosis developing later, but only if exposure is maintained for a considerable length of time.

Results

1 *Acute attacks* – Though clinically distressing and alarming, single attacks seldom have sequelae of lung damage.
2 *Repeated attacks* – There is an increasing risk of progressive pulmonary fibrosis and functional impairment.
3 *Removal from exposure* – This is normally effective in preventing serious damage.

ALVEOLAR LIPO-PROTEINOSIS

Nature

A rare pulmonary disease which is of unknown aetiology, though experimental and other studies clearly indicate that it results from hyperplasia of type 2 pneumocytes with subsequent excess production of phospholipid and protein.

Appearances

The lungs appear widely consolidated and microscopically this is found to be due to distension of alveoli by a lipid-rich proteinaceous material which is strongly PAS-positive, alcian blue negative and stains metachromatically with toluidine blue.

Results

Most cases resolve spontaneously though about one-third have progressed to death from respiratory failure.

Other types of pulmonary fibrosis

IDIOPATHIC INTERSTITIAL FIBROSIS – FIBROSING ALVEOLITIS

Nature

A wide spectrum of clinical pulmonary diseases in which there is interstitial fibrosis of the lung without any identifiable aetiology.

This infers exclusion of known causes of interstitial fibrosis such as bacterial and virus pneumonia, radiation lung, chemical fumes and dusts, metabolic disorders and immunologically-mediated disorders such as the fibrosis of connective tissue disease (see p. 673).

Types

1 *Acute – Hamman-Rich lung*. This acute and frequently rapidly progressive type of interstitial fibrosis may extend for a few days or months before death from respiratory failure occurs or may become less acute and proceed to a chronic course.

Histologically, oedema, desquamation of lung cells and hyaline membrane formation is followed by accumulation of large numbers of histiocytes and subsequently by fibroblasts with abundant interstitial reticulin increase and later collagen. The severely desquamative variant has been sometimes incorrectly identified as '*desquamative interstitial pneumonia*'.

2 *Chronic – Diffuse interstitial fibrosis*. This may arise following the acute type above or *de novo* as a more insidious clinical and pathological disorder in which there is progressive interstitial fibrosis with obliteration of alveoli, alveolar ducts and bronchioles. This often leads to cyst formation and honeycomb lung with associated smooth-muscle hyperplasia and sometimes foci of calcification and even ossification – *microlithiasis pulmonum*. A wide spectrum of changes may be found in biopsy tissue from the single patient. A rare variant is *giant-cell interstitial pneumonia* in which foreign body type giant cells are numerous but inclusion bodies, as in measles pneumonia (see p. 662), are not seen.

Epithelial metaplastic changes are common.

Course

The clinical course is very variable in respect of the speed of progression.

The aetiology is unknown but, not uncommonly, serum rheumatoid factor is positive and moderate numbers of patients have low titres of ANA.

Some cases have responded to corticosteroid therapy with apparent arrest of progression but the clinical course of individual cases varies very widely and is rather unpredictable.

There appears to be a real increase in the development of peripheral lung cancer in long-standing cases of fibrosing alveolitis.

'HONEYCOMB LUNG'

Nature

This is a purely descriptive term applied to a localized or generalized, trabeculated, cystic or 'honeycomb' appearance of the lungs.

Macroscopical

The affected area or areas show a firm sponge-like appearance with a coarse texture due to cystic spaces which are thick-walled. This differentiates the appearances from those of emphysema.

Microscopical

The fibrous-walled, cystic spaces are lined by cuboidal or flattened cells and there is an increase in the smooth muscle. The cystic spaces are probably alveolar ducts which have become distended. In addition, there is obliteration of many alveolar spaces, whilst sometimes the specific cause of this alveolar obliteration may be histologically apparent, e.g. tuberculosis, sarcoidosis.

Aetiology

The cystic spaces are probably derived by distension of the alveolar ducts which follows obliteration of alveolar spaces. The causes of the alveolar destruction and thus of 'honeycomb lung' are:
1 *Fibrosing alveolitis* (see p. 672).
2 *Non-specific inflammation.*
3 *Specific granulomas and other lesions.* Previous tuberculosis, sarcoidosis, berylliosis, scleroderma, leiomyomatosis, eosinophil granuloma.

Results

Progressive pulmonary dysfunction and cor pulmonale.

LUNG CHANGES IN THE CONNECTIVE TISSUE DISEASES

In several of the connective tissue diseases (see p. 280–287), involvement of the lungs may be a prominent feature.

1 *Rheumatoid lung – Caplan's syndrome.* Rheumatoid nodules in the lungs in the general population have been described from time to time but they are exceedingly rare. What Caplan showed was that the pneumoconiotic lung is particularly vulnerable to this nodular rheumatoid disease. Caplan's syndrome, therefore, is 'rheumatoid pneumoconiosis'. In the general population, diffuse interstitial inflammation with fibrosis in the lung is a more common finding in rheumatoid disease than are nodules in the lung.

2 *Polyarteritis nodosa.* The pulmonary arteries are not uncommonly involved by this necrotizing arteritis (see p. 282). Ischaemic changes and infarcts may result.

In the allied condition of Wegener's granuloma (see p. 640) the lungs are invariably involved. Cavitating granulomas with necrotic centres and containing giant cells of Langhans' type are associated with fibrinoid necrosis in arteries and interstitial tissue.

3 *Systemic lupus erythematosus.* Pleural involvement is very common in this disease (see p. 281) but the lung parenchyma is only rarely affected.

4 *Scleroderma.* In the generalized type of this disease – *progressive systemic sclerosis* – fibrosis commonly occurs in the lungs with 'honeycomb' lung a frequent sequel (see above).

Causes of pulmonary fibrosis

The following diseases are the commoner causes of lung fibrosis:
1 *Inflammatory* – Bronchopneumonia (occasionally lobar pneumonia); chronic bronchitis with emphysema; tuberculosis; sarcoidosis; mycotic diseases; irradiation.
2 *Mechanical* – Bronchiectasis; collapse.
3 *Vascular* – Chronic passive venous congestion; infarction.
4 *Connective tissue diseases* – Scleroderma; rheumatoid lung.
5 *Pneumoconioses* – Including extrinsic allergic alveolitis.
6 *Fibrosing alveolitis.*

Chapter III
Respiratory System – Carcinoma of the Bronchus: Other Tumours: Diseases of Pleura

Carcinoma of bronchus

Incidence
There has been a great increase in incidence of primary carcinoma of the bronchus in recent years and there is little doubt that the increase is absolute. Deaths in England and Wales from lung cancer have increased from 7640 in 1946 to 35 000 in 1976. This latter figure represents approximately 35 per cent of all cancer deaths and 7 per cent of deaths from all causes.

Age
Fifteen to eighty years of age; with an average of 55 years.

Sex
Marked but falling male preponderance – M:F 3.5:1 in this country.

Aetiological factors
1 *Smoking*. This is undoubtedly the major factor. A definite statistical relationship has been estab-

674

lished between heavy cigarette smoking (more than twenty a day) and carcinoma of the bronchus. Such smokers have a ten times greater liability than light smokers or non-smokers, but the incidence in pipe and cigar smokers is much less. Furthermore, previously heavy smokers who give up the habit return to a non-smoker risk pattern at about 10 years. Carcinogenic hydrocarbons have been found in the tar from cigarette tobacco which, when applied to skin of animals, produce tumours and there is other supportive experimental evidence.

2 *Irradiation.* The very high incidence of carcinoma of the lung in the cobalt miners at Schneeberg and the radium miners at Joachimsthal (more than 50 per cent die from lung cancer) is associated with the presence of radioactive matter in the form of radon. This is believed to be the operative aetiological agent.

3 *Occupational lung cancers.* There is a high incidence in workers exposed to nickel carbonyl (nickel refiners) and arsenic (weed killers). Haematite quarry workers (haematite lung) and persons working with asbestos and with chromates also have an increased incidence.

4 *Atmospheric pollution.* City dwellers have a higher lung cancer rate than those who live in the country and although known carcinogens from industrial and diesel fumes are present in the atmosphere of cities, there is no direct evidence of a statistically significant increased incidence of carcinoma of the lung, if one corrects for cigarette smoking in the two localities.

Sites

1 *Central.* Approximately 55 per cent of the tumours arise in relation to main, lobar or segmental bronchi. The trachea is only very rarely a site of origin, although it may be invaded by extension of tumour arising in a main bronchus.

2 *Peripheral.* Approximately 40 per cent arise from smaller bronchi or from bronchioles; a macroscopic bronchial connection is commonly difficult to establish.

3 *Diffuse.* In 5 per cent the origin is either indeterminate or multifocal.

Macroscopical

Bronchus. Invasion of the bronchial wall with ulceration of the surface and narrowing or obliteration of the lumen at the site of origin is usually found. Occasionally, polypoid tumour tissue may fill the lumen.

Lung. Centred around the bronchus of origin, the tumour invades extensively in the lung tissue forming a pale, firm mass which may reach enormous sizes, e.g. 15 cm in diameter, and replace the entire lung. Areas of necrosis and haemorrhage are common, together with abscess formation within necrotic tumour.

Effects on the lung. Occlusion of bronchi leads to collapse and infection beyond the tumour with resulting bronchiectasis, abscess formation and fibrosis. Disturbance of vascular supply by the tumour may cause areas of infarction, a sinister sign which is usually indicative of vascular invasion.

Microscopical

1 *Squamous cell carcinoma.* Forty per cent of surgically removed tumours. This arises as a result of squamous metaplasia of bronchial epithelium. Metaplasia occurs frequently in chronic inflammatory conditions of the lungs but in these circumstances it is regular and does not progress to cancer; indeed, there is no increased incidence in these conditions. Atypical squamous metaplasia is nearly always found adjacent to squamous lung cancers and may be seen in other bronchi of the same patient. This may be sufficiently atypical and dysplastic to be designated 'carcinoma *in situ*'. These changes are widespread in the bronchi and trachea in patients with lung cancer and are also seen more frequently in smokers than in non-smokers dying of unrelated conditions. It has been suggested that areas of atypical squamous metaplasia may progress after a period of time, perhaps 10 years or more, to invasive carcinoma, but the occurrence of similar changes in the trachea makes the interpretation of the significance of these findings less certain.

The squamous cell tumours are mostly poorly differentiated with little keratin formation but they retain definitive squamous features.

2 *Adenocarcinoma.* Fifteen per cent of surgically removed tumours. This is a mucus-secreting adenocarcinoma in which tubule formation is often present. It is relatively more common in females.

3 *Bronchiolar (alveolar cell) carcinoma.* Approximately 0.5 per cent. This type of papillary mucus-secreting adenocarcinoma has certain distinguishing features. There is abundant mucus secretion and, from its origin in bronchioles, the cells spread widely using the alveolar framework of the lung which commonly remains. This type often appears to be multifocal in origin and is usually bilateral

with massive tumourous consolidation of the lungs. Whether the multiple nodules are of multifocal origin or spread via the air passages is debatable. The tumour bears a close resemblance to an infective condition which occurs in sheep – *Jagziekte*.

It is possible that some of the described cases of this tumour are in fact examples of secondary deposits of carcinoma within the lung which behave in this curious manner, e.g. from the pancreas.

4 *Small cell and oat cell carcinoma*. Fifteen per cent of surgically removed tumours but a much higher proportion of all lung cancers are of this cell type. The cells are hyperchromatic, elongated, closely packed and sometimes arranged in a rosette-like manner. Individual cells contain *neurosecretory granules* and are argyrophilic but not argentaffinic. They arise from bronchial mucosal cells of the '*diffuse endocrine system*' (see p. 145) and may produce a wide range of peptide hormones, particularly ACTH, ADH and calcitonin, sometimes clinically apparent (see p. 159).

5 *Large cell undifferentiated carcinoma*. Thirty per cent of surgically removed tumours. The cells are large and polygonal, arranged in solid sheets or with an alveolar arrangement. None of the distinguishing histological features described above are seen but this group probably represents undifferentiated forms of squamous cell carcinomas and adenocarcinomas.

Spread

These are usually rapidly growing tumours and metastasize early.

Direct. From its most common situation near the hilum of the lung the tumour invades lung and mediastinal tissues. The pericardium and heart are commonly invaded producing an haemorrhagic pericardial effusion and cardiac arrhythmias. Extension alongside pulmonary vessels is common and the oesophagus may likewise be involved with broncho-oesophageal fistula as a complication. Pleural invasion with the production of an effusion, often bloodstained, occurs frequently and this may become infected to produce an empyema. The chest wall may be invaded across the pleural cavity together with vertebrae and the tissues adjacent to the apex, where involvement of the cervical sympathetic chain and brachial plexus roots may give rise to the superior sulcus syndrome – *Pancoast's tumour*.

Lymphatic. These occur early in the natural history of the disease with invasion firstly of the regional intrapulmonary hilar lymph nodes and thence the extrapulmonary tracheobronchial and other groups of mediastinal lymph nodes. From this situation, lymphatic spread may occur to the cervical, supraclavicular and axillary nodes superiorly and to the para-aortic, iliac and inguinal groups caudally.

Massive mediastinal lymph node invasion may be the presenting feature of the disease with compression of the superior vena cava – *superior vena caval syndrome*, or the trachea – asphyxia.

Blood. At the time of surgical resection, examination of operative specimens may show vascular invasion in up to 70 per cent of cases. This propensity for early vascular invasion is the most important factor prognostically, reflecting the high inherent malignancy of the tumour. Metastases may occur in any organ, but are most frequently seen in the liver, bones, brain and adrenals. The lung is the commonest site of origin of secondary tumours in both the brain and the adrenals.

Transcoelomic. Multiple tumour deposits in the pleura may occur as a result of pleural invasion and subsequent transcoelomic spread.

Diagnosis

Biopsy. Bronchoscopic biopsy is the most satisfactory diagnostic procedure and its range has been extended by flexible fibre-optical instruments and transbronchial biopsy of alveolar tissue. Brushing and bronchial aspiration techniques are also very useful.

Sputum. Cytological examination of smears of sputum for malignant cells from cases of lung cancer may give positive results in as many as 85 per cent of cases and is thus an invaluable diagnostic aid. Many very small carcinomas, unseen radiologically, may be diagnosed in this way.

Pleural fluid. Malignant cells may be identified in aspirates from pleural effusions, particularly when they are haemorrhagic.

Lymph node biopsy. Enlarged cervical or axillary lymph nodes may, on histological examination, confirm the diagnosis. 'Blind' biopsy of scalene lymph nodes shows invasion by tumour in a surprisingly high number of cases.

Results

The course of the disease is generally rapidly progressive due to the high inherent malignancy and early lymphatic and vascular metastases.

Twenty per cent have distant metastases when first seen, many presenting with symptoms related to these. Untreated, the average survival time from diagnosis is 4 months, although 15 per cent may survive from 2 to 7 years. Most patients die from carcinomatosis. Adenocarcinomas are particularly unresponsive to therapy and there is little purpose in surgical treatment of oat-cell carcinoma.

Surgical treatment. Pneumonectomy and lobectomy yield 5-year survival figures of about 30 per cent, but when the number of cases which prove inoperable are included, the overall 5-year survival is 7–10 per cent.

Radiotherapy. The average survival time is prolonged to 14 months by radiotherapy, but only occasional long-term cures have been reported.

Cytotoxic chemotherapy. This may be particularly useful for palliation of oat-cell carcinomas.

Other lung tumours

BRONCHIAL CARCINOID

Nature
These are rare tumours of large bronchi forming less than 1 per cent of lung neoplasms but are important to identify because of their slow growing, late metastasizing behaviour, often in relatively young persons.

They resemble intestinal carcinoids (see p. 212) and arise from the Kultschitzsky cells in bronchial mucosa.

Macroscopical
A cherry-red, rounded swelling projecting into the lumen and covered by intact mucosa but with a greater proportion of the circumscribed tumour deep in the wall – 'iceberg' phenomenon.

Microscopical
The cells are small, eosinophilic, regular and typical of carcinoids elsewhere. They are arranged in a mixture of columns, rosettes or lacework patterns and are argyrophilic but only rarely argentaffinic or diazo-positive. Neurosecretory granules are present, ultrastructurally.

Effects
Bronchial obstruction with pulmonary collapse, infection and bronchiectasis. Clinical hormonal effects due to excess 5-hydroxytryptamine produc-

tion (see p. 145) is unusual, but occasional cases of the carcinoid syndrome from bronchial tumours have been recorded. Some secrete ACTH.

Results
Usually amenable to surgical resection and cure. Occasionally, the tumour has metastasized by the time of diagnosis but, even so, the fatal course is very protracted.

ADENOID CYSTIC CARCINOMA

Nature
Arises rarely in trachea and main bronchi as an infiltrating, late metastasizing tumour of mucous gland origin identical in other respects to similar tumours in salivary glands (see p. 180).

Behaviour
Locally, this produces luminal narrowing and progressive obstruction and also shows an 'iceberg' effect, like the carcinoid tumour. Ulceration is more common as is invasion of large blood vessels by direct extension.

Surgical resection may be impossible for anatomical reasons but it may be possible to prevent asphyxia by bronchoscopic resection of tumour over many years. Metastases are a late manifestation and the course is often in excess of 10 years.

OTHER EPITHELIAL TUMOURS

Occasional examples of mucoepidermoid and other mucous gland tumours (see p. 179) have been described in the major air passages. There is also a very rare benign bronchial papilloma of respiratory or squamous epithelium.

HAMARTOMA – ADENOCHONDROMA

Definition
A mass formed by tumorous overgrowth of a mixture of adult tissues normally present in the organ of origin.

Site
Almost all are subpleural lesions.

Macroscopical

The tumours are usually not more than 3 cm in diameter. They are spherical, easily shelled out, encapsulated, lobulated and hard. The majority are gritty on section due to areas of calcification and present a glistening cartilaginous cut surface. No bronchial connection is demonstrable.

Microscopical

The commonest type is composed predominantly of cartilaginous nodules separated by epithelial clefts. In addition, variable amounts of fibrous tissue, nerves, smooth muscle and blood vessels may be present.

Results

Cure follows enucleation of the tumour.

CONNECTIVE TISSUE TUMOURS

Fibroma
Haemangioma
Lipoma } All are extremely rare and benign.
Leiomyoma
Neurofibroma

Occasional cases of fibrosarcoma, neurofibrosarcoma and leiomyosarcoma have been recorded.

SECONDARY TUMOURS

The lungs are very frequently the site of metastases from tumours in many organs. Large solitary or multiple nodules of variable size may occur as a result of vascular spread via the systemic venous drainage, e.g. from the breast, bones, kidneys. A further type of widespead parenchymal invasion spreading fan-wise from the hilar region occurs as a result of retrograde lymphatic spread from mediastinal lymph nodes invaded by secondary tumour – *lymphangitis carcinomatosa*.

Diseases of the pleura

PLEURAL EFFUSIONS

TRANSUDATES

Appearances

This is a non-inflammatory collection of fluid in the pleural cavity, clear and straw-coloured with a relative density of less than 1.012 and a protein content of 0.3 g/100 ml or less.

The only cells present are occasional lymphocytes and mesothelial cells.

Causes

1 *Cardiac failure*. Associated with pulmonary oedema.
2 *Renal disease*. Hypoproteinaemic type in the nephrotic syndrome; renal failure.
3 *Liver disease*. Particularly cirrhosis.
4 *Meigs' syndrome*. Fibroma of the ovary associated with right-sided hydrothorax (see p. 437).

Effects

The volume of fluid may attain very large proportions – 2–3 litres, and is usually bilateral. The lungs are compressed, causing peripheral collapse and interference with respiratory function. The pleura remains glistening except in longstanding cases.

EXUDATES

Serous, sero-fibrinous and fibrinous

Appearances. All are examples of inflammatory exudates of straw-coloured fluid with varying amounts of pale fibrin. The relative density is 1.016–1.020 and the protein content is usually greater than 3 g/100 ml. In addition to exfoliated mesothelial cells a variable mixture of lymphocytes and polymorphs is present.

Causes. Most are secondary to inflammatory diseases of the underlying lung, e.g. tuberculosis, pneumonia, lung abscess and bronchiectasis. Organisms may be found, usually in small numbers, in the fluid.

Pleural exudates may also be associated with systemic infections, uraemia, pulmonary infarction, rheumatic fever and disseminated lupus erythematosus.

Effects. The fluid collects rapidly and often in large amounts causing collapse of lung by compression. The pleural surface is dull and covered by an inflammatory exudate of varying amounts.

Results. Alleviation of the cause leads to absorption of the fluid but some degree of adhesion formation is usual, especially when fluid persists for a considerable time. When longstanding this may cause fibrous thickening or obliteration of the pleural space. Progression of the inflammation in the underlying lung tissue may lead to empyema.

Empyema

Appearances. The fluid is characteristically creamy pus of yellow-green colour and contains large numbers of polymorphs in addition to the causative organisms.

Causes. Most commonly a complication of intra-pulmonary suppuration. Other causes include: extension of subdiaphragmatic infection, e.g. subphrenic abscess; spread from distant foci by lymphatic or haematogenous pathways; due to bronchopleural fistula; from mediastinitis, particularly due to perforation of the oesophagus or following leakage of surgical anastomoses.

The commonest bacteria causing empyema are: staphylococci, streptococci, pneumococci and *Mycobacterium tuberculosis*.

Effects

1 *Local.* The volume may be large with pressure effects on the lung. There is marked thickening of the pleura by fibrin, and adhesions form which usually lead to early localization or loculation of the pus.

2 *General.* Marked toxaemia is evident and there is a considerable polymorph leucocytosis.

Results. Rarely, the empyema may resolve, but nearly always there is organization of the exudate in spite of drainage or aspiration of the pus. This may lead to total obliteration of the pleural space or to a grossly thickened fibrotic pleura in which areas of calcification may subsequently occur. Expansion of the lung may be considerably hampered by such a layer and may require surgical decortication before the residual lung can re-expand. Some resulting disability is then inevitable.

Haemorrhagic

True haemorrhagic inflammatory exudates must be distinguished from haemothorax and from traumatic blood contamination of other exudates. They are found occasionally in haemorrhagic diatheses and in metastatic tumour involvement in the pleural cavity.

HAEMOTHORAX

This occurs when pure arterial or venous blood escapes into the pleural cavity. In addition to operative bleeding, direct injury to the chest wall with penetrating injuries of the lung or spontaneous rupture of diseased arteries, e.g. aortic aneurysm, dissecting aneurysm, are the common causes.

CHYLOTHORAX

The presence of milky-white fluid, containing large amounts of finely emulsified fat, in the pleural cavity usually reflects tumour obstruction of thoracic or cervical lymphatics. It may occasionally be traumatic in origin.

PNEUMOTHORAX

Air or gas in the pleural cavities.

1 *Spontaneous.* Occurs as a result of pulmonary disease with communication to the pleural space. It is most commonly associated with emphysematous bullae, cysts, abscess of the lung or tuberculosis.

2 *Traumatic.* Perforating injuries to the chest wall which allow air to enter the space from outside or following laceration of the lung substance.

3 *Therapeutic.* A largely discontinued method of lung deflation to promote rest and healing of tuberculosis was to introduce air into the pleural space with replenishment as absorption occurred.

Effects

In all cases, collapse of lung ensues and is maintained unless the communication seals. A valve-like action of tissue at the site of communication may lead to positive pressure in the space – tension pneumothorax, massive collapse of the lung and mediastinal shift.

TUMOURS

SECONDARY

The great majority of pleural tumours are metastatic deposits, particularly from breast and lung carcinomas. Numerous nodules scattered over visceral and parietal layers are seen, associated with effusions, often haemorrhagic.

PRIMARY

Primary pleural tumours are rare. Benign connective tissue tumours, e.g. fibromas and haemangiomas occur, as does also a benign tumour of fibrous tissue and mesothelial cells – *benign mesothelioma.*

Mesothelioma

This specifically pleural and peritoneal tumour is almost always associated with exposure to asbestos particularly the 'blue' type – *crocidolite* but at a dosage less than that which causes asbestosis (see p. 670). The gross appearances are characteristic of a very dense sheet of hard tumour tissue encasing one or both lungs and histologically showing cleft-like spaces surrounded by PAS-negative malignant mesothelial cells in a dense fibroblastic stroma. The course is rapidly fatal. Asbestos bodies are almost always found in lung parenchymal tissue.

Chapter 112
Skeletal System – Congenital: Traumatic

Bone structure

Bone is a connective tissue with specialized features which are relevant to an understanding of its pathology.

CORTEX

There is a cortex composed of dense (compact) bone with Haversian systems.

MEDULLA

The centre of the bone is the medulla with trabeculae of cancellous bone between which there is marrow, active or fatty depending on the site.

PERIOSTEUM

External to the cortex is the periosteum which has an outer fibrous layer and an inner osteogenic layer.

BLOOD SUPPLY

The blood supply is derived from the nutrient artery which penetrates through to the medulla and supplies the inner portion of the cortex as well as the medulla. Periosteal vessels supply the outer layers of the cortex.

REGIONS

In growing bone there are the following regions which are illustrated in Fig. 83.
1 *Diaphysis* or shaft.
2 *Metaphysis* – the zone adjacent to, and on the shaft side of, the epiphyseal line.
3 *Epiphyseal line* – the zone of enchondral ossification.
4 *Epiphysis* – the portion of bone at the end of a long bone which ossifies separately.

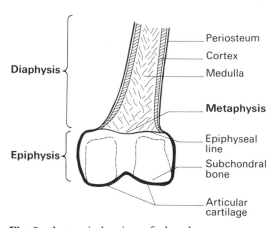

Fig. 83. Anatomical regions of a long bone.

BONE MATRIX

The organic matrix of bone – osteoid tissue, is composed of collagenous fibres separated by a mucopolysaccharide, chondroitin sulphate. The fibres are characteristically arranged in sheets – *lamellar bone*, which can be visualized with polarized light. In the embryo, young child and a range of pathological conditions irregular arrangement of fibres is a '*woven*' or *non-lamellar* pattern. There are three types of cell closely associated with osteoid tissue:

1 The mononuclear osteoblasts which lay down the osteoid tissue.
2 The multinucleated osteoclasts which are associated with bone resorption (see Fig. 6 on p. 26).
3 The osteocytes which are osteoblasts incorporated in lacunae in the bone matrix as bone cells, but which are no longer active in the formation of bone.

In health, bone matrix is not a static tissue, but is constantly changing due to osteoblasts laying down osteoid tissue and a balanced amount being removed by osteoclasts.

BONE MINERAL

This is the inorganic content of bone – 'bone salt', which is composed of a complex of calcium and phosphates known as *hydroxyapatite*. This mineral is deposited in the osteoid tissue and renders it hard. Thus:

osteoid tissue + mineral = bone.

However, bone is not simply a rigid static structure, as there is a constant exchange of calcium and phosphates between the bones and the body fluids and tissues.

OSSIFICATION

There are many factors involved in the formation of bone including:
1 An adequate blood level of calcium and phosphorus.
2 Vitamin D in adequate amounts.
3 The bone matrix must be present.
4 The skeletal mesenchyme must be normal.
5 Weight-bearing and exercise stimulate bone growth.
6 Alkaline phosphatase, derived from osteoblasts, probably releases phosphates from organic combination and thus promotes the precipitation of the calcium × phosphate complex.
7 Parathormone is a major factor in the control of serum calcium levels and indirectly of the phosphate levels. Calcitonin is also important (see p. 304).
8 Hormones, especially thyroxine, adrenal hormones, oestrogens and pituitary hormones should be present in normal balance.
9 The pH of the tissue is important; normal ossification occurs in a slightly alkaline medium.

BONE GROWTH

Growth of bone occurs by ossification of pre-existing tissues in two distinct ways:

OSSIFICATION IN MEMBRANE

Osteoid tissue is formed in connective tissue by osteoblastic activity without the intervention of preformed cartilage, e.g. membrane bones of the vault of the skull.

ENCHONDRAL OSSIFICATION

Ossification in preformed cartilage at epiphyseal lines and in the numerous separate ossification centres of bones, before and after birth.

NORMAL EPIPHYSEAL LINE

This is the site of enchondral ossification at the ends of long bones; enchondral ossification produces growth in length.

Macroscopical
A straight regular line with a white appearance due to a zone of calcification of cartilage and with a red vascular layer on the metaphyseal side.

Microscopical
An orderly structure composed of zones:
1 *Resting cartilage*. Columns of regular, small, cartilage cells.
2 *Proliferating cartilage*. Columns of large, hypertrophic, cartilage cells.
3 *Provisional calcification*. A zone of calcification of the cartilaginous stroma, the cartilage cells disappearing.
4 *Osteoid zone*. Osteoblasts grow in from the vascular metaphysis to lay down osteoid tissue on the calcified matrix.
5 *Mineralization*. The osteoid tissue becomes mineralized to form bone.
6 *Remodelling*. The bone is altered by remodelling to produce compact cortical and cancellous medullary bone.

Congenital diseases of bone

ACHONDROPLASIA

Nature
A congenital disease of dominant inheritance affecting all the bones in which enchondral ossification occurs, e.g. the long bones, the base of the skull and the pelvis.

Macroscopical
Achondroplastic dwarfs are approximately 137 cm tall with normally developed trunks but short limbs.
   Long bones. Approximately two-thirds of the normal length with a 'dumb-bell' appearance due to a short shaft but normally developed epiphyseal bone.
   Spine. Lordosis.
   Pelvis. Reduced in all diameters.
   Head. The base of the skull is small but the calvarium, which forms by ossification in membrane, is normal.

Microscopical
The abnormality is at the epiphyseal line where the epiphyseal cartilage is narrowed due to absence of the proliferating zone. As a result diminished growth in length occurs, the shaft is short but the epiphyseal bone is normally formed.

DYSCHONDROPLASIA

Nature
Developmental abnormalities of the epiphyseal line may result in persistence of cartilage inside or outside the bone.

Pathogenesis
There is persistence of epiphyseal cartilage into adulthood so that islands of cartilage are present within the bone – *enchondromas*, or on the cortical surface as cartilaginous masses growing away from the epiphyseal line – *ecchondromas*.

Macroscopical
1 *Enchondromas*. Single or multiple masses of cartilage in any bone, e.g. femur, but most commonly found in the fingers – *Ollier's disease*.
2 *Ecchondromas*. Cartilaginous nodules, frequently multiple, which are directed away from

their epiphyseal line of origin; the most common site is adjacent to the knee joint. The disease has a familial tendency and is variously named – *diaphyseal aclasia*, *multiple exostoses*, or *cancellous osteomas*. The cartilage ossifies from the base to leave only a cap of cartilage covering the cancellous bone; this also eventually ossifies.

Results

1 *Enchondromas*. May slowly ossify with disappearance of the cartilage or may become cystic due to degeneration; some grow to produce benign chondromas within the bone. It is this type of lesion which is the probable site of origin of many chondrosarcomas.

2 *Ecchondromas*. Produce protruberances, pain and deformity; a bursa may be formed superficial to the mass. Rarely, a chondrosarcoma may arise from the cartilage, an osteosarcoma from the bony base or a fibrosarcoma from the overlying fibrous tissues.

GARGOYLISM – LIPOCHONDRODYSTROPHY

Nature
A rare autosomal or sex-linked recessive disease combining a chondrodystrophy with the storage of lipid material in the brain and viscera.

Appearances
There are irregularities of enchondral ossification with variation of the size, shape and density of the long bones and kyphosis due to deformed vertebrae with posterior displacement. The accumulation of gangliosides and cerebrosides in the nerve cells of the brain results in mental retardation and convulsions and similar lipid storage in the viscera produces hepatosplenomegaly and cardiomegaly.

CHONDRO-OSTEODYSTROPHY – MORQUIO'S DISEASE

Nature
A rare congenital autosomal recessive disease affecting predominantly the epiphyses and spine.

Appearances
There is a severe kyphosis due to wedge-shaped vertebrae with irregular calcification and deformity

of the epiphyseal cartilages of the long bones resulting in enlargement of the ends of these bones.

MELORHEOSTOSIS

Nature
A rare congenital disease manifested by cortical hyperostoses, which begins in childhood and slowly progresses.

Appearances
One or more bones of the limbs shows thickened, flat, bony outgrowths from the cortex reminiscent of the appearance of wax solidifying from a candle. The causation of the disease is unknown but sometimes this extracortical bone has a cartilaginous cap, and the condition may thus be analogous to diaphyseal aclasia (see above).

MARFAN'S SYNDROME

Nature
A developmental autosomal dominant disease affecting mesenchymal tissues and especially involving the skeleton, eyes and cardiovascular tissues.

Appearances
The affected individuals are tall and thin with long tapering fingers – *arachnodactyly*, subluxations of the lenses of the eyes, defects of the cardiac atrial septum and a predisposition to develop medionecrosis of the aorta and thus a dissecting aneurysm (see p. 273). The basic defect appears to be a biochemical abnormality of the connective tissue cement substance.

MARBLE BONE DISEASE – OSTEOPETROSIS; ALBERS-SCHÖNBERG'S DISEASE

Nature
An inherited disease, in severe form autosomal recessive, and in mild form dominant with increased density of all bones ossified from cartilage, especially the vertebrae, pelvic bones and ribs.

Macroscopical
The bones are extremely hard and yet brittle so that

fractures readily occur. On section, the cortical compact bone extends into the medulla which is thus devoid of cancellous bone.

Microscopical
The abnormality starts at the epiphyseal line where there is prominence and persistence of the zone of calcification. This becomes surrounded by dense compact bone and there is a failure of remodelling into a cortex and medulla.

Results
In spite of the hardness, the bone is brittle and fractures are common. The encroachment of compact bone on the medulla results in a leuco-erythroblastic anaemia by displacement of haemopoietic tissues (see p. 448).

DRUG INDUCED – PHOCOMELIA

Nature
Failure or incomplete development of limbs due to interference with limb bud formation, e.g. as in thalidomide therapy during pregnancy.

Traumatic

SLIPPED EPIPHYSIS

Trauma is probably an important factor in the aetiology of slipped epiphysis but the precise mechanism remains unknown. Trauma may also affect the epiphyseal bone to cause osteochondritis juvenilis.

OSTEOCHONDRITIS JUVENILIS

Nature
This is a general term used to describe a number of lesions at different sites but which have pathological features in common.

Aetiology
There is usually a history of trauma which probably interferes with the epiphyseal blood supply. This is then followed by an avascular bone necrosis.

Sites
The disease affects epiphyseal bone prior to epiphyseal line fusion.

Macroscopical
The epiphyseal bone is irregularly sclerotic and rarefied with fragmentation and deformity. In a weight-bearing site the deformity involves the articular cartilage, producing characteristic radiological appearances upon which the diagnosis is usually made.

Microscopical
The initial lesion is an avascular necrosis of bone and the subsequent changes are those of attempted repair, with bone regeneration, haemorrhages, organization, sequestration and callus formation.

Results
The lesion produces pain and the condition clinically mimics joint tuberculosis. The articular cartilage may become deformed as a result of the alteration of shape of the underlying bone and thus predisposes to osteoarthritis, which is a common sequel, particularly in the hip.

Types
Named clinical types include:
1 Legg–Calvé–Perthes – Hip.
2 Osgood–Schlatter – Tibial tuberosity.
3 Sever – Calcaneum.
4 Kienböck – Lunate.
5 Köhler – Navicular.
6 Preiser – Carpal scaphoid.

FRACTURES

Nature
A fracture is a break in the continuity of the bone and it may be complete or partial – greenstick, simple or compound, comminuted or impacted. A pathological fracture is one through an area of previously abnormal bone, e.g. through a tumour, cyst, etc.

Stages of healing
1 *Haematoma formation.* The fracture severs the blood vessels in the medulla, cortex and periosteum so that a haematoma is produced.
2 *Organization.* Within 24 hours, capillary loops and fibroblasts begin to grow into the haematoma accompanied by an inflammatory cell infiltration. Thus, the area of blood clot is converted into vascular fibroblastic granulation tissue.
3 *Provisional callus.* By about the seventh day,

islands of cartilage and osteoid tissue appear in this granulation tissue. The cartilage probably arises from metaplasia of fibroblasts and the osteoid tissue is laid down by osteoblasts growing in from the adjacent bone ends. The osteoid tissue, in the form of irregular spicules and trabeculae, mineralizes to form the provisional callus which is in three zones:

(a) External callus – subperiosteal.
(b) Internal callus – medullary.
(c) Intermediate callus – cortical.

This irregular new bone is rapidly formed and the provisional callus is largely complete by about the twenty-fifth day.

4 *Definitive callus.* The disorderly provisional callus is gradually replaced by orderly bone with Haversian systems – definitive callus.

5 *Remodelling.* The normal contour of the bone is reconstituted by the process of remodelling due to both osteoblastic bone formation and osteoclastic resorption. This occurs relatively slowly over a variable period of time but eventually all the excess callus is removed, and the original appearances and structure of the bone reconstituted.

Abnormalities of healing

Bones show great facility for healing but certain complications may occur:

1 *Malunion.* Poor anatomical alignment of the fracture results in deformity, angulation or displacement.

2 *Delayed union.* This is common and is due to a large number of factors, many of which have in common the features of continued hyperaemia and decalcification:

(a) *Infection.* Occurs most commonly following compound fracture with retardation of all stages of the repair process.

(b) *Foreign bodies,* e.g. missiles, clothing, etc.

(c) *Dead bone fragments.* Especially in comminuted fractures.

(d) *Inadequate immobilization.* Results in damage to the reparative tissues.

(e) *Distraction of the fractured ends.* Increasing the volume of repair tissue required.

(f) *Avascularity.* Relative or absolute, e.g. avascular bone necrosis of the carpal scaphoid, head of the femur, etc.

(g) *Pathological fracture,* e.g. through tumours and cysts.

(h) *Age.* Rapid healing occurs in young persons but is often retarded in the elderly. This is due in part to the presence of decreased vascularity and also from slowing of all metabolic processes.

(i) *Nutritional and metabolic disorders.* Especially those affecting the basic materials required, e.g. calcium and phosphate; hypovitaminosis D; renal disease; parathyroid disorders; protein starvation, malabsorption syndromes or excessive protein loss as in albuminuria.

3. *Non-union.* Bony union does not occur, the defect being filled by fibrous tissue. Occasionally, a false joint may form at this site – *pseudo-arthrosis.* The following factors may be responsible for non-union:

(a) Lack of immobilization.
(b) Interposition of soft tissues, e.g. muscle.
(c) Wide separation of fragments, e.g. patella.
(d) Pathological fracture, e.g. through a malignant tumour.

Chapter 113
Skeletal System – Infections: Miscellaneous Bone Disorders

Bone infections

PYOGENIC

ACUTE OSTEOMYELITIS

Organisms
Most commonly *Staphylococcus pyogenes*, but may be caused by any pyogenic organism.

Mode of infection
Usually blood-borne from a septic focus, e.g. boil, although this may not be obvious; sometimes it occurs due to direct spread, e.g. from a septic finger, infected wound or compound fracture.

Age
The haematogenous form of the disease mostly occurs in children.

Sites
May involve any bone at any site but most frequently the metaphysis of long bones.

Macroscopical
The infection usually starts in the medullary cavity or in the subcortical bone and spreads up the medulla, or bursts through the cortex to produce elevation of the periosteum. At this stage there is bone destruction with pus formation and, in severe cases, the cortex dies due to deprivation of the

endosteal and periosteal blood supply resulting in the formation of a *sequestrum*.

This is strictly the end of the acute stage but in progressive cases it merges with chronic osteomyelitis.

In progressive cases, subperiosteal bone formation produces a sheath of new bone – the *involucrum*, in which there are defects – *cloacae* or sinuses, which allow exit of pus, necrotic debris and sequestra.

Microscopical

There is an acute inflammatory reaction within the bone with pus formation and bone destruction. Vascular thrombosis may be apparent, resulting in areas of dead bone.

Results

This description applies to the florid cases now seldom seen. The following may, however, result:
1 *Extensive destruction of the bone*. Sometimes with pathological fracture.
2 *Chronic osteomyelitis*. With osteoclerosis of surrounding bone and subperiosteal new bone formation.
3 *Resolution*. This only occurs if antibiotic treatment is given at an early stage. Minor degrees of bone destruction frequently result in sequestrum formation and complete healing is retarded until these fragments are removed.
4 *Suppurative arthritis*. By extension to neighbouring joints, e.g. hip joint where the epiphyseal line is intracapsular.
5 *Amyloid disease*. This may follow prolonged suppuration.
6 *Death*. From septicaemia or pyaemia.

CHRONIC OSTEOMYELITIS

Nature
In addition to the chronic phase following acute osteomyelitis described above, a chronic osteomyelitis may arise *de novo* due to localized bone infection with few organisms or with bacteria of low-grade pathogenicity.

Age
Most frequently seen in adults but may occur in children.

Organisms
Staph. pyogenes is the most common organism and is blood-borne. Other organisms, e.g. *Salmonella typhi* and brucella, are occasionally responsible.

Macroscopical
An area of dense sclerotic bone with an osteolytic centre expanding the shaft of the affected bone. This is known as a *Brodie's abscess* and the upper tibia is a favoured site.

Microscopical
The centre is composed of pus with surrounding inflammatory granulation tissue and fibrous tissue and with dense sclerotic bone due to reactive new bone formation. The subperiosteal tissues are also thickened with new bone formation.

Results
This tends to remain as a localized chronic inflammation which does not heal until the pus has been evacuated. The adjacent periosteum shows reactive new bone formation, resulting in thickening and increased density of the affected bone. Occasionally, chronic sinus formation may occur which in longstanding cases, may by complicated by amyloid disease.

NON-SUPPURATIVE OSTEOMYELITIS – GARRÉ'S OSTEOMYELITIS

A rare condition usually producing enlargement and increased density of the shaft of a long bone. Microscopically, there is a chronic non-specific granulomatous reaction in the bone and associated new bone formation but no pus is formed.

GRANULOMATOUS

BONE TUBERCULOSIS

Mode of infection
Haematogenous spread from a tuberculous focus elsewhere, most commonly from the lungs where the lesion may be either clinically active or healed.

Age
Maximal in children up to 10 years of age; rare in adults.

Sites

The vertebral bodies are the commonest site (see p. 717) but long bones, fingers and joints (see p. 709) are also involved. In a long bone, the tuberculous focus may start in the mid-shaft, at the metaphysis or in the subchondral bone.

Macroscopical

The bone becomes progressively and irregularly destroyed and shows extensive caseous material with rarefaction but no new bone formation – *caries*.

Microscopical

The bone is destroyed and replaced by active caseous tuberculous granulation tissue.

Results

As long as the infection remains, active bone destruction continues. With antituberculous chemotherapy, healing occurs, firstly by fibrosis and subsequently by new bone formation.

Complications

These are frequent and include:
1 Extension through the periosteum into the soft tissues sometimes with the production of a 'cold abscess'.
2 Sinus formation through the overlying skin.
3 Pathological fracture through the caseous material.
4 Joint involvement, especially with a subchondral focus (see p. 709).
5 Haematogenous spread to involve other organs.
6 Amyloid disease in very chronic cases.

SYPHILIS OF BONE

This is now a rare disease but the following types still occur:

Congenital

1 *Osteochondritis or epiphysitis*. The epiphyseal line becomes widened, soft and yellow in appearance.
2 *Periostitis*. The lesions may affect the periosteum producing a diffuse periostitis with new bone formation e.g. '*Sabre tibia*'.

Acquired

1 *Periostitis*. As in the congenital type, the perio-steum may be involved to produce irregular new bone formation.
2 *Gumma*. Solitary or multiple gummata may occur.

Miscellaneous bone disorders

FIBROUS DYSPLASIA – ALBRIGHT'S DISEASE

Nature

In the complete and relatively uncommon syndrome there is a triad of fibrous dysplasia of bone, skin pigmentation and precocious puberty. This complete syndrome is rarely seen, but single bone involvement – monostotic fibrous dysplasia, is common.

Aetiology

Probably due to a developmental defect of mesenchyme with excess fibrous tissue in the bone. This disease is unrelated to Paget's disease or to hyperparathyroidism.

Age

Young adults up to 40 years of age.

Sites

In the monostotic form, the mandible or maxilla are the most common sites but any bone may be involved. In the polyostotic type, the jaw may be involved bilaterally but in the long bones the multiple lesions are usually unilateral.

Macroscopical

The bone is expanded by firm, white, fibrous tissue containing palpable spicules of bone which fills the medulla and results in thinning of the cortex, so that pathological fracture is common.

Microscopical

The lesion is composed of comparatively avascular and acellular fibrous tissue which replaces the bone. There are no inflammatory cells present but a few fine bone trabeculae usually traverse the fibrous tissue and some osteoclastic activity may also be evident.

Biochemical

The serum alkaline phosphatase is raised, but calcium and phosphate levels are normal.

Results
In severe cases, pathological fractures, swellings and deformities result. Rarely, a fibrosarcoma may arise in an affected area.

PAGET'S DISEASE OF BONE – OSTEITIS DEFORMANS

Nature
A disease of unknown aetiology, occurring in both sexes above the age of 60 and associated with irregular thickening and softening of the bones.

Bones affected
Isolated solitary lesions of the spine or pelvis are common radiological findings on routine examinations, but clinical disease produced by lesions in many bones is uncommon.

Skull. Progressive increase in the size of the skull due to thickening of the bone which, on section, shows gross thickening of both tables and obliteration of the diploe. The base may also be involved to produce platybasia and pressure on nerves in their foramina.

Spine. Thickening and softening of the bones resulting in kyphosis, shortening of the trunk and pressure on nerves in the intervertebral foramina.

Femur. Increased in thickness with coxa vara and anterior bowing.

Pelvis. The bones are irregularly thickened, especially the iliac bones.

Tibia. Anterior bowing with gross thickening and palpable irregularity of the bone contour.

Clavicle. Thickened and unduly prominent.

On section, all the involved bones show gross and irregular thickening of cortical bone with loss of the normal sharp line of distinction between the cortex and medulla. The cortical bone encroaches upon the medulla in an irregular manner and there is softening and marked vascularity.

Microscopical
There is increased osteoclastic activity absorbing bone on one side of bone trabeculae, but more dominant is marked osteoblastic activity laying down new bone on the other side. This new bone is irregular and there are well marked 'cement lines' visible in the bone, producing the 'mosaic' or 'crazy-paving' appearance. The spaces between the thickened bone trabeculae are occupied by fibrous tissue containing large vascular channels. This latter feature is responsible for the marked vascularity evident macroscopically. The serum alkaline phosphatase is raised (see p. 696).

Results
This disease, which is slowly progressive but which, in severe cases, may be symptomatically improved by calcitonin, may produce:

1 *Deformities.* Of all the bones involved.
2 *Pain.* Due to stretching of the periosteum.
3 *Pressure on nerves.* As they pass through bony foramina, e.g. deafness, blindness, etc.
4 *Cardiac hypertrophy.* Due to the grossly increased vascularity of the bones.
5 *Sarcomatous change.* In approximately 1 per cent of cases (see p. 699).

HYPERTROPHIC PULMONARY OSTEO-ARTHROPATHY

Nature
Clubbing of the fingers associated with thickening of the terminal limb bones.

Aetiology
Usually associated with chronic pulmonary disease or cyanotic heart disease but occasionally occurs in ulcerative colitis and other abdominal conditions.

Appearances
There is marked periosteal fibrosis and subperiosteal new bone formation of the distal phalanges to produce the clubbing. In severe cases this may also involve other bones of the hands, wrists or feet.

Pathogenesis
The cause of the bone thickening remains unknown but may be due to anoxia or it may follow oedema of the affected areas.

HISTIOCYTOSIS X

Nature
A range of disorders with a common histiocytic factor and usually systemic in distribution but with particular clinical effects in bones.

The aetiology is unknown and there is overlapping between the types identified below.

Types

1 *Eosinophil granuloma of bone.* This presents in children and young adults as solitary or multiple foci of bone rarefaction particularly in skull, pelvis and vertebrae. The lesions are composed of histiocytes, fibroblasts and large numbers of eosinophils. Local lesions may require curettage and bone chips, but most regress spontaneously. Occasionally, lesions are present in non-skeletal tissues, e.g. lung, gastrointestinal tract, subcutaneous tissues. Some patients show a mixture of this lesion and changes of Hand–Schüller–Christian disease.

2 *Hand–Schüller–Christian disease.* This normocholesterolaemic lipid storage disease of children and young adults also presents as multiple, punched out, radiolucent areas of bones, particularly skull. The predominant cell is a foamy cholesterol-laden histiocyte with some fibroblasts and eosinophils present. Deposits in the skull often occur in the orbit causing proptosis and hypothalamic region producing hypopituitarism. Visceral deposits may cause hepatosplenomegaly. The disorder is rapidly fatal in children, more protracted in adults.

3 *Letterer–Siwe disease – Non-lipid reticuloendotheliosis.* Usually, this is a rapidly progressive fatal disease of childhood in which deposits of atypical and often primitive and bizarre histiocytic cells are found in many organs, particularly skin, lymph nodes, spleen, liver, lung and bones. No lipid is present in these malignant-appearing cells, but foci of typical Hand–Schüller–Christian disease lesions are also often present.

Chapter 114
Skeletal System III – Bone Rarefaction

Nature
Rarefaction of bone is seen radiologically as decreased density and can be due to three completely different processes:
1 A deficiency of the bone matrix – *osteoporosis*.
2 Defective mineralization – *rickets and osteomalacia*.
3 Hyperparathyroidism – *osteitis fibrosa cystica*.

Osteoporosis

Definition
Osteoporosis is a reduction in the quantity of the bone matrix; the matrix which remains is fully mineralized.

In osteoporosis, the blood levels of calcium, phosphate and alkaline phosphatase are all within normal limits (see Fig. 76 on p. 696), although there is evidence of increased urinary calcium excretion.

Macroscopical
Osteoporotic bones are lighter in weight, less dense on radiography and show thinning of the cortex. This osteoporotic bone is weaker than normal and is, therefore, prone to fracture, e.g. in the spine.

Microscopical

The bone trabeculae are thinner than normal, but are fully mineralized. Usually there is a decrease in the number of osteoblasts resulting in a failure to lay down new bone matrix, although in some instances there may be an excess of osteoclastic activity absorbing the bone matrix.

Osteoporosis is found in the following conditions:

SCURVY

Nature

A generalized disease due to lack of vitamin C.

Aetiology

Ascorbic acid is water-soluble and is derived from the diet. It is rapidly absorbed and there is a long time-lag before the appearance of signs of deficiency as there are large stores in many organs of the body. Scurvy arises due to inadequate intake of fresh fruit and vegetables, which are the main dietary source of the vitamin.

Action of ascorbic acid

Vitamin C is essential for:
1 The formation of collagen.
2 The formation of osteoid tissue.
3 The production of intercellular cement substances and maintenance of the integrity of blood vessels.

Thus, in scurvy, there is poor collagen formation, e.g. poor healing of wounds, lack of osteoid tissue so that normal bone matrix cannot be formed and haemorrhages from the abnormal blood vessels.

Macroscopical

Calcification is normal in scurvy and the zone of provisional calcification persists as a thick white line visible macroscopically and radiologically. There is decreased osteoid formation and haemorrhages occur in the vascular metaphysis and in the subperiosteal regions.

Microscopical

At the epiphyseal line, the resting and proliferating zones are normal. The zone of provisional calcification is pronounced to form the 'scorbutic lattice', but osteoid deposition in this zone is deficient. Instead, there is a vascular, haemorrhagic and oedematous zone of myxomatous tissue. The bones also become generally osteoporotic as normal amounts of osteoid tissue cannot be formed by the osteoblasts, so that the whole skeleton becomes progressively deficient in bone matrix.

DISUSE

Normal muscular activity is a stimulus for the preservation of normal bone structure, so that any prolonged immobilization or muscular paralysis induces osteoporosis. In the early stages, there is increased osteoclastic bone resorption resulting in thinning of the bone which may be associated with excessive mobilization of calcium, hypercalciuria and renal stone formation. Later, the bone becomes quiescent with diminution of both osteoclastic and osteoblastic activity. The bones return to normal when the patient resumes normal activity.

HYPERTHYROIDISM

Thyrotoxicosis may be associated with mild osteoporosis, apparently due to increased osteoclastic activity.

OSTEOGENESIS IMPERFECTA

A congenital dominant disease in which the bones are slender and the trabeculae thinner than normal although normally mineralized. When severe, the condition may result in multiple fractures and gross deformities in the neonatal period.

A similar condition, producing multiple fractures and associated with blue sclerotics and otosclerosis, is known as *fragilitas ossium*.

CUSHING'S SYNDROME

Osteoporosis is a constant finding in this syndrome and is believed to be due to the suppression of osteoblastic activity by the excess glucocorticoids (see p. 291).

CORTICOSTEROID THERAPY

The prolonged administration of prednisone and allied steroids frequently produces osteoporosis in a similar manner to Cushing's syndrome.

IMPAIRED SUPPLY OF PROTEINS

Excessive loss of protein, e.g. the nephrotic syndrome; deficient production, e.g. cirrhosis of the liver; or malabsorption, e.g. malabsorption syndromes, may all result in osteoporosis. This is due to the inability to form osteoid tissue in protein-deficient states.

PRIMARY, INVOLUTIONAL, SENILE OSTEOPOROSIS

Nature
The commonest type of osteoporosis with no known cause but with increasing frequency with age and presenting the features of an involutionary process.

Aetiology
Unknown mechanism but recent studies suggest a relative calcium deficiency to be important, perhaps with a failure of osteoblastic activity, through the involutionary process of the ageing body, to keep pace with skeletal loss. The widely held view that oestrogen deficiency, as in post-menopausal women, was important, has no support when unselected material is examined in which the sex incidence of porotic changes is roughly equal.

Sites
All bones except skull may be affected but particularly spine and upper femur.

Macroscopical
Affected bones are excessively fragile and prone to fracture or collapse, e.g. *codfish spine*, and very frequent fractures of femoral neck in the elderly.

Microscopical
The bone trabeculae are thinned and reduced in number but appear fully mineralized. The osteoblasts show little activity.

Demineralization

Definition
This second group of conditions causes bone rarefaction due to abnormalities of mineralization. The skeleton therefore contains osteoid tissue which is deficient of its mineral content. The group

is characterized by lowered serum calcium and phosphate levels, the calcium × phosphate solubility product is reduced and the alkaline phosphatase is raised (see Fig. 84 on p. 696).

RICKETS

Nature
A generalized bone disease due to deficiency of vitamin D and affecting the epiphyseal line and all other skeletal tissues.

Aetiology
Usually due to dietary deficiency, but sometimes may be caused by failure of absorption of vitamin D or by a low intake of calcium or phosphate.

Action of Vitamin D
This fat-soluble vitamin has several actions including:
1 Aids in the absorption of calcium and phosphate from the intestine.
2 Utilization of calcium and phosphate and its deposition to mineralize osteoid tissue.
3 Excretion of phosphate.

Age
Young children, including infants more than 6 months old.

Incidence
The disease is now very rare in this and many other countries, but remains important in economically backward areas.

Macroscopical
1 *Enlarged epiphyseal lines.* These are widened, lengthened and irregular. This produces a clinical deformity commonly seen in the ribs where it is referred to as 'rickety rosary'.
2 *Softening of the bones.* The skeleton generally is poorly mineralized and soft. The resulting deformities vary according to the stresses at different sites, e.g. coxa vara, flattened pelvis, scoliosis, 'pigeon chest', etc.
3 *Stunted growth.*
4 *'Craniotabes'.* Bossed appearance of the skull due to persistence of suture lines and fontanelles.
5 *Delayed dentition.*

Microscopical

The basic abnormality is a failure of full mineralization of osteoid tissue at all sites. The changes are thus:

1 The zone of provisional calcification is deficient, but there is continuation of growth of the proliferating cartilage cells so that areas of cartilage are found in the diaphysis away from the epiphyseal line.

2 The proliferating cartilage continues to grow to produce a thick, broad and irregular line.

3 Osteoid is laid down on the irregular foci of poorly calcified cartilage to produce a completely haphazard and irregular mass instead of the orderly arrangement of cells at the normal epiphyseal line.

4 The shafts of the bones are formed by osteoid tissue with gross deficiency of mineralization so that there is little true bone; this is the cause of the softening and resulting deformities.

OSTEOMALACIA – ADULT RICKETS

Nature

This is the adult form of rickets and is very uncommon in this country when due to dietary deficiency, but cases occur associated with the malabsorption syndromes (see p. 208).

Aetiology

Vitamin-D deficiency and reduced calcium intake in adults, especially in women during pregnancy and lactation, when excessive demands are made upon relatively inadequate dietary supplies of calcium. Rickets or osteomalacia may occur in coeliac disease or idiopathic steatorrhoea, where there is failure to absorb both vitamin D and calcium. A gluten-free diet may markedly improve all aspects of the condition which is described on p. 209.

Appearances

There is an excessive amount of osteoid tissue surrounding the thin bone trabeculae with little evidence of mineralization. The lack of mineral results in softened bones and produces many of the changes seen in rickets, particularly the deformities. Some cases may also show areas of osteitis fibrosa cystica presumed to be due to secondary parathyroid hyperplasia following a lowering of the serum ionized calcium level (see p. 317). The biochemical changes are summarized in Fig. 84 on p. 696.

RENAL OSTEODYSTROPHY

Nature

The kidney is intimately involved in calcium and phosphate metabolism and, just as primary disturbances of mineral metabolism, e.g. in hyperparathyroidism, can cause renal disease, e.g. nephrocalcinosis, so some cases of renal disease will manifest skeletal changes. The part played by the kidney in maintenance of normal levels of calcium and phosphorus in the body is largely a tubular function. It follows, therefore, that skeletal abnormalities are most likely to occur in renal lesions associated with loss of tubular mass or with defective tubular function.

The bone changes due to renal disease, however, vary very widely according to the nature of the renal lesion, its duration and age of the patient, and renal rickets is not a term which describes the condition sufficiently accurately. Renal osteodystrophy is a preferred name for these secondary skeletal changes.

It should be noted that the changes are often patchily distributed and that the several types of change may occur together even in the same bone. In many cases of chronic renal disease significant bone abnormalities never occur but in a small proportion, particularly in progressive renal failure in childhood, the skeletal deformities may be the most striking clinical abnormality.

Bone changes

1 *Osteitis fibrosa* – due to reactive hyperplasia of the parathyroids, *secondary hyperparathyroidism*.

2 *Rickets or osteomalacia* – due to disturbance of vitamin-D metabolism, probably due to an acquired insensitivity to its action.

3 *Osteosclerosis* – the cause of which is obscure but may be an unusual manifestation of parathyroid overactivity. In these cases there is markedly increased radiodensity of affected bones, particularly of the vertebrae. The bone adjacent to the intervertebral discs is affected in the first place – *rugger-jersey spine*. The cancellous trabeculae are grossly thickened with reduction of marrow space, remaining areas having a fibrocellular content.

Classification

URAEMIC OSTEODYSTROPHY
Juvenile form (renal dwarfism, renal rickets).
Adult form.

ASSOCIATED WITH FAILURE OF TUBULAR
REABSORPTION

1 *Phosphaturia* – vitamin-D-resistant rickets. A
Mendelian dominant hereditary tubular disease
characterized by defective tubular reabsorption of
phosphates and hence increased urinary output.
The bone changes are those of rickets or osteomalacia depending on the age of the patient and are
resistant to normal dosage of vitamin D but respond
to high dosage, which needs to be maintained in
spite of the risk of hypercalcaemia and subsequent
nephrocalcinosis.

2 *Renal tubular acidosis.* An intrinsic functional
abnormality of renal tubules causing an inability to
secrete an acid urine with resulting acidosis, high
urinary calcium excretion and excess phosphate
loss. The skeletal changes are those of osteomalacia.
Potassium depletion also occurs and requires correction together with the acidosis: vitamin-D therapy improves the bone disorder. Osteomalacic
changes may also be produced by the hyperchloraemic acidosis due to implantation of ureters in the
colon.

3 *Fanconi syndrome.* A congenital autosomal
recessive disorder of renal tubular function with a
variety of effects notably aminoaciduria, phosphaturia and glycosuria. The bone changes are those of
osteomalacia. In some cases cystine crystals are
deposited in the tissues – *Lignac–Fanconi syndrome.*

There is a *swan-neck* deformity of the proximal
convoluted tubules which are shorter than normal.
Treatment is by large doses of vitamin D together
with correction of potassium depletion and acidosis.

Biochemical changes
These are summarized in Fig. 84 below.

SUMMARY

Thus, bone matrix which is not fully mineralized is
characteristic of osteomalacia and rickets. This may
be due to:

1 *Dietary causes.* Vitamin-D deficiency.

2 *Intestinal malabsorption,* e.g. coeliac disease and
idiopathic steatorrhoea.

3 *Renal causes.* Congenital tubular defects;
acquired loss of tubules.

When there is an associated lowering of serum

	Blood				Urine		
	Ca	P	Alk. Ph	Urea etc.	Ca	P	Protein etc.
Osteoporosis	N	N	N	N	N or Sl+	N	Nil
Osteomalacia	N or Sl. low	Low	Raised	N	Low	Low	Nil
Hyperparathyroidism (uncomplicated)	Raised	Low	Raised or N	N	++	Raised	Nil
Uraemic osteodystrophy	N or Sl. low	Raised	N or raised	Raised	N or low	Low	Protein+
Phosphaturia	N	Low	N	N	Low	Raised	Nil
Tubular acidosis	N	Low	N	Low CO$_2$ High Cl. Low K	Raised	Raised	Nil Raised K
Fanconi syndrome	N or Sl. low	Low	N	N	Low	Raised	Protein+ Amino acid+ Glucose+
Paget's disease	N	N	Raised+	N	N	N	N

Fig. 84. Metabolic changes in bone disease.

ionized calcium level, the histological picture of osteomalacia may be complicated by secondary hyperparathyroidism with, in severe cases, osteitis fibrosa cystica.

Hyperparathyroidism

OSTEITIS FIBROSA CYSTICA – VON RECKLINGHAUSEN'S DISEASE OF BONE

PRIMARY HYPERPARATHYROIDISM

Aetiology
Hypersecretion of parathormone by an adenoma, an adenocarcinoma or, more rarely, by hyperplastic parathyroid tissue (see p. 316).

Pathogenesis
The excess parathormone mobilizes mineral from the bone, followed by removal of matrix and subsequently by fibrous replacement and cysts.

Bone changes
Detectable bony changes occur in only 25 per cent of cases of hyperparathyroidism.

Macroscopical
The bones become demineralized and, in advanced cases, so soft that they can be cut with a knife.

Deformities follow the softening. In addition, there may be single or multiple expanded, haemorrhagic and cystic tumour-like areas in the bone – '*brown tumours*' (see p. 703).

Microscopical
The demineralized bone is removed by osteoclastic activity and replaced by vascular and cellular fibrous tissue containing many osteoclastic giant cells with cysts and areas of haemorrhage.

Effects
The appearances of the parathyroid glands, the nephrocalcinosis, metastatic calcification and the blood changes are described on p. 317. The important and diagnostic biochemical feature is a rise in the serum ionized calcium level.

SECONDARY HYPERPARATHYROIDISM

As described above many examples of rickets and osteomalacia may contain areas of osteitis fibrosa cystica in the bones. This appearance is the result of excess parathormone due to secondary hyperplasia of the parathyroid glands induced by a low ionized serum calcium level. The conditions may thus follow disturbances of vitamin-D metabolism, renal tubular lesions or malabsorption syndromes.

Chapter 115
Skeletal System – Tumours of Bone

INTRODUCTION

Secondary tumours in bone are common but primary tumours of bone are comparatively rare. Malignant bone tumours account for approximately 0.6 per cent of deaths from malignant disease, killing some 600 people annually in England and Wales.

In spite of their comparative rarity, a large number of types occur and no completely satisfactory classification has yet emerged. The following account covers many of the relatively more common tumours which are encountered and the variants from which they have to be differentiated.

Bone tumours

These are osteoblastic tumours, i.e. tumours of osteoblasts.

OSTEOMA

Two types of benign osteoma are described:

CANCELLOUS OSTEOMA

This is not a true tumour but is a manifestation of diaphyseal aclasia (see p. 684). The outgrowth of cancellous bone has a cartilaginous cap from which chondrosarcoma may rarely develop.

IVORY OSTEOMA

A rare but true tumour of bone which almost always occurs in the skull. It is usually a spheroid of dense, compact bone and may cause pressure effects within the cranial cavity or in a nasal air sinus. Histologically, there is compact bone with Haversian systems. Symptoms are produced by pressure or by infection which may result in osteomyelitis of the adjacent bone.

OSTEOSARCOMA – OSTEOGENIC SARCOMA

Age
Maximal between 10–25 years of age but the tumour also occurs in an older age group when it may arise in relationship to Paget's disease of bone.

Sites
May occur in any bone but is most commonly found in the neighbourhood of the knee joint. They mostly arise near the ends of long bones and rarely are multifocal in origin.

Predisposing factors
1   Paget's disease of bone.
2   Long-term effects of radioactive substances, e.g. painters of luminous watch dials.

In the majority of cases the causation remains completely unknown and trauma is almost certainly in no way an aetiological factor.

Macroscopical
An haemorrhagic, variegated tumour expanding the bone and destroying both medulla and cortex; spicules of bone may be palpable within the tumour substance. The periosteum is frequently raised to produce 'Codman's triangle' at the junction of the raised periosteum and the cortex. This is, however, in no way specific for an osteosarcoma and may be produced by any lesion which lifts the periosteum and is followed by subperiosteal new bone formation.

Microscopical
The essential feature is the presence of malignant osteoblasts which lay down spicules of irregular osteoid tissue. This osteoid tissue may or may not calcify and this variable feature will determine the radiological appearances as being either osteolytic or osteosclerotic. The tumour osteoblasts are atypical, bizarre, show mitotic activity and frequently giant-cell forms. Small areas of cartilage may be present and secondary necrosis and haemorrhage are also frequently seen. It is common to find microscopical evidence of vascular invasion within the tumour tissue.

Spread
These tumours are rapidly growing, destroy bone locally and often penetrate the periosteum to involve soft tissues. Lymphatic spread is unusual but vascular spread is common and early.

Prognosis
This tumour has a most sinister prognosis and a 10 per cent 5-year survival is optimistic. Widespread

blood-borne metastases occur, especially in the lungs. A better differentiated variant of improved prognosis which develops on the external surface of a bone is the *juxtacortical osteosarcoma*.

OTHER OSTEOBLASTIC TUMOURS

OSTEOID OSTEOMA

Nature. A rare lesion occurring in the subcortical areas of any bone but especially in the femur and tibia. It arises in patients between 15–25 year of age and causes severe pain, especially at night.

Macroscopical. A central, pink, fleshy nidus of soft tissue of about 1 cm or less in diameter is surrounded by dense sclerotic bone.

Microscopical. The central nidus is composed of vascular tissue in which there is osteoblastic activity forming osteoid tissue and bone. A few osteoclasts may also be present.

Results. Incomplete removal may lead to a recurrence but complete removal is curative. When the lesion is very small, it is helpful to X-ray the specimen to ascertain the correct area to section.

BENIGN OSTEOBLASTOMA – OSTEOGENIC FIBROMA – GIANT OSTEOID OSTEOMA

Sites. Although most commonly seen in the neural arches of vertebrae, other bones in young adults may be the site of this very rare lesion.

Macroscopical. There is expansion of the bone of origin by a mass with a translucent centre containing specks of calcification.

Microscopical. The appearances are somewhat similar to those of an osteoid osteoma but there is a more prominent fibrous stroma and the lesions are larger.

Results. Expansion of the bone of the vertebral arch may result in spinal cord compression (see p. 719). The histological appearance has to be distinguished from that of an osteosarcoma. The prominent fibrous stroma with areas of active ossification is responsible for the descriptive name of osteogenic fibroma.

Cartilage tumours

These are tumours of cartilage cells.

CHONDROMA

Two types of chondroma are described:
1 *Ecchondroma.*
2 *Enchondroma.*

The ecchondroma is the cartilaginous outgrowth which occurs in diaphyseal aclasia (see p. 684) and the enchondroma is the cartilage which persists within the bone in dyschondroplasia (see p. 683). The latter are single or multiple cartilaginous areas which may:
1 Ossify and disappear.
2 Remain as islands of cartilage.
3 Slowly grow as chondromas.

The most frequent site is the phalanges of the fingers, where they are usually multiple, but similar tumours may occur elsewhere, e.g. in the femur. Histologically, they are formed by regular, mature and comparatively acellular cartilage, with areas of ossification or mucoid degeneration in the stroma.

Results

Regression may occur at any stage or the lesions may continue to grow, producing pain or deformity. Pathological fracture through an enchondroma may occasionally occur and there is a risk of chondrosarcoma developing subsequently.

CHONDROSARCOMA

Nature

This tumour of cartilage cells is probably the most frequently encountered primary malignant tumour of bone.

Age

All ages are affected although there is a slight predilection for young persons.

Sites

Pelvis and long bones, especially in the area of the knee.

Predisposing factors

Most of the tumours probably arise in pre-existing enchondromas or ecchondromas but some have been reported as occurring in association with Paget's disease in the older age groups.

Macroscopical

Bulky, lobulated, glistening and semitranslucent

tumours. The tumour may be entirely within the bone but more usually extends outside or away from the bone to indent or invade adjacent soft tissues. White, gritty areas of calcification and areas of cystic degeneration are commonly seen.

Microscopical

A malignant tumour composed of cellular atypical cartilage with irregularity of the cells, many of which have double nuclei. Mitotic figures are usually scanty but areas of cystic change, calcification or ossification are frequently seen in the stroma.

Spread

These are more slowly growing than osteosarcomas and compress adjacent soft tissues in the early stages. Later, direct invasion occurs and blood, and occasionally lymphatic, spread may also be manifest.

Prognosis

Surgical extirpation results in approximately a 50 per cent 5-year survival. In fatal cases, the lungs are the most common site of metastases.

OTHER CARTILAGINOUS TUMOURS

BENIGN CHONDROBLASTOMA – CODMAN'S TUMOUR

A rare tumour occurring at the age of 20 or younger. Epiphyseal bone with involvement of the epiphyseal line is the site of choice, especially at the knee or in the upper end of the humerus. Microscopically, this is a cellular tumour composed of chondroblasts. The cells frequently show mitoses and giant cells which, however, are much smaller than those seen in a giant cell tumour. In addition, there are areas of cartilage which may calcify and often areas showing some bone formation.

This is a benign tumour, but its chief importance is that the cellularity of the stroma may lead to a false diagnosis of malignancy, usually being designated as a malignant giant-cell tumour.

CHONDROMYXOID FIBROMA

An equally rare tumour occurring below the age of 30 and involving the epiphyseal line, especially at the upper end of the tibia; however, the epiphysis is spared. The tumour is firm and lobulated and composed of lobules of fibrous tissue separated by myxomatous tissue containing cells in lacunae, thus mimicking the appearances of cartilage.

This is also a benign tumour and yet the cellularity and atypicality of some of the areas may result in an incorrect histological interpretation as a chondrosarcoma.

Fibrous tumours

There are a number of fibrous tissue lesions in bone:

FIBROMA OF BONE

A rare lesion in bone producing a localized area of rarefaction with a clear-cut margin. Microscopically, it is composed of inactive, acellular, fibrous tissue, but its precise differentiation from fibrous dysplasia (see p. 689) is difficult to determine. The stroma may ossify to result in an 'ossifying fibroma' and the chief complication is pathological fracture.

FIBROSARCOMA

Age
Occurs particularly in young adults and those of middle age although the elderly are not exempt.

Sites
The ends of long bones are the sites of election but they may less commonly occur in the mid-shaft regions.

Macroscopical
Two types:

1 *Periosteal*. A rare form which produces a white, firm, fibrous tumour firmly attached to the periosteum and involving the adjacent soft tissues to a greater extent than the bone.

2 *Endosteal*. The endosteal or medullary fibrosarcoma produces expansion of the bone with destruction due to replacement by firm, white, fibrous tumour extending within the medullary cavity.

Microscopical
Both are fibrosarcomas showing variable collagen

formation. The medullary type destroys the bone as it progresses along the shaft and there is usually microscopic extension well beyond the macroscopic margins.

Spread
Spread occurs by direct invasion and also by lymphatics and by the blood stream.

Prognosis
The periosteal form has a better prognosis than the more common medullary type, which has a 25 per cent 5-year survival.

OTHER FIBROUS TUMOURS

MALIGNANT FIBROUS HISTIOCYTOMA

Rather high-grade malignant bone tumours containing a mixture of spindle-shaped fibroblasts with histiocytic cells, some multinucleated. A '*storiform*' pattern is characteristic.

OSTEOGENIC FIBROMA

This is a synonymous term for 'benign osteoblastoma' which has been considered on p. 700.

NON-OSTEOGENIC FIBROMA OF BONE – METAPHYSEAL FIBROUS DEFECT

This also is a rare lesion which presents as a tumour in the subcortical region of the metaphysis of patients in the 12–20 age group. The tumours are firm, fibrous and of yellow or brown coloration. They are composed of whorled fibrous tissue containing a variable number of foam cells and giant cells which contain haemosiderin pigment, but there is no bone formation. This is probably not a true tumour but is a failure of bone remodelling. The lesion, if followed radiologically over a period of time, gradually 'grows away' from the metaphysis towards the mid-shaft and eventually disappears. This, therefore, is a benign condition which was previously regarded as a regressing, fibrous or xanthomatous 'variant' of a giant-cell tumour.

CHONDROMYXOID FIBROMA

This is regarded by some authorities as essentially a benign fibrous tumour of bone displaying unusual myxomatous characteristics which simulate the appearance of cartilage. The lesion is described on p. 701.

Giant-cell tumour – Osteoclastoma

A tumour with many histological and clinical imitators – *giant-cell variants*.

TRUE GIANT-CELL TUMOURS

Age
The common age is 20–35 years; they are rare below the age of 20. Most of the 'giant-cell variants' occur in younger persons.

Origin
This is unknown, but is considered to be a tumour of osteoclasts, hence the name osteoclastoma.

Sites
The ends of long bones are the sites of election. They do not occur in mid-shaft regions nor in the jaw but the pelvis and vertebrae are rare sites. Bones around the knee joint account for over 50 per cent of cases.

Predisposing factors
Apart from the few cases which arise from Paget's disease in the older age groups, there are no known predisposing factors.

Macroscopical
Present as eccentric expanding tumours destroying the bone and with little or no reactive bone formation. On section, the tumour is red and fleshy and expands the bone with thinning of the cortex. The tumour remains confined within the periosteum in most cases.

Microscopical
The essential diagnostic features are the presence of two types of cells:
1 The mononuclear cells which form the stroma of the tumour.

2 Giant cells of osteoclast type (see Fig. 6 on p. 24).

Fibrous tissue, cartilage and bone are not present in the stroma and areas of haemorrhage and foam cells are only seen as secondary changes after trauma, fracture or attempted treatment. The mononuclear cells are tumour cells and are oval, round or spindle-shaped, often showing pleomorphism and mitoses. The giant cells contain up to 250 nuclei, do not show mitoses and are not phagocytic. It should be emphasized that the presence of significant amount of bone, cartilage, foam cells, fibrous tissue or large vascular spaces, excludes the diagnosis of a true-giant-cell tumour; these are the features of many of the 'variants'.

Spread
All giant-cell tumours are locally malignant and untreated will progressively destroy the surrounding bone and may even penetrate a joint or surrounding soft tissue. Moreover, untreated, about 15 per cent will eventually metastasize, still as a giant-cell tumour, via the blood stream to the lungs.

Prognosis
These tumours almost always recur after local curettage. Wide local excision is usually necessary to prevent a recurrence but this is often only possible by amputation. The 5-year survival figure is approximately 80 per cent.

GIANT-CELL VARIANTS

It has already been stated that the giant-cell tumour has many impersonators and the following are some of these 'giant-cell variants', the common feature being the presence of osteoclast-like giant cells within the lesion.

SIMPLE BONE CYST – UNICAMERAL BONE CYST

Simple cysts occur before the age of 20 years and they frequently produce pathological fractures. Histologically, the fibrous wall contains giant cells of osteoclast type. They are not true tumours and, although their origin is obscure, they are probably congenital disorders.

ANEURYSMAL BONE CYST

Large and often rapidly expanding lesions of long bones and vertebrae of young persons. Because of their rapidly increasing size they clinically imitate a malignant tumour. Macroscopically, they are extremely vascular lesions which microscopically show numerous, large vascular channels lined by a cellular fibrous tissue containing giant cells. Although superficially resembling osteoclasts, these giant cells are phagocytic and contain haemosiderin. The lesions are of uncertain origin but are often cured by curettage.

'BROWN TUMOURS'

These are the localized bone lesions of osteitis fibrosa cystica. The elevated serum calcium in this condition assists in arriving at the correct interpretation of these tumour-like masses containing giant cells, cysts and fibrous tissue (see p. 697).

NON-OSTEOGENIC FIBROMA

This fibrous lesion has been described on p. 702. It was formerly regarded as a fibrous, regressing or xanthomatous variant of giant-cell tumour.

BENIGN CHONDROBLASTOMA

The cellularity and the presence of giant cells in this tumour has resulted in misinterpretation of the appearances as those of a giant-cell tumour. However, the presence of fibrous tissue, cartilage or bone in the stroma and the smaller size of the giant cells permits its exclusion. The condition is described on p. 701.

GIANT-CELL REPARATIVE GRANULOMA

This benign lesion of the jaw contains giant cells and has frequently been misinterpreted as a true giant-cell tumour. This accounts for the jaw being frequently quoted as a common site of giant-cell tumour. The condition is described on p. 177.

EXCESSIVE OSTEOCLASTIC
ACTIVITY

Any area of marked osteoclastic bone resorption
may mimic a giant-cell tumour. This appearance
may be associated with osteoid osteoma, benign
chondroblastoma, or with the edge of any rarefying
bone lesion, e.g. fibrous dysplasia, in which osteoclasts may be profuse.

Summary
It will be noted that all the lesions mentioned above
are benign and if these are removed from any series
of 'giant-cell tumours' the remainder, which are the
true giant-cell tumours, only form a comparatively
uncommon but important group. In all these
variants, examination of the whole 'tumour' enables
a correct diagnosis to be made, but considerable
difficulties may occur in the interpretation of some
biopsy material, expecially if only small amounts
are available for examination.

Fatty Tumours

Lipomas can occur in bone, especially subperios-
teally, but they are rare. Liposarcoma, which is
described as occurring in the medullary cavity, is
extremely rare.

Vascular tumours

Haemangiomas are common and are malformations
most commonly seen in the bodies of vertebrae (see
p. 718). The malignant vasoformative tumour –
angiosarcoma, is rare and produces a large, very
vascular tumour of high malignancy. Microscopically, it is composed of primitive and atypical blood
vessels of capillary calibre and metastasizes rapidly.

Nerve tumours

Tumours of nerve tissue, neurofibroma, and neurofibrosarcoma, are occasionally found in bone but
are extremely rare, except in the jaw (see p. 177).

Tumours of bone marrow cells

Nature
Tumours arising in haemopoietic and lymphoreticular cells of the bone marrow.

LEUKAEMIA

This is by far the most common and is described on
pp. 462–468.

EWING'S TUMOUR OF BONE

Nature
A tumour of characteristic appearance but of unknown cell type.

Age
Children, nearly all below the age of 10 years.

Sites
The mid-shaft region of long bones is the site of
election, but it occasionally occurs in the pelvis and
other flat bones.

Macroscopical
Fleshy, non-bone-forming tumours in the mid-
shaft with reactive bone formation externally, producing the radiological 'onion-skin' appearance.

Microscopical
The tumour is composed of sheets of uniform,
hyperchromatic, round cells, with little cytoplasm
and virtually no stroma. Reticulin staining is negative and there is absence of fibrous tissue, cartilage
or bone within the tumour matrix. The tumour
cells contain abundant glycogen.

Spread
Local with destruction of bone. Early blood spread
and pulmonary metastases are common.

Prognosis
This is almost always a fatal tumour but a few cases
have been cured by radical operation at an early
stage.

Differential diagnosis

A secondary deposit in bone from a neuroblastoma of the adrenal or other sites in the sympathetic nervous system may closely simulate a Ewing's tumour and no example is acceptable unless an exhaustive search has excluded such a primary. A lymphoma may also show a similar picture, but in such a tumour reticulin is usually present.

PRIMARY LYMPHOMA OF BONE

A rare primary tumour of bone which typically occurs in young adults aged about 30 and presents as a radiotranslucent lesion in the shaft of a long bone. Histologically, the tumour shows features of immunoblastic or, more rarely, histiocytic, lymphoma (see p. 583). These are radiosensitive tumours and the prognosis is relatively good. This is almost always an isolated lesion and appears to differ from the generalized disease.

MULTIPLE MYELOMA – MYELOMATOSIS

This uncommon tumour of marrow plasma cells is described on pp. 470–471.

Chordoma – Tumour of the notochord

This only occurs in relation to notochord remnants and is described on p. 719.

'Adamantinoma' of the tibia

This is a very rare primary tumour in bone, of epithelial appearance and which mimics an adamantinoma of the jaw (see p. 175). The origin of this tumour is debatable, but many are probably basal-cell carcinomas in bone derived from misplaced accessory skin structures.

Classification of bone tumours

Thus, primary bone tumours may be classified as shown below.

Secondary tumours in bone

Incidence

Secondary tumours are found in bones in 15–20 per cent of all fatal cases of malignant disease; they are

Bone tumours	Cartilage tumours	Fibrous tumours	Giant-cell tumours
B. Osteoma	B. Chondroma	B. Fibroma	M. True giant-cell tumour
B. Osteoid osteoma	B. Benign chondroblastoma	B. Osteogenic fibroma	
B. Benign osteoblastoma	B. Chondromyxoid fibroma	B. Non-osteogenic fibroma	B. Giant-cell 'variants'
M. Osteosarcoma	M. Chondrosarcoma	M. Fibrosarcoma	
		M. Malignant fibrous histiocytoma	
Fatty tumours	**Vascular tumours**	**Nerve tumours**	**Bone marrow tumours**
B. Lipoma	B. Haemangioma	B. Neurofibroma	M. Leukaemia
M. Liposarcoma	M. Angiosarcoma	B. Neurinoma	M. Ewing's tumour
		M. Neurofibrosarcoma	M. Primary lymphoma
			M. Multiple myeloma
Notochord tumour	**Epithelial tumour**		
M. Chordoma	M. 'Adamantinoma' of tibia		

B Benign
M Malignant

Fig. 85. Bone tumour classification.

thus much more common than all the primary bone tumours.

Sources
Metastases in bone most commonly arise from primary tumours of the prostate, breast, bronchus, kidney, stomach and thyroid or from a malignant lymphoma.

Macroscopical
Single or multiple, soft or hard deposits of tumours in bones; pathological fractures are common. In the spine, there may be collapse of the vertebral bodies, but the discs are usually spared until an advanced stage.

Microscopical
Similar in appearance to the primary tumour but the bone reaction is variable:

1 In the early stages, the tumour grows between the bone trabeculae with no bone destruction and no visible radiological changes.

2 The tumour destroys and replaces the bone, producing the more usual appearance of osteolytic deposits.

3 The tumour cells may evoke an osteoblastic response resulting in osteosclerotic deposits. This occurs especially with prostatic carcinoma, but breast secondaries, Hodgkin's disease and other tumours may occasionally produce the same appearance.

Chapter 116
Skeletal System – Diseases of Joints

NORMAL JOINTS

A synovial joint has a lining of flattened synovia cells. The articular cartilages are normally closely apposed, smooth, resilient structures which glide over each other with every movement of the joint and are lubricated by the slightly viscid synovial fluid. The articular cartilage is an avascular structure which is demarcated from the subchondral bone by a calcified line and yet is moored to the underlying bone by fibres. The articular cartilage derives its essential nutrients from the synovial fluid.

OSTEOARTHROSIS – OSTEOARTHRITIS

Nature
An extremely common degenerative process of articular cartilage.

Age
Occurs spontaneously in the older age groups and is thus very common above the age of 60 years. It may also occur in the joints of younger persons following any form of previous mechanical derangement, e.g. trauma, congenital dislocation of the hip, osteochondritis, etc.

Sites
Usually the large weight-bearing joints, e.g. the hip and knee.

Macroscopical
Loss of joint space due to thinning of the cartilage which shows loss of lustre and a velvety appearance from *fibrillation*. Later, the cartilage disappears in areas to produce ulceration and to expose the underlying subchondral bone. The bone becomes thickened as a buttressing effect and extends beyond the articular margins to form bony outgrowths – *osteophytes*. In some areas the subchondral bone is not thickened and may allow entry of the synovial fluid into the underlying bone to produce a radiological cystic appearance. The end result is an articular surface denuded of cartilage and formed by a highly polished surface of eburnated bone with marginal osteophytes, some of which may break off to form loose bodies in the joint.

Microscopical
The normal blue-staining cartilage (on haematoxylin and eosin staining) degenerates and becomes pink-staining with loss of mucopolysaccharide ground substance. The degenerate cartilage splits along the lines of the fibres, tangentially at the surface but vertically as the splits extend into the deeper layers, to produce fronds of degenerate cartilage – fibrillation. This cartilage falls off and the subchondral bone becomes thickened and compact. The osteophytes at the joint margins are formed by reactive new bone. The synovial membrane often shows fibrous thickening and may also contain small foci of degenerate cartilage. At a later stage no cartilage remains, articulation occurring between the two faces of eburnated, thickened, subchondral bone.

Results
The loss of cartilage results in radiological narrowing of the joint space; the osteophytes are also prominent radiologically. Pain is usually present and commonly severe and is due in part to the synovial reaction associated with phagocytosed fragments of degenerate cartilage. The end result is commonly a stiff and painful joint.

RHEUMATOID ARTHRITIS

Nature
Although a generalized disease of connective tissues (see p. 285), the polyarthritis due to disease of the synovial tissues is usually the dominant clinical and pathological feature.

Age
Usually presents in females between the ages of 20 and the menopause, and rather later in men. Children are not exempt – *Still's disease*.

Sites
Many of the small joints, particularly those of the fingers, hands and wrists are most commonly involved but the larger joints at the ankle, hip and knee are also frequently affected.

Macroscopical
The joints are painful, swollen and tender. The synovial membrane is thickened, with villous overgrowth, increased vascularity and a *pannus* or plate which grows over and replaces the articular cartilage.

Microscopical
The synovial membrane shows villous proliferation with an intense lymphocytic and plasma cell infiltration of the oedematous and vascular fronds. The subsynovial and the periarticular collagen shows swelling with oedema and degenerative changes in the collagen, including foci of fibrinoid necrosis. The proliferated synovial tissues extend over the surface of the articular cartilage as a pannus of fibrous tissue containing lymphocytes, eroding and gradually replacing the articular cartilage by a fibrous mass. This unites with similar fibrous tissue on the opposite side of the joint space to produce fibrous ankylosis.

Results

The periarticular collagenous changes produce pain and the fusiform joint swelling. The pannus and the fibrous ankylosis result in pain and limitation of joint movement. There is a disuse atrophy of the bone and muscles working affected joints. Any other connective tissue, especially muscles and blood vessels, may be involved by the rheumatoid process and subcutaneous nodules, composed of circular areas of necrotic collagen surrounded by histiocytes and giant cells, may also occur.

SUPPURATIVE ARTHRITIS

Nature

Pyogenic inflammation of the joints arising as a result of blood-borne infection or by extension from osteomyelitis of the adjacent bone.

Age

When associated with osteomyelitis, the disease is usually in children and is especially common in the hip. The septicaemic type occurs in both adults and children.

Sites

The hip is the commonest joint involved due to the presence of the epiphyseal line within the joint capsule, but no joint is exempt.

Macroscopical

The joint space is distended by pus and the synovial membrane shows acute inflammatory hyperaemia. The underlying bone may show evidence of an osteomyelitis spreading into the joint and the articular cartilage is irregularly eroded and frequently completely destroyed.

Microscopical

There is an acute polymorph pyogenic reaction in the bone, joint space and synovial membrane. The articular cartilage disappears rapidly due to its dissolution by proteolytic ferments in the pus.

Results

The articular surface is denuded of cartilage and replaced by inflammatory granulation tissue. This organizes to fibrous tissue and fibrous ankylosis results, which may later progress to bony ankylosis. Intra-articular and periarticular ligaments are also commonly destroyed or damaged to increase the disability.

TUBERCULOUS ARTHRITIS

Nature

A blood borne tuberculous infection involving either bone or joint or both together. The primary origin of the infection is frequently pulmonary, less commonly intestinal.

Age

Mostly occurs in children up to the age of 10 years.

Sites

The commonest site of bone and joint tuberculosis is the spine – Pott's disease (see p. 717), but the hip, knee, wrist, ankle and shoulders may also be involved.

Macroscopical

The involvement may be due to extension from a subchondral focus, or in the synovial membrane, or both together, but the end result is likely to be the same. The synovial membrane is thick, grey and gelatinous, filling and distending the joint space and a pannus of tuberculous granulation tissue grows over the articular cartilage. The subchondral focus or tissue from the synovial membrane spreads subjacent to the cartilage as subchondral granulations. The pannus and the subchondral granulations then sandwich the articular cartilage, which becomes separated from its underlying bone and dies, forming a sheet of sequestrated cartilage. Later, fibrous tissue, containing areas of calcification and caseous material, develops.

Microscopical

Typical tuberculous giant-cell lesions with caseation.

Results

The sequestrated cartilage eventually breaks up with the formation of loose bodies. When healing occurs the joint shows inactive caseous material, fibrous tissue, fibrous ankylosis and eventually bony ankylosis.

In some cases of tuberculosis small firm elongated bodies are found – 'melon seed' bodies. These are usually composed of fibrin, but they are not specific for tuberculosis as they are rather more commonly observed in cases of rheumatoid arthritis and in non-specific synovitis.

GOUT

Nature
A disease due to abnormal purine metabolism whereby sodium biurate is deposited in many tissues, but particularly as subcutaneous tophi or in the periarticular tissues. The latter may involve the joint, producing mechanical derangements (see p. 111).

Age
Usually in middle-aged or elderly men although females may be affected, especially when there is a family history of gout.

Sites
The first metatarso-phalangeal joint is the predominant site but many other joints, including those of the hands, may be affected.

Macroscopical
The joint is swollen and red and shows white 'chalky' patches in the skin, through which sodium biurate crystals can often be expressed. The periarticular tissues are distended by the deposition of these crystals and similar deposits may extend into the joint with disruption of bone and articular cartilage.

Microscopical
The affected areas show multiple foci of sodium biurate crystals surrounded by a fibrous and foreign body giant-cell reaction.

Results
Joint function is disturbed by the presence of deposits and stiffness and pain result. Acute exacerbations are common which are exquisitely painful and are often associated with considerable constitutional upset. Deposition of the crystals in the kidney may lead to impaired renal function. Prophylactic treatment by allopurinol or related substances is very effective.

NEUROPATHIC ARTHRITIS – CHARCOT'S JOINT

Nature
A degenerative joint disease which occurs due to loss of the sensory nerve supply.

Aetiology
This occurs most frequently in the knee or hip joints in tabes dorsalis and in the shoulder or elbow in syringomyelia. It may also follow nerve destruction in leprosy, but only rarely occurs with other causes of sensory nerve loss.

Appearances
The joint is swollen due to a large effusion and there is a rapid degeneration of the articular cartilage. The underlying bones show a mixture of decalcification and osteophyte formation and in some cases the capsular tissues may calcify.

Results
The large effusion associated with the loss of the subchondral bone results in stretching of the joint ligaments and in gross deformity. The deterioration is usually rapid and the joint becomes completely disorganized and unstable. Frequent dislocations occur but the condition remains painless throughout its course.

OSTEOCHONDRITIS DISSECANS

Nature
Due to necrosis of a segment of subchondral bone which sequestrates and is extruded into the joint space as a loose body. The aetiology is unknown, but trauma leading to an area of avascular necrosis is the most probably cause.

Age
Usually in children or young adults.

Macroscopical
There is a bony loose body in the joint with a cap of cartilage and a corresponding defect in the articular surface.

Microscopical
The loose body, usually triangular, is composed of dead bone but viable cartilage, as the cartilage continues to derive its metabolic needs from the synovial fluid.

Results
The condition predisposes to osteoarthrosis by trauma from the loose body and by the unevenness in the articular surface caused by the defect.

'GANGLION'

Nature

A cystic swelling most commonly found at the wrist, or less frequently at the ankle or foot, and always in close relationship to synovial membrane or tendon sheath.

Macroscopical

Small cystic swellings which may have a visible connection with the synovial membrane or tendon sheath and which contain mucoid, glairy fluid.

Microscopical

All contain a myxomatous centre which originally may have been surrounded by synovial-type cells and a fibrous wall. By the time of removal synovial cells are usually not present and the mucinous material merges with the fibrous tissue.

Pathogenesis

The majority are probably herniations of tendon sheath or synovial membrane which then become distended by modified synovial fluid to form the cystic spaces. The examples which show no synovial cells may be due to post-traumatic extravasation of synovial fluid into the adjacent fibrous tissue.

CYST OF SEMILUNAR CARTILAGE

Nature

Multilocular cysts which occur in the semilunar cartilage of the knee joint, more commonly in the lateral cartilage.

Macroscopical

A multilocular cystic swelling containing mucoid material at the rim of the meniscus.

Microscopical

The cystic spaces are lined by synovial cells and the mucoid contents may extend through the cyst wall in between the fibres of the fibrocartilage.

Pathogenesis

These are probably due to islands of synovial cells incorporated in the meniscus. The production of synovial fluid results in cyst formation.

Results

They produce a gradually enlarging mass, which is cured by excision.

SYNOVIAL OSTEOCHONDROMATOSIS

Nature

The presence of multiple nodules of cartilage in the synovial membrane.

Macroscopical

The synovial membrane, usually of the knee, shoulder or elbow is studded by multiple nodules of translucent cartilage. Many of these protrude into the joint space on a narrow pedicle or lie free within the joint cavity where they form loose bodies, sometimes several hundred in number.

Microscopical

The synovial tissues contain multiple foci of benign cartilage, some of which show areas of ossification. The cartilaginous loose bodies are viable and may continue to grow as they obtain their nutritional requirements from the synovial fluid.

Pathogenesis

This remains unknown; it is regarded by some authorities as a true tumour, but it is more probably a metaplastic or developmental abnormality of the synovial tissues.

Results

The condition produces progressive swelling of the joint with 'locking' due to the loose bodies. Synovectomy may be followed by recurrence but the lesion is entirely benign.

'Synovioma'

The 'synoviomas' are a group of space-occupying lesions arising from joint and tendon sheath synovial membranes, both of which have a common origin and structure. It is very doubtful if the benign lesions described below are true tumours.

BENIGN 'SYNOVIOMA' – TENDON SHEATH TUMOUR – GIANT-CELL TUMOUR OF TENDON SHEATH

Nature

These are almost certainly not neoplasms but a localized peripheral nodular form of pigmented villo-nodular synovitis.

Age
Occur most commonly at about 30 years of age but no age group is exempt.

Sites
The fingers are by far the most common sites; they may also occur on the toes, rarely elsewhere.

Macroscopical
These are rounded, lobulated, yellow-brown, firm tumours, usually with a poorly formed capsule.

Microscopical
Composed of mononuclear cells similar in appearance to the normal lining cells of a tendon sheath or synovial membrane. There is a variably collagenous stroma with foam cells, haemosiderin-laden macrophages and giant cells which also frequently contain haemosiderin.

Results
These are slowly growing lesions and complete excision is curative. However, local recurrence occurs in up to 20–30 per cent of cases due to incomplete excision resulting from their poor encapsulation.

PIGMENTED VILLO-NODULAR SYNOVITIS

Nature
A pigmented villous overgrowth of synovial membrane which nearly always occurs in the knee or hip joints. The lesion is self-limiting and benign and shows no real neoplastic features. The features indicate an inflammatory reactive process.

Macroscopical
The joint is swollen and painful due to fronded, brown-coloured, seaweed-like material filling and distending the joint space. Extension into neighbouring tissues and bone may occasionally be seen. Sometimes a few or solitary nodules are the only features.

Microscopical
The synovial membrane shows villous overgrowth with nodules formed by fusion of the fronds. The villi are covered by synovial cells and the core is composed of mononuclear cells, foam cells, giant cells and haemosiderin pigment, i.e. the cellular components are identical to those of a tendon

sheath 'tumour' described above, indeed the lesions are almost certainly the same.

Results
The condition is benign and, after a variable slowly progressive course, inevitably regresses. Although treatment may be required on symptomatic grounds there is no evidence that surgery or radiotherapy significantly alter the natural course of the disorder.

SYNOVIAL SARCOMA – MALIGNANT SYNOVIOMA

Nature
A group of rare malignant tumours, mostly of high malignancy, arising from the synovium and showing biphasic cellular characteristics.

Age
Usually present between 30–40 years of age.

Sites
The knee and hip joints are the commonest sites and they only very rarely occur in other joints.

Macroscopical
Firm, solid and usually pale tumours which arise from the synovial membrane and invade surrounding bone and soft tissues, usually extensively.

Microscopical
Extremely variable. The well differentiated type shows definite biphasic features with cuboidal cells lining cleft-like spaces thus imitating joint spaces. The least well differentiated are spindle-cell sarcomas with scanty cleft-like spaces and there are many intermediate forms.

Spread
The tumours tend to grow away from the joint of origin and they invade the adjacent soft tissues and bone widely. Early blood borne metastases are common in all but the well differentiated type.

Prognosis
The differentiated forms are slowly growing and wide local resection is curative. The more anaplastic tumours, which are more common, are extremely rapidly growing and produce pulmonary metastases at an early stage, so that there is only about a 5–10 per cent 5-year survival.

Chapter 117
Skeletal System – Diseases of the Spine

Degenerative diseases
Nature

SYNOVIAL
   JOINTS – OSTEOARTHROSIS
Sites
Appearances
Results

INTERVERTEBRAL
   DISCS – DEGENERATION

Vertical herniation

Posterior herniation

Annular herniation

Osteophytosis – Spondylosis

Adolescent kyphosis

Senile kyphosis

VERTEBRAL BONE DISORDERS

Primary, senile, involutional
   osteoporosis

Scoliosis
Definition
Causes
Results

Kyphosis
Definition

SMOOTH KYPHOSIS
Causes

ANGULAR KYPHOSIS
Causes

Ankylosing spondylitis
Nature
Aetiology
Incidence
Appearances
Results

Infections

PYOGENIC OSTEOMYELITIS
Organisms
Mode of infection
Macroscopical
Microscopical
Results

SPINAL TUBERCULOSIS
Nature
Incidence
Sites
Route of infection
Age
Appearances
Results

Primary tumours of
   vertebrae
Incidence
Types

Benign tumours

HAEMANGIOMA
Nature
Incidence
Sites

Macroscopical
Microscopical
Results

ANEURYSMAL BONE CYST
Nature
Origin
Age
Macroscopical
Microscopical
Results

BENIGN OSTEOBLASTOMA
Nature
Age
Sites
Macroscopical
Microscopical
Results

Malignant tumours

CHORDOMA
Origin
Incidence
Age
Sex
Sites
Macroscopical
Microscopical
Spread
Results

MYELOMATOSIS

Secondary Tumours

Degenerative diseases

Nature
Degenerative changes commonly occur in the spine with advancing age and may affect the synovial joints of the spine, the intervertebral discs or the bones.

SYNOVIAL JOINTS – OSTEOARTHROSIS

Sites
The posterior and lateral spinal joints which have articular cartilages and synovial membranes, i.e. not the intervertebral discs.

Appearances
These joints are commonly affected by osteoarthrosis. There is degeneration of the articular cartilage with fibrillation and osteophyte formation is prominent (see p. 708).

Results
This degenerative joint disease may be associated with root pain and limitation of spinal movement, especially in the cervical region (see Fig. 86).

INTERVERTEBRAL DISCS – DEGENERATION

The central part of the intervertebral disc is composed of a myxoid, fluid-containing material – nucleus pulposus. This is bounded externally by the fibrocartilaginous annulus fibrosus and confined above and below by the vertebral bodies. The central nucleus pulposus is under constant pressure; if it escapes from its normal confines, pathological changes may result:

VERTICAL HERNIATION

Herniation vertically results in protrusion of the nuclear tissue into the vertebral body above or below the disc. This becomes radiologically visible when reactive new bone surrounds the protrusion. This is extremely common and is called a *Schmorl's node* (see Fig. 87).

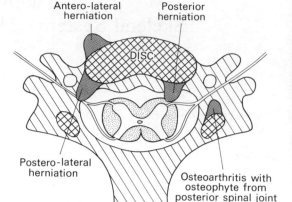

Fig. 86. Spine – sites of degenerative lesions.

POSTERIOR HERNIATION

Posterior herniation of disc tissue produces bulging of the posterior longitudinal ligament which may cause pressure on the spinal cord. More frequently, the disc tissue herniates postero-laterally to one side of the mid-line to produce unilateral neurological pressure signs (see Fig. 86).

ANNULAR HERNIATION

As a result of desiccation of the nucleus pulposus, which is common with advancing years, the disc space becomes narrowed with resulting bulging of the fibres of the peripheral portion of the annulus fibrosus beyond the bony margins. This may occur posteriorly to produce the pressure symptoms of a disc syndrome, but more commonly occurs laterally or antero-laterally and eventually results in osteophytosis of the spine (see Fig. 87).

OSTEOPHYTOSIS OR SPONDYLOSIS

Osteophytosis of the spine is the condition of marginal bony lipping of the vertebral bodies at the disc margins. The disc tissue becomes narrowed following vertical prolapse or desiccation and the

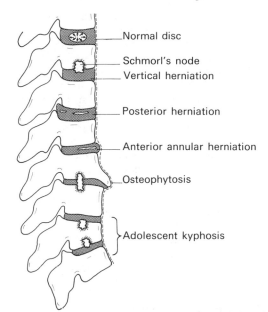

Normal disc

Schmorl's node
Vertical herniation

Posterior herniation

Anterior annular herniation

Osteophytosis

Adolescent kyphosis

Fig. 87. Spine – diagrammatic representation of the effects of disc degeneration.

annulus fibrosus protrudes at the periphery thus raising the overlying periosteum from the adjacent vertebral margins. Reactive subperiosteal new bone formation results in bony spurs or osteophyte production but the line of the annulus fibrosus separates the bony spurs from each other. The osteophytes produced cause no clinical manifestations except in the postero-lateral position where they may press on the spinal cord or nerve roots (see Fig. 86).

ADOLESCENT KYPHOSIS

The primary condition is herniation of the nucleus pulposus to produce Schmorl's nodes and narrowing of the disc space. The posterior portions of the vertebral bodies are supported by the posterior spinal joints but the anterior portions have no such support, so forward tilting of the vertebrae occurs leading to kyphosis. This deformity then interferes with normal growth of the vertebral bodies so that a permanent wedge-shaped deformity ensues. It was formerly considered that epiphysitis of the vertebral bodies produced this wedge-shaped deformity and this disease is still sometimes known as *Scheuermann's disease* (see Fig. 87).

SENILE KYPHOSIS

This is a common disease in the over-60 age group in which there is disc degeneration, especially of the anterior portion. The discs protrude in all directions with osteophyte formation and bony union occurs through the thinned anterior portions of the disc. Ossification then occurs between the vertebral bodies and the kyphosis is permanent.

VERTEBRAL BONE DISORDERS

PRIMARY, INVOLUTIONAL, SENILE OSTEOPOROSIS

This common type of osteoporosis causes decreased density of the vertebral bodies and predisposes to fractures. Many cases remain asymptomatic but pain, collapse and pressure on nerves at the intervertebral foramina may occur (see p. 714).

Scoliosis

Definition
Lateral curvature of the spine associated with rotation of vertebrae.

Causes
1 *Congenital.* Defects in development, or of ossification, of one or more vertebrae, may cause scoliosis, e.g. hemivertebra, absence of intervertebral disc with fusion of vertebral bodies, anomalies of ribs, etc.
2 *Paralytic.* Following nerve paralysis there may be imbalance of the trunk muscles.
3 *Neurofibromatosis.* Generalized neurofibromatosis is sometimes associated with other congenital abnormalities, including scoliosis or kyphoscoliosis due to failure of development of one side of the vertebral body (see p. 620).
4 *Neuropathic and myopathic.* Rare causes of scoliosis are syringomyelia, Friedreich's ataxia and the muscular dystrophies.
5 *Pulmonary causes.* Extensive unilateral pulmonary fibrosis following empyema or tuberculosis may produce scoliosis. Pneumonectomy or thoracoplasty may have similar effects.
6 *Vertebral destruction.* Destruction or deformity of a vertebra by disease, e.g. rickets, tuberculosis, osteomyelitis, tumour or trauma.

7 *Compensatory*. Scoliosis may follow compensatory rotation or tilting of the pelvis due to shortening of the leg bones, lesions of the hip, etc.

8 *Idiopathic*. This is the commonest variety of scoliosis and is not associated with any known or detectable disease; the diagnosis is made by a process of exclusion of the known causes.

Results

The vertebral bodies become deformed with a wedge-shaped appearance, the apices of which are directed towards the concavity. The intervertebral discs protrude and, by elevation of the periosteum, result in osteophytosis at the disc margins. In long standing cases, fusion between the osteophytes across the disc tissue may produce permanent bony fixation of the spine in its deformed position.

Kyphosis

Definition
Flexion deformity of the spine. It may be associated with scoliosis – *kyphoscoliosis*.

SMOOTH KYPHOSIS

A gradual exaggeration of the normal dorsal curvature of the spine.

Causes
1 *Disc disease*. Adolescent and senile kyphosis (see p. 715).
2 *Faulty posture*. A doubtful aetiology.
3 *Early ankylosing spondylitis* (see below).
4 *Tuberculosis*. Rarely.
5 *Paget's disease* (see p. 690).

ANGULAR KYPHOSIS

Sharp angulation of the spine produces a hump – *gibbus*.

Causes
1 *Congenital*. Due to congenital 'wedge-shaped' vertebrae, to the narrowed 'cushion-shaped' vertebrae of Morquio's chondro-osteodystrophy or to gargoylism (see p. 684).
2 *Calvé's disease*. This was formerly regarded as a form of 'osteochondritis', but is now considered

more likely to be a healed area of eosinophil granuloma (see p. 691) producing a plate of sclerotic bone in one vertebral body – *vertebra plana*.

3 *Trauma*. Crush fracture may produce an acute angular kyphosis or the angulation may occur more slowly in Kümmell's disease. This occurs after trauma followed by bone rarefaction of the vertebra leading to collapse of the anterior portion of the body with wedge deformity. The process is probably due to progressive collapse of bone from weight-bearing at the site of a vertebral fracture.

4 *Vertebral body infection*. Tuberculosis, or less frequently a pyogenic infection (see p. 717).

5 *Bone rarefaction*. Rickets, osteomalacia, osteoporosis (see p. 692).

Results of kyphosis
The kyphosis results in deformity of the spine with compensatory curves above and below.

Ankylosing spondylitis – Rheumatoid spondylitis

Nature
A disease characterized by a rigid spine due to ossification of the spinal joints and ligaments.

Aetiology
This remains unknown although it is regarded by some authorities as a variant of rheumatoid arthritis. A very large proportion of patients with the disease and close relatives have HLA antigen B27 present.

Incidence
A rare disease, predominantly of young males between 15 and 35 years at the age of onset.

Appearances
There is a multiple arthritis affecting the spinal, costo-vertebral and sacro-iliac joints. It starts as a proliferating synovitis with eventual fibrous replacement of the articular cartilages, fibrous ankylosis and subsequently bony ankylosis.

The intervertebral discs are of normal thickness but there is marginal ossification of the outer fibres of the annulus fibrosus. This results in fusion of the vertebral bodies at the periphery of the disc space – *'bamboo-spine'* appearance. Similar changes affect the spinal ligaments and sacro-iliac joints, adding to the spinal rigidity.

Sometimes there is involvement of other joints, especially the hip and knee, by changes which are identical to those found in rheumatoid arthritis; indeed, it is these findings which lend support to the concept of rheumatoid disease of the spine.

Results
There is marked pain, stiffness of the spine and ultimately complete rigidity, often in a grossly deformed position. Rheumatoid aortitis may develop in longstanding cases (see p. 286).

Infections

PYOGENIC OSTEOMYELITIS

Organisms
Staphylococcus pyogenes is by far the most common, but other pyogenic organisms e.g. *S. typhi*, may be implicated (see p. 199).

Mode of infection
The infection is usually blood borne from a septic focus elsewhere, e.g. boil, whitlow, etc. Occasionally, infection from adjacent soft tissue, e.g. retropharyngeal abscess, may extend into the spine.

Macroscopical
One or more vertebrae may be involved in the acute stage with rarefaction and destruction of the body, pedicles or transverse processes.

Microscopical
Acute suppurative osteomyelitis with bone destruction.

Results
1 *Healing*. This is the usual result if the diagnosis is made early and the disease treated adequately by chemotherapy.
2 *Bone destruction*. Leading to collapse of the vertebrae, cord compression or kyphosis. In the cervical region the pressure effects are sometimes fatal.
3 *Abscess formation*. This may be restricted to the bone – Brodie's abscess, or extend posteriorly from the vertebral body as an extradural abscess producing cord compression. The pus may track along fascial or muscle planes as in tuberculosis and thus present at remote sites.
4 *Disc destruction*. May occur rarely, with direct extension of the disease into adjacent vertebrae.

SPINAL TUBERCULOSIS – POTT'S DISEASE OF THE SPINE

Nature
Tuberculous osteomyelitis of one or more vertebrae.

Incidence
Tuberculous involvement of the spine accounts for 30–50 per cent of all cases of bone and joint tuberculosis.

Sites
The thoracic vertebrae, especially D. 11, but any may be affected.

Route of infection
Haematogenous spread, almost always from a pulmonary focus which may be clinically active or healed.

Age
The disease is commonest in the first 10 years of life but adults are occasionally affected.

Appearances
The disease starts in the vertebral body which histologically shows progressive destruction of the bone and replacement by active caseous tuberculous granulation tissue: the discs are commonly destroyed. Whilst the tuberculous infection is active there is no new bone formation; the spinal bone is progressively destroyed and collapse with angular kyphosis follows.

Results
1 *Collapse*. The vertebral body will collapse unless suitably supported by orthopaedic measures. In spite of adequate treatment, however, a kyphosis frequently follows.
2 *'Cold abscess'*. The abscess is a collection of caseous material which extends outside the bone to form a mass anterior or lateral to the vertebral bodies. This material remains at the site until the pressure increases to such a degree that it is forced along fascial and muscle planes to produce a retropharyngeal or a cervical abscess, rib or mediastinal lesions, or tracks down the spine into the psoas sheath from whence it may eventually present as a cold abscess in the inguinal region.
3 *Pott's paraplegia*. Cord paralysis may ensue from pressure of extradural caseous material or by

producing endarteritis in the spinal blood vessels with cord ischaemia and degeneration. If thrombosis of the thickened, segmental, spinal vessels occurs, paraplegia will be permanent. It is probable that angulation of the spine *per se* can also produce paraplegia.

4   *Meningitis.* The spinal dura is remarkably resistant to infection and is only rarely spontaneously penetrated. Tuberculous meningitis, may, however, follow operative procedures in the area.

Primary tumours of vertebrae

Incidence
With a few notable exceptions, primary tumours of the spine are extremely rare.

Types
All the primary bone tumours that are encountered elsewhere in the skeleton have been reported as occurring in the spine, e.g. osteosarcoma, chondrosarcoma, etc. These are considered on pp. 698–706 but certain lesions occur in the spine with sufficient frequency to merit special mention.

Benign tumours

HAEMANGIOMA

Nature
Probably best regarded as vascular hamartomatous malformations rather than true neoplasms.

Incidence
Common lesions; approximately 10 per cent of the population have a vertebral haemangioma, although most are of small size.

Sites
Usually solitary, predominantly affecting a lumbar vertebra.

Macroscopical
Vary in size from a minute microscopical lesion to one which expands the whole of a vertebral body and replaces it by a vascular mass.

Microscopical
Composed of large cavernous, blood-filled spaces lined by endothelium; areas of organized thrombus are commonly seen. The bone of the vertebra is largely replaced but the surviving trabeculae are arranged as vertical bands which buttress the bone and prevent collapse.

Results
Most are completely asymptomatic and are chance radiological findings. A small minority may produce cord compression by posterior bulging of the vertebral body; vertebral collapse only rarely occurs.

ANEURYSMAL BONE CYST

Nature
An uncommon bone lesion which occurs in the spine and long bones. Many examples of so-called giant-cell tumour of the spine have been shown on subsequent review of the histological material to be aneurysmal bone cysts.

Origin
This is obscure, but they are probably a form of angiomatous malformation.

Age
Fifteen to thirty age group.

Macroscopical
Expansion and destruction of one or more vertebrae by an haemorrhagic or brown, soft, tumour-like mass.

Microscopical
A fibrous-walled cyst with the centre of the lesion formed by large vascular channels and fibrous septa. The fibrous tissue contains a profusion of giant cells, haemosiderin and fragments of new bone.

Results
The lesion distorts and destroys the vertebral body and may spread to involve adjacent vertebrae. The resulting deformity may produce cord compression or vertebral collapse. This is a benign lesion, however, and the small lesions are curable by thorough curettage.

BENIGN OSTEOBLASTOMA – OSTEOGENIC FIBROMA – GIANT OSTEOID OSTEOMA

Nature
A rare condition which affects the spine and occasionally other bones.

Age
Mostly between 15–25 years of age.

Sites
The neural arch is the usual spinal site.

Macroscopical
A comparatively small fleshy area within the expanded bone.

Microscopical
A spindle cell or fibroblastic and vascular stroma in which there is formation of osteoid tissue with areas of mineralization; osteoclasts may be prominent.

Results
The lesion expands the bone and may cause cord or root compression, but is entirely benign and excision is curative.

Malignant tumours

CHORDOMA

Origin
Arises from the remnants of the notochord.

Incidence
A very rare tumour.

Age
No age is exempt but the cranial cases tend to present at a younger age group (35 years) than the sacral cases (50 years).

Sex
M:F 2:1.

Sites
Sacro-coccygeal 50 per cent; base of skull (sphenoid and basi-occiput) 35 per cent; vertebral column at various levels 15 per cent. This tumour does not occur at any other site.

Macroscopical
Large, soft, mucoid, lobulated, locally destructive tumours. They extend by direct spread into adjacent tissues to produce large masses in the nasopharynx, retroperitoneal tissues, pelvis, buttocks or thighs. Frequently there are haemorrhagic, cystic or calcified areas in the tumour.

Microscopical
The tumour has a mucoid stroma in which there are clumps of polyhedral cells arranged in irregular groups. The cells have a characteristic vacuolated appearance – '*physalipherous cells*'. Multinucleate cells and foci of calcification are also commonly present.

Spread
Chordomas are slowly growing but invade directly into adjacent tissues:
1 Destroy the base of the skull and present as an intracranial space-occupying lesion.
2 Cord compression.
3 Produce sacral destruction and a pelvic mass.

Results
Unless diagnosed at a very early stage, these tumours are not readily amenable to surgery but, because of their slow growth, many patients have lived for 5 years or more although long-term survivors are very few in number. A small minority, probably less than 10 per cent, do metastasize to lymph nodes and via the blood to the lungs and liver.

MYELOMATOSIS – MULTIPLE MYELOMA

The spine is the most common site of this usually generalized tumour of bone which is described on p. 470.

Secondary tumours

Secondary malignant deposits of tumour in the spine are common and approximately 4 per cent of all spines examined at autopsy from elderly patients contain metastatic tumour.

Chapter 118
Diseases of the Skin

NORMAL SKIN

The epidermis has four layers. See Fig. 88.

1 *Horny layer.* The surface layer is composed of flattened anuclear scales of keratin.

2 *Granular layer.* Composed of two to three layers of flattened cells, which contain kerato-hyaline granules.

3 *Stratum malpighii or prickle-cell layer.* Polygonal-shaped cells which form a mosaic pattern, several cells in depth, the spaces between the cells being traversed by prickles or intercellular bridges. Towards the surface the cells become flattened.

4 *Basal cell layer.* Normally, a single layer of columnar-shaped cells which lie on the basement membrane and form the junction between the epidermis and the underlying dermis.

The dermis contains:

1 Collagen.
2 Elastic fibres.

3 Reticulin fibres, which are probably immature collagen fibres.

4 Nerves and nerve end-organs, e.g. Pacinian and Meissner end-organs.

5 Blood vessels – arterioles, dermal capillaries and venules.

6 Lymphatics.

7 Muscle of the arrectores pilorum, which is smooth muscle.

The dermis also contains the epidermal appendages:

1 *Sweat glands.* Distributed throughout the body, but maximal in the skin of the soles of the feet and palms of the hands. They have a coiled secretory portion and the epithelial cells are surrounded by myo-epithelial cells which are contractile and thus propel the secretion into the duct, from which it is expelled through the epidermis to the skin surface.

2 *Apocrine glands.* These are vestigial scent glands which occur in the axilla, genital folds and around the nipples. The glands are formed by eosinophilic

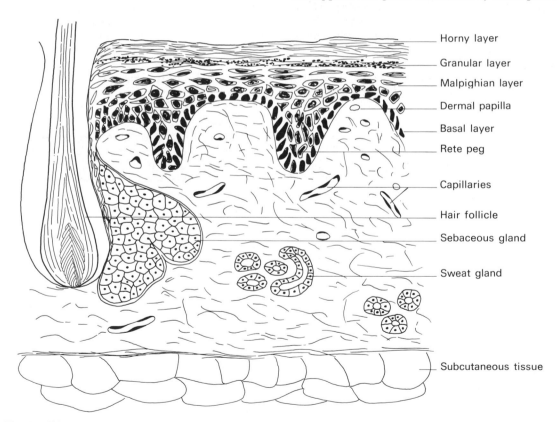

Fig. 88. Skin – normal structure.

epithelium and their secretion passes into the pilo-sebaceous follicles and not directly through the epidermis.

3 *Sebaceous glands*. These are present everywhere except in the soles and palms. The lobulated gland structure of clear cells produce sebaceous material which passes along the sebaceous duct and is discharged into the pilo-sebaceous follicles and thence on to the surface.

4 *Hair follicles*. These produce the keratinized structures, hairs.

Terminology

There are a number of common pathological processes which occur in the skin tissues. The following are some of the pathological terms in common use:

1 *Acantholysis*. Dissolution of the intercellular bridges between the prickle cells with the subsequent formation of vesicles or bullae.

2 *Acanthosis*. Proliferation of the prickle cell layer, resulting in increased thickening of the epidermis.

3 *Bulla*. A fluid-containing space, either intra-epidermal or subepidermal in position.

4 *Dyskeratosis*. Disorderly keratinization of the skin with premature keratin formation. This often occurs in the deeper layers of the skin or within individual cells.

5 *Hyperkeratosis*. Excessive thickness of the horny layer of keratin.

6 *Lichenification*. Irregular areas of thickened skin with exaggerated skin markings.

7 *Liquefaction of basal cells*. Vacuolization and subsequent dissolution of the cells in the basal layer.

8 *Micro-abscess*. Small collections of inflammatory cells within the epidermis.

9 *Parakeratosis*. Disorderly keratin formation on the surface with persistence of nuclei in the horny layer.

10 *Rete pegs*. Downgrowth of the squamous epithelium indenting the dermis and resulting, therefore, in prolongation of the dermal papillae, i.e. the dermal tissue between these epithelial downgrowths.

11 *Spongiosis*. Oedema fluid between the prickle cells.

12 *Vesicle*. A small bulla.

In the ensuing account of the more common skin diseases, these pathological terms will be used without further explanation.

Congenital diseases

XERODERMA PIGMENTOSA

Appearances

An autosomal recessive disease in which there is hypersensitivity to ultraviolet light so that the lesions are maximal on the exposed skin surfaces. Early changes include erythema, scaling and patchy pigmentation, whilst later, there is a mixture of atrophy, patchy pigmentation and warty excrescences which may eventually form squamous cell carcinomas.

Microscopical

1 Hyperkeratosis.
2 Patchy atrophy of the prickle cell layer.
3 Patchy acanthosis.
4 Patchy basal cell melanin pigmentation.
5 Dermal oedema.
6 Dermal foci of chronic inflammatory cells.

Later, the hyperkeratosis increases with the development of atypical acanthosis and ultimately squamous cell carcinoma develops.

HYDROA VACCINIFORME AND HYDROA AESTIVALE

Appearances

A papulo-vesicular eruption occurring usually in boys during the summer months and associated with photosensitivity and congenital porphyria (see p. 117). The milder form, hydroa aestivale, ends at puberty and does not produce scarring but hydroa vacciniforme persists throughout life and results in fibrous dermal scars.

Microscopical

1 Intra-epidermal vesicle formation.
2 Dermal inflammation with vascular thrombosis.
3 Dermal necrosis followed by scarring although this is minimal in hydroa aestivale.

ICHTHYOSIS

Appearances

Dry rough 'fish-scale' skin maximal on the extensor surfaces.

Microscopical
1 Marked hyperkeratosis.
2 Hair follicle plugging by keratin – follicular plugging.
3 Atrophy of the prickle cell layer.

Inflammatory skin conditions

ECZEMATOUS LESIONS

Nature
An inflammatory reaction in the skin, usually of allergic aetiology and caused by a large number of agents including proteins, organisms and chemical substances. These allergens may be externally and locally applied or be more distant in origin as manifestations of a generalized hypersensitivity reaction and produce many and varied skin lesions which may be acute, subacute or chronic.

ACUTE ECZEMA

Appearances
A common example is contact dermatitis, in which there is a variable rash of macules, papules and vesicles later coalescing to produce a diffuse erythematous reaction.

Microscopical
1 Intra-epidermal vesicles and bullae containing serous fluid and inflammatory cells.
2 Spongiosis.
3 Dermal oedema.
4 Acute inflammatory cell infiltration of the dermis.

SUBACUTE ECZEMA

Appearances
This is exemplified by nummular eczema and is intermediate between the acute and chronic forms. It frequently shows features of both, but the typical finding is the formation of pin-point vesicles.

Microscopical
1 Scanty intra-epidermal vesicles which are smaller and sparser than in the acute stage.
2 Spongiosis.
3 Acanthosis resulting in epidermal thickening.

4 Patchy parakeratosis.
5 Dermal infiltration of acute and chronic inflammatory cells.

CHRONIC ECZEMA

Appearances
In atopic eczema or chronic neurodermatitis, there is thickening of the skin with mixtures of scaling, lichenification, crust and fissure formation.

Microscopical
1 Hyperkeratosis.
2 Parakeratosis.
3 Acanthosis.
4 Prolongation of the rete pegs.
5 Dermal infiltration by lymphocytes.
6 Variable dermal fibrosis.

EXFOLIATIVE DERMATITIS

Nature
A condition of generalized epidermal peeling which may be associated with severe fluid loss and is occasionally fatal. It commonly occurs as a severe drug hypersensitivity reaction following penicillin, sulphonamides, arsenicals, etc.

Macroscopical
There is a generalized exfoliation of the epidermis resulting in extensive weeping erythematous areas.

Microscopical
1 Parakeratosis.
2 Severe spongiosis and intracellular oedema.
3 Acanthosis.
4 Dermal inflammatory cell infiltration.
5 Exfoliation of the prickle cell layer to a variable depth.

Miscellaneous conditions

PEMPHIGUS VULGARIS

Appearances
A bullous eruption affecting any skin surface, but especially the groins, axilla and mouth and which, before cortisone therapy was available, was often fatal.

Microscopical

1 Acantholysis with 'acantholytic cells'. These degenerate epidermal cells are visible on a stained smear of the contents of the bullae – *Tzanck test*.
2 Intra-epidermal bullae – a layer of basal cells persists in the floor of the bulla.
3 Dermal oedema.
4 Dermal inflammatory cell infiltration with polymorphs and some eosinophils.

PEMPHIGUS VEGETANS

Appearances
Similar to pemphigus vulgaris, but the bullae are followed by the formation of warty excrescences and by pustules.

Microscopical
Similar to pemphigus vulgaris but additionally shows:
1 Acanthosis.
2 Epithelial downgrowths.
3 Papillary overgrowth of the epidermis forming the 'warts'.
4 Intra-epidermal abscesses containing almost 100 per cent eosinophils.

BULLOUS PEMPHIGOID

Appearances
A self-limiting bullous disorder of more or less generalized distribution. Involvement of the mouth is usually mild or absent. Clinical differentiation from dermatitis herpetiformis and pemphigus may be difficult.

Microscopical
1 Sub-epidermal bullae.
2 No acantholysis.
3 Variable; usually slight inflammatory cell infiltration of the base of the bullae but occasionally eosinophils may be numerous.

BENIGN MUCOUS MEMBRANE PEMPHIGOID

Nature
A further type of sub-epidermal bullous lesion of benign course with no acantholysis.

Bullous lesions and denuded areas are present on mucous membranes and, in half the cases, on the skin. Scarring of considerable extent may develop on the conjunctiva which is often involved.

PSORIASIS

Appearances
A common chronic dermatosis with dry, sharply demarcated plaques covered with layers of silvery scales. On scraping, the scales are removed to expose multiple fine bleeding points.

Microscopical
1 Parakeratosis.
2 Acanthosis.
3 Prolongation of the rete pegs.
4 Elongation of the dermal papillae which are of increased vascularity.
5 Thinning of the prickle cell layer over these papillae. This accounts for the 'bleeding points' following scraping.
6 Foci of inflammatory cells in the epidermis – micro-abscesses of Munro.

ACNE VULGARIS

Nature
An extremely common disease, usually maximal in adolescence, and affecting young males more commonly than young females, in which the sebaceous glands are predominantly involved.

Aetiology
The precise aetiology is unknown, but the following factors may be contributory:
1 *Hormonal.* Androgens cause hypertrophy of sebaceous glands, and oestrogens result in their atrophy. It has also been noted that some patients on corticosteroids in high dosage develop acne. Conversely, acne may be controlled by large dosage of oestrogens.
2 *Dietary.* Some patients with acne find that certain foodstuffs, e.g. chocolate, produce clinical exacerbations of the condition, but the precise role of dietary substances is obscure.
3 *Vitamins.* Vitamin-A deficiency may produce hyperkeratosis and follicular plugging and thus promote acne, but there is rarely any vitamin-A deficiency demonstrable in cases of acne.

Sites
Predominantly the face, upper chest, and back of the trunk and neck.

Macroscopical
The basic lesion is the 'blackhead' – *comedo*. This produces a tissue reaction in the plugged pilo-sebaceous follicle and forms a papule. Secondary infection, frequently by staphylococci, produces the pustule or pimple and the ensuing suppuration is followed by a variable degree of scarring.

Microscopical
Early. Plugging of the pilo-sebaceous follicles by keratin and inspissated sebaceous material – *comedo*.

Later. A folliculitis and peri-folliculitis forms the papule and secondary infection results in suppuration in and around the hair follicle and sebaceous gland. The disrupted glandular material may then evoke a foreign body giant-cell reaction.

Late. The local lesion heals by fibrosis and the degree of scarring will depend upon the amount of tissue destruction.

Results
The florid case shows lesions in all stages of development with blackheads, papules, pustules and scarred areas. Eventually, the disease tends to wane spontaneously but, in severe cases, disfiguring and permanent scarring will remain.

SEBORRHOEIC DERMATITIS

Nature
An extremely common condition in its mild form – *seborrhoea or dandruff*. The 'scales' of dandruff are desquamated keratin matted together by sebaceous material. In the more florid form there is an actual dermatitis present.

Macroscopical
Seborrhoeic dermatitis shows as raised erythematous scaly plaques involving the scalp, eyebrows and eyelids, face, ears and sometimes the chest.

Microscopical
The picture is not specifically diagnostic and is that of a chronic dermatitis (see p. 723) showing:
1 Hyperkeratosis
2 Parakeratosis } Forming the scales.

3 Acanthosis.
4 Rete peg downgrowths.
5 Mild spongiosis.
6 Mild inflammatory cell infiltration of the dermis.

LICHEN PLANUS

Appearances
A chronic dermatitis in which violaceous, flat-topped papules form, usually on the extensor surfaces and frequently involving the mouth.

Microscopical
1 Hyperkeratosis.
2 Acanthosis.
3 Irregular rete peg prolongation to produce 'saw-tooth' downgrowths into the dermis.
4 Basal cell layer liquefaction.
5 A dense lymphocytic dermal infiltration which 'hugs' the undersurface of the epidermis.

DERMATITIS HERPETIFORMIS

Appearances
A chronic, recurrent, itching condition of symmetrical distribution on the shoulders, buttocks and extensor extremities, consisting of vesicles and papules on an erythematous base.

Microscopical
1 Subepidermal vesicles containing albuminous fluid and abundant eosinophils.
2 Dermal oedema.
3 Dermal eosinophil infiltration.

Connective tissue diseases

GRANULOMA ANNULARE

Appearances
Groups of small, red, firm nodules on the hands and feet.

Microscopical
1 Collagen necrosis in the mid-dermis.
2 Increased mucin in the collagen.
3 A radiate arrangement of inflammatory cells around the foci of necrotic collagen.
4 Scanty foreign body giant cells.

SCLERODERMA

Appearances

A diffuse induration of the skin which becomes thin, pale and firmly adherent to the underlying tissues, decreasing limb mobility and affecting especially the arms, hands and face. The condition may progress to affect the oesophagus, heart, lungs, intestines, etc. (see p. 283).

Microscopical

1 Slight mucoid degeneration of dermal collagen.
2 Increased collagen in the dermis.
3 Extension of collagen into the underlying subcutaneous fat.
4 Disappearance of the sebaceous glands and hair follicles.
5 Preservation of the sweat glands until the disease is advanced, as they lie deeper in the dermis.
6 Vascular thickening and sometimes thrombosis.
7 Sparse lymphocytic infiltration in the perivascular areas and around the skin appendages.
8 Atrophy of the overlying epidermis.

CHRONIC DISCOID LUPUS ERYTHEMATOSUS

Appearances

This occurs typically on the face of young women as an infiltrated erythematous rash of 'butterfly' distribution which is frequently scaly and shows follicular plugging. Systemic lupus erythematosus may follow (see p. 281).

Microscopical

1 Hyperkeratosis.
2 Follicular plugging by keratin.
3 Atrophy of the prickle cells with epidermal thickening.
4 Liquefaction of the basal cells.
5 Basophilic degeneration of the dermal collagen.
6 A perivascular and focal lymphocytic infiltration of the dermis.

Lesions involving subcutaneous fat – panniculitis

ERYTHEMA NODOSUM

Appearances

Multiple, raised, red, tender nodules, typically on the anterior surfaces of the legs, which may be associated with rheumatic disease, tuberculosis or sarcoidosis.

Microscopical

1 Infiltration of the subcutaneous fat by polymorphs and lymphocytes in a patchy distribution.
2 Infiltration of the walls of the veins, which show endothelial proliferation, by similar inflammatory cells.
3 Later, small collections of histiocytes and scanty foreign body giant cells form in the dermis and subcutaneous tissues.
4 Abscess formation and necrosis do not occur.
5 In addition, some cases will show the histiological features of the underlying aetiology, e.g. tuberculous or sarcoid granulomas.

NODULAR VASCULITIS

Appearances

Multiple painful nodules occurring on the legs and sometimes on the neck, usually in females.

Microscopical

1 A vasculitis is present involving both veins and arteries. These show thickening of their walls and obliteration of the lumen in all the affected vessels in the dermis and subcutaneous tissues.
2 Increased fibrosis of the subcutaneous fat.
3 A mild non-specific inflammatory cell infiltration of the fat.
4 Numerous foreign body giant cells.

ERYTHEMA INDURATUM

Appearances

Multiple, recurrent, deep-seated infiltrations on the calves of women, which slowly extend to the surface as bluish-red plaques and often ulcerate. These are due to tuberculous infection and the organisms may be isolated from the lesions.

Microscopical

1 The subcutaneous fat contains tuberculous granulomas.
2 The dermal tissues show a non-specific inflammatory infiltration.
3 The arteries and veins are infiltrated by inflammatory cells and show obliterative changes.
4 Later, extensive caseation and necrosis follow

the vascular lesions with tissue destruction and overlying ulceration.

WEBER-CHRISTIAN DISEASE – NODULAR, NON-SUPPURATIVE, RELAPSING, FEBRILE PANNICULITIS

Appearances
Multiple, indurated, tender nodules in the subcutaneous fat, which usually heal by fibrosis leaving depressed scars. Visceral lesions occasionally occur and may lead to a fatal outcome.

Microscopical
There are three histological stages:
1 An acute inflammatory cell infiltration with polymorphs between the fat cells of the subcutaneous tissue.
2 Later, the predominant cell is the macrophage which phagocytoses fat and has a foamy cytoplasm; some of these macrophages form giant cells. Polymorphs, lymphocytes and plasma cells are also present.
   Stages 1 and 2 form the nodule.
3 The area becomes replaced by fibrous tissue and this forms the scars. There are residual cellular foci similar in appearance to stage 2 above.

DUPUYTREN'S CONTRACTURE

Nature
A thickening and contracture of the palmar fascia.

Macroscopical
Variable amounts of the palmar fascia are densely fibrous and thickened, frequently with nodular areas.

Microscopical
There is marked fibroblastic proliferation of the palmar fascial tissues, extremely cellular areas alternating with dense bands of hyaline fibrous tissue.

Pathogenesis
The causation of this condition remains unknown. Trauma may be a factor as the right hand is more commonly affected than the left, but the condition occurs as frequently in sedentary workers as in labourers. There is frequently a family history of the disease, of autosomal dominant type with variable penetrance and earlier onset in men, but see other fibromatoses (p. 148).

Results
The condition leads to contracture of the fingers with resulting disability.

Chapter 119
Skin Tumours

Epidermal tumours

BENIGN

SQUAMOUS CELL PAPILLOMA

Macroscopical
A fronded, pigmented or non-pigmented, hyper-keratotic, papillary lesion. If the hyperkeratosis is excessive it may form a cutaneous 'horn'.

Microscopical
Papillary overgrowth of the squamous epithelium which is regular and forms an excess of keratin on the surface. The squamous cells may show melanin pigmentation and there is frequently an inflammatory cell infiltration at the base but no invasion is demonstrable.

OTHER PAPILLARY SKIN LESIONS

Warts

AETIOLOGY
All are probably caused by virus infection, which may be transmitted by direct contact or by auto-inoculation.

TYPES
1 *Verruca vulgaris*. The common wart showing a papillomatous appearance.
2 *Verruca plantaris*. The plantar wart, where the effect of pressure forces the lesion into the underlying dermis.
3 *Verruca plana juvenilis*. The flat warts which are usually multiple and occur especially on the hands and face of children.
4 *Condyloma acuminata*. So-called 'venereal warts' which occur in the anogenital region. The 'venereal' aspect is based on the fact that sometimes the 'partner' will also have similar warts in the same region.

MICROSCOPICAL
1 Hyperkeratosis.
2 Papillary overgrowth of the squamous epithelium.
3 Acanthosis.
4 Spongiosis.
5 Prominence of the granular cell layer.

6 Vacuolization of the epidermal cells which may contain viral inclusion bodies.
7 An intact basal cell layer.
8 A dermal inflammatory cell infiltrate.

Molluscum contagiosum (see p. 730)

Corns

NATURE
Horny thickening with a broad base on the skin surface and apex in the dermis.

SITES
At any point of long continued pressure.

MICROSCOPICAL
A compressed mass of keratin producing atrophy of the adjacent epidermis and indenting the underlying dermis in which there is an inflammatory cell reaction.

Seborrhoeic wart – Seborrhoeic keratosis – Basal cell papilloma – Verruca senilis

NATURE
Benign surface growths which are usually multiple and pigmented, occurring particularly in elderly subjects and especially on the trunk, face and arms.

MACROSCOPICAL
Sharply circumscribed, yellow or brown, roughened and raised lesions, varying from a few millimeters to several cm in diameter.

MICROSCOPICAL
The lesion extends outwards, away from the surface epithelium and shows:
1 Hyperkeratosis.
2 Marked basal cell proliferation forming the epidermal thickening, hence the name 'basal cell papilloma'.
3 The keratin extends into the epithelium to form circular keratin-filled cysts – 'horn cysts'.
4 Melanin pigmentation of the epithelium.

RESULTS
This is a benign condition and does not predispose to malignancy. However, it requires clinical differentiation from carcinoma and malignant melanoma.

Kerato-acanthoma – Molluscum sebaceum

MACROSCOPICAL
A rapidly enlarging lesion which typically occurs on the face of elderly subjects and which presents as a raised plaque with a central keratin plug. The lesion grows rapidly and thus mimics a malignant tumour and yet the vast majority of these lesions are self-healing within a few months.

MICROSCOPICAL
A central core of laminated keratin producing a 'volcano' appearance. This keratin is surrounded by active but benign squamous epithelium which extends downwards and beneath the adjacent skin epithelium at the margins of the central core. A small biopsy specimen frequently leads to a false impression of invasion by carcinoma, but if the lesion is seen as a whole, the structure of the tumour is distinctive and diagnostic.

This lesion should not be confused with *molluscum contagiosum* which is a papillary warty hyperkeratotic mass on the skin surface. The overgrowth of the squamous epithelium is due to a virus and virus inclusion bodies can be seen in the squamous cells.

Leukoplakia

MACROSCOPICAL
This condition has already been described in the mouth (p. 171). It may occur at other sites on the skin surface where it presents as thickened, white, fissured plaques.

MICROSCOPICAL
Hyperkeratosis, acanthosis and prominence of the rete pegs which form atypical downgrowths into the chronically inflamed dermis. This is a pre-malignant condition wherever it is found, with ultimate progression to squamous cell carcinoma in a high percentage of untreated cases.

Senile keratosis

MACROSCOPICAL
Appears on the face and hands of elderly subjects as small, hard and often scaly lesions on an erythematous base.

MICROSCOPICAL
A localized area of hyperkeratosis with acanthosis and dyskeratosis showing individual cell keratin formation. The rete pegs are thickened and extend into the dermis. In addition, many of the cells in the prickle layer are atypical and show mitotic activity. Squamous cell carcinoma ultimately develops in some of these lesions.

MALIGNANT

Bowen's disease – Intra-epidermal carcinoma – 'Carcinoma-in-situ'

MACROSCOPICAL
Usually a solitary, slightly thickened, scaly or brown lesion which slowly extends.

MICROSCOPICAL
Hyperkeratosis, parakeratosis, spongiosis and dyskeratosis. The basal cell layer is intact but the prickle cells show marked atypicality, with loss of polarity, individual cell keratinization, mitotic activity with bizarre forms, giant cells and other nuclear irregularities. This is not a pre-malignant condition, it is already malignant. The basement membrane is intact but, if left untreated, invasion as a squamous cell carcinoma will occur.

Erythroplasia of Queyrat is a similar condition occurring on the glans penis (see p. 407).

Paget's disease of the skin
The thickening of the epidermis associated with the presence of Paget's cells has already been described in the breast section on p. 230. It should be reiterated that Paget's disease of the nipple is secondary to a carcinoma of the underlying breast ducts, but a similar lesion may also occur in extra-mammary situations in the vulva, axilla and anal regions. When occurring in these sites, it is also secondary to a carcinoma, usually of the underlying apocrine glands.

Squamous cell carcinoma

INCIDENCE
This is difficult to assess as a significant proportion of cases are cured and the patients eventually die from completely unrelated diseases. As a cause of death, malignant disease of the skin accounts for about 1 per cent of all cancers, but the lesion may possibly be responsible for about 10 per cent of all cases of malignant disease.

AGE

The majority of cases occur in the elderly, but some cases, especially those with predisposing skin lesions or following irradiation in youth, develop at an earlier age

SEX

M:F 4:1.

SITES

These tumours occur at any site on the skin surface but exposed parts, particularly the face, neck and hands, are most frequently involved.

PREDISPOSING FACTORS

1 *Skin diseases.* Leukoplakia, senile keratosis, Bowen's disease, lupus erythematosus, lupus vulgaris and xeroderma pigmentosa.

2 *Actinic cancers.* There is a prevalence in farmers, fishermen, sailors, gardeners and other outdoor workers, especially those living in sunny climates and in fair-skinned individuals.

3 *Carcinogenic hydrocarbons.* Workers in pitch, tar, paraffin, creosote and soot may, after a long latent period of many years, develop skin cancers in a significant proportion of cases (see p. 157).

4 *Arsenic.* Prolonged administration of arsenic, e.g. Fowler's solution, produces an arsenical keratosis which may be followed by squamous cell or basal cell cancer. Workers handling arsenic are similarly prone to tumour formation.

5 *Irradiation.* Squamous cell and basal cell cancers may arise in therapeutically irradiated areas or in X-ray workers who have been subjected to prolonged and repetitive exposures.

6 *Chronic ulceration.* Marjolin's ulcer – chronic ulceration, e.g. chronic sinuses, scars, varicose ulcers, burns and wounds, may undergo malignant change. Kangri basket burns are also in this category.

7 *Pre-existing sebaceous cysts.* If is often alleged that simple sebaceous cysts undergo malignant change. This undoubtedly does occur but is excessively rare.

MACROSCOPICAL

Some appear as proliferative papillary lesions, but the majority are indolent ulcers with a scab in the centre and raised, rolled, nodular and everted edges. Invasion of underlying tissue, together with local fixation and surrounding induration, also occurs.

MICROSCOPICAL

Vary in their degree of differentiation from the fully keratinized well-differentiated Grade I tumour with well-developed keratin, prickle cells and basal cells closely imitating skin, through all degrees of de-differentiation to an anaplastic, non-keratinizing carcinoma of Grade IV malignancy. The vast majority show some keratin formation and are thus readily recognizable as being of squamous cell origin.

SPREAD

Very variable in their speed of invasiveness and this is usually related to their degree of histological differentiation. They infiltrate locally and eventually metastasize to the regional lymph nodes. In fatal cases, blood dissemination is usually seen.

PROGNOSIS

With modern therapy, either irradiation or surgery, or both, the prognosis is reasonably favourable and an overall 5-year survival rate of 80 per cent can be anticipated. It should be remembered, however, that, until recent years, many reported series included examples of the self-limiting kerato-acanthoma among the numbers of their therapeutic successes (see p. 730).

Basal cell carcinoma – Rodent ulcer

AGE

Occur maximally between 60–80 years of age.

SEX

M:F 2:1.

ORIGIN

The precise cell of origin remains debatable but the basal cells of the hair follicles are the most probable; the tumours are sometimes multifocal in origin.

SITES

The majority occur on the face above a line joining the angle of the mouth to the ear, especially around the eye, about the naso-labial folds and in the scalp. Any other region of the skin which possesses hair follicles may also be a site of origin.

PREDISPOSING FACTORS

Sunlight, ultraviolet light, previous radiation and prolonged contact with arsenic all predispose to subsequent development of rodent ulcers.

MACROSCOPICAL

Present as pearly papules which eventually ulcerate and develop a scab. The edge is slightly raised and is slowly advancing.

MICROSCOPICAL

Composed of solid sheets of uniform, darkly staining basal type cells which invade the dermis. Mitotic figures, melanin pigment, cystic areas and mucus are frequently seen, but prickle cells and keratin are absent. The cells at the periphery of the epithelial sheets have a characteristic palisaded arrangement and an almost columnar appearance.

SPREAD

They spread by direct infiltration and, because of their frequent origin on the face, invade the subjacent bone or cartilage, the tumour cells often spreading well beyond the macroscopic tumour margin. Metastases to lymph nodes or via the blood stream are exceptionally rare.

PROGNOSIS

The most frequent cause of recurrence is inadequate removal at the first operation, tumour cells having spread beyond the margins of excision; this is particularly common when bone or cartilage are invaded.

In a recent series, approximately 15 per cent recurred following the initial treatment and, although some of these recurrences were subsequently cured, approximately 5 per cent died with active basal cell carcinoma present; most of these cases were either initially more than 2.5 cm in diameter or were facial lesions invading bone or cartilage.

Variant – Baso-squamous carcinoma

Some predominantly basal cell carcinomas contain areas of prickle cells, i.e. squamous cells. Such baso-squamous tumours, however, still behave as basal cell carcinomas and not as squamous cell cancers.

Tumours of skin appendages

SEBACEOUS GLANDS

Sebaceous naevus

A developmental overgrowth of sebaceous glands, usually on the scalp. A basal cell carcinoma may occasionally arise in one area of the tumour.

Adenoma sebaceum

An increase in the number of sebaceous glands to form tumour-like masses on the face – *epiloia*. The lesions are usually multiple and are frequently associated with other abnormalities of growth in the viscera and with glial nodules in the brain, as manifestations of tuberose sclerosis (see p. 593).

Sebaceous adenoma

This true tumour of sebaceous glands is very rare and is composed of sebaceous lobules of irregular size and shape. A basal cell carcinoma containing areas of sebaceous differentiation may arise in this lesion.

SWEAT GLANDS

Tumours of sweat glands are adenomas or adenocarcinomas; special names often used are *syringoma* for tumours arising from the ducts, *hidradenoma* from the acini and *syringocystadenoma* when cystic. The tumours are well differentiated and form papillary, cystic or solid, slowly growing lesions, histologically very similar to sweat ducts or acini and containing secretions. The duct-like forms have a double layer of cells lining the tubules, the basal layer being composed of myo-epithelial cells. Sometimes, the solid type of tumour is composed of this cell type and is then called *myoepithelioma*. Malignant tumours of sweat gland origin are very rare and are usually basal cell in type, less commonly they may be adenocarcinomas.

A cylindroma occurs in the scalp and is composed of columns or cylinders of clear cells surrounded by a layer of myo-epithelial cells enclosed in a hyaline membrane. They are benign, are probably of sweat or apocrine gland origin and are not related to cylindromas of mucous glands (see p. 180).

HAIR FOLLICLES

Basal cell carcinomas probably arise from the hair follicles. In addition, there is a locally destructive lesion composed of a mixture of horn cysts showing abortive hair formation and lined by squamous epithelium with basal cell areas – *trichoepithelioma* or *epithelioma adenoides cysticum*.

Dermal tumours

FROM COLLAGEN – FIBROMA, CELLULAR FIBROMA AND FIBROSARCOMA

The appearances are very variable, ranging from mature fibrous tissue to spindle cell sarcoma.

FROM NERVES – NEUROFIBROMA, AND NEUROFIBROSARCOMA

These tumours may all occur in the dermis.

FROM BLOOD VESSELS – HAEMANGIOMAS

A large variety of vascular lesions may arise in the dermis most of which have been described on p. 155. The lesions include:
1 Capillary haemangioma.
2 Cavernous haemangioma.
3 Sclerosing haemangioma.
4 Glomus tumour (see p. 278).
5 Haemangiopericytoma (see p. 279).
6 Angiosarcoma.
7 Kaposi's sarcoma.

Kaposi's sarcoma
A rare disease presenting as multiple haemorrhagic nodules and plaques. Some regress and disappear whilst others enlarge and new lesions appear. Microscopically, the early lesions show overgrowth of the vascular channels in the dermis with the formation of new capillaries and an infiltration of the dermis by lymphocytes, red cells, plasma cells, histiocytes, fibroblasts and haemosiderin pigment. At a later stage, the vascularity diminishes. The lesion behaves in the majority of cases (approximately 90 per cent) in a self-limiting benign manner but, in the remainder, widespread systemic lesions occur with a fatal outcome. This is particularly likely in homosexual males with the 'acquired immune deficiency syndrome'. An oncogenic virus seems to be the likely aetiological agent.

FROM LYMPHATICS – LYMPHANGIOMAS

Lymphangiomas have been described on p. 155. The following types may occur in the dermis:
1 Simple lymphangioma.
2 Cavernous lymphangioma.
3 Cystic – cystic hygroma.
4 Lymphangiosarcoma.

FROM MUSCLES – LEIOMYOMA

The smooth muscle of the arrectores pilorum or of the blood vessel walls may be the site of origin of a dermal leiomyoma. Single or multiple lesions present as small nodules composed of regular, smooth muscle fibres commonly associated with a prominent vascular pattern.

Tumours of naevus cells

CELL OF ORIGIN
The cell of origin of these tumours is the naevus cell, a DOPA-positive cell (see p. 117). It is almost certainly of neuroectodermal origin.

Intradermal naevus – mole
This is the most frequently encountered naevus and is present in variable numbers is virtually all individuals. The lesions may be flat or raised, brown or black, scaly, hairy, hyperkeratotic, or inflamed. Histologically, there are many variable features. The naevus cells are usually confined to the dermis, are regular in shape, size and staining and contain pigment, especially noticeable in the superficial portions. This is the *intradermal naevus* and the overlying epidermis is free from naevus cells. A modification of this appearance – the *junctional naevus*, shows marked proliferative activity of the naevus cells at the junction of dermis and epidermis. The cells at the junction are plump, active and appear in clumps. The process is known as junctional activity and is a constant feature of many naevi in childhood and up to the age of puberty – *juvenile melanoma*, which is a benign lesion. However, in adult life this junctional activity is of more sinister significance, as it is a precursor of malignancy. Thus, it is important to know the age of the patient when assessing the significance of junctional activity. A further modification is the

presence of naevus cells in the dermis and at the junctional area – *compound naevus*.

Malignant melanoma

INCIDENCE
Unlike naevi, which are present in virtually all individuals, malignant melanomas are uncommon, causing about 0.5 per cent of deaths from malignant disease in England and Wales.

AGE
Very rare before puberty and most occur above the age of 30 years. As described above, a juvenile melanoma should not be confused with a malignant melanoma.

SITES
Any part of the skin surface may be involved but the more common sites are the hands, feet (subungual), face and neck.

PREDISPOSING FACTORS
Most if not all, malignant melanomas originate in a pre-existing benign mole. The signs of malignancy in adult life are usually:
1   Increase in size.
2   Deepening pigmentation.
3   Ulceration.
4   Bleeding.
5   Satellite lesions.

MACROSCOPICAL
Usually deeply or variably pigmented and rapidly growing tumours sometimes ulcerated or showing small outlying tumour nodules and a surrounding pigmented flare.

MICROSCOPICAL
The appearances are very diverse but the presence in the adult of junctional activity, pleomorphism of the cells, giant cells, mitoses, marked irregularity of pigment distribution and especially pigment in the depths of the lesion, all point to malignancy. Some of the lesions show no pigment – *amelanotic melanomas*, but the cells are still DOPA-positive.

SPREAD
1   *Direct*. Local spread produces an enlarging lesion with extension of the pigmented area.

2   *Lymphatic*. Spread to regional lymph nodes may be found at the time of presentation and there is a marked tendency for nodules of tumour to develop along the course of the intermediate dermal lymphatics.
3   *Blood*. Metastases may occur early in the disease and be situated in virtually any organ of the body, but especially in the liver, lungs and brain.

PROGNOSIS
If the juvenile melanomas are excluded, the malignant melanoma of adult life has a poor prognosis with a 5-year survival of about 25 per cent. Most of the fatal cases show invasion of the regional lymph nodes and blood-borne metastases. Even after many years of freedom from tumour following treatment, clinical recurrence may occur.

In assessing prognosis of a surgically excised melanoma the most important factor is depth of penetration of tumour cells in the dermis.

OTHER PIGMENTED TUMOURS

'Blue naevus'
Blue or brown lesions which cause palpable thickening of the dermis. Histologically, the epidermis is normal but the dermis contains a collection of pigment-containing phagocytes – *melanophores* (see p. 117), which give a brown colour if situated just beneath the epidermis or a blue colour if in the deeper layers of the dermis. These lesions are not pre-malignant, do not contain naevus cells and produce cosmetic problems only.

Lentigo
In this condition there is a flat melanotic pigmented lesion associated with naevus cell activity and rete peg downgrowths. The vast majority occur in older age groups, usually on exposed parts and remain benign. However, a small minority progressively enlarge with increasing pigmentation and, whilst remaining flat, show histological evidence of excessive, atypical naevus cell activity – *lentigo maligna*. If left untreated some of these lesions will progress to frankly invasive malignant melanoma.

Chapter 120
Diseases of the Spleen

Structure
The spleen is the largest single collection of lymphoid tissue in the body. It normally weighs between 150–200 g, is enclosed in a fibrous capsule and is supplied by the large splenic artery. The artery divides and ultimately forms arterioles within the spleen which are surrounded by lymphoid tissue – *Malpighian bodies*. The blood from the arterioles may then circulate through to the splenic veins – closed circulation, or more usually passes into the splenic pulp – open circulation. The splenic pulp is a fibrous sponge-like structure with spaces lined by lymphoreticular cells and the blood percolates slowly through this meshwork before passing out on the venous side.

Functions
These are described in the section on hypersplenism on p. 456.

Congenital abnormalities
Rarely, the spleen may be absent; more common is the presence of multiple accessory spleens in adjacent areas – *splenunculi*.

Atrophy
With increasing age there is a progressive atrophy of the lymphoid tissue, so that, in the elderly, the organ is much reduced in size, to 50–100 g or less.

Perisplenitis

NATURE
A fairly frequent incidental post-mortem finding in which an inflammatory process has previously involved the splenic capsule. The condition has no practical clinical significance.

AETIOLOGY

Any intra-abdominal infection, e.g. peritonitis, which may be due to pyogenic organisms but also follows a tuberculous peritonitis. In addition, similar appearances occur following any non-infective exudate in the peritoneum, e.g. ascites in cirrhosis of the liver.

MACROSCOPICAL

The spleen may be of normal size or slightly enlarged and the capsular surface is covered with a thick, shiny, white, fibrous covering – 'sugar-icing' spleen.

MICROSCOPICAL

The capsule shows dense hyaline fibrosis, but minimal inflammatory cells.

Splenic enlargement – splenomegaly

The majority of the clinically significant diseases of the spleen result in its enlargement and some of the more important of these are listed below. Many of these conditions have been described under their appropriate sections, so only the diseases where the splenic abnormality is of special significance will be described here.

INFECTIONS

NON-SPECIFIC

AETIOLOGY

The spleen commonly enlarges with any bacteraemia or septicaemia.

MACROSCOPICAL

Enlarged, soft and red, with a diffluent pulp – *septic spleen*.

MICROSCOPICAL

There is marked hyperplasia of the lymphoreticular elements with pulp proliferation and a diffuse infiltration of polymorphs. Organisms may be isolated by culture.

RESULTS

This is the appearance in septicaemia, endocarditis, etc., and once the infection has been successfully treated, the spleen returns to normal.

SPECIFIC

The spleen is enlarged in a large number of specific inflammatory processes of which the following are the more important examples.

Enteric fever

MACROSCOPICAL

Enlarged, soft, deep red in colour, the pulp sometimes simulating blood clot.

MICROSCOPICAL

There is a diffuse lymphoreticular cell proliferation with a mononuclear cell infiltration and erythrophagocytosis. Organisms of the enteric group, e.g. *Salmonella typhi*, are present (see p. 199).

Malaria

MACROSCOPICAL

Acute. Enlarged, soft and haemorrhagic (see p. 64). *Chronic*. Grossly enlarged, firm, deep brown or almost black in colour.

MICROSCOPICAL

Acute. Marked congestion with pigmentation and the presence of malarial parasites in the lymphoreticular cells.
Chronic. Marked splenic fibrosis with lymphoreticular cell overgrowth and pigmentation.

Kala-azar – visceral leishmaniasis

MACROSCOPICAL

The spleen is grossly enlarged, firm and congested with fibrous thickening of the capsule.

MICROSCOPICAL

There is lymphoreticular cell proliferation with distension of these cells by the parasites *Leishmania donovani* (see p. 62).

Brucellosis

MACROSCOPICAL

Firm, congested and enlarged spleen.

MICROSCOPICAL

The diagnostic feature is the presence of focal granulomas consisting of lymphoreticular cells, lymphocytes, fibroblasts, scanty giant cells and a small area of central necrosis. This 'brucella granuloma' has to be distinguished from sarcoidosis, tuberculosis and Hodgkin's disease.

Syphilis

This is a very rare cause of splenomegaly but the spleen may be palpable in the secondary stage due to reactive hyperplasia of the lymphoid tissue and in the tertiary stage due to the presence of a gumma.

Tuberculosis

The spleen may be palpable in miliary tuberculosis, but is rarely very large in this condition. On section the splenic pulp is studded with pinhead-sized tubercles.

Rarely, the spleen may be involved in a chronic form of abdominal tuberculosis which may be associated with haematological disorders, e.g. pancytopenia or a leukaemoid bone marrow reaction (see p. 448).

Sarcoidosis

The spleen is enlarged in sarcoidosis in 13 per cent of cases – Stengel-Wolbach splenomegaly, and the pulp contains the typical sarcoid granulomas (see p. 57).

CIRCULATORY DISORDERS

Cardiac failure

Passive right-sided venous congestion mainly affects the liver, but the spleen may be slightly enlarged, firm and dark red due to the congestion.

Portal hypertension

AETIOLOGY

The commonest cause is cirrhosis of the liver (see p. 560) but portal vein obstruction by tumour or thrombus is occasionally responsible and in some cases this condition is idiopathic.

MACROSCOPICAL

The spleen is grossly enlarged, firm, dark red or brown in colour and the capsule may show fibrous thickening.

MICROSCOPICAL

There is marked increase in the fibrous tissue due to thickening of both the trabeculae and of the sinusoid walls, so that the whole of the spleen becomes a thick, fibrous-walled sponge in the interstices of which are red cells and haemosiderin-laden phagocytes – 'brown induration' of the spleen (see p. 120). The more longstanding the condition the greater is the degree of fibrosis and the lymphoid tissue elements disappear. In very chronic cases *siderotic nodules* are present.

RESULTS

As the portal hypertension increases, anastomotic channels with the systemic circulation open through the splenic capsule to the diaphragm where very vascular adhesions between the spleen and the diaphragm may develop. The enlargement of the spleen may be associated with anaemia and leucopenia – *hypersplenism* (see p. 457).

Infarcts

INCIDENCE

The spleen is a relatively common site for both bland and septic infarcts, being the site of lodgement of emboli from infective endocarditis, mural and atrial thrombi. Infarcts also occur in enlarged spleens due to thrombosis of splenic vessels, e.g. in leukaemia (see p. 465).

MACROSCOPICAL

The infarcts appear as wedge-shaped pale areas involving the capsule. Later, there is a depressed fibrous scar with puckering of the capsular surface.

INFILTRATIONS

Amyloid

This may occur in a localized or in a diffuse form (see p. 109).

1 *Localized.* Produces the 'sago' spleen due to the nodular deposition of amyloid material around the arterioles of the Malpighian bodies.

2 *Diffuse.* There is a diffuse deposition of amyloid material in the walls of the sinusoids of the pulp.

Lipid storage diseases

In Gaucher's disease and Niemann–Pick disease, the spleen is enlarged due to infiltration by lymphoreticular cells containing the particular lipid diagnostic of the disease (see p. 113). In Hand–Schüller–Christian disease, the spleen is frequently spared, the majority of the lesions being prominent in the bones (see p. 691).

**Non-Lipid Reticuloendotheliosis –
Letterer–Siwe Disease**
A disease of the lymphoid system which has many
of the characteristics of the lipid storage diseases,
but the bizarre histiocytes which form tumour
masses do not contain lipid. It is a disease of infants
and young children and is characterized by skin
rashes, hepatomegaly, splenomegaly, lymphadenopathy, a progressive anaemia and bone lesions (see
p. 691). All the involved organs show an infiltration
of the abnormal histiocytes and the condition is
rapidly fatal.

CONNECTIVE TISSUE DISEASES

In many of the connective tissue diseases, the
spleen may show moderate enlargement. These
include:
1   Systemic lupus erythematosus (see p. 281).
2   Polyarteritis nodosa (see p. 282).
3   Still's disease (see p. 708).
4   Felty's syndrome (see p. 286).

TUMOURS

Benign
These are all very rare and include hamartomatous
malformations as well as true tumours. The more
common types are simple, unilocular cysts replacing the splenic pulp and causing splenomegaly;
fibroma, lymphangioma and haemangioma also
occur.

Malignant
These are much more common and include:

MALIGNANT LYMPHOMAS
The spleen is frequently involved by Hodgkin's and
non-Hodgkin's lymphomas (see p. 580). Variable
sized pale nodular deposits are present.

SECONDARY CARCINOMA
Secondary carcinoma in the spleen is rare. It is
sometimes seen as a result of direct invasion from an
adjacent carcinoma of the stomach or from the
splenic flexure of the colon, but is only rarely seen
following blood dissemination.

BLOOD DISEASES

Splenomegaly is a prominent feature of many
haematological disorders especially:

Red cells
Congenital and acquired haemolytic anaemias (see
pp. 486–507).
Polycythaemia rubra vera (p. 459).
Pernicious anaemia (p. 482).

White Cells
Leukaemias (pp. 462–468).

Pancytopenia
'Hypersplenism' (see p. 457).

Appendices

Length and weight of foetus

Month	Weight (grams)	Length (cm)
2	4	3
3	5–20	7–9
4	120	10–17
5	280	18–27
6	430	28–34
7	1220	35–38
8	1550	39–41
9	2000	42–44

Average normal weights of adult organs (in grams)

Heart	F.	250–280
	M.	270–360
Lungs	Rt.	480–680
	Lt.	420–600
Spleen		150–200
Liver		1400–1700
Kidneys	Rt.	140
	Lt.	150
Brain	F.	1250
	M.	1400
Adrenals (combined)		12–14
Parathyroids (combined)		0·1
Pituitary		0·3–0·6
Thyroid		30–40

Adult normal values

The following values are intended as a guide only. There is considerable variation between laboratories according to the different methods that they use.

Blood, plasma or serum

Acid phosphatase	
Total	0–11 IU/l
Tartrate labile (prostatic)	0–4 IU/l
Adrenocorticotrophic hormone (ACTH) 0900 hours	< 100 ng/l
Alkaline phosphatase	100–280 IU/l
Albumin	27–45 g/l
Alanine aminotransferase (GPT)	5–40 IU/l
Aldolase	0·5–3·1 IU/l
Ammonia	50–80 μmol/l
Amylase	70–300 IU/l
Aspartate aminotransferase (GOT)	4–40 IU/l
Bicarbonate	
Total CO_2	24–32 mmol/l
'True'	23–31 mmol/l
Bilirubin	5–17 μmol/l
Calcium	
Total	2·2–2·6 mmol/l
Ionized	1·1–1·3 mmol/l
Chloride	96–109 mmol/l
Cholesterol	
Total	3·6–7·8 mmol/l
HDL	1–2 mmol/l★
Cortisol	
0900 hours	140–700 nmol/l
Midnight	< 140 nmol/l
Creatine kinase (CK)	10–80 IU/l
Creatinine	60–120 μmol/l
Ferritin	M 45–200 μg/l
	F 15–80 μg/l
Follicle stimulating hormone (FSH)	M 2–9 U/l
	F 2–30 U/l†
Menstruating	F 38–167 U/l
Post-menopausal	M 10–50 IU/l
γ Glutamyl transferase (γGT)	F 8–40 IU/l
Globulins	
α1	1–4 g/l
α2	3–8 g/l
β	7–12 g/l
γ	7–14 g/l
Glucose	
Blood	3·0–7·0 mmol/l
Plasma	3·5–7·5 mmol/l
Growth hormone (hGH)	< 10 mU/l
Human placental lactogen (HPL)	
24 weeks gestation	2–4 mg/l
34 weeks gestation	4–9 mg/l
40 weeks gestation	4–10 mg/l
Hydrogen ion	36–44 nmol/l
α Hydroxybutyrate dehydrogenase (αHBD)	55–140 IU/l

17α Hydroxyprogesterone	M 1·6–7·6 nmol/l
Menstruating	F 1–13 nmol/1†
Post menopausal	F 0·9–5·1 nmol/l
Insulin	6–25 mU/l
Iron	M 14–34 μmol/l
	F 11–30 μmol/l
Iron binding capacity (TIBC)	45–72 μmol/l
Lactate	0·5–1·5 mmol/l
Lactate dehydrogenase	120–140 IU/l
Luteinizing hormone (LH)	M 0·5–12 U/l
Menstruating	F 0–100 U/l†
Post menopausal	F 30–90 U/l
Magnesium	0·7–1·0 mmol/l
Oestradiol	M < 220 pmol/l
Menstruating	F 75–1500 pmol/l†
Post menopausal	F < 220 pmol/l
Oestriol	
32 weeks gestation	120–820 nmol/l
36 weeks gestation	200–1200 nmol/l
39 weeks gestation	250–2000 nmol/l
Osmolality	285–295 mosm/kg
$PaCO_2$	4·5–6·1 kPa
PaO_2	12–15 kPa
pH	7·36–7·44
Phosphate (inorganic)	0·8–1·4 mmol/l
Potassium	3·5–5·5 mmol/l
Progesterone	M 0·32–1·27 nmol/l
Menstruating	F 0·5–80 nmol/l†
Pregnant	F 30–800 nmol/l
Post menopausal	F 0·32–1·27 nmol/l
Prolactin	100–400 mU/l
Sodium	135–145 mmol/l
Testosterone	M 8–27 nmol/l
	F 0–2·8 nmol/l
Thyroid function tests	
Tri-iodothyronine (T3)	1·25–2·75 nmol/l
Thyroxine (T4)	50–160 nmol/l
'T3 resin uptake'	120–85
Free tri-iodothyronine index	1·7–2·7
Free thyroxine index	70–125
Free thyroxine	9–23 pmol/l
Thyroid stimulating hormone (TSH)	Less than 7 mU/l
Transferrin	2–4 g/l
Triglycerides	0·3–1·8 mmol/l
Urate	100–400 μmol/l

* Normally more than 20 per cent of total.
† Varies greatly with different stages of the menstrual cycle.
‡ As tested at the bedside with commercial 'stix'.

Urea	1·0–6·0 mmol/l
Zinc	11–20 μmol/l

Urine

Amylase	170–2000 IU/l
Bilirubin	Nil
Catecholamines	
Total	50–1600 nmol/24 h
Free	50–700 nmol/24 h
Creatinine	6–17 mmol/24 h
Glucose	Nil
11 Hydroxycorticosteroids (Free cortisol)	100–330 nmol/24 h
17 Hydroxycorticosteroids	M 17–73 μmol/24 h
	F 14–55 μmol/24 h
5 Hydroxy indoleacetic acid (5 HIAA)	< 50 μmol/24 h
Metanephrines	< 5 μmol/24 h
Oestrogens (non-pregnant)	M 25–80 nmol/24 h
Menstruating	F 25–360 nmol/24 h†
Post menopausal	F 7–55 nmol/24 h
Oestriol	
30 weeks gestation	24–92 μmol/24 h
35 weeks gestation	43–135 μmol/24 h
40 weeks gestation	69–226 μmol/24 h
17 Oxosteroids	
20–40 year	M 15–97 μmol/24 h
70 year	M 1·5–25 μmol/24 h
20–40 year	F 10–70 μmol/24 h
70 year	F 0–17 μmol/24 h
Potassium	Normally equals intake
Protein	< 0·07 g/24 h
Sodium	Normally equals intake
Urea	150–250 mmol/24 h
Urobilinogen	No excess‡
Vanillylmandelic acid (VMA)	15–25 μmol/24 h

Faeces

Fat	< 18 mmol/24 h

Staining Reactions

Amongst the more commonly used stains are the following but many persons have alternative favourites

Material	Stain	Result
Routine for most tissues	Haematoxylin and eosin	Nuclei – blue Cytoplasm – pink
Amyloid	Sirius red, Congo red Thioflavine T	Red Yellow-green fluorescence in U.V. light
Argentaffin granules	Diazo Lead haematoxylin	Orange-red granules (Formalin fixed only) Blue-black granules
Argyrophilia	Grimelius silver Bodian's protargol	Black granules Black granules
Blood films and bone marrow	Romanowsky stains May–Grunwald–Giemsa	Nuclei – blue Eosinophil granules – pink-red Basophil granules – blue Erythrocytes – salmon pink
Cytological smears	Papanicolaou	Nuclei – blue Cytoplasm – green to orange
Calcium	von Kossa	Black
Chromaffin	Giemsa Schmorl reaction	Blue-green granules (dichromate fixed only) Blue granules
Elastic tissues	Weigert elastin or modifications	Blue-black
Fat (neutral)	Oil red O	Red (frozen sections only)
Fibrin	M.S.B. trichrome	Red
Fibrous tissue	van Gieson	Collagen fibres red (Muscle fibres yellow-orange)
Fungi	Periodic acid-Schiff (P.A.S.) Methenamine silver	Red Black
Glycogen	P.A.S. (with diastase)	Before diastase – red After diastase – nil
Immune substances, peptide hormones and tumour products	Peroxidase anti-peroxidase (P.A.P.) using specific antisera	Brown granules
Iron (free)	Prussian blue reaction (Perls')	Blue
Mast cells	Toluidine blue	Red-purple granules
Melanin	Masson-Fontana silver	Black
Muco substances: acid Neutral	Alcian blue at low pH P.A.S.	Blue Red
Muscle	van Gieson	Muscle fibres yellow-orange
Muscle stripes	Phosphotungstic acid haematoxylin (P.T.A.H.)	Stripes – black Cytoplasm – blue
Myco. tuberculosis	Ziehl–Neelsen (Z.N.)	Tubercle bacilli – red

Myelin – normal	Solochrome cyanin (Page)	Blue
– early degenerate	Marchi	Black
Nerve cells and fibres	Bielschowsky or modifications	Black
Neuroglial fibres	Phosphotungstic acid haematoxylin (P.T.A.H.)	Blue
Nissl granules	Pyronin-Methyl green (Unna Pappenheim)	Red
Organisms – bacteria	Gram	Gram positive – blue Gram negative – red
Parasites	Giemsa	Red – blue
Plasma cells	Pyronin-Methyl green	Cytoplasm (R.N.A.) – red Nuclei (D.N.A.) – green-blue
Renal basement membranes	Periodic acid-Schiff (P.A.S.) Methenamine silver	Red Black
Reticulin fibres	Gordon and Sweet's silver stain	Black

Index

743